Dental Composite Materials for Direct Restorations

Vesna Miletic
Editor

Dental Composite Materials for Direct Restorations

Springer

Editor
Vesna Miletic
DentalNet Research Group
University of Belgrade
School of Dental Medicine
Belgrade, Serbia

ISBN 978-3-319-60960-7 ISBN 978-3-319-60961-4 (eBook)
https://doi.org/10.1007/978-3-319-60961-4

Library of Congress Control Number: 2017959660

Printed on acid-free paper

This Springer imprint is published by Springer Nature
The registered company is Springer International Publishing AG
The registered company address is: Gewerbestrasse 11, 6330 Cham, Switzerland

Preface

Contemporary restorative dentistry is unthinkable without composite materials. Continuous improvements of these materials have expanded their indications for use and contributed to excellent clinical results in terms of function and esthetics.

This book covers basic scientific and clinically relevant aspects of dental composites for direct restorations with a view to meeting the needs of researchers and practitioners. It is divided into eight parts and its 19 chapters cover such topics as development and composition, curing reactions, monomer conversion, the importance of the dental curing light, properties of current materials giving emphasis to new formulations, new classification criteria, esthetic appearance, and biological potential. Clinically relevant aspects include bonding to tooth tissues, polymerization shrinkage stress, secondary caries, repair, and longevity of composite restorations. Future perspectives discuss avenues for potential advancement of composite materials. Finally, clinical application is presented focusing on shade selection, techniques for material placement and management, and finishing and polishing procedures.

I would like to express my sincere gratitude to all the authors for their contribution to this book, their dedication, and hard work which made the final outcome possible. Indeed, it has been a privilege to collaborate with colleagues whose work has pushed the boundaries of knowledge and who continuously strive for excellence.

Belgrade, Serbia — Vesna Miletic

Contents

Part I

Development and Composition

1 Development of Dental Composites

Vesna Miletic

The era of dental composites began about 1954 when silicate cements and unfilled methyl methacrylate resins were the only esthetic direct filling materials. Adhesive epoxy resins became available, and their use to bind together a maximum volume of very small fused silica particles was evaluated. The slow hardening of epoxy formulations led to the synthesis of Bis-GMA in 1956.
—R.L. Bowen, personal communication, Fig. 1.1

Dental composites have come a long way over the last five decades with continuous improvements to become the material of choice for most anterior and posterior restorations. The aim is to esthetically and functionally replace the missing tooth tissue and ensure long-term stability of the tooth-restoration complex in the oral environment.

The term "composite material" refers to a material made up of at least two distinct components, insoluble in each other, which produce a material with different, often better, characteristics than the components alone. Three main components of dental composites are (1) the organic resin matrix in which (2) inorganic filler particles are distributed and (3) the silane coupling agent that coats the filler particles for chemical bonding to the resin matrix. Dental composites contain other important ingredients, such as initiators for the onset of polymerization reaction, inhibitors that prevent spontaneous polymerization, and pigments for tooth-matching color range.

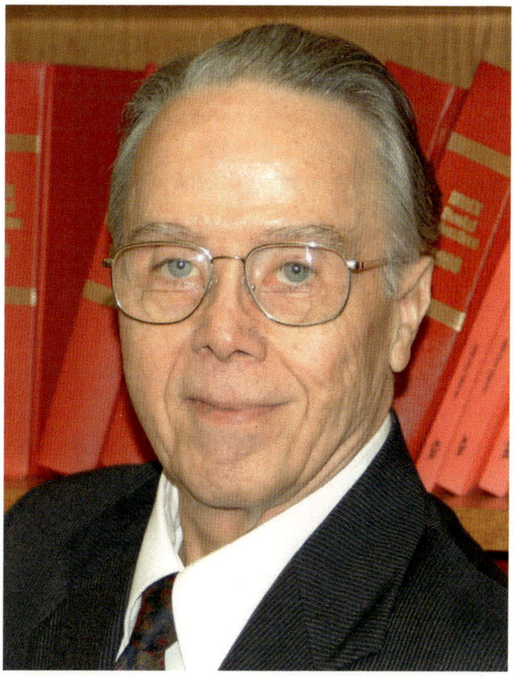

Fig. 1.1 Rafael L. Bowen, D.D.S., D.Sc., inventor of Bis-GMA (bisphenol A glycidyl methacrylate)

Hundreds of millions of composite restorations are placed each year worldwide. However, there is a discrepancy in affordability and accessibility to composite-based dental care around

V. Miletic
DentalNet Research Group, School of Dental Medicine, University of Belgrade, Belgrade, Serbia
e-mail: vesna.miletic@stomf.bg.ac.rs

V. Miletic (ed.), *Dental Composite Materials for Direct Restorations*,
http://doi.org/10.1007/978-3-319-60961-4_1

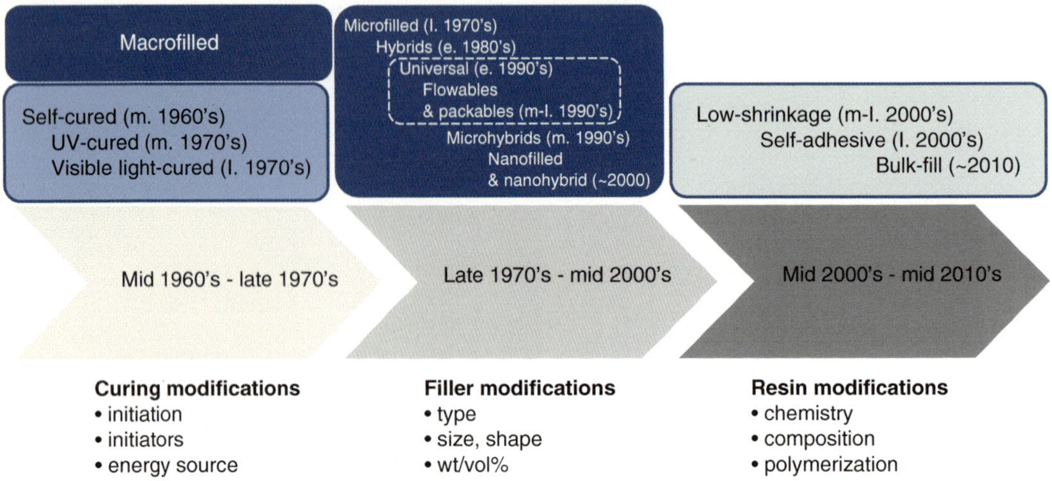

Fig. 1.2 Development of dental composite materials for direct restorations. Abbreviations: *m* mid, *l* late, *e* early

the world. A recent WHO document states that amalgam restorations are still prevalent in most low- and middle-income countries [1]. High cost of dental care based on amalgam alternatives has been identified as the most important factor for this finding. It includes high cost of tooth-colored materials, equipment and facilities, the lack of manpower, and proper training of dental personnel as well as unfavorable public health policies. Clearly the material properties are not among these concerns, although the manufacturers are urged to continue to improve the existing and develop new materials and reduce the cost of tooth-colored materials. One could argue that clinical procedure related to dental composites remains an important avenue for simplification, an aspect that is affected by material properties.

The aim of this chapter is to provide an overview of the development of dental composites. Key elements of product optimization are presented and discussed.

The synthesis of BisGMA in 1956 was followed by US patents for dental filling materials in 1962 and 1965 [2–4]. Commercial dental composites, indicated for restoring anterior teeth, were introduced in the mid-1960s [5]. The following five decades of composite development can be broadly divided into three main periods (Fig. 1.2).

There is little available information in the literature on dental composites in those early years. In part this is due to the fact that material composition was rarely reported as it is done today but also because past research is no way near the extent of contemporary research in this field. Also early research papers are not readily available through today's medical libraries making it more difficult for today's researchers to get a glimpse into history of dental composites.

1.1 Curing Modifications

Early composites consisted of two pastes which initiated the curing reaction on mixing. As no external factor was involved in the curing process, these composites were called "self-cured" or "chemically cured." The two pastes were based on BisGMA resin matrix diluted with liquid monomers, primarily TEGDMA,[1] with suspended 70–80 wt% of quartz, borosilicate, ceramic, or glass particles, irregularly shaped and up to 100 μm in diameter [6, 7]. Because of low wear resistance leading to the loss of anatomic form, the use of such macrofilled composites in posterior teeth was not recommended [8, 9]. Indications for the use of macrofilled composites were primarily Class III and V and limited Class I and IV restorations. Another problem with self-cured composites was hand-mixing which could lead to errors in paste concentrations and inclu-

[1] Triethyleneglycoldimethacrylate.

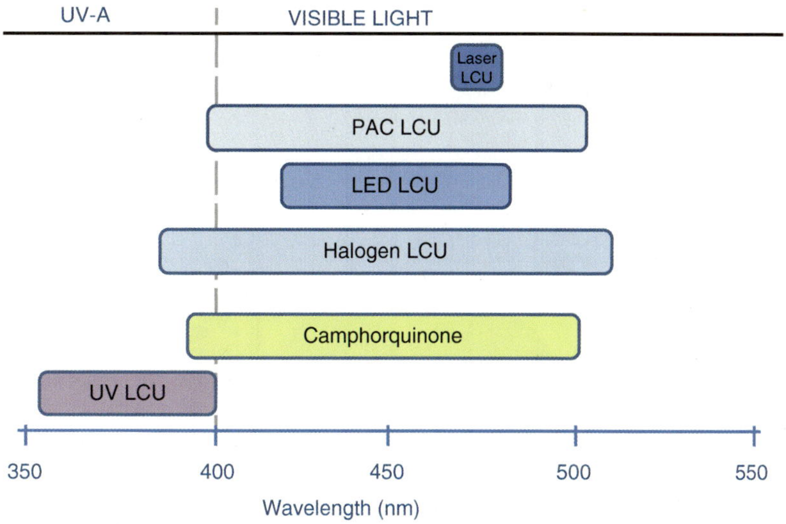

Fig. 1.3 The range of emission spectra of early UV and later visible light-cured units and the range of the absorption spectrum of camphorquinone. Abbreviations: *UV* ultraviolet, *LCU* light-curing unit, *LED* light-emitting diode, *PAC* plasma arc

sion of air bubbles in the polymer, resulting in compromised material properties.

In mid-1970s a milestone change occurred as light-cured composites were introduced. This allowed composites to be prepared as one paste with precisely defined composition by the manufacturers. The first light-cured composites required UV light sources, operating between 360 and 400 nm, to initiate polymerization. The drawbacks of UV lights included health hazard to eye and oral tissue, rapid deterioration of light intensity, as well as shallow penetration resulting in inferior depth of cure of *UV-cured composites* [10].

In the late 1970s, *visible light-cured composites* were introduced with the potential to overcome the drawbacks of UV-cured composites. The new photoinitiator system based on camphorquinone in tandem with tertiary amine coinitiator provided higher monomer-to-polymer conversion than that of self-cured composites with no drawbacks associated with UV lights (Fig. 1.3) [6].

1.2 Filler Modifications

As mentioned earlier, the first developed composites contained filler particles in the range of 10–50 μm even up to 100 μm and were labeled *macrofilled composites*. The late 1970s marked another important milestone in the development of dental composites—the introduction of *microfilled composites* (Fig. 1.4).

Hydrolysis and precipitation were employed to grow fine silica microfiller particles 0.04 μm in size (average) instead of milling/grinding larger quartz, glass, or ceramic particles. It is now clear that the term "microfiller" was not appropriate as the particles were in the "nano" range. It is likely that this term "microfiller" was coined to imply substantially smaller particle range compared to the previously used macrofillers, but also because the concept of "nano" did not exist at the time. Higher polishability and better color stability of microfilled than macrofilled composites allowed superior esthetics required for anterior restorations [11, 12]. Conversely, microfiller particles exerted extremely high surface area limiting the filler load. Lower filler load resulted in inferior mechanical properties and higher coefficient of thermal expansion of microfilled than macrofilled composites [13].

One way to increase the filler content, and hence mechanical properties, was the addition of microfiller-based complexes [6] or prepolymerized resin fillers [14] into the resin matrix of microfilled composites. These organic-inorganic fillers were produced by milling the prepolymerized microfilled composite into splintered particles (1–200 μm) or by incorporating silica microfillers into prepolymerized spherical particles (20–30 μm). The third type was purely

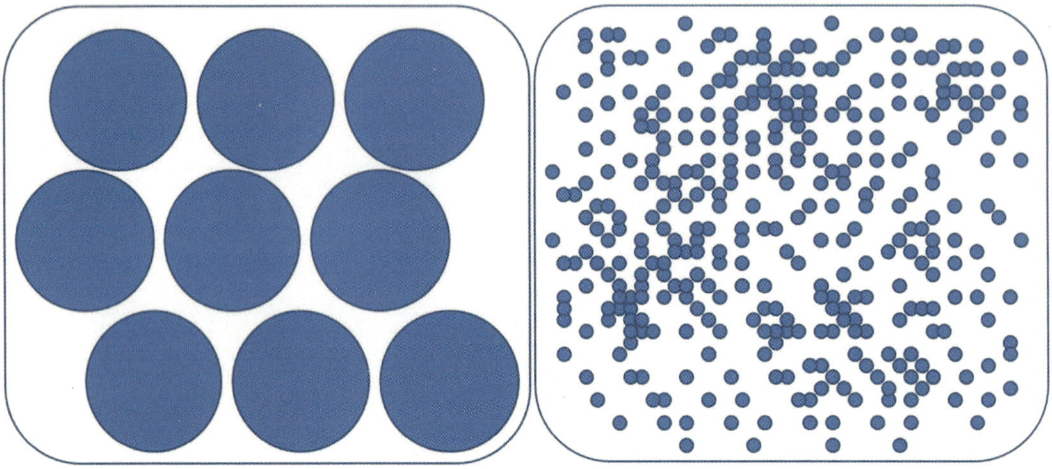

Fig. 1.4 The concept of macrofilled (*left*) and microfilled (*right*) composites. The original ratio of "particles" in this schematic is 1:10, suggesting that individual filler particles in microfilled composites were even smaller than presented in this figure

inorganic agglomerated microfiller complexes (1–25 μm) [6]. Prepolymers were able to increase the filler content in microfilled composites up to 60 wt%. However, prepolymers could not be covalently bonded to the resin matrix due to the lack of available C=C bonds at their surface resulting in low wear resistance in load-bearing areas [7].

Shortly afterwards, in the early 1980s, *hybrid composites* were introduced as a true combination of macrofilled and microfilled composites. They contained macrofiller quartz, glass, or Ba/Sr/Al/Zr-silicate particles (1–50 μm) with amorphous silica microfiller particles (0.04 μm). The tendency over the 1980s was to further reduce the size of macrofiller particles to an average of 1–5 μm (midifills) or 0.6–1 μm (minifills) [7]. Hybrid composites were considered an optimal combination of macrofilled and microfilled predecessors for favorable mechanical and optical properties and improved wear resistance [6]. Quartz was being replaced with other types of fillers due to its high abrasiveness toward enamel and lack of radiopacity. Ba-glass and ytterbium/yttrium trifluoride fillers were added for radiopacity and potential fluoride release. However, it was shown that trifluoride-containing composite released significantly lower amounts of fluoride than a glass-ionomer cement [15] excluding anticariogenic potential of such composites.

When hybrid composites were introduced, there was a difference in anterior and posterior composites in that anterior composites satisfied high esthetics requirements at the expense of high strength and vice versa. However, in the late 1980s, this gap was closing, and in the early 1990s, *universal composites* were introduced on the market. Small filler particles in hybrid composites allowed the decrease in interparticle distances which in turn improved wear resistance and mechanical properties in general and maintained good polishability and esthetic properties of microfilled composites. Therefore, universal composites were recommended for restoring both anterior and posterior teeth. Also, the term "microhybrid composite" was invented to refer to the hybrids containing 0.4–1 μm glass, zirconia, or ceramic filler particles in combination with smaller 0.04 μm-sized amorphous silica particles.

In mid- and late 1990s, two very different "classes" of composite materials were developed, based on their consistency—*flowables* and *packables*. Flowable composites were designed for better adaptation in deep or undercut areas of the cavity. Their low viscosity is achieved by either lowering the filler content or adding surfactants to reduce the viscosity but maintain the filler content. The mechanical properties of flowables were significantly worse than those of universal composites [16, 17] which restricted their field of indications to cavity lining, small restorations at load-free areas (e.g., Class V), or restoration repair.

Packable composites were designed specifically for posterior teeth as a potential amalgam replacement. The intention was to simplify the clinical procedure by introducing a harder material which would be condensed in a similar matter as amalgam. High viscosity was achieved in different ways maintaining the filler content in the range of 75–85 wt%: (1) fused particle agglomerates, (2) fibrous fillers, and (3) narrow distribution of midi-, mini-, and microfillers [18]. The mechanical properties of packable composites were not improved nor the polymerization shrinkage reduced as would be expected of high-density materials [18].

Around the year 2000, nanotechnology allowed further improvement of dental composites and the launch of nanofilled and nanohybrid composites. *Nanofilled composites* contain silica and/or zirconia particles (5–20 nm) in the form of discrete/non-agglomerated particle and fused/agglomerated nanoclusters (avg. size = 0.6–10 μm). *Nanohybrid composites* contain silica/zirconia nanoparticles and larger 0.6–1 μm glass/zirconia/silica particles. Nanohybrid composites also contain prepolymerized resin fillers and nanoclusters. The new sol-gel technology used to create nano-sized filler particles allowed greater nanofiller content compared to the traditional microfilled composites. High overall filler content in excess of 80 wt% of ultrafine particles is responsible for excellent optical properties, polishability, and gloss though mechanical properties, hardness, strength, and wear resistance did not surpass microhybrid composites [19–22]. Furthermore, volumetric shrinkage of nanofilled and nanohybrid composites was not substantially reduced, being between 1.5 and 2.5 vol% as claimed by the manufacturers and confirmed by independent researchers [23].

1.3 Resin Modifications

For the most part of the five decades of composite development, the focus was on the filler content, whereas the resin matrix changed very little. Until the mid-1990s, 80–90% of all marketed composites contained BisGMA. Other monomers were mostly TEGDMA, UDMA,[2] and BisEMA,[3] while other methacrylate monomers or other types of monomers (tricyclodecane or linear polyurethane) were rarely used in commercial composites [7]. Research shows that methacrylate-based composites are characterized by incomplete cure and cross-linking with most pendant C=C double bonds remaining within the polymer network and up to 10% of leachable uncured monomers [5, 7]. Methacrylate-based composites are prone to water sorption and hydrolysis. Enzymes such as cholesterol esterase may also hydrolyze methacrylate polymers [24].

Polymerization shrinkage is a downside of methacrylate-based composites attracting most research efforts. It occurs due to the shortening of distances between monomeric units in the polymer compared to intermolecular distances of uncured monomers. Considerable efforts were made over the 1990s and 2000s regarding resin modifications to reduce polymerization shrinkage and the associated stress. Experimental formulations contained oxybismethacrylates, highly branched methacrylates, silsesquioxane, and cyclic siloxane monomers [25]. Ring-opening molecules attracted attention as Stansbury [26] developed spiro-orthocarbonate monomers which polymerize via double-ring opening for potential use in dental composites. Ring-opening polymerization is based on opening of a cyclic structure resulting in expansion rather than shrinkage during monomer bonding and cross-linking. Thiol-ene methacrylate systems were also investigated as potential shrinkage stress reducers but, at the same time, maintaining strength and conversion over the usual curing time [27].

[2] Urethane dimethacrylate.

[3] Ethoxylated bisphenol A dimethacrylate.

As a result of these efforts, *low-shrinkage composites* were introduced in the mid-2000s. Methacrylate-free Filtek Silorane (3M ESPE) contained silorane resin and microhybrid quartz and yttrium fluoride fillers. Cationic ring-opening polymerization involved multiple oxirane groups facilitating cross-linking with the polymer. Polymerization shrinkage was shown to be below 1% and mechanical properties similar to methacrylate-based composites [28]. Other low-shrinkage composites that followed were based on long-chain monomers with higher molecular weight than BisGMA. In vitro studies showed similar or lower shrinkage and shrinkage stress of low shrinkage than universal composites [29–32]. However, there is a lack of clinical studies, and the available data suggest no significant improvements of posterior restorations with low-shrinkage composites [33, 34].

The demand for simplification of the clinical procedure with resin-based composites led to the development of the so-called *self-adhesive (self-adhering) composites* which are applied to tooth tissue without prior use of an adhesive system. Though the first two materials from this group (Vertise Flow, Kerr and Fusio Liquid Dentin, Pentron) were introduced on the market in late 2000s, there have not been any further additions. In vivo and in vitro research data indicate inferior performance of the current self-adhesive composites questioning their routine clinical application [35–37]. The addition of acidic monomers to the existing self-adhesive methacrylate-based composition does not seem to provide sufficient adhesion to enamel and dentin. It seems reasonable to assume that self-adhesive composites will remain an attractive possibility, but material improvement is clearly required.

Around 2010, the options for posterior restorations were expanded with a new "class" of composite materials—*bulk-fill composites*. Bulk-fills are indicated for 4–5 mm thick layers meaning that cavities as deep as 4–5 mm may be restored using the "bulk" instead of "layering" technique. This approach has a clear advantage in that it saves time especially with large posterior restorations. There are two major types of bulk-fills: (1) flowable bulk-fills which require a universal composite capping layer and (2) sculptable bulk-fills which may be used to restore the entire cavity. An exception is the fiber-reinforced composite EverX Posterior (GC) which, although sculptable, requires the capping layer because 1–3 mm glass fibers hinder finishing and polishing. The primary mechanisms of shrinkage and stress control in bulk-fill composites, as claimed by the manufacturers, are high molecular weight monomers which reduce the number of reacting groups similarly to low-shrinkage composites and the so-called stress modulators, resin monomers with cleavage sites for stress relief during polymerization. Though shrinkage and shrinkage stress of bulk-fill composites have been shown to be similar [38], their mechanical properties are mostly inferior to nanohybrid composites requiring further improvements [39–41].

References

1. WHO. Future use of materials for dental restoration: report of the meeting convened at WHO HQ, Geneva, Switzerland, 16–17 Nov 2009. 2010.
2. Bowen RL. Dental filling material comprising vinyl silane treated fused silica and a binder consisting of the reaction product of Bis-phenol and glycidyl acrylate. US Patents No. 3066112. 1962.
3. Bowen RL. Method of preparing a monomer having phenoxy and methacrylate groups linked by hydroxy glyceryl groups. United States Patents No. 3179623. 1965.
4. Bowen RL. Silica-resin direct filling material and method of preparation. United States Patents No. 3194783 and No. 3194784. 1965.
5. Peutzfeldt A. Resin composites in dentistry: the monomer systems. Eur J Oral Sci. 1997;105:97–116.
6. Lutz F, Phillips RW. A classification and evaluation of composite resin systems. J Prosthet Dent. 1983;50:480–8.
7. Ferracane JL. Current trends in dental composites. Crit Rev Oral Biol Med. 1995;6:302–18.
8. Phillips RW, Avery DR, Mehra R, Swartz ML, McCune RJ. Observations on a composite resin for class II restorations: three-year report. J Prosthet Dent. 1973;30:891–7.
9. Osborne JW, Gale EN, Ferguson GW. One-yer and two-year clinical evaluation of a composite resin vs. amalgam. J Prosthet Dent. 1973;30:795–800.

10. Santini A, Gallegos IT, Felix CM. Photoinitiators in dentistry: a review. Prim Dent J. 2013;2:30–3.
11. Dennison JB, Fan PL, Powers JM. Surface roughness of microfilled composites. J Am Dent Assoc. 1981;102:859–62.
12. Powers JM, Fan PL, Raptis CN. Color stability of new composite restorative materials under accelerated aging. J Dent Res. 1980;59:2071–4.
13. Raptis CN, Fan PL, Powers JM. Properties of microfilled and visible light-cured composite resins. J Am Dent Assoc. 1979;99:631–3.
14. Ferracane JL. Resin composite—state of the art. Dent Mater. 2011;27:29–38.
15. Young A, von der Fehr FR, Sonju T, Nordbo H. Fluoride release and uptake in vitro from a composite resin and two orthodontic adhesives. Acta Odontol Scand. 1996;54:223–8.
16. Attar N, Tam LE, McComb D. Flow, strength, stiffness and radiopacity of flowable resin composites. J Can Dent Assoc. 2003;69:516–21.
17. Schultz S, Rosentritt M, Behr M, Handel G. Mechanical properties and three-body wear of dental restoratives and their comparative flowable materials. Quintessence Int. 2010;41:e1–10.
18. Leinfelder KF, Bayne SC, Swift EJ Jr. Packable composites: overview and technical considerations. J Esthet Dent. 1999;11:234–49.
19. Jin J, Takahashi R, Hickel R, Kunzelmann KH. Surface properties of universal and flowable nanohybrid composites after simulated tooth brushing. Am J Dent. 2014;27:149–54.
20. Melander J, Dunn WP, Link MP, Wang Y, Xu C, Walker MP. Comparison of flexural properties and surface roughness of nanohybrid and microhybrid dental composites. Gen Dent. 2011;59:342–7. quiz 8-9
21. Ilie N, Hickel R. Investigations on mechanical behaviour of dental composites. Clin Oral Investig. 2009;13:427–38.
22. Takahashi H, Finger WJ, Endo T, Kanehira M, Koottathape N, Komatsu M, et al. Comparative evaluation of mechanical characteristics of nanofiller containing resin composites. Am J Dent. 2011;24: 264–70.
23. Sideridou ID, Karabela MM, Vouvoudi E. Physical properties of current dental nanohybrid and nanofill light-cured resin composites. Dent Mater. 2011;27:598–607.
24. Finer Y, Santerre JP. The influence of resin chemistry on a dental composite's biodegradation. J Biomed Mater Res A. 2004;69:233–46.
25. Chen M-H. Update on dental nanocomposites. J Dent Res. 2010;89:549–60.
26. Stansbury JW. Synthesis and evaluation of new oxaspiro monomers for double ring-opening polymerization. J Dent Res. 1992;71:1408–12.
27. Cramer NB, Stansbury JW, Bowman CN. Recent advances and developments in composite dental restorative materials. J Dent Res. 2011;90:402–16.
28. Weinmann W, Thalacker C, Guggenberger R. Siloranes in dental composites. Dent Mater. 2005;21:68–74.
29. Van Ende A, Mine A, De Munck J, Poitevin A, Van Meerbeek B. Bonding of low-shrinking composites in high C-factor cavities. J Dent. 2012;40:295–303.
30. Aleixo AR, Guiraldo RD, Fugolin AP, Berger SB, Consani RL, Correr AB, et al. Evaluation of contraction stress, conversion degree, and cross-link density in low-shrinkage composites. Photomed Laser Surg. 2014;32:267–73.
31. Ilie N, Jelen E, Clementino-Luedemann T, Hickel R. Low-shrinkage composite for dental application. Dent Mater J. 2007;26:149–55.
32. Marchesi G, Breschi L, Antoniolli F, Di Lenarda R, Ferracane J, Cadenaro M. Contraction stress of low-shrinkage composite materials assessed with different testing systems. Dent Mater. 2010;26:947–53.
33. Baracco B, Perdigao J, Cabrera E, Ceballos L. Two-year clinical performance of a low-shrinkage composite in posterior restorations. Oper Dent. 2013;38:591–600.
34. Walter R, Boushell LW, Heymann HO, Ritter AV, Sturdevant JR, Wilder AD Jr, et al. Three-year clinical evaluation of a silorane composite resin. J Esthet Restor Dent. 2014;26:179–90.
35. Kucukyilmaz E, Savas S. Evaluation of different fissure sealant materials and Flowable composites used as pit-and-fissure sealants: a 24-month clinical trial. Pediatr Dent. 2015;37:468–73.
36. Pinna R, Bortone A, Sotgiu G, Dore S, Usai P, Milia E. Clinical evaluation of the efficacy of one self-adhesive composite in dental hypersensitivity. Clin Oral Investig. 2015;19:1663–72.
37. Poitevin A, De Munck J, Van Ende A, Suyama Y, Mine A, Peumans M, et al. Bonding effectiveness of self-adhesive composites to dentin and enamel. Dent Mater. 2013;29:221–30.
38. Al Sunbul H, Silikas N, Watts DC. Polymerization shrinkage kinetics and shrinkage-stress in dental resin-composites. Dent Mater. 2016;32:998–1006.
39. Ilie N, Bucuta S, Draenert M. Bulk-fill resin-based composites: an in vitro assessment of their mechanical performance. Oper Dent. 2013;38:618–25.
40. Leprince JG, Palin WM, Vanacker J, Sabbagh J, Devaux J, Leloup G. Physico-mechanical characteristics of commercially available bulk-fill composites. J Dent. 2014;42:993–1000.
41. Miletic V, Pongprueksa P, De Munck J, Brooks NR, Van Meerbeek B. Curing characteristics of flowable and sculptable bulk-fill composites. Clin Oral Investig. 2017;21:1201–12.

Composition of Dental Resin-Based Composites for Direct Restorations

2

Luc D. Randolph, William M. Palin, and Julian G. Leprince

Ever since the introduction of light-curable resin-based composites in the 1970s, these mixtures of organic and inorganic phases have continuously evolved to meet the increasing requirements of material design and dental practitioners. However, fundamentally, the chemistry of composite phases has not significantly changed, with material design that commonly involves particle dispersion within a resin matrix. Such matrix is typically based on (di)methacrylate chemistry and a camphorquinone system to initiate polymerization upon light activation. The lack of any substantial shift in the use of conventional manufacturing approaches is, in part, testament to the relative success of resin composites as restorative dental filling materials. Current research focuses on strategies that would allow bulk-curing or bioactive and adhesive properties, which may lead to an improved longevity.

Among the current key requirements for modern resin-based composites (Fig. 2.1), shorter curing times and maximized depth of cure with user-friendly shading systems and handling properties have increased in popularity. To meet these requirements, minor alterations to the composition are made, changing the bulk properties of resin-based composites. Hence, an understanding of the fundamental compositional changes is required in order to grasp the trade-offs and limitations that may arise. As one property is usually pushed forward by manufacturers, practitioners must be provided the opportunity to understand any compromise in other key characteristics. For example, depth of cure may be greatly improved at the cost of increased translucency and reduced cosmetic results and/or mechanical properties.

This Chapter aims to provide a comprehension of modern dental resin composite composition in

L.D. Randolph (✉)
Advanced Drug Delivery and Biomaterials, Louvain Drug Research Institute, Université Catholique de Louvain, Brussels, Belgium

Institute of Condensed Matter and Nanosciences, Bio- and Soft-Matter, Université Catholique de Louvain, Louvain-la-Neuve, Belgium
e-mail: luc.randolph@uclouvain.be

W.M. Palin
College of Medical and Dental Sciences, Institute of Clinical Sciences, Birmingham Dental School and Hospital, University of Birmingham, 5 Mill Pool Way, Birmingham B5 7EG, UK

J.G. Leprince
Advanced Drug Delivery and Biomaterials, Louvain Drug Research Institute, Université Catholique de Louvain, Brussels, Belgium

Institute of Condensed Matter and Nanosciences, Bio- and Soft-Matter, Université Catholique de Louvain, Louvain-la-Neuve, Belgium

School of Dentistry and Stomatology, Cliniques universitaires St Luc, Université Catholique de Louvain, Brussels, Belgium

V. Miletic (ed.), *Dental Composite Materials for Direct Restorations*, http://doi.org/10.1007/978-3-319-60961-4_2

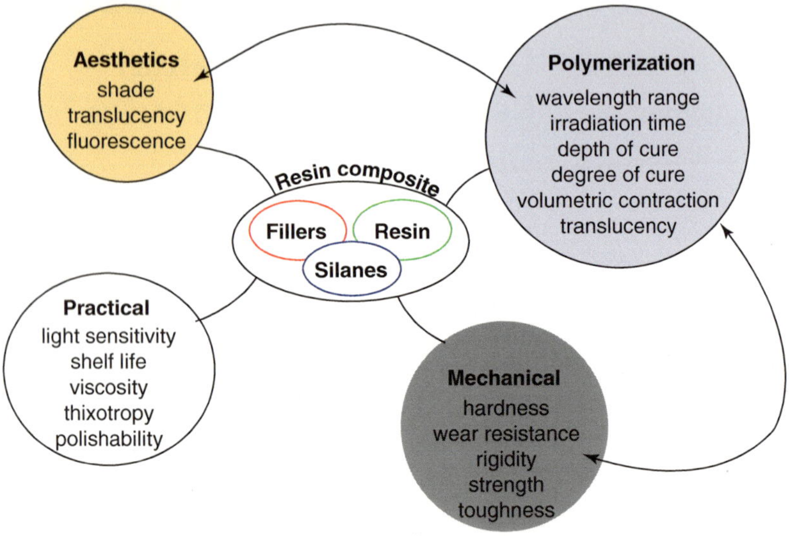

Fig. 2.1 Technical and practical requirements for resin-based composites used in dentistry

relation to brief historical perspectives and recent innovations, in terms of (a) resin chemistry, (b) chemical and photoinitiator chemistry, (c) inorganic particulate or fibrous filler phase, and (d) silane functionalization.

2.1 Monomers

The resin phase of dental resin composites is composed of reactive monomers, some providing rigidity or reduced shrinkage, while others, less viscous, are used as diluents to accommodate high filler particle loads and appropriate handling properties. Monomers that can be used in resin composites must display an activity of functional groups allowing for fast curing in the ambient, oxygen-rich environment. Further, the polymerization reaction proceeds in a filled paste system that necessarily displays a high viscosity and, hence, limited molecular mobility.

Historically, the monomers used have relied on the methacrylate group for functionality and a core of varying flexibility and hydrophilicity to match that of surface functionalized fillers (Fig. 2.2). The methacrylate-functional monomers satisfy the requirements for fast, in situ free-radical polymerization. The "Bowen" monomer bisphenol A glycidyl methacrylate (BisGMA) synthesized from bisphenol A and glycidyl methacrylate was patented in 1961 (patent US3179623 A). Due to its highly rigid core and relative hydrophobicity, it remains widely used in resin-based composites. BisGMA is however highly viscous (η = 1200 Pa.s [1]) which prevents the addition of large amounts of fillers. A comonomer blend based on BisGMA and triethylene glycol dimethacrylate (or TegDMA, η = 0.006 Pa.s [2]) is hence often used. Such blend displays an improved conversion and cross-linking compared to BisGMA alone [3]. As detailed in Chap. 5, much effort has been directed at improving the degree of polymer conversion, which averages 60% in paste-like composites [4]. The classical BisGMA/TegDMA blend has progressively been replaced or complemented with other molecules in an attempt to overcome the associated drawbacks. Most notably, molecules leading to a reduced "polymerization stress" have been proposed: silorane and thiol-ene systems are two examples of alternative functional chemistries to methacrylates (Fig. 2.2). Few materials based on silorane or thiol-ene systems have been marketed however. One material, the Filtek Silorane (3 M ESPE), was introduced in recent years but removed due the need of a specific bonding agent. This, by some accounts, posed too much confusion. Most validated strategies selected methacrylate monomers of greater flexibility: for example, ethoxylated bisphenol-A dimethacrylate

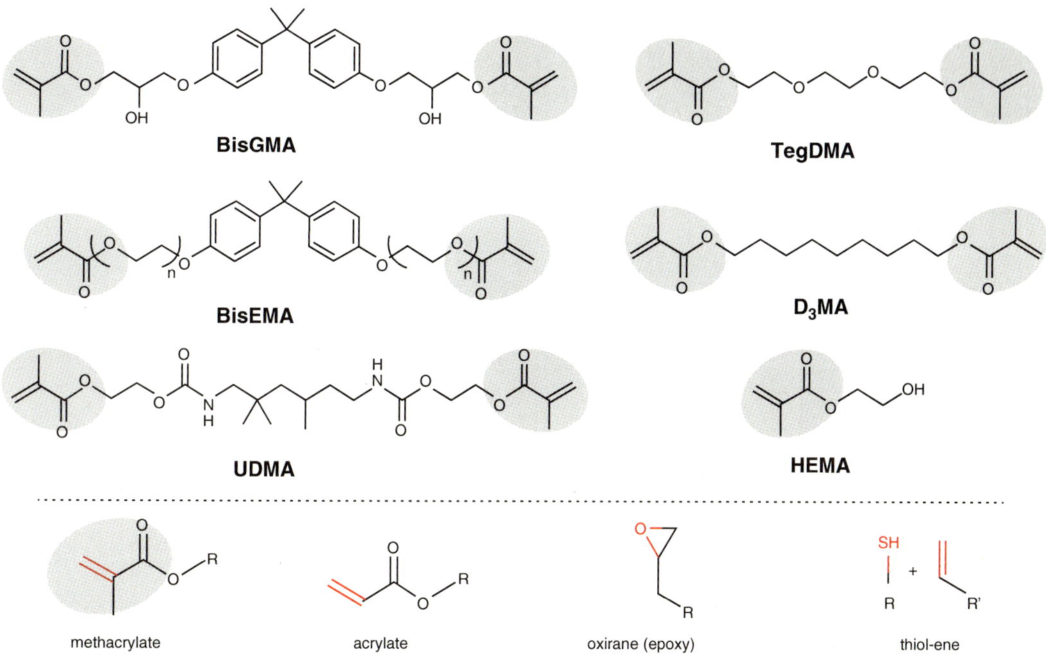

Fig. 2.2 Molecular structure of typical dimethacrylate monomers used in resin-based dental composites. The methacrylate group is highlighted in *gray* and compared to acrylate, silorane (epoxy), and thiol-ene functionalities

(BisEMA) is a type of monomer with BisGMA core moieties but displaying flexible ethylene glycol spacers. The addition of BisEMA can reduce the viscosity of a blend, improve conversion [5], and decrease polymerization stress, at the cost of a general decrease in mechanical properties [6].

Due to doubts about the stability of BisGMA and release of bisphenol A (the biological risk of which remains controversial, though very unlikely considering the concentrations observed [7, 8]), monomers such as urethane dimethacrylate (UDMA) have been introduced. The molecule, as shown in Fig. 2.2, has a lower molecular weight (M = 470 g/mol) and is more flexible than BisGMA. Resin blends composed of UDMA as replacement of BisGMA typically are less viscous, hence reducing the need for a diluent [3]. Further, the monomer to polymer conversion and mechanical strength are generally greater when replacing BisGMA with UDMA ([3, 9], respectively). However, the molecule presented in Fig. 2.2 (CAS registry number CAS 72869-86-4) is not the only one referred to as UDMA: the denomination is misleading as a variety of molecules are labeled with the "urethane" short name [10]. In fact, while urethane groups (–NH–(C=O)–O–) can be observed in "UDMA" molecules, entirely different structures exist (Fig. 2.3). Hence, modern dental composites that contain "urethane" monomers may display advantageous properties, although it remains difficult to associate these to specific molecules.

Some years ago, organic/inorganic oligomer-based materials were introduced to the market, termed "Ormocers" (ORganically MOdified CERamics). Generally, Ormocers can still be considered as glass-filled composites. The main departure from conventional chemistries lies in the nature of the resin phase. Oligomers within Ormocer materials consist of condensed (silane) molecules similar to those used to functionalize the surface of fillers in conventional resin composites. By hydrolyzing and condensing silanes, oligomers of specific composition and structure may be obtained (Fig. 2.4). The main goal of Ormocer molecules is to increase the amount of silicium in resin composites, a change marketed as an increase in filler content. Furthermore, the oligomers can replace BisGMA, TegDMA, and

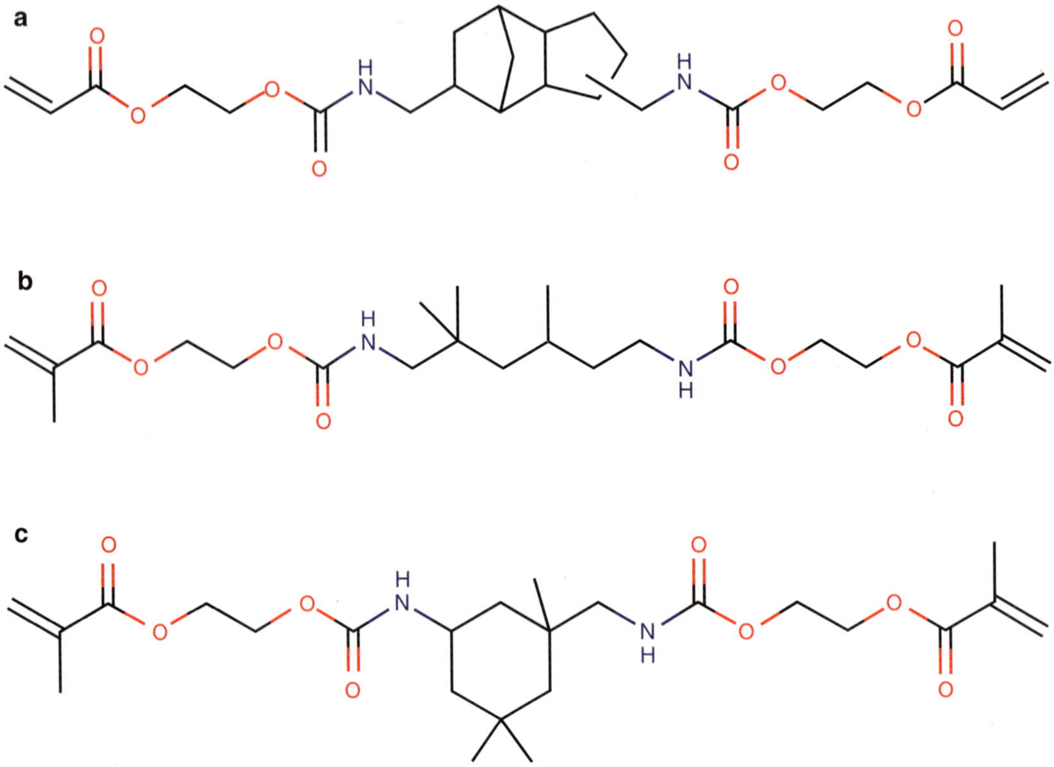

Fig. 2.3 "Urethane" di(meth)acrylate monomers used in dental composites, as described in patent US 2010/0076115 A1 (**a**) and manufacturer information (**b** and **c**)

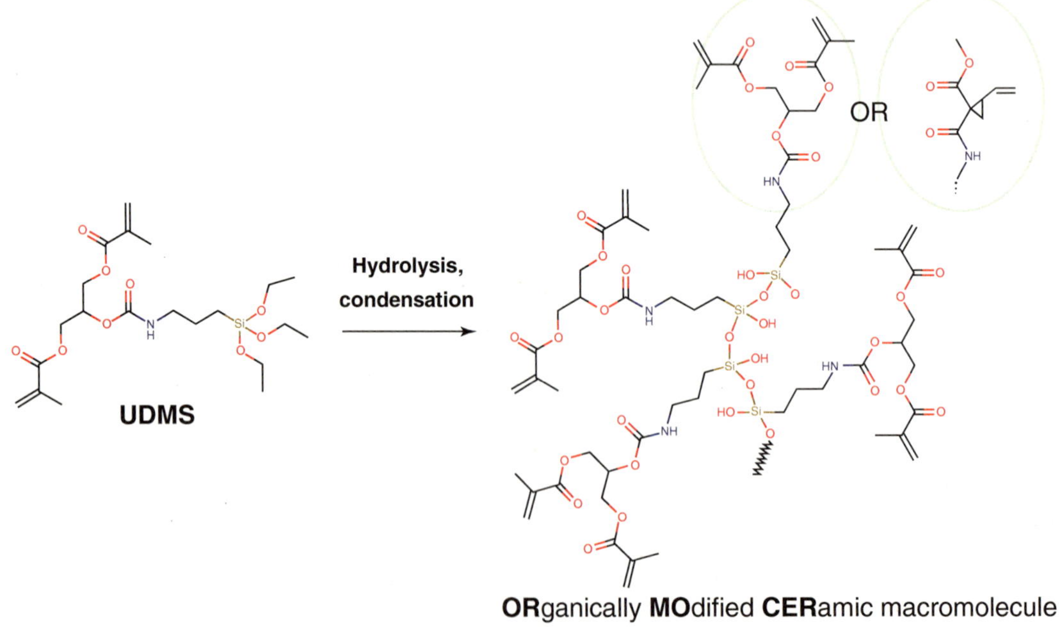

Fig. 2.4 Scheme exemplifying silane condensation to prepare an organic-inorganic macromolecule, where the functionality available for polymerization can be methacrylate, vinylcyclopropane, etc. UDMS stands for Urethane DiMethacrylate Silane

other conventional dimethacrylates so long as their viscosity and hydrophilicity allow for appropriate handling properties and filler loading [11]. The organic/inorganic oligomers may maintain the methacrylate functionality or switch to ring-opening chemistries [12]. In the latter case, a lower volumetric shrinkage could be expected due to an inherently lower molar shrinkage coefficient [13]. The oligomers may constitute the whole resin phase so long as the viscosity and hydrophilicity allow for appropriate handling properties and filler loading. However, little is known about the actual design of the organic/inorganic molecules in commercial materials, and further characterization is required in order to correlate compositional changes to clinical results. A commercial Ormocer material was shown to perform as well as other clinically validated resin composites after 3 years [14]. Additional studies will determine the long-term performance of current Ormocers.

Further efforts have focused on the development of self-adhesive composites, whose composition should provide adhesion to dental tissues without the use of a separate bonding layer. While the strength of such self-adhesion remains quite low [15], the resin composite utilizes monomers presenting acid groups capable of reacting with calcium groups in hydroxyapatite ($Ca_{10}(PO_4)_6(OH)_2$). Several different monomers were produced based on carboxylic or phosphoric acid groups as with chemistries used for self-etching or so-called 'universal' dental adhesives. Self-adhesive composites must display a pH low enough ($\approx$2–3) to etch the smear layer and bind to exposed mineralized collagen fibers [16]. At such pH, the hydrolytic stability of conventional dimethacrylates is severely compromised, and designing self-adhesive resin composites with a suitable shelf life is complex [17]. Further, self-adhesive composites must display a low viscosity and be amphiphilic in order to wet dentin but also prevent phase separation in the material. Unfortunately, as with Ormocers, information regarding developments and the composition of the commercial self-adhesive resin composites is scarce. One study did investigate the nanostructuring of the interface between an experimental two-part self-adhesive resin composite containing a phosphoric acid ester molecule and mineralized tissues [18]. Results showed the formation of a hybrid layer typical of relatively high-pH self-etch adhesives (pH > 2). The interaction was limited, and authors indicated acceptable bond strength to dentin but not to enamel. In vitro, the bonding effectiveness of current self-adhesive resin composites to enamel and dentin remains suboptimal, with adhesion values lower than that of one-step (and most simple) adhesives [15, 19]. The technology is still evolving and improving and, in many ways, following closely to the development of self-adhesive resin cements and resin composite bonding systems.

2.2 Initiators in Conventional Photopolymerization

The in situ photopolymerization of dental resin composites requires the use of a molecule or system capable of inducing optimal polymerization throughout a significant depth (several millimeters) of pigmented material, with clinically compatible irradiation times ($\approx$20 s). Historically, and typical of most commercialized materials today, the type II photoinitiator camphorquinone, combined with a co-initiator, usually a tertiary amine, is used. On absorbing of corresponding photons, the photoinitiator system starts a free-radical polymerization (FRP) process. Camphorquinone absorbs over the 400–500 nm range with a peak of absorption located at 470 nm (Fig. 2.5). Alternative and simpler type I photoinitiator molecules have been suggested, such as phosphine oxides or germanium-based molecules. Such systems absorb at lower wavelength, with an absorption maximum located around 400 nm. While manufacturers provide little information on composition, the introduction of LED light-curing units provides two discrete outputs usually located at approximately 410 nm and 470 nm, which confirms the use of different photoinitiators [20, 21].

As the different absorption profiles suggest (Fig. 2.5a), CQ imparts a yellowish color to resin composite bulk, while the molecule phenylbis(2,4,6-trimethylbenzoyl) phosphine oxide (TPO) appears as a white powder (Fig. 2.5b), and Ivocerin™, a germanium-based photoinitiator, is standing in between. This is of importance as resin composites for anterior applications, for example, "enamel" shades, can require high translucency with minimal pigmentation. Besides the absorption spectra, the chemistry of initiators also affects color. Experimentally, nonpigmented resin composites based on phosphine oxides show better color stability than those using CQ [22, 23], associated to differences in polymer networks. Phosphine oxide-containing resin composites may present a more cross-linked polymer network [24, 25], making it less susceptible to pigment diffusion (such as tannins) and color variations.

The efficiency of initiators depends on several characteristics, including the absorption yield efficiency (ε, in L/mol.cm) [26], which describes how many photons can be absorbed per initiator molecule at a given wavelength. When comparing TPO and CQ in terms of absorption, the data shown in Fig. 2.5 highlights the greater efficiency of TPO at lower concentration (10x lower). The greater absorption maxima of TPO are related to the aromatic rings, or chromophores, present in TPO (Fig. 2.6). In addition, the TPO molecule upon excitation yields two active radicals [27], while a type II photoinitiator system such as CQ/amine yields one [28]. The overlap between the absorption spectra and the light-curing unit (LCU) emission spectrum also greatly influences polymerization efficiency. Modern LED LCUs display narrow outputs (approx. 40 nm wide) located around the absorption maxima of initiator molecules, which ensures that emitted photons

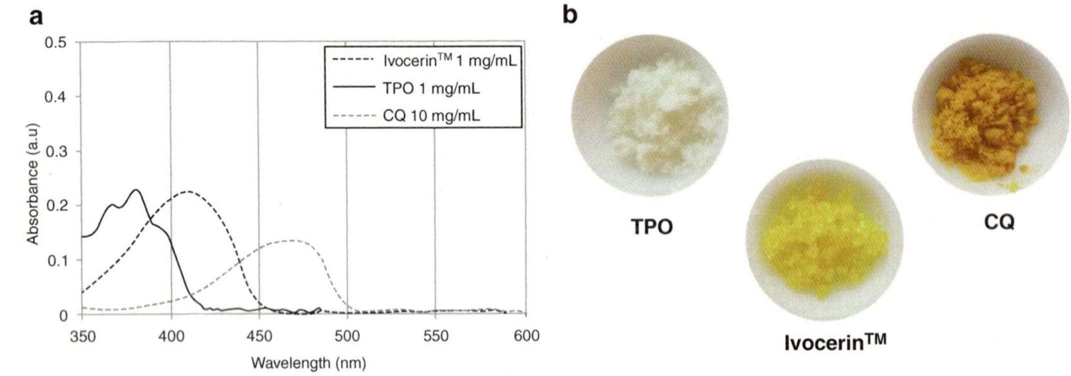

Fig. 2.5 Absorption spectra (**a**) of diphenyl(2,4,6-trimethylbenzoyl) phosphine oxide (TPO), camphorquinone (CQ), or benzoyl germanium (Ivocerin™) photoinitiators in the range 350–600 nm. Note the differences in absorption range, absorption maxima, and absorption taking into account the concentrations. Visual aspect of initiators in powder form (**b**)

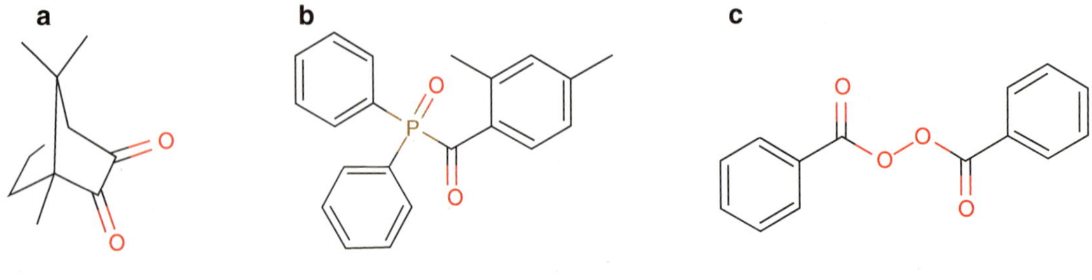

Fig. 2.6 Initiators used in dental composites for photo or "self" polymerization. (**a**) Camphorquinone, (**b**) TPO, and (**c**) benzoyl peroxide (BPO)

can be absorbed and utilized to initiate polymerization rather than contributing to the exotherm of polymerizing material and heating the surrounding tissues, such as the dental pulp.

Finally, in some resin composites, the polymerization is not light initiated but rather starts upon mixing two pastes. This may be needed for resin composite materials used for cementation of indirect restorations or root filling in the placement of posts or other applications where light transmission might be problematic. Such "auto" polymerization typically results from the reaction of benzoyl peroxide (BPO, Fig. 2.6) with a tertiary amine contained within separate pastes. In order to accommodate an appropriate working time, inhibitor molecules are added to the composite to prevent premature hardening following mixing. These, such as butylated hydroxytoluene (BHT) or 4-methoxyphenol (MEHQ), are antioxidants and consume active radicals, and the polymerization reaction only starts once they have been depleted.

2.3 Fillers

2.3.1 General Description

In order to increase mechanical properties of resin-based dental restorative materials, fillers must be optimally loaded and dispersed in the resin matrix. The inorganic filler particles act as reinforcing phase, increasing the elastic modulus of the resin composite, providing resistance to wear, and improving fracture toughness, and, prior to curing, influence handling properties that must be adapted for shaping and sculpting by the practitioner. Fillers, composed of inorganic oxides and glasses, can be described by their type (glass composition), morphology (size distribution and shape), density, radiopacity, refractive index, and surface porosity [29–33]. These characteristics, used as basis for classification and categorization of dental resin composites, along with their evolution are reviewed in Chap. 6.

Two "classes" of particles used in modern dental resin composites may be distinguished based on manufacturing processes and size, i.e., micro- and nanoscale particles (Fig. 2.7, orange and green boxes, respectively). While the latter, with, by definition, an average particle size smaller than 100 nm, are produced using a bottom-up approach, the micro-sized particles are usually milled, ground, and sieved from larger sizes. Historically, the first fillers to be introduced were large (> 10 μm) micron-sized particles. The need for improved cosmetic results, polishability, and higher filler loading to improve mechanical properties led to a decrease in average particle size (1–10 μm) and more refined particle size distribution. In recent years, resin composites with submicron average particle sizes have been marketed (0.2–1 μm). The nanoparticles, typically fumed silica, act in part as viscosity modifiers and display sizes in the range of 10–40 nm but are rarely observed as discrete, non-agglomerated particles. Weak physical interactions at the nanometer scale promote agglomeration, and nanoparticles often appear as agglomerates. In order to aid dispersion, particles must be properly silanated (Sect. 2.4).

The morphology of microparticles may be controlled through the grinding process and greatly influences packing and hence maximal

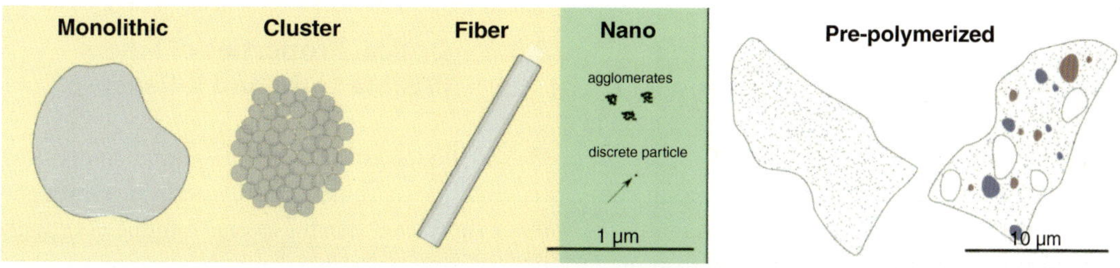

Fig. 2.7 Filler classes and possible geometries and composition. The pre-polymerized fillers can be composed of ground composite using nanoparticles and/or glass particles, which may vary in composition

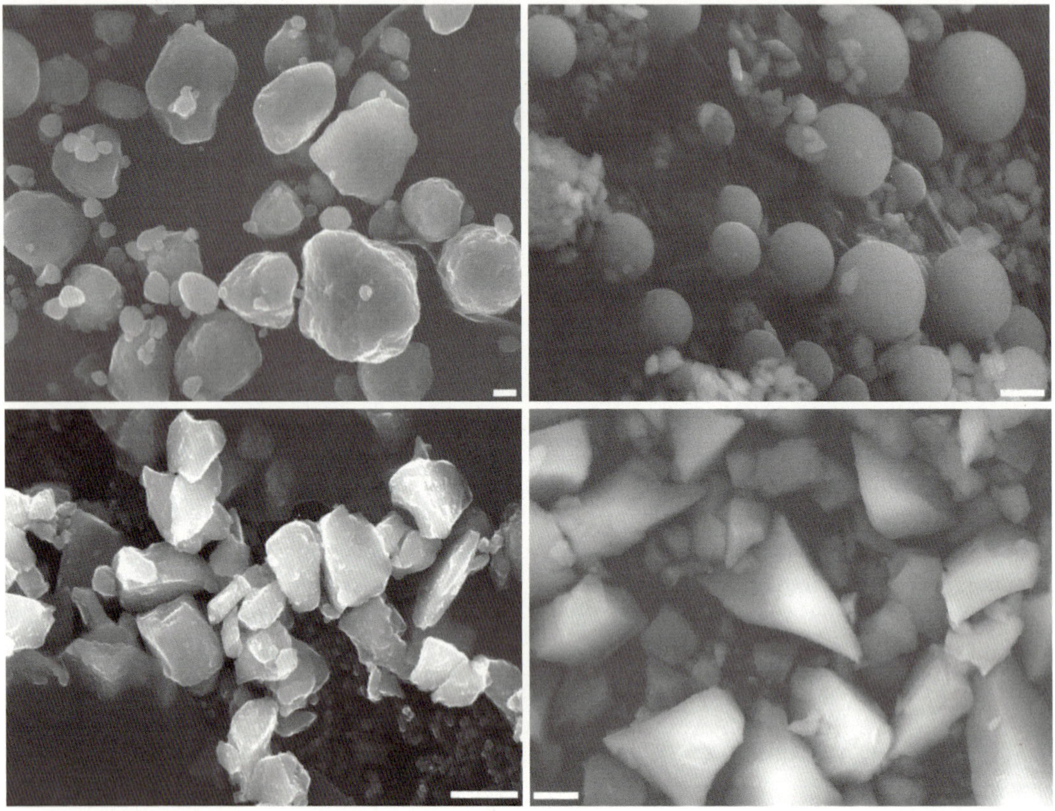

Fig. 2.8 Morphology of fillers—microparticles—separated from the resin phase in four different commercial resin composites. The scale bar indicates 1 μm in all SEM pictures

filler loading. Filler morphology varies greatly (Fig. 2.8) but is difficult to relate to packing and the bulk properties of a material. Resin composites often contain more than one size distribution (bimodal) to allow for more efficient packing where smaller particles can occupy interstices between larger fillers [29, 33].

Filler content is negatively correlated with the volumetric shrinkage and polymerization stress [34]. While several strategies have been investigated to limit stress development during curing, increasing the filler content appears as an efficient solution. In modern resin composites, this content is invariably higher than 35 vol%, even in "flowables."

The composition of fillers varies among commercial composites and is optimized to match the refractive index of the resin but also to provide radiopacity (Sect. 2.3.2). Conventional monolithic microparticles (Fig. 2.7) are composed of silica-rich glasses, with doping oxides such as alumina and barium oxide (Al_2O_3 and BaO), which are commonly used for radiopacity [35]. Less common elements such as Sr, Yb, or Zr can also be found. Few changes in terms of composition were observed over the last two decades, but efforts rather went to generating particular structures and microstructures (Chapter 2c.iii, Specific Fillers).

2.3.2 Optical Properties of Fillers (Visible Light and X-Rays)

Photopolymerization of dental resin composites requires a design enabling polymerization throughout a significant depth (several millimeters), with limited irradiation time. Light penetration depends on the transmission of light or how much light reaches the deeper resin composite layers.

Table 2.1 Representative refractive indices for several resin blends and fillers. Information extracted from manufacturers' websites and reference [36]

Resin blend		Fillers	
Type, description	Refractive index	Type, description	Refractive index
TegDMA/BisGMA 30/70	1.524 → 1.556[a]	Barium borosilicate glass, Esstech Inc.	1.553
TegDMA/BisGMA 90/10	1.474 → 1.538[a]	Aluminosilicate glass ceramic, Esstech Inc.	1.54
TegDMA, Esstech Inc.	1.4595	Barium borosilicate glass "IS 50 1102 dental glass 1,0"; Ferro Corp.	1.52
HEMA, Sigma-Aldrich	1.453	–	

[a]Refractive index variation after polymerization (the value increases)

Ideally, fillers should transmit light in the visible range so that color is mainly controlled through the addition of a selection of pigments. Loss of light with depth is mainly due to refraction: the law of refraction describes the extent light deviates at an interface from its original direction, which is related to the difference in the refractive index of each phase. In resin composites, each filler particle represents an interface with the resin matrix. It is assumed that a similar refractive index of fillers to that of the resin blend will increase light transmission and depth of cure.

Refractive index of the polymer increases with increasing cross-linking density of the resin, i.e., most manufacturers design resin composites with a filler refractive index close to that of the cured copolymer blend (Table 2.1). It follows that most current commercial resin composites increase in translucency as polymerization proceeds. However, some modern so-called "bulk-fill" materials exhibit a reduction in light transmission, and increased opacity, as the resin cures in order to better mimic the aesthetic properties of enamel. There is no current consensus on how light transmission changes throughout polymerization affect degree of conversion with depth.

The light emitted from a resin composite, perceived by the eye, is a mixture of light reflecting off its surface and emitted from the bulk after scattering and absorption. In order for a resin composite to blend with surrounding mineralized tissues, optical properties should be optimized to match that of dentin and enamel. Particle size and filler content, for example, influence optical characteristics. A decrease in particle size is associated with an increase in transmittance, related to a decrease in scattering [37]. Further, the higher the filler content, the higher the scattering coefficient [38] and hence the lower the transmission [37]. It follows that more translucent resin composites, for example, "enamel" shades, generally have a lower filler content. Modern resin composites still fail to match the optical properties of enamel, including the absorption and scattering over the visible range of light [39]. Further research in composition, including that of fillers, is required to reach optimal material blending with tissues.

Opacity to X-rays (high-energy photons) or radiopacity is a crucial requirement for resin composites. In order to properly diagnose secondary carries, a dental practitioner must be able to clearly distinguish a restorative material from degraded tissues. The main tool for diagnosis is X-ray imaging, where carious tissues appear more radio-transparent as they are demineralized. This is explained by X-ray absorption being directly related to the atomic number of atoms encountered. ISO 4049 specifies the minimal radiopacity for resin composites, with the standard chosen as the absorption of a 1 mm-thick layer of pure aluminum (atomic number, $Z = 13$) [40]. The resin phase of resin composites contributes very little to X-ray absorption. Consequently, resin composites must incorporate a high fraction of radiopaque fillers composed of heavy elements such as strontium ($Z = 38$), zirconium ($Z = 40$), barium ($Z = 56$), lanthanum ($Z = 57$), Ytterbium ($Z = 70$), or bismuth ($Z = 83$), the most common being barium [32, 35]. Modern resin composites meet the ISO requirement for radiopacity [41, 42].

2.3.3 Specific Fillers

The geometry and microstructure of fillers can be engineered to provide specific properties and improvements with regard to bulk and surface properties. To date, the modifications and specificities can be grouped as follows: fibers or fiber-like particles, clusters, and pre-polymerized fillers.

2.3.3.1 Fibers

To improve the fracture toughness of resin composites, particles with a high length to diameter ratio have been used, both experimentally [43] and in commercial materials [44]. When silanized, fibers may increase the strength of a composite due to the additional "pullout" that must occur for a crack to progress around them. The fibers in dental composite are typically silica-based (SiO_2). The glass fibers were adapted or directly taken from industrial applications and are denoted E (E for "electrical") or S type depending on their origin: the former was originally developed for insulation in electronics and contains a mixture of SiO_2, alumina (Al_2O_3), calcium, magnesium, and boron oxides (CaO, MgO, and B_2O_3). The S-glass (S for "stiff") fibers are composed of SiO_2, Al_2O_3, and MgO. Both types of glasses are amorphous and resistant to deformation compared to the polymer matrix: their elastic moduli are greater than 60 GPa [45].

Given the morphology of glass fibers, their use in resin composites is complicated and often limited to nonaesthetic but functional materials, e.g., composites in prosthodontics (dentures) or orthodontics (retainers). The introduction of fibers is difficult as the length of fibers usually exceeds the millimeter, and their diameter is in the tens of micrometers (Fig. 2.9). The random orientation of fibers prevents packing, resulting in potential voids. In resin composites, the presence of fibers is associated with rough surfaces [46] and poor wear resistance [47].

2.3.3.2 Clusters

So-called (nano)clusters are fillers composed of submicron particles that are agglomerated after sintering or chemical binding. These clusters are

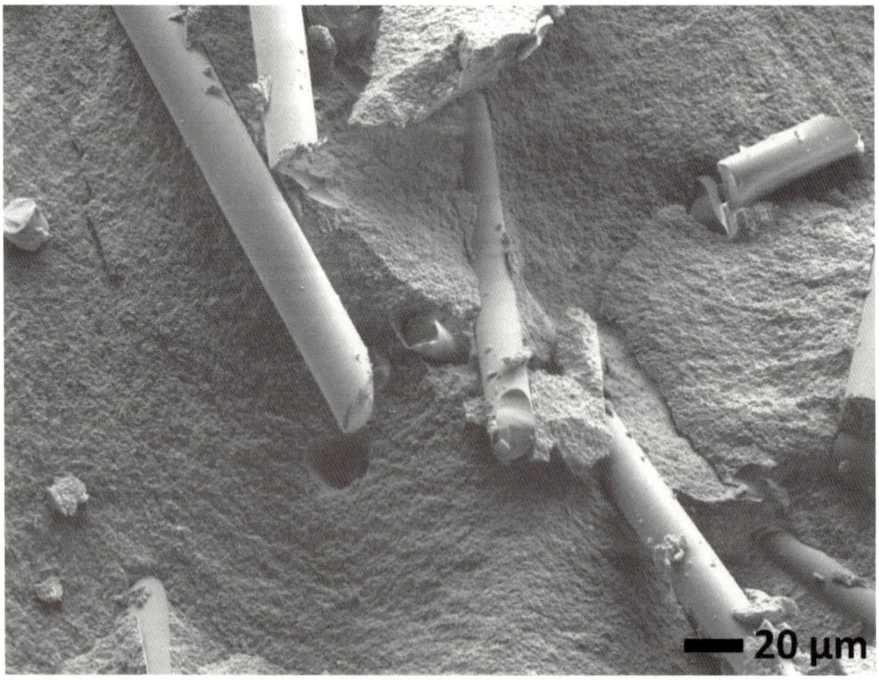

Fig. 2.9 Fracture interface after 3-point bending testing of a fiber-reinforced dental composite (Xenius, GC)

proposed as a solution to improve the strength of composites: upon meeting a cluster, a growing crack would have to physically separate the clusters into aggregates of smaller size to progress, an energy-consuming mechanism. Thermally processed clusters, sintered particles, can be viewed as ceramic fillers. Depending on the glass composition of the particles, some amount of crystallinity could be expected [31].

2.3.3.3 "Pre-polymerized" Fillers

The aesthetic quality of a composite relies on several factors, most noted previously and related directly to fillers. Maintaining high filler contents can also prove difficult due to issues with filler dispersion. Manufacturers have introduced pre-polymerized particles as early as the 1980s to solve these problems.

Pre-polymerized fillers (PPFs) are ground, cured resin composites, which may be originally filled with nano- and/or micron-sized particles (Figs. 2.7 and 2.10). These PPFs are clearly distinguishable from "structural" fillers (see EDX map in Fig. 2.10), which are added in the final resin composite along with PPFs [48]. The size of PPFs usually exceeds 10 μm (Fig. 2.10) and can serve to increase light scattering and diffuse reflection for an improved optical matching with dentin and enamel tissues. Resin composites containing PPFs are also known to exhibit higher polishability and luster and usually designed for anterior application [48]. Adding PPFs however decreases the elastic

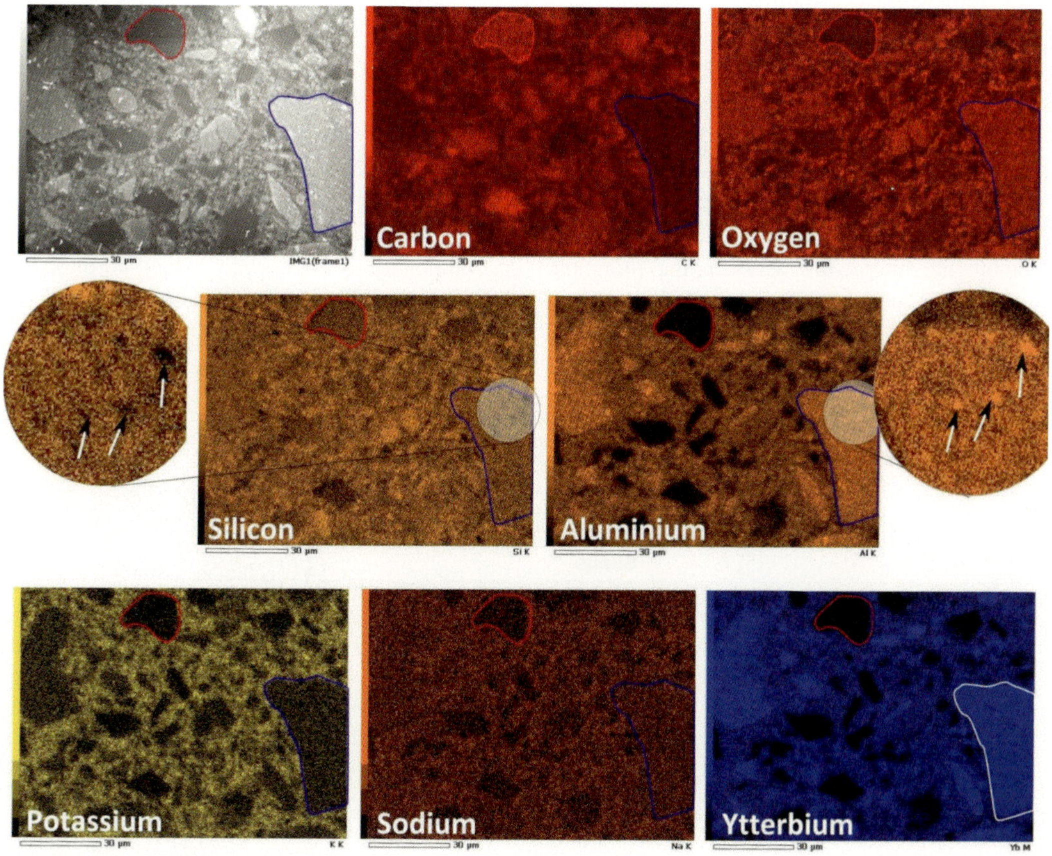

Fig. 2.10 EDX analysis of a polished resin composite commercial material containing pre-polymerized fillers (PPF). Two different types of PPF are outlined in the micrograph. In *red* is a nano-filled particle (carbon-rich, with some silicon but no glass, i.e., Al, K, Na, Yb-poor), and in *blue* is a nano- and micro-filled particle (from a hybrid resin composite, i.e., carbon-poor and composed of glasses containing silica, alumina, sodium, and ytterbium oxides). The *arrows* in magnified areas point to alumina particles. The scale bar is 30 μm in all pictures

moduli and resin composites with PPFs that typically absorb more water than those which do not [29]. Further, the PPF integration in the resin is poor without treatment as the functional groups already reacted during their preparation.

2.4 Functional Silane Chemistry

The mechanical performance of dental resin composites depends largely on the interaction, or lack thereof, between filler particles and the resin matrix. When stressed, the phases in a composite share the forces applied to different extents depending on their relative intrinsic mechanical properties. Stress distribution and transfer between phases are crucial in the performance of resin composites. In dental composites, the disparity in elastic modulus between the fillers (≫10 GPa) and that of the resin (1–3 GPa) indicates that under iso-stress, i.e., a homogeneously distributed stress, the matrix will deform to a greater extent [49]. This may compromise particle-resin cohesion, creating voids and/or accelerating the deterioration of the material. To promote the interaction between the inorganic and organic phases, fillers are silanized, to enhance particle wetting and chemical binding to the matrix. Silanization increases the overall strength of a resin composite by about 50% [50].

Most silanes used in dentistry are difunctional molecules: one end presents one or more reactive groups (methacrylate, acrylate, epoxy, etc.) to bind with the resin phase, while the other end can bind to –OH groups at the surface of the glass (oxides, mostly silica) or metals. A typical structure of a methacrylate-functional silane is presented in Fig. 2.11.

Both the core and ends of silanes can be modified to adapt their suitability with regard to resin or filler composition:

– Regarding the resin phase, the chemistry of silanes greatly influences particle wetting and is hence a crucial parameter. For relatively hydrophobic resin blends such as BisGMA/TegDMA, the silane γ-MPS has been deemed suitable for decades. A longer alkyl spacer, more hydrophobic, may be even better suited. Extending chain length to ten carbons was associated with improved flexural strength and, equally important, higher filler loading due to improved wetting by the resin [51]. Further, the structure of silanes influences water sorption and potentially the stability of a composite. For example, water sorption of experimental resin composites based on γ-MPS is lesser than with UDMS (shown in Fig. 2.4) [52]. Reducing the hydrophilicity of

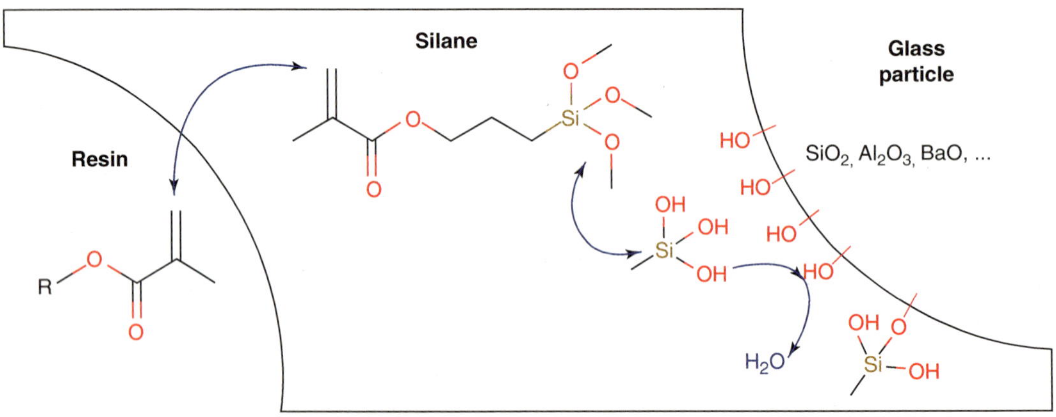

Fig. 2.11 γ-(methacryloxy)propyltrimethoxy silane (γ-MPS), a typical molecule used in dental materials, with one methacrylate end to react with the resin phase and another, hydrolysable $Si(OCH_3)_3$, that can react with conventional silica-based glass particles

the silane layer may be associated with increased durability [53].

– In order to improve the efficiency of silanes, the number of functional groups per molecule can be increased such as with UDMS (Fig. 2.4). This higher functionality and cross-linking potential may be associated with composite that is less prone to swelling [52].

Acknowledgments L.D. Randolph is a FRIA (F.R.S-FNRS) scholar.

References

1. Davy KWM, Kalachandra S, Pandain MS, Braden M. Relationship between composite matrix molecular structure and properties. Biomaterials. 1998;19:2007–14.
2. Feng L, Suh BI. Exposure reciprocity law in Photopolymerization of multi-functional acrylates and Methacrylates. Macromol Chem Phys. 2007;208:295–306.
3. Dickens SH, Stansbury JW, Choi KM, Floyd CJE. Photopolymerization kinetics of methacrylate dental resins. Macromolecules. 2003;36:6043–53.
4. Hadis M, Leprince JG, Shortall AC, Devaux J, Leloup G, Palin WM. High irradiance curing and anomalies of exposure reciprocity law in resin-based materials. J Dent. 2011;39:549–57.
5. de Godoy Fróes-Salgado NR, Gajewski V, Ornaghi BP, Pfeifer CSC, Meier MM, Xavier TA, Braga RR. Influence of the base and diluent monomer on network characteristics and mechanical properties of neat resin and composite materials. Odontology. 2015;103:160–8.
6. Boaro LC, Goncalves F, Guimaraes TC, Ferracane JL, Versluis A, Braga RR. Polymerization stress, shrinkage and elastic modulus of current low-shrinkage restorative composites. Dent Mater. 2010;26:1144–50.
7. Polydorou O, Konig A, Hellwig E, Kummerer K. Long-term release of monomers from modern dental-composite materials. Eur J Oral Sci. 2009;117:68–75.
8. Sevkusic M, Schuster L, Rothmund L, Dettinger K, Maier M, Hickel R, Van Landhuyt KL, Durner J, Hogg C, Reichl FX. The elution and breakdown behavior of constituents from various light-cured composites. Dent Mater. 2014;30:619–31.
9. Asmussen E, Peutzfeldt A. Influence of UEDMA BisGMA and TEGDMA on selected mechanical properties of experimental resin composites. Dent Mater. 1998;14:51–6.
10. Polydorou O, König A, Hellwig E, Kümmerer K. Uthethane dimethacrylate: a molecule that may cause confusion in dental research. J Biomed Mater Res B Appl Biomater. 2009;91B:1–4.
11. Moszner N, Völkel T, Cramer von Clausbruch S, Geiter E, Batliner N, Rheinberger V. Sol-Gel materials, 1. Synthesis and hydrolytic condensation of new cross-linking alkoxysilane methacrylates and light-curing composites based upon the condensates. Macromol Mater Eng. 2002;287:339–47.
12. Klapdohr S, Moszner N. New inorganic components for dental filling composites. Monatshefte für Chemie. 2004;136:21–45.
13. Contreras PP, Tyagi P, Agarwal S. Low volume shrinkage of polymers by photopolymerization of 1,1-bis(ethoxycarbonyl)-2-vinylcyclopropanes. Polym Chem. 2015;6:2297–304.
14. Mahmoud S, El-Embaby A, AbdAllah A. Clinical performance of Ormocer, Nanofilled, and Nanoceramic resin composites in class I and class II restorations: a three-year evaluation. Oper Dent. 2014;39:32–42.
15. Poitevin A, De Munck J, Van Ende A, Suyama Y, Mine A, Peumans M, Van Meerbeek B. Bonding effectiveness of self-adhesive composites to dentin and enamel. Dent Mater. 2013;29:221–30.
16. Van Meerbeek B, Yoshihara K, Yoshida Y, Mine A, De Munck J, Van Landuyt KL. State of the art of self-etch adhesives. Dent Mater. 2011;27:17–28.
17. Moszner N, Salz U, Zimmermann J. Chemical aspects of self-etching enamel-dentin adhesives: a systematic review. Dent Mater. 2005;21:895–910.
18. Hanabusa M, Mine A, Kuboki T, Momoi Y, Van Landuyt KL, Van Meerbeek B, De Munck J. TEM interfacial characterization of an experimental self-adhesive filling material bonded to enamel/dentin. Dent Mater. 2011;27:818–24.
19. Vichi A, Margvelashvili M, Goracci C, Papacchini F, Ferrari M. Bonding and sealing ability of a new self-adhering flowable composite resin in class I restorations. Clin Oral Investig. 2013;17:1497–506.
20. Neumann MG, Miranda WG Jr, Schmitt CC, Rueggeberg FA, Correa IC. Molar extinction coefficients and the photon absorption efficiency of dental photoinitiators and light curing units. J Dent. 2005;33:525–32.
21. Price RB, Felix CA. Effect of delivering light in specific narrow bandwidths from 394 to 515nm on the micro-hardness of resin composites. Dent Mater. 2009;25:899–908.
22. Albuquerque PPAC, Moreira ADL, Moraes RR, Cavalcante LM, Schneider LFJ. Color stability, conversion, water sorption and solubility of dental composites formulated with different photoinitiator systems. J Dent. 2013;41(Suppl 3):e67–72.
23. Manojlovic D, Dramićanin MD, Lezaja M, Pongprueksa P, Van Meerbeek B, Miletic V. Effect of resin and photoinitiator on color, translucency and color stability of conventional and low-shrinkage model composites. Dent Mater. 2016;32:183–91.
24. Randolph LD, Steinhaus J, Moginger B, Gallez B, Stansbury J, Palin WM, Leloup G, Leprince JG. Photopolymerization of highly filled dimethacrylate-based composites using type I or type II photoinitiators and varying co-monomer ratios. Dent Mater. 2016;32:136–48.

25. Palin WM, Hadis MA, Leprince JG, Leloup G, Boland L, Fleming GJP, Krastl G, Watts DC. Reduced polymerization stress of MAPO-containing resin composites with increased curing speed, degree of conversion and mechanical properties. Dent Mater. 2014;30:507–16.
26. Neumann MG, Schmitt CC, Ferreira GC, Corrêa IC. The initiating radical yields and the efficiency of polymerization for various dental photoinitiators excited by different light curing units. Dent Mater. 2006;22:576–84.
27. Jockusch S, Koptyug IV, McGarry PF, Sluggett GW, Turro NJ, Watkins DM. A steady-state and picosecond pump-probe investigation of the photophysics of an acyl and a Bis(acyl)phosphine oxide. J Am Chem Soc. 1997;119:11495–501.
28. Cook WD. Photopolymerization kinetics of dimethacrylates using the camphorquinone/amine initiator system. Polymer. 1992;33:600–9.
29. Randolph LD, Palin WM, Leloup G, Leprince JG. Filler characteristics of modern dental resin composites and their influence on physico-mechanical properties. Dent Mater. 2016;32:1586–99.
30. Leprince J, Palin WM, Mullier T, Devaux J, Vreven J, Leloup G. Investigating filler morphology and mechanical properties of new low-shrinkage resin composite types. J Oral Rehabil. 2010;37:364–76.
31. Curtis AR, Palin WM, Fleming GJ, Shortall AC, Marquis PM. The mechanical properties of nanofilled resin-based composites: characterizing discrete filler particles and agglomerates using a micromanipulation technique. Dent Mater. 2009;25:180–7.
32. Scougall-Vilchis RJ, Hotta Y, Hotta M, Idono T, Yamamoto K. Examination of composite resins with electron microscopy, microhardness tester and energy dispersive X-ray microanalyzer. Dent Mater J. 2009;28:102–12.
33. Willems G, Lambrechts P, Braem M, Celis JP, Vanherle G. A classification of dental composites according to their morphological and mechanical characteristics. Dent Mater. 1992;8:310–9.
34. Goncalves F, Azevedo CL, Ferracane JL, Braga RR. BisGMA/TEGDMA ratio and filler content effects on shrinkage stress. Dent Mater. 2011;27:520–6.
35. Kim KH, Ong JL, Okuno O. The effect of filler loading and morphology on the mechanical properties of contemporary composites. J Prosthet Dent. 2002;87:642–9.
36. Hadis MA, Tomlins PH, Shortall AC, Palin WM. Dynamic monitoring of refractive index change through photoactive resins. Dent Mater. 2010;26:1106–12.
37. Arikawa H, Kanie T, Fujii K, Takahashi H, Ban S. Effect of filler properties in composite resins on light transmittance characteristics and color. Dent Mater J. 2007;26:38–44.
38. Lim YK, Lee YK, Lim BS, Rhee SH, Yang HC. Influence of filler distribution on the color parameters of experimental resin composites. Dent Mater. 2008;24:67–73.
39. Li R, Ma X, Liang S, Sa Y, Jiang T, Wang Y. *Optical properties of enamel and translucent composites by diffuse reflectance measurements*. J Dent. 2012;40(Suppl 1):e40–7.
40. ISO 4049:2009. Dentistry–Polymer-based restorative materials. 4th ed; 2009. p. 28.
41. Ergucu Z, Turkun LS, Onem E, Guneri P. Comparative radiopacity of six flowable resin composites. Oper Dent. 2010;35:436–40.
42. Dukic W, Delija B, Derossi D, Dadic I. Radiopacity of composite dental materials using a digital X-ray system. Dent Mater J. 2012;31:47–53.
43. Bocalon ACE, Mita D, Narumyia I, Shouha P, Xavier TA, Braga RR. Replacement of glass particles by multidirectional short glass fibers in experimental composites: effects on degree of conversion, mechanical properties and polymerization shrinkage. Dent Mater. 2016;32:e204–10.
44. Garoushi S, Sailynoja E, Vallittu PK, Lassila L. Physical properties and depth of cure of a new short fiber reinforced composite. Dent Mater. 2013;29:835–41.
45. Fu SY, Lauke B, Mäder E, Yue CY, Hu X. Tensile properties of short-glass-fiber- and short-carbon-fiber-reinforced polypropylene composites. Compos A: Appl Sci Manuf. 2000;31:1117–25.
46. van Dijken JW, Sunnegardh-Gronberg K. Fiber-reinforced packable resin composites in class II cavities. J Dent. 2006;34:763–9.
47. Manhart J, Kunzelmann KH, Chen HY, Hickel R. Mechanical properties and wear behavior of light-cured packable composite resins. Dent Mater. 2000;16:33–40.
48. Angeletakis C, Nguyen MDS, Kobashigawa AI. *Prepolymerized filler in dental restorative composite*. 2005. Google Patents.
49. Darvell, B.W. Chapter 6 – Resin restorative materials. In: Materials science for dentistry. 9th ed. Sawston, Cambridge: Woodhead; 2009. p. 128–62. https://www.elsevier.com/books/materials-science-fordentistry/ darvell/978-1-84569-529-3.
50. Arksornnukit M, Takahashi H, Nishiyama N. Effects of silane coupling agent amount on mechanical properties and hydrolytic durability of composite resin after hot water storage. Dent Mater J. 2004;23:31–6.
51. Antonucci JM, Dickens SH, Fowler BO, Xu HHK, McDonough WG. Chemistry of silanes: interfaces in dental polymers and composites. J Res Natl Inst Stand Technol. 2005;110:541–58.
52. Karabela MM, Sideridou ID. Effect of the structure of silane coupling agent on sorption characteristics of solvents by dental resin-nanocomposites. Dent Mater. 2008;24:1631–9.
53. Nihei T. Dental applications for silane coupling agents. J Oral Sci. 2016;58:151–5.

Part II

Polymerization

Curing Reaction and Kinetics

3

Ana Paula Piovezan Fugolin, Ataís Bacchi,
and Carmem S. Pfeifer

3.1 Introduction

The study of polymerization kinetics is of great interest in dentistry, particularly for restorative composites. Most commonly, those materials are composed of multimethacrylate monomers, photopolymerized to give a cross-linked polymer network. The rate at which that reaction takes place influences not only the final degree of conversion (extent of polymerization) but also some of the important physical and mechanical properties of the final material. Understanding how the polymerization progresses is important for researchers developing new materials and for clinicians to obtain the best performance out of the final restoration. In this chapter, the different types of polymerization will be discussed, so to contextualized the mechanisms involved in the polymerization of methacrylates and chain-transfer reactions induced by the presence of thiols. Emphasis will also be given to particular aspects of the photoinitiation reaction.

A.P.P. Fugolin • C.S. Pfeifer (✉)
Biomaterials and Biomechanics,
Oregon Health and Science University,
3181 SW Sam Jackson Park Road,
Portland, OR 97239, USA
e-mail: pfeiferc@ohsu.edu

A. Bacchi
Meridional Faculty—IMED,
School of Dentistry, Prosthodontics and
Dental Materials, Av. Senador Pinheiro, 304,
Passo Fundo, RS 99070-220, Brazil

3.2 Principles of Polymer Chemistry

3.2.1 Types of Polymers and Polymerization Reactions

Polymers are formed by a large number of small molecules—*monomers*—linked with each other building up macromolecules. Polymers and polymerization reactions may be classified following the criteria presented in Table 3.1. Frequently, the terms condensation and step polymerization and addition and chain polymerization are used interchangeably because the majority of addition polymers are obtained by chain-growth polymerization reaction and, in turn, condensation polymers by step-growth polymerization. However, it is not always the case, because the terms "condensation" and "addition" are based on the polymer composition and structure, and "step" and "chain" are characterized by mechanisms of polymerization reaction. Therefore, different aspects are considered for those classifications.

Methacrylates polymerize through vinyl bonds, via a chain-growth mechanism. When combined with chain-transfer agents, such as thiols, or in thiol-ene monomer systems, a combination of chain and step-growth reactions takes place, with profound impact on reaction kinetics and the final polymer structure. Chain-transfer reactions are used as a strategy to control

V. Miletic (ed.), *Dental Composite Materials for Direct Restorations*,
http://doi.org/10.1007/978-3-319-60961-4_3

Table 3.1 Classification criteria for polymers, polymer chains, and polymerization reactions

Criteria	Classification
Polymer structure—Composition	Condensation polymers Addition polymers
Polymer chain configuration	Linear Branched Cross-linked
Polymerization mechanism	Step-growth polymerization Chain-growth polymerization

molecular weight in linear polymers and control gelation in cross-linked networks. These aspects will be discussed in more detail in the section on Chain-Transfer Reactions and their effect on kinetic chain length.

3.2.1.1 Polymer Structure

The polymer structure classification is based on compositional differences between the polymer and the monomers from which it was synthesized. According to this criterion, the polymers may be divided in condensation and addition.

Condensation Polymers

Condensation polymers are synthesized from polyfunctional monomers through condensation reactions involving organic chemistry and, in general, elimination of small molecules. Generally, the eliminated molecule is water, but hydrogen chloride (HCl), ammonia (NH_3), hydrogen cyanide (HCN), or alcohol (–OH), among others, may also be eliminated. An example of condensation polymer is the polyamides:

$$\underset{\text{Diamide}}{nH_2N-R-NH_2}+\underset{\text{Diacids}}{nHO_2C-R'-CO_2H}\rightarrow \underset{\text{Polyamides}}{H-\left(-NH-R-NHCO-R'-CO-\right)_n-OH}+\underset{\text{Water}}{\left(2n-1\right)}$$

The parentheses indicate the *repeating unit*, i.e., unit that repeats itself several times in the polymer chain. It is important to mention that one determined condensation polymer can be obtained from different reactions (e.g., polyamides may be synthesized from the reaction between diamides and diacids (or diacyl chlorides), but the self-condensation of amino acids is also able to produce polyamides).

It is noteworthy that some condensation reactions do not eliminate by-products, such as is the case in click reactions between alcohols or thiols and isocyanates [1–3]. Those are useful for the formation of several polycarbamates, such as polyurethanes and polythiourethanes, both with several uses in coating industry and, more recently, in dentistry [4–6].

Addition Polymers

Addition polymers are synthesized without the loss of small molecules, resulting in polymers with the same chemical composition as the monomers. The majority of the addition monomers present carbon-carbon double bonds (C=C), which convert from pi to sigma bonds during polymerization. Each pi bond that is broken originates two other sigma bonds, and those form the polymer chains. Note that the C=C bonds most commonly involved in chain-growth polymerizations are of the vinyl type, which implies a CH_2=C-group linked to some constituent. One example of addition polymer is polyethylene:

$$\underset{\text{Ethylene}}{nCH_2=CH_2}\rightarrow \underset{\text{Polyethylene}}{-\left(CH_2-CH_2-\right)_n}$$

Condensation Polymers Versus Addition Polymers

The classification proposed by Wallace Carothers considers only two aspects to classify a polymer as addition or condensation: (1) elemental composition of the polymer and (2) elimination or not of any small molecule. However, in some cases if only those two aspects are observed, an incorrect classification may be achieved. Therefore, the term *condensation polymers* is attributed to polymers constituted by repeating units linked by functional units of ester (–COO–), amide (–NHCO–), urethane (–OCONH–), sulfide (–S–), and ether linkages (–O–). It is also possible that their repeating units lack certain atoms that are present in the monomer, which could have been degraded (i.e., poly(p-xylene) produced by the dehydrogenation of p-xylene), or, as seen previously, their synthesis involved the elimination of small molecules. On the other hand, when the polymer does not fulfill any of those requirements, it is classified as an *addition polymer.*

3.2.1.2 Polymer Chain Configuration

The configuration of a polymer refers to the physical arrangement of monomers along the backbone of the chain. It strongly influences the properties of a polymer. The breaking of covalent bonds is required to change the polymer structure. Depending on the polymeric chain structure, polymers can be classified as linear, branched, or cross-linked (Fig. 3.1).

Linear Polymers

When the monomer molecules are linked together in one continuous chain of repeated units, it is classified as *linear polymer*. Examples are polyethylene, polyvinyl chloride, polystyrene, and nylon. In the case of addition polymers, those are formed by monofunctional monomers, such as mono-vinyls (e.g., methyl methacrylate), which are not capable of forming cross-links. They are also known as thermoplastic polymers (meaning they can be shaped by heat) and can be dissolved by solvents. Some mono-methacrylate monomers are used in the composition of dental adhesives, and their reaction kinetics is markedly different from those of cross-linking multimethacrylates. The speed of reaction and the swell ability of such materials influence their structure, particularly in the case of dentinal adhesives, which polymerize in a moist environment and are subject to phase separation during polymerization.

The size or length of the chain has significant impact on the polymer's physical properties. For example, the longer is the chain length, the higher is the material boiling and melting temperature. The increase of chain length furthermore tends to decrease chain mobility and increase strength, toughness, viscosity, and glass transition temperature (T_g).

Branched Polymers

In some reactions, side branches of linked monomer molecules protruding from various central branch points along the main polymer chain can be observed. In this case, *branched polymer* is the more appropriate definition. These polymers show decreased crystallinity because the side chains sterically hinder polymer folding and packing. It is important to point out that the term branched polymer does not refer to linear polymers containing side groups that are part of the monomer structure, such as pendant groups. Only those polymers that contain side branches composed of complete monomer units are termed branched polymers.

Hyperbranched polymers are a special type of branched molecule, formed via controlled, sequential polymerizations [7]. RAFT (reversible addition fragmentation chain-transfer) mechanisms are very common to synthesize branched polymer structures. Those find applications in drug delivery systems, as well as to reinforce other polymer structures [7].

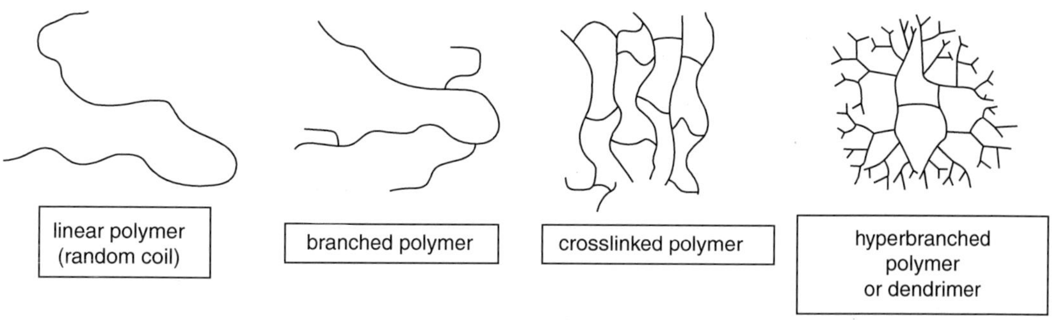

Fig. 3.1 Representation of polymeric chain types. (*1*) Linear polymer, (*2*) branched polymer, and (*3*) cross-linked polymers

Cross-Linked Polymers

Polymer molecules linked to each other by covalent bonds at points other than their ends are defined as *cross-linked.* Light cross-linking is used to impart good recovery (elastic) properties to polymers to be used as rubbers. High degrees of cross-linking are used to impart high rigidity. Cross-linking tends to increase T_g and increase strength and toughness. Cross-linking is necessarily a product of polymerization of multifunctional monomers, may it happen via a condensation or chain-growth mechanism. Cross-linked polymers are also known as thermosets, as they do not present a melting temperature and cannot be shaped by heat, nor dissolved by solvents. Depending on the degree of cross-linking, as already mentioned, physical properties can be tailored, including flexural properties, fracture toughness, T_g, and swell ability in aqueous or organic solvents. The nature of the cross-links themselves dictates polymer properties and free volume, may they come from flexible monomers such as triethylene glycol dimethacrylates or from more rigid structures such as bisphenol A diglycidyl dimethacrylate (BisGMA), two monomers commonly used in composites. A representation of the two types of cross-links is show in Fig. 3.2.

3.2.1.3 Polymerization Mechanisms

A polymer chain buildup might occur by two distinct polymerization mechanisms: step- or chain-growth polymerizations. Those mechanisms differ in the types of monomers involved, as well as on the stages of polymerization at which the development of high molecular weight species is observed. Mainly, in step-growth polymerizations, the molecular weight (in the case of linear polymers) or the polymer network (in the case of cross-linked polymers) does not develop until very high degrees of conversion. This has profound effects on gelation behavior and final stress development, as will be explored further in the following sections.

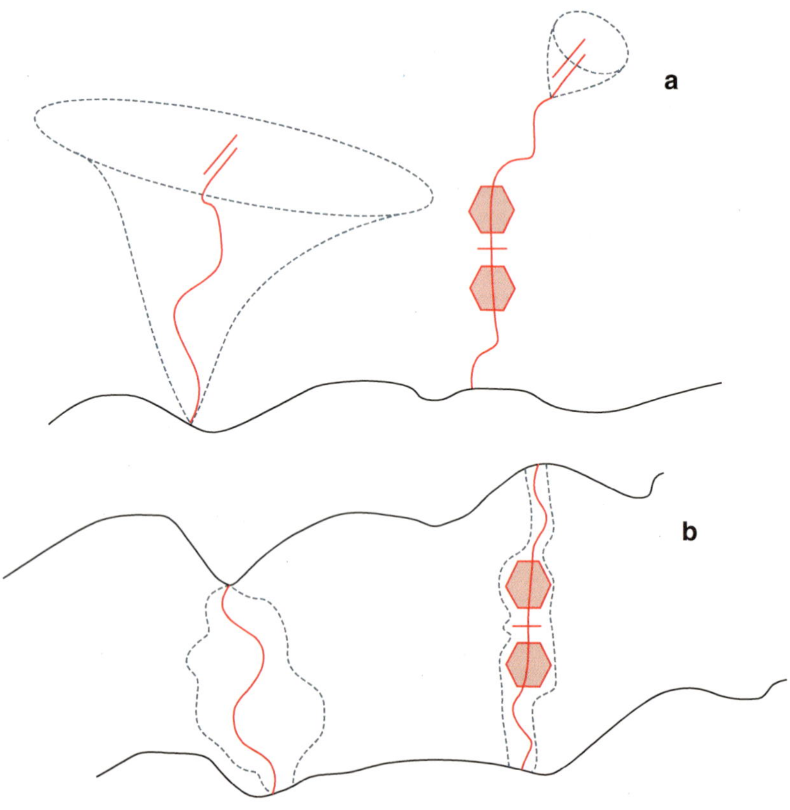

Fig. 3.2 Degrees of freedom of (**a**) pendant groups and (**b**) cross-links formed by the aliphatic TEGDMA and the aromatic BisGMA (in *red*). The *dotted lines* show the space occupied by each molecule's motion (modified from [8])

In step-growth polymerization, the reaction proceeds between two different functional groups, whether they are on the same molecule or different molecules. Examples include the reactions of hydroxyl and carboxyl groups, or isocyanate and hydroxyl groups, or thiol and ene monomers. Step-growth polymerizations include esterification, amidation, aromatic substitutions, the formation of urethanes, and others. In fact, step-growth polymerizations can be divided in two subgroups:

(a) Two different bifunctional and/or polyfunctional monomers, but each monomer shows only one type of functional group.

Example: nA–A + nB–B → –(–A–AB–B–)–$_n$, where A and B are different types of functional groups.

(b) Only one monomer with both types of functional groups.

Example: nA–B → –(–A–B–)–$_n$

Importantly, in this reaction mechanism, several chains of different sizes are built, originating dimers, trimers, tetramers, pentamers, and hexamers, which then finally are linked together at the tail end of the reaction to form large molecular weight polymers (Fig. 3.3).

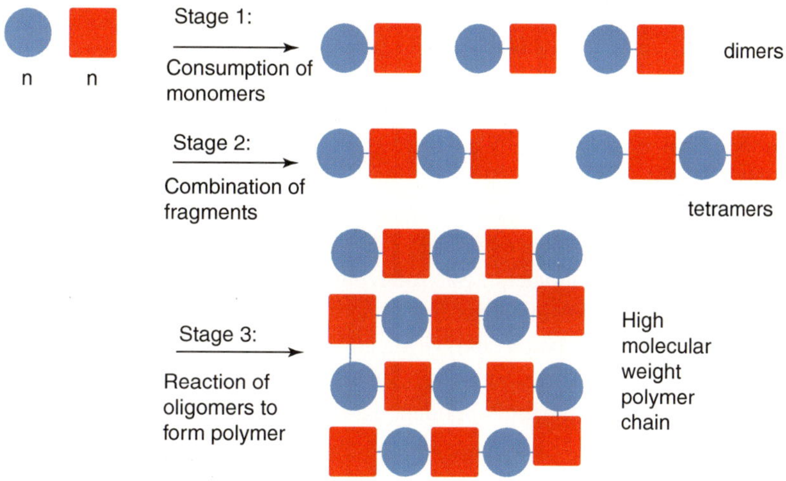

Fig. 3.3 Representation of the stages of a step-growth polymerization. Modified from http://www.slideshare.net/guest32ca93/polymer-course

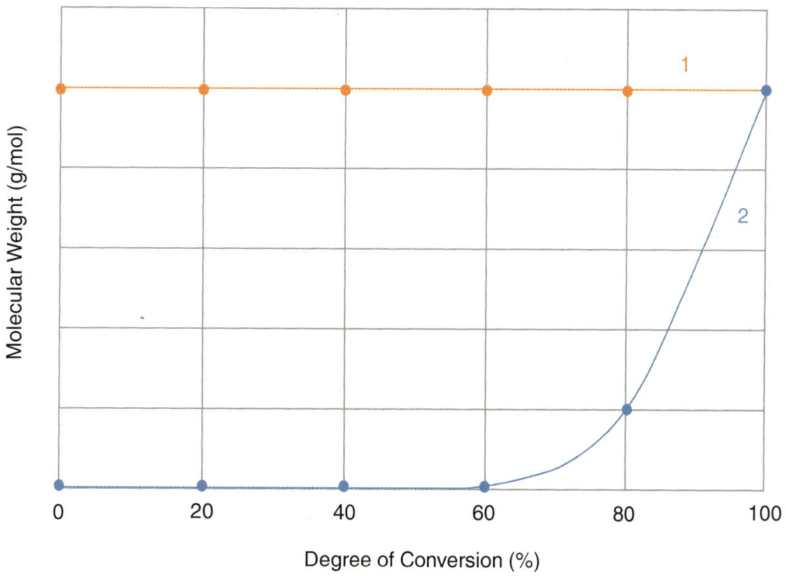

Fig. 3.4 Graphic representation of molecular weight (g/mol) in function of the degree of conversion (%). (*1*) Characteristic curve for chain-growth polymerization reaction and (2) for step-growth polymerization reaction. Modified from [9]

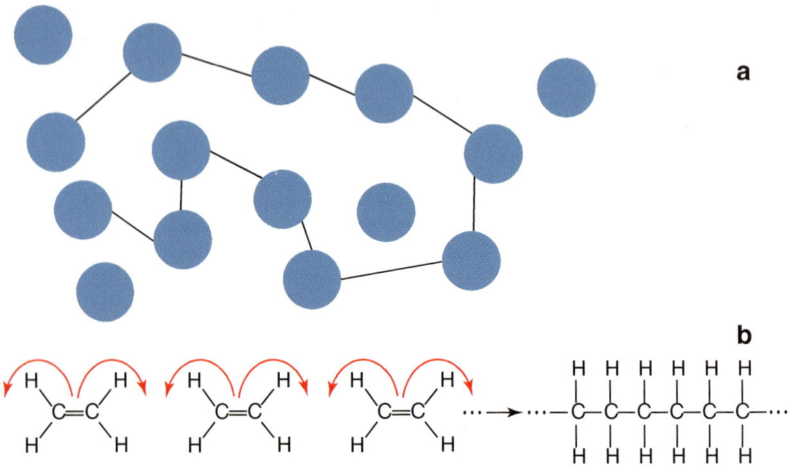

Fig. 3.5 Representation of mechanisms in a chain-growth polymerization. (**a**) Formation of high molecular weight chains immediately after polymerization starts. (**b**) Example of chain-growth polymerization of polyethylene

The polymer molecular weight increases gradually during the reaction, at relatively slow speed (Fig. 3.4—curve 2), and only near the end of the reaction are high molecular weight specimens found. In other words, the molecular weight does not build up until later in conversion. The main practical consequence of this fact is that, for multifunctional monomers polymerizing via step-growth (i.e., forming cross-linked networks via step growth), gelation and vitrification are delayed to very late stages in conversion and that affects the onset of modulus buildup, as well as stress development [5, 10, 11].

By contrast, in chain-growth polymerizations, the final size and weight of polymer chain are reached almost immediately after the beginning of the reaction (Fig. 3.4—curve 1). The reaction occurs from the propagation of reactive species (free radical, cation, or anion) produced from an initiator, which promotes successive additions of monomer molecules in a chain reaction. In other words, very large chains or complex networks are formed at relatively low degrees of conversion and, especially for cross-linked systems, cause incomplete monomer conversion and early stress buildup [12]. Chain-growth reactions take place between monomers containing a single type of functional group, commonly a carbon-carbon double bond. The reactive species open the π-bond forming a new radical (a macroradical) and allowing the addition to a monomer molecule. In this case, monomers do not react with other monomers and different sized chains; the monomers react only with the reactive center allowing the addition of more monomer molecules in the polymer chain. The polymer chain growth is interrupted when the center is destroyed by an appropriate reaction depending on the type of reactive center and the reaction conditions. This is the mechanism through which methacrylates polymerize and will receive the most emphasis on this chapter for its importance in the polymerization of dental composites (Fig. 3.5).

In general, chain polymerization shows three phases: initiation, propagation, and termination.

1. Initiation: The initiator is activated by an influx of energy (thermal, photoactive, or redox mechanism) producing reactive centers.

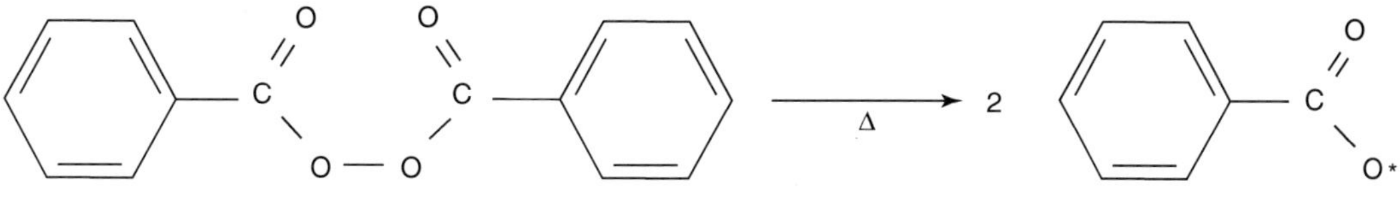

The reactive centers will react with the monomer molecule, breaking carbon double bonds leading to the formation of a macroradical:

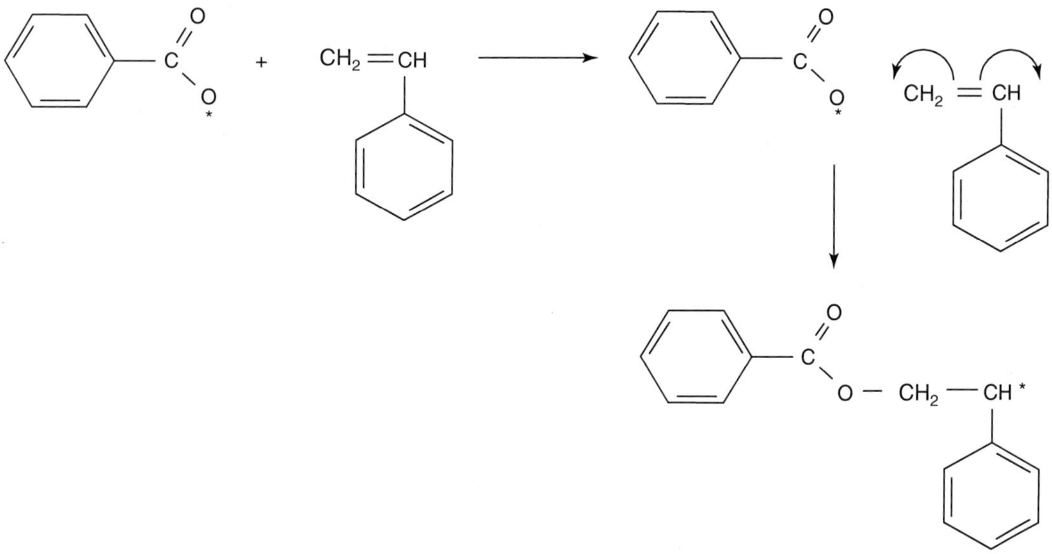

2. *Propagation*: The reactive center is continuously transferred between the monomer molecules, and each monomer molecule addition creates a new reactive center. The polymer chain grows in high speed:

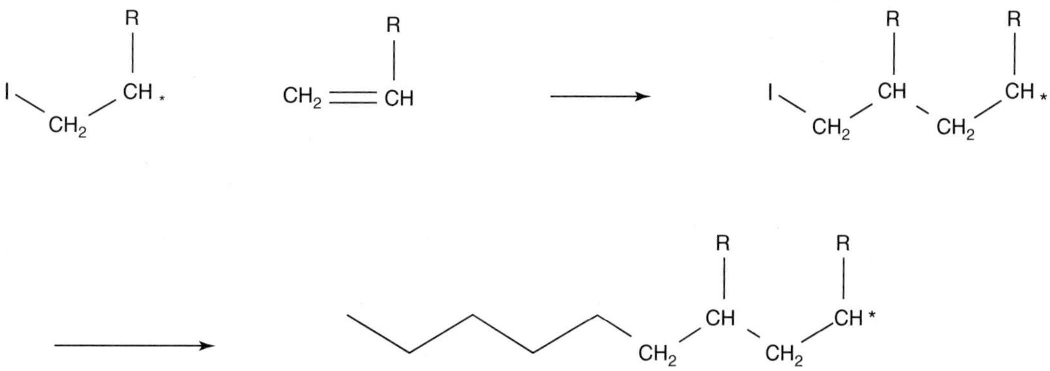

3. *Termination*: Reactive centers are destroyed (by combination of macroradicals or disproportionation reactions), and the addition of new monomer molecules is limited.

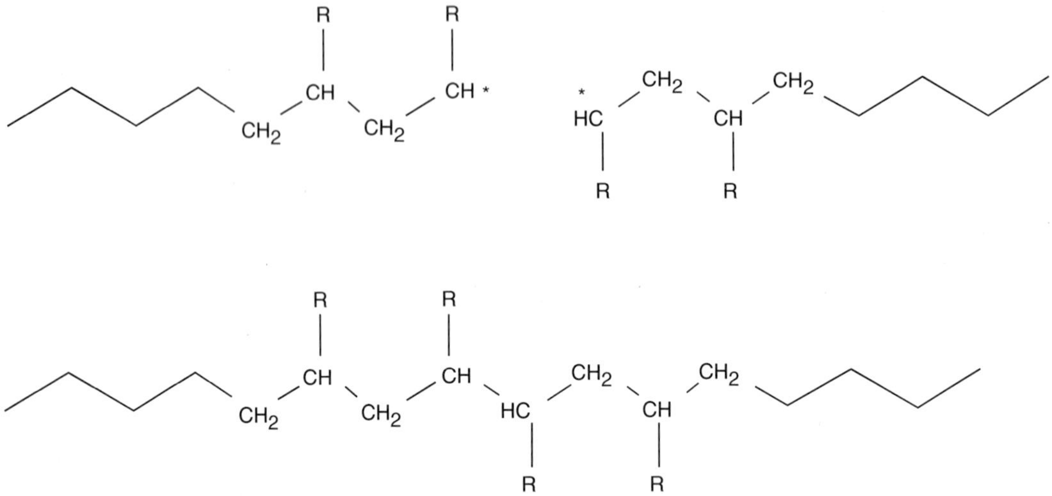

Combination between two macroradicals

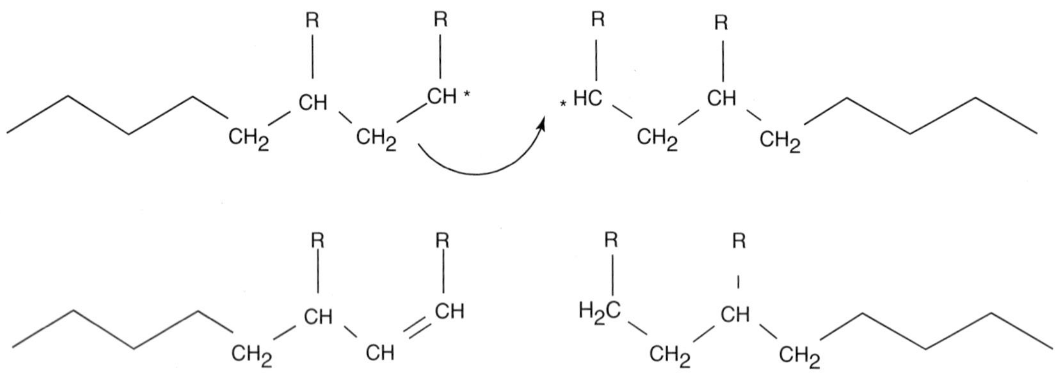

Disproportionation reaction

It is worth mentioning that the chain polymerization reaction may be classified according to the selectivity in relation to the type of reactive center. Some monomers will undergo polymerization with any reactive species, while others show high selectivity toward ionic (cationic or anionic) or radical initiator. Methacrylates are not particularly selective and can react either via radical or ionic mechanisms.

3.2.2 Kinetics of Radical Chain Polymerizations: Fundamental Aspects

The majority of monomers used in dental materials polymerize through a chain-growth mechanism, more specifically, a radical chain polymerization. As seen previously, the chain-growth polymerization reaction shows three different phases that are controlled by some factors which affect directly the reaction kinetics. These phases are presented in more detail in the following paragraphs.

Initiation—This phase involves two important reactions:

1. Generation of free radicals—A homolytic dissociation of an initiator species **(I)** occurs (via a photo, thermal, or redox mechanism) to yield two radicals **(R*)** – ***initiator radical or primary radical***—and there is a rate constant, $\boldsymbol{k_d}$, for this catalyst dissociation:

$$1 \xrightarrow{k_d} 2R\cdot$$

2. Interaction between the free radical **(R*)** and the first monomer molecule **(M)** to produce the chain-initiating radical **(M_1*)**. There is a rate constant for the initiation step—$\boldsymbol{k_i}$—acting on this process:

$$R\cdot + M \xrightarrow{k_i} M_1\cdot$$

Propagation—This phase consists of the growth of **M_1*** by the successive additions of a large numbers of monomer molecules, creating a new radical with the same identity in each addition:

$$M_1\cdot + M \xrightarrow{k_P} M_2\cdot$$

$$M_2\cdot + M \xrightarrow{k_P} M_3\cdot$$

$$M_3\cdot + M \xrightarrow{k_P} M_4\cdot$$

$$M_n\cdot + M \xrightarrow{k_P} M_{n+1}\cdot$$

In this reaction, there is a rate constant for propagation $\boldsymbol{k_p}$.

Termination—At some point, the polymer chain stops to grow and the reaction is terminated. For this to happen, the radical centers have to be destroyed by a *combination reaction* (two radicals react with each other) or a *disproportionation reaction* (a beta hydrogen radical from one radical center is transferred to another radical center). As in previous reactions, the termination reaction occurs under a rate—termination rate $\boldsymbol{k_t}$.

$$M_n\cdot + M_m\cdot \xrightarrow{k_t} \text{dead polymer}$$

In practice, these three phases happen concomitantly during polymerization, with predominance of one versus another phenomenon depending on the extent of polymerization and reaction medium mobility. Several factors contribute to the progression of the reaction, among which the radical concentration, the initial viscosity of the medium, the relative reactivity of the monomer species, the difference between cure temperature and glass transition temperature [13–15], etc. Those will be discussed in the following sections, with emphasis on methacrylate polymerizations.

3.2.2.1 Reaction Kinetics (and Its Relationship with Network Development)

For the purposes of the polymerization of dental composites and adhesives, this section will concentrate on the photoactivated reaction of methacrylates. In general terms, at the beginning of the reaction, the radicals that are generated by the excitation of the photosensitive molecule proceed to interact with the monomers and attack the first vinyl double bonds. The reaction is *chemically controlled* at this stage, which means the rates of propagation (k_p) and termination (k_t) are largely dependent on the supply of monomers and radicals, since there are not enough high molecular weight species that can contribute to the increase in viscosity of the medium and hinder diffusional mobility. At this stage, propagation and termination reactions occur concomitantly and at similar rates. As the reaction progresses, and more of high molecular weight species and cross-linking starts to occur, viscosity starts to increase, and the reaction becomes *diffusion-controlled*. This means that molecular mobility becomes more difficult, especially so for larger molecules. In turn, this leads to a decrease in termination events, because it becomes increasingly unlikely for bimolecular termination or disproportionation to take place. With the consequent decrease in the termination events, the propagation is favored, leading to **autoacceleration** of the reaction (*Trommsdorff effect*). The *gelation* of the network is defined as the point in conversion at which one macromolecule spans the whole

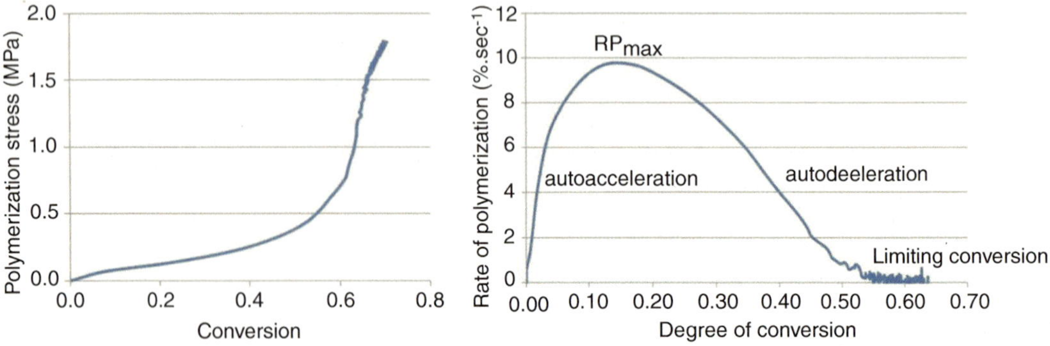

Fig. 3.6 Polymerization stress and rate of polymerization as a function of conversion for a typical multifunctional methacrylate (ethoxylated bisphenol A). Polymerization stress and degree of conversion were followed simultaneously on the same specimen. Note that the conversion at which stresses start to more markedly build up (inflection point on the stress vs. conversion curve) coincides with the end of the deceleration shown in the rate vs. conversion curve

specimen [9]. The propagation continues to dominate until the maximum rate of polymerization (Rp_{max}) is reached (Fig. 3.6). Even though it is not possible to precise the onset of gelation from this curve alone (rheology experiments are more suitable for that measurement), sometime before the Rp_{max} is reached, gelation of the forming network is observed. The gelation of methacrylates has been shown to occur at around 5% conversion, as determined by IR-coupled rheology experiments [16], while the Rp_{max} is usually observed at around 5–20% conversion, even though this second landmark is a lot more dependent on the reaction conditions [17]. The conversion at gelation and the conversion registered at the end of the autoacceleration (or at Rp_{max}) greatly influence the limiting conversion achieved by a monomer system, as well as the final polymerization stress development.

With the progression of the polymerization reaction, the restriction to molecular mobility increases even further, to the point that even small molecule diffusion is affected. This leads to a decrease in the rate of propagation from Rp_{max} (propagation also becomes diffusion-controlled), and the rate vs. conversion curve shows a **deceleration** slope (Fig. 3.6). The onset of deceleration coincides with the onset of network vitrification and that also means that opportunities for network rearrangement to compensate for shrinkage are limited, and stresses start to more significantly build up [12]. At the end of the auto-deceleration slope, the network has reached almost complete vitrification, which means any additional conversion translates into a sharp increase in stress, as has been demonstrated in simultaneous conversion vs. stress experiments [11]. One example is shown in Fig. 3.7, where for the same specimen, stress vs. conversion and polymerization rate vs. conversion plots are presented. In summary, before the network reaches vitrification, there is still opportunity for stress relaxation [11]. This is the reason why delayed gelation and vitrification strategies have gained so much attention in the development of low-stress materials [4–6], but it is important to point out that, for them to be effective, the delay has to occur in terms of conversion and not time.

The rate of polymerization (**R_p**) or rate of monomer disappearance is the speed at which monomer molecules are converted to polymer. This rate is based on **k_p**, **k_t**, monomer concentration **[M]** and rate of initiation (**R_i**), according to the following equation:

$$R_p = k_p[\mathrm{M}]\left(\frac{R_i}{2k_t}\right)^{1/2}$$

It can be observed that the rate of propagation is directly proportional to the square root of the rate of initiation (R_i).

Particularly for the resin composites used in dentistry, which are for the most part

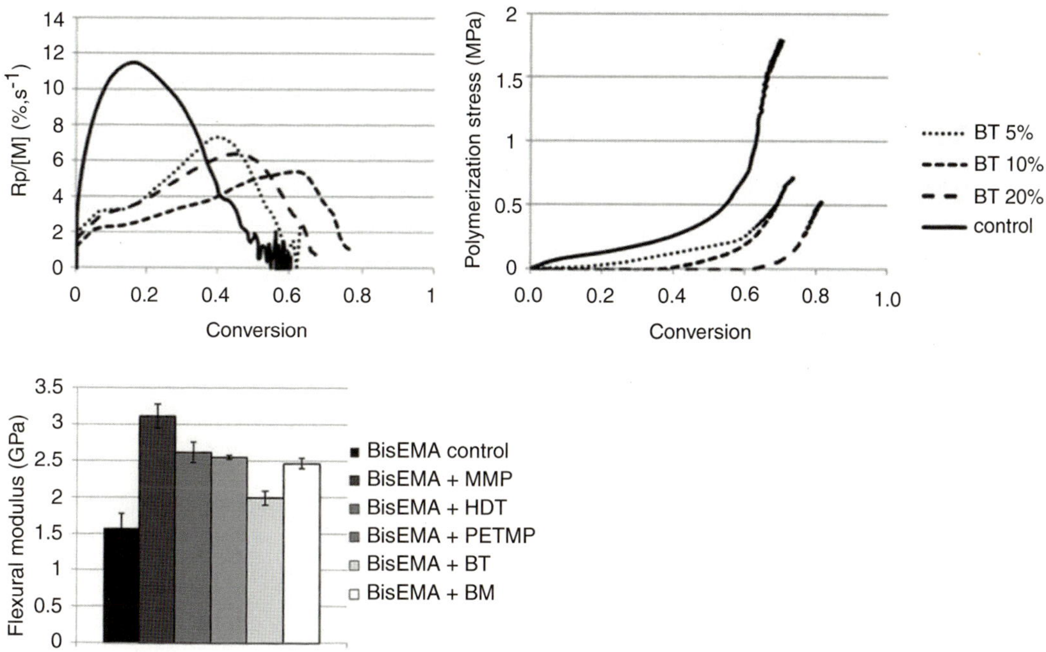

Fig. 3.7 Evidence for delayed gelation/vitrification in methacrylate networks containing up to 20 wt% thiols. Polymerization stress is significantly decreased without prejudice to mechanical properties. In this specific case, the increased conversion achieved with these materials led to increased flexural strength. Modified from [11]

photoactivated, it is important to consider the intensity of absorbed light—I_a (or irradiance, in moles of light quanta for liter-second)—as shown in the following equation:

$$R_p = k_p[M]\left(\frac{\phi I_a}{k_t}\right)^{1/2}$$

This equation makes it clear that the rate of polymerization is dependent on the square root of the irradiance, with the implication that the overall rate of reaction cannot be reduced significantly unless the irradiance is reduced by at least two orders of magnitude [9]. This makes the effectiveness of so-called soft-start irradiation protocols questionable [18, 19].

Degree of Conversion

Degree of conversion is the percentage of carbon double bonds converted in single bonds or, in other words, the extent of conversion of monomer to polymer. In reactions with only one type of monomer, this percentage is obtained by the following equation:

$$DC = 1 - \frac{[M]}{[M_0]}$$

where M_0 is the initial monomer concentration. In copolymerizations, where more than one type of monomer are reacting, the concentration of each constituent is considered. On the kinetics graph, the final degree of conversion is shown at the very end portion of the curve. A high degree of conversion is important for composite resins in order to increase general chemical and physical properties, as well as to reduce the effects of residual monomer in the organism. As already explained, the limiting conversion of methacrylates is typically around 70%. The fact that multimethacrylates do not reach complete conversion at room temperature is due to trapped radicals in the network, which in turn, stems from the fact that gelation and vitrification are reached at relatively low conversions. Also as mentioned, after deceleration, steep diffusional limitations preclude any additional conversion from taking place. This is true at least for the conditions at which methacrylates are usually polymerized in the clinical situation (room temperature at relatively high irradiances) [9, 12].

Kinetic Chain Length

Kinetic chain length (v) is the average number of monomer molecules polymerized for each free radical that initiates a polymer chain. This average is in function of the ratio of polymerization and termination/initiation rates, as per the following equation:

$$\nu = \frac{k_p^2[\mathrm{M}]}{2k_t R_p}$$

Kinetic chain length at constant rate of polymerization is a particular characteristic of the monomer and independent of initiation method (thermal, redox, or photochemical).

The chain length plays an important role in the kinetics process. Long chains are less mobile than short chains, and during the polymerization reaction, they reduce the termination rate. This reduction is responsible for increasing the rate of polymerization and potentiating the autoacceleration process. However, when shorter kinetic chain lengths are induced, the termination rate is increased, and then the termination-propagation rate is also increased before the vitrification point. The effect of this on the kinetics reaction is that instead of the rate of polymerization increasing too fast, it increases gradually allowing for higher degrees of conversion before the reaction reaches gelation/vitrification. In other words, shorter kinetic chain lengths are responsible for delaying the phase at which the reaction starts to become diffusion-controlled due to the mobility restriction imposed by the increased molecular weight or cross-linking. Any mechanism that is able to delay the onset of gelation and vitrification as a function of conversion has a very significant impact on polymerization stress development, since stress can be easily relaxed in the pre-gel and pre-vitrification phases. This is the mechanism through which stress reduction in methacrylates is obtained with chain-transfer reactions using thiols or in thiol-ene polymerizations [1, 11]. It is worth mentioning that kinetic chain length is inversely dependent on the radical concentration or the polymerization rate. It has a special importance because any attempt to increase the polymerization rate by increasing the radical concentration comes at the expense of producing smaller polymers.

Chain-Transfer Reactions

The effect of chain-transfer on polymerization kinetics and ultimately network development has been extensively studied [9, 12]. Chain-transfer reactions are radical displacement events, as shown below:

$$M_n^{\ *} + XA \xrightarrow{k_{tr}} M_n X + A^*$$

where XA may be a monomer, initiator, solvent, or another substance and X is the atom or species transferred.

The rate of chain-transfer reaction is given by:

$$R_{tr} = k_{tr}\left[M^*\right]\left[XA\right]$$

where k_{tr} is the chain-transfer constant. In other words, chain transfer is a chain breaking mechanism in which the new radical formed through the transfer is considered to be a new initiation site [9].

Some compounds, named chain-transfer agents, are known to facilitate this process, with thiols being by far the most commonly used and the most studied compounds. The chain-transfer constant depends on the molecular structure, but in general, even at low concentrations, thiols are capable of reducing the rate of polymerization and the radical chain length significantly [12]. When the radical from a propagating chain is transferred to a thiol, that molecule transfers the charge to another unreacted monomer and "caps" the growing polymer chain, which in turn becomes a "dead polymer." The implication for this is the molecular weight and cross-linking (or network formation) are delayed in relation to the consumption of vinyl double bonds, and ultimately, the polymerization stress can be decreased. However, the potentially decreased overall cross-linking density may also impart poorer mechanical properties [3]. This is unlikely for lower thiol concentrations, and in fact, up to 10 wt% small molecule thiols have been added to methacrylate networks to delay gelation/vitrification, reducing stress without prejudice to final mechanical properties [11], as can be seen in Fig. 3.7. At higher thiol concentrations, the reaction with the methacrylate monomer becomes a more important factor in network development [10, 20], and the transfer rate constant (k_{tr}) is significantly higher than the propagation rate constant (k_p), accompanied by a delay in the autoacceleration [10].

Thiol-ene Reactions: Radical-Assisted Step-Growth Polymerization

For typical thiol-ene systems, the predominant polymerization mechanism is step growth [21], as long as the stoichiometric ratio is kept at 1:1 thiol to ene and that the ene monomer does not preferentially undergo homopolymerization via chain growth (ene monomers contain vinyl polymerizable functionalities, but methacrylates are not good candidates for this kind of reaction) [1, 21]. There are a couple of disadvantages with thiol-ene systems, including low T_g due to the presence of flexible thioether bonds incorporated in the polymer backbone through chain-transfer reactions to the methacrylate, issues with shelf-life stability as the monomers can undergo Michael addition reactions and spontaneously polymerize in the bottle, and the malodor of low molecular weight thiol species [20]. However, when these are combined with methacrylates in ternary systems, some of these drawbacks can be overcome [11]. In this case, the reaction can be initiated via a photoactive event, which generates the first radical. In general terms, that radical can undergo transfer to another methacrylate or chain-transfer to another vinyl (from the methacrylate or the ene) by the thiol. There is, therefore, competition between chain and step-growth mechanisms as the methacrylate can undergo both homopolymerization and chain transfer with the thiol in addition to the thiol-ene reaction [21, 22]. Because the methacrylate is more likely to undergo homopolymerization, in thiol-ene/methacrylate systems, the ene consumption has been demonstrated to be delayed until the methacrylate-thiol reaction is largely complete [23], shown in Fig. 3.8. The methacrylate conversion still progresses at a slower rate, as already explained, due to the chain-transfer reactions with the thiol, which delay gelation/vitrification and consequently reduce stress (Fig. 3.8). It is important to note that the delayed gelation in this case also leads to more homogeneous networks, whose polymerization progresses further in terms of conversion because of the extended opportunity for viscous flow which, incidentally, is also capable of alleviating part of the polymerization stress [3].

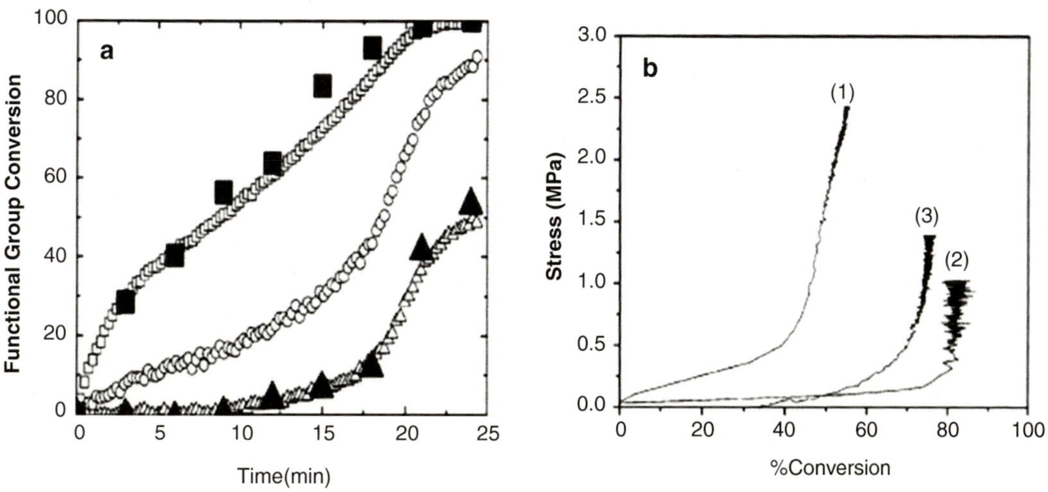

Fig. 3.8 (**a**) Functional group conversion vs. time plots of a dithiol (HDT, *circle*), a triene (TATATO, *triangle*), and a dimethacrylate (HDDMA, square) ternary mixtures. (**b**) Shrinkage stress of (*1*) BisGMA/TEGDMA 70/30, (*2*) thiol-ene, and (*3*) thiol-ene-methacrylate as a function of the overall double bond conversion. Modified from [23]

3.2.3 Factors Influencing the Polymerization

3.2.3.1 Initiators of Polymerization

Initiators can be defined as chemical substances that produce free radicals and start chemical reactions. Radicals are reactive chemical species possessing a free (unbonded or unpaired) electron. Energy is necessary to generate radicals from an initiator. Light or redox components (or a combination) are traditionally utilized as energy source for polymerization of composite dental materials. Once formed, radicals undergo two basic types of reactions: propagation reactions and termination reactions. In a propagation reaction, a radical reacts to form a covalent bond and to generate a new radical. In a termination reaction, two radicals interact in a mutually destructive reaction in which both radicals form covalent bonds and reaction ceases. The polymerization rate depends on the concentration of photosensitizer (initiator) and co-initiator [24], as well as on the interaction with specific monomer species [25].

3.2.3.2 Monomer Structure and Copolymerization

The monomer structure plays a crucial role during the polymerization reaction. The degree of conversion is directly dependent on the spacer group flexibility between the phenyl ring core and the methacrylate functional group. However, when ethylene glycol groups are added to BisGMA to increase the flexibility, this monomer shows an opposite behavior due to the hydrogen bonding in its network which reduces the mobility and the degree of conversion [26]. Considering that all resin composites commercially available are composed at least of two different monomers, the interaction between them determines the mixture performance. BisGMA and TEGDMA are frequently copolymerized to improve the viscosity, reactivity, and final degree of conversion of these materials. In Fig. 3.9, it is possible to see the rate of polymerization as a function of the degree of conversion for BisGMA, TEGDMA, and a mixture 50% BisGMA and 50% TEGDMA. These are the most common monomers of dental composites. The synergistic effect is clear for the mixture of monomers. It is possible to see that the polymerization rate is increased significantly and the final degree of conversion is similar to pure TEGDMA. This can be explained by the high reactivity of BisGMA when mixed to TEGDMA—a reactive diluent able to improve the mobility of the system and hence the carbon double bond conversion [9, 15].

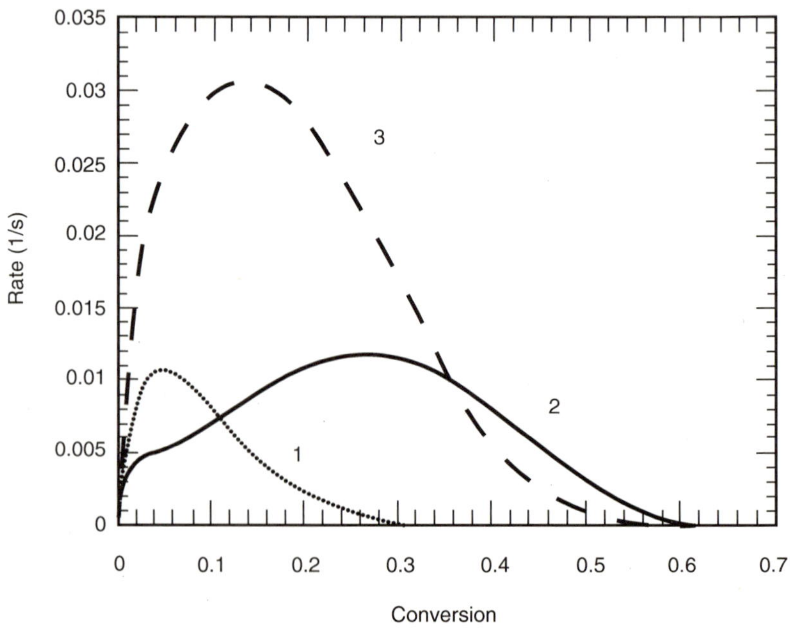

Fig. 3.9 Rate of polymerization in function of degree of conversion for (*1*) BisGMA, (*2*) TEGDMA, and (*3*) BisGMA + TEGDMA. Modified from [15]

3.2.3.3 Cross-Linking and Cyclization

Cross-linkers are monomers with functionality necessarily equal to or greater than two, capable of joining two or more molecules by a covalent bond, establishing inter- and intramolecular cross-links. Cross-links formed by BisGMA and TEGDMA are shown in Fig. 3.2b, earlier in the chapter. The concentration of cross-linkers interferes on the cyclization process. Cyclization is defined as the formation of one or more rings in a chemical compound, mainly a hydrocarbon. In free-radical cross-linking polymerizations, there are primary and secondary cyclizations. Primary cyclization happens when the free radicals attack pendant double bonds in the same chain. Secondary cyclization happens when the free radicals attack pendant double bonds on other chains already incorporated in the polymer network. Both types of cyclization processes have effects on the termination rate in copolymerization systems containing up to 4 mol% cross-linker. The effect in this case is an increase of coil size of macroradicals and hence increase of termination rate. However, during reaction development, the cross-links formed inside the macroradical coil decrease the mobility and then the termination rate. In higher concentrations, the cross-linkers show an increase in cyclization process leading to compact primary particle formation which limits the access of the radical centers and pendant vinyl groups to other polymer molecules. The result of this process is a diffusion-controlled termination rate decreased and cross-linker concentration increased. In BisGMA/TEGDMA copolymerizations, the relative ratio of each monomer has been shown to greatly interfere with the resulting polymer packing and free volume [8], as well as with the sol-gel composition of the resulting material [27].

3.2.3.4 Inhibitor and Catalyst

A chemical inhibitor is a reactant that slows down or delays the start of a chemical reaction. Inhibitors react with the initiating and propagating radicals, converting them to either non-radical species or radicals of reactivity too low to undergo the propagation process. In general, there are two kinds of inhibitors: reversible and irreversible inhibitors. Reversible inhibitors slow down a chemical reaction but do not stop it completely. Irreversible inhibitors prevent an unwanted reaction from occurring. The effect of the addition of inhibitors is to stop every radical, and polymerization is completely halted until they are completely consumed. In polymer chemistry, reaction inhibitors are used to modify the properties of the final polymer product as well as to prolong usefulness. The catalyst is in general a molecule used in polymers to increase the rate of a chemical reaction. Catalysts work by providing an alternative mechanism involving a different transition state and lower activation energy. Consequently, more molecular collisions have the energy needed to reach the transition state. Hence, catalysts can enable reactions that would otherwise be blocked or slowed by a kinetic barrier. The catalyst may increase reaction rate or selectivity or enable the reaction at lower temperatures.

3.2.3.5 Cure Temperature Versus Glass Transition Temperature

In general terms, the closer the cure and the glass transition temperature of a polymer are, the more likely it is for the material to reach full conversion [28]. This is explained by the diffusion-limited reactions in cross-linked networks described in detail in previous sections. If a material undergoes polymerization at a temperature where the translational capability of its molecular chains is high (close to its T_g), it is far more likely that all chains will be able to react, with little to no unreacted/trapped monomers. In contrast, let us consider, for example, a polymeric material presenting as glassy at room temperature (with, hypothetically, T_g = 100 °C), being polymerized at room temperature. By the time the conversion reaches 20 or 30%, the network has already developed enough to increase the modulus and the T_g from the monomeric state by a considerable amount. This, as already explained, undermines molecular mobility (particularly, larger molecule mobility) and impedes complete conversion. This is the reason high T_g polymers generally present lower limiting conversions when polymerized at room temperature, as is the case with many dimethacrylates used in dentistry [29].

References

1. Hoyle CE, Bowman CN. Thiol-ene click chemistry. Angewandte Chemie – International Edition. 2010;49(9):1540–73.
2. Li Q, Zhou H, Wicks DA, Hoyle CE. Thiourethane-based thiol-ene high T g networks: preparation, thermal, mechanical, and physical properties. J Polym Sci A Polym Chem. 2007;45(22):5103–11.
3. Senyurt AF, Hoyle CE, Wei H, Piland SG, Gould TE. Thermal and mechanical properties of cross-linked photopolymers based on multifunctional thiol-urethane ene monomers. Macromolecules. 2007;40(9):3174–82.
4. Bacchi A, Dobson A, Ferracane JL, Consani R, Pfeifer CS. Thio-urethanes improve properties of dual-cured composite cements. J Dent Res. 2014;**93**(12):1320–5.
5. Bacchi A, Nelson M, Pfeifer CS. Characterization of methacrylate-based composites containing thio-urethane oligomers. Dent Mater. 2016;32(2):233–9.
6. Bacchi A, Pfeifer CS. Rheological and mechanical properties and interfacial stress development of composite cements modified with thio-urethane oligomers. Dent Mater. 2016;32(8):978–86.
7. Voit BI, Lederer A. Hyperbranched and highly branched polymer architectures--synthetic strategies and major characterization aspects. Chem Rev. 2009;109(11):5924–73.
8. Pfeifer CS, Shelton ZR, Braga RR, Windmoller D, Machado JC, Stansbury JW. Characterization of dimethacrylate polymeric networks: a study of the crosslinked structure formed by monomers used in dental composites. Eur Polym J. 2011;47(2):162–70.
9. Odian G. Principles of polymerization. Staten Island, NY: Wiley-Interscience; 2004. p. 198–349.
10. Lecamp L, Houllier F, Youssef B, Bunel C. Photoinitiated cross-linking of a thiol-methacrylate system. Polymer. 2001;42(7):2727–36.
11. Pfeifer CS, Wilson ND, Shelton ZR, Stansbury JW. Delayed gelation through chain-transfer reactions: mechanism for stress reduction in methacrylate networks. Polymer (Guildf). 2011;52(15):3295–303.
12. Berchtold KA, Lovestead TM, Bowman CN. Coupling chain length dependent and reaction diffusion controlled termination in the free radical polymerization of multivinyl (meth)acrylates. Macromolecules. 2002;35(21):7968–75.
13. Lovell LG, Berchtold KA, Elliott JE, Lu H, Bowman CN. Understanding the kinetics and network formation of dimethacrylate dental resins. Polym Adv Technol. 2001;12(6):335–45.
14. Lovell LG, Newman SM, Bowman CN. The effects of light intensity, temperature, and comonomer composition on the polymerization behavior of dimethacrylate dental resins. J Dent Res. 1999;78(8):1469–76.
15. Lovell LG, Stansbury JW, Syrpes DC, Bowman CN. Effects of composition and reactivity on the reaction kinetics of dimethacrylate/dimethacrylate copolymerizations. Macromolecules. 1999;32(12):3913–21.
16. Cook WD, Brockhurst P. The oscillating rheometer – what does it measure? J Dent Res. 1980;59(5):795–9.
17. Dickens SH, Stansbury JW, Choi KM, Floyd CJE. Photopolymerization kinetics of methacrylate dental resins. Macromolecules. 2003;36(16):6043–53.
18. Hasegawa T, Itoh K, Yukitani W, Wakumoto S, Hisamitsu H. Effects of soft-start irradiation on the depth of cure and marginal adaptation to dentin. Oper Dent. 2001;26(4):389–95.
19. Yap AU, Ng SC, Siow KS. Soft-start polymerization: influence on effectiveness of cure and post-gel shrinkage. Oper Dent. 2001;26(3):260–6.
20. Cramer NB, Couch CL, Schreck KM, Carioscia JA, Boulden JE, Stansbury JW, Bowman CN. Investigation of thiol-ene and thiol-ene-methacrylate based resins as dental restorative materials. Dent Mater. 2010;26(1):21–8.
21. Cramer NB, Bowman CN. Kinetics of thiol-ene and thiol-acrylate photopolymerizations with real-time Fourier transform infrared. J Polym Sci A Polym Chem. 2001;39(19):3311–9.
22. Reddy SK, Cramer NB, Bowman CN. Thiol-vinyl mechanisms. 2. Kinetic modeling of ternary thiol-vinyl photopolymerizations. Macromolecules. 2006;39(10):3681–7.
23. Lee TY, Carioscia J, Smith Z, Bowman CN. Thiol-allyl ether-methacrylate ternary systems. Evolution mechanism of polymerization-induced shrinkage stress and mechanical properties. Macromolecules. 2007;40(5):1473–9.
24. Musanje L, Ferracane JL, Sakaguchi RL. Determination of the optimal photoinitiator concentration in dental composites based on essential material properties. Dent Mater. 2009;25(8):994–1000.
25. Vaidyanathan TK, Vaidyanathan J, Lizymol PP, Ariya S, Krishnan KV. Study of visible light activated polymerization in BisGMA-TEGDMA monomers with type 1 and type 2 photoinitiators using Raman spectroscopy. Dent Mater. 2017;33(1):1–11.
26. Cook WD. Thermal aspects of the kinetics of dimethacrylate photopolymerization. Polymer. 1992;33(10):2152–61.
27. Stansbury JW, Dickens SH. Determination of double bond conversion in dental resins by near infrared spectroscopy. Dent Mater. 2001;17(1):71–9.
28. Wisanrakkit G, Gillham JK. The glass transition temperature (Tg) as an index of chemical conversion for a high-Tg amine/epoxy system: chemical and diffusion-controlled reaction kinetics. J Appl Polym Sci. 1990;41(11–12):2885–929.
29. Sideridou I, Tserki V, Papanastasiou G. Effect of chemical structure on degree of conversion in light-cured dimethacrylate-based dental resins. Biomaterials. 2002;23(8):1819–29.

The Dental Curing Light

4

Richard B. Price

Light-cured dental resins have revolutionized modern dentistry, and the dental curing light has become an indispensable piece of equipment in almost every dental office [1–3]. Despite its routine use, the importance of the curing light and how it is used is poorly understood by most operators [4–6]. Every study that has evaluated curing lights used in dental offices has shown that they often deliver an inadequate light output [7–13], and a study published in 2017 reported that 14.5% of dentists did not carry out any regular maintenance on their curing lights [6]. In many offices, the dentists were unaware that their lights were not delivering an adequate light output or that their resins were not achieving the manufacturer's specifications [7]. This is most likely because the dentist can only test the top surface of the resin. Here, the resin appears hard and well cured, yet the bulk of the resin underneath may be undercured.

This chapter will discuss dental curing lights and their use in dentistry. The International System of Units (SI) radiometric terminology will be used to describe the output from a curing light instead of terms such as lux, power density, energy density, or intensity.

R.B. Price
Department of Dental Clinical Scietnces, Dalhousie University, Halifax, NS, Canada, B3H 4R2
e-mail: Richard.Price@dal.ca

4.1 Radiometric Terminology

The appropriate SI radiometric terms to describe the output from a curing light are provided in Table 4.1 [3].

In keeping with the low output from dental curing lights and their size, values are usually reported in milliwatts (mW) rather than watts and in millimeters (mm) or centimeters (cm) rather than meters.

4.1.1 Radiant Exitance (Irradiance) Vs. Radiant Power

When reporting the output from curing lights, manufacturers commonly report an irradiance value (mW/cm^2) that was measured at the tip of the light. When the curing light tip is in direct contact with the detector of a meter or the surface of the resin, this irradiance value is effectively the same as the radiant exitance. However, this irradiance value gives no indication how powerful a light is because the irradiance received by the resin restoration is greatly influenced by both the diameter of the light tip and the distance from the light tip to the resin. For example, some curing lights use a small tip diameter of 7 mm, compared to others that have a tip diameter of 10 mm or more. While a 3-mm reduction in tip diameter may seem insignificant,

V. Miletic (ed.), *Dental Composite Materials for Direct Restorations*,
http://doi.org/10.1007/978-3-319-60961-4_4

Table 4.1 Radiometric terminology used to describe the output from a light source [3]

Term	Units	Symbol	Notes
Radiant power or radiant flux	Watt	W	Radiant energy delivered per unit time (J/s)
Radiant energy	Joule	J	This describes the energy from the source (W/s)
Radiant exposure	Joule per square centimeter	J/cm^2	This describes the energy received per unit area. Sometimes this is incorrectly described as "energy density"
Radiant energy density	Joule per cubic centimeter	J/cm^3	This is the energy in a defined volume (cm^3)
Radiant exitance or Radiant emittance	Watt per square centimeter	W/cm^2	Radiant power (flux) that is emitted from a surface, e.g., the tip of a curing light
Irradiance (incident irradiance)	Watt per square centimeter	W/cm^2	Radiant power (flux) incident on a known surface area. This is an averaged value over the surface area
Spectral radiant power	Watt per nanometer	W/nm	Radiant power at each wavelength of the electromagnetic spectrum in nanometers (nm)
Spectral irradiance	Watt per square centimeter per nanometer	$W/cm^2/nm$	Irradiance at each wavelength of the electromagnetic spectrum in nanometers (nm)

it changes the area of the light tip from 78.5 mm^2 (10-mm diameter) to 38.5 mm^2 (7-mm diameter). This doubles the radiant exitance (irradiance) at the tip. Thus, just by changing the tip diameter, two curing lights can deliver the same irradiance, but very different radiant power outputs [14]. Consequently, in the era of bulk filling and bulk curing of large restorations, the radiant power (in mWatts), the active tip diameter (mm), and the irradiance (mW/cm^2) should all be reported. Otherwise, the clinician may not recognize that they are actually using a low-powered curing light that uses a small diameter light tip to boost the irradiance.

4.1.2 Spectral Radiant Power

To the human eye, all dental curing lights appear to deliver the same blue light, but this is not the case. Instead, the emission spectrum from dental curing lights can be very different (Fig. 4.1 A-D), and thus the lights will have very different effects on the photoinitiators found within the resins used in dentistry. Consequently, it is important that the spectral radiant power from the curing light be reported so that the user can judge if the light they are using is ideal for the resin they are trying to photocure (Fig. 4.1).

4.1.3 Light Beam Uniformity

A laser beam profiler records the spatial intensity profile of a light beam, and can be used to measure the beam uniformity from dental curing lights [14–19]. A digital camera records an image of the light output on a specified diffusing screen. The light received by each camera pixel is then displayed as a color-coded two- or three-dimensional image. Such images of curing lights show that many curing lights have "hot spots" of high irradiance and "cold spots" where the irradiance is lower [14–19]. Examples of inhomogeneous distributions of irradiance across the emitting tips of different dental light curing units are seen in Fig. 4.2.

The beam profile images show that the irradiance homogeneity depends on the design of the curing light and that using a single irradiance value does not describe the irradiance across the entire light tip. Instead this is an average of the high and low irradiance values that are present across the light tip. In addition, the use of multiple LED pads, each producing a different color, in order to produce a broad spectral range in multi-peak or polywave® curing lights can cause problems of spectral inhomogeneity as well as irradiance inhomogeneity across the light tip [16].

The beam profile images also show that unless the operator is careful, the irradiance and radiant

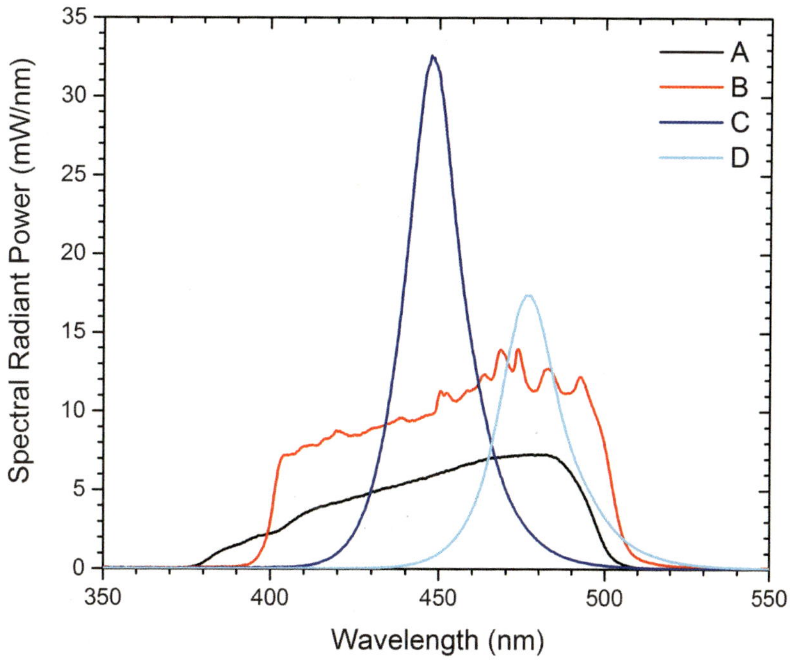

Fig. 4.1 Emission spectra from four contemporary curing lights. Note the differences between the lights

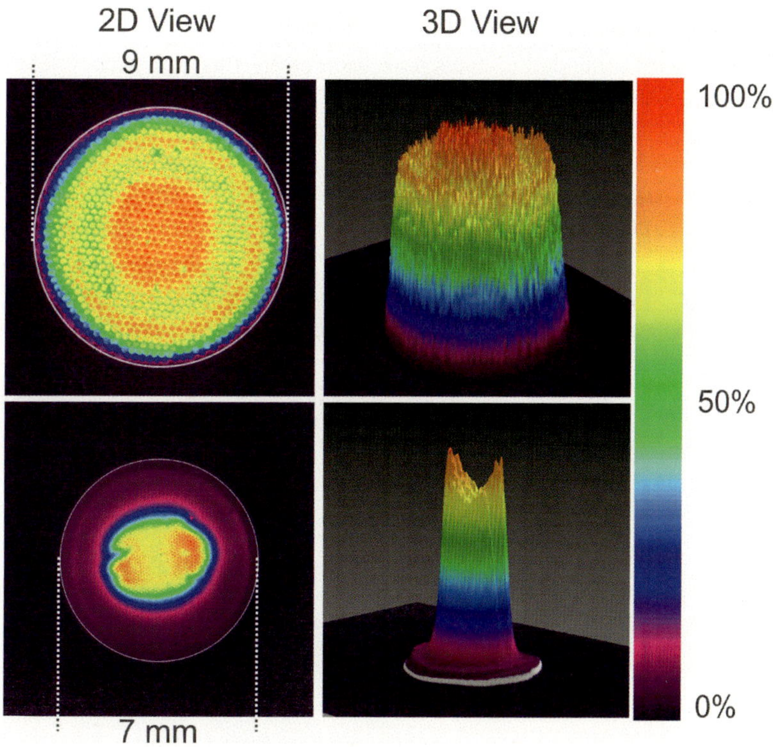

Fig. 4.2 Image of the beam profiles from two contemporary curing lights. The left sets of images are scaled 2-D representations of the irradiance distribution. The right side views are 3-D representations of the same lights with all images scaled to their own maximum irradiance value. Note the differences in the beam diameters and the inhomogeneous irradiance distribution across the light tips

exposure received at the gingival margins of the proximal boxes from some curing lights may be insufficient to adequately polymerize the adhesive or the resin restoration at the bottom of the proximal boxes [14, 18, 19]. Not only are these regions the most difficult to reach with the curing light, they are also the furthest away from the light source [20, 21]. Consequently, resin at these locations will receive the least amount of light and may well be under-polymerized, unless the operator pays close attention to ensure that they position the light tip properly and use the light for long enough so that the resin receives an adequate amount of light.

4.2 Development of Dental Curing Lights

Four types of blue light sources have been used in dentistry: quartz-tungsten-halogen (QTH), plasma arc (PAC), argon-ion laser, and light-emitting diodes (LED). Examples of PAC, QTH, and LED curing lights are shown below (Fig. 4.3), General guidelines for using curing lights have been proposed [1–3, 22–24].

4.2.1 Quartz-Tungsten-Halogen (QTH) Lights

Blue light-emitting curing lights initially used a quartz-tungsten-halogen (QTH) light bulb that produced a broad spectrum of electromagnetic energy, from near ultra violet (UV) and into the infrared region. To deliver just the blue light required to photocure the resin, the light from the QTH bulb was aggressively filtered to remove the UV and infrared wavelengths of light.

Inside the QTH bulb is a halogen gas and a tungsten filament [1, 25]. When electrical current passes through the filament, the tungsten wire becomes incandescent and atoms are vaporized from its surface. This releases a large amount of electromagnetic energy, most of which is emitted in the infrared region. When the current is turned off, the filament cools, and the halogen gas redeposits the vaporized tungsten atoms back onto the filament surface [25]. This process is called "the halogen cycle." A fan inside the unit cools the reflector, bulb, and filters, but the surfaces still become very hot. Vapors from solvents, cleaning agents, or moisture in the operatory air can all be deposited onto the reflector surface. This dulls the reflector surface and gradually reduces the amount of light delivered by the curing light. All this can occur without any outward sign of a decrease in light output, thus it is essential to monitor the light output on a regular basis. Under ideal conditions, the QTH bulb should last about 50 h before it burns out [1, 2], but the lifespan of the bulb will be shortened if the user turns the power supply off immediately after light curing in order to stop the noise from the cooling fan. This occurs because the filament inside the bulb

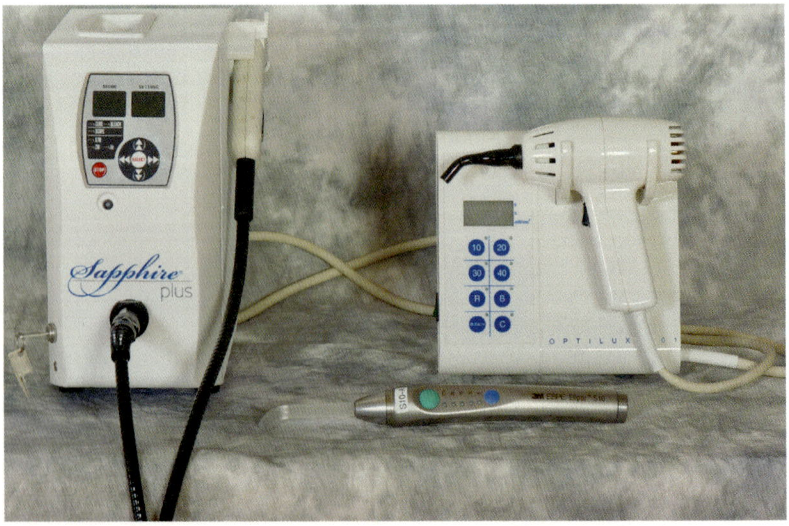

Fig. 4.3 Examples of contemporary QTH, PAC, and LED curing lights. Note the different designs and form factors

must be allowed to cool down at a controlled rate for the halogen cycle to occur; otherwise, the vaporized tungsten atoms are not redeposited onto the filament surface, thus shortening the lifetime of the bulb [25].

The light from the QTH bulb is first directed toward a relatively large silverized parabolic reflector. This reflector allows some of the infrared wavelengths to pass through so that they are not reflected forward. The reflected light is projected forward through bandpass filters so that only wavelengths of light between approximately 400 and 500 nm reach the proximal surface of the light guide [25]. As much as 70% of the power going into the QTH bulb is converted to heat, with only 10% of the power producing visible light. Only 0.5–2% of the input is emitted as useful blue light [24, 26].

Although QTH lights deliver a broad emission spectrum, the units deliver a relatively low radiant power, and they require an exposure time of between 30 and 60 s to adequately polymerize a 2-mm-thick increment of resin composite. The majority of these lights are mains-powered, and the cooling fan was noisy.

4.2.2 Plasma Arc (PAC) Lights

In an attempt to reduce light exposure times, high-power PAC lights were introduced. These lights claimed to deliver a very high irradiance and only required a short 3–5-s exposure time to light cure a 2-mm-thick increment of resin composite. In contrast to an incandescent filament, PAC lights produce light from two tungsten electrodes that are surrounded by xenon gas. When a high voltage is applied, a spark is formed that ionizes the xenon gas to produce an electrically conductive gaseous medium (a plasma) that maintains the spark [1, 25]. Intense optical filtering is required within PAC lights to prevent the emission of unwanted ionizing radiation and infrared light that would produce an unacceptable temperature increase.

Although they are excellent curing lights, PAC lights are expensive, they have a noisy fan, they are large, and they cannot be battery operated. Consequently, they have become less popular in recent years.

4.2.3 Argon-Ion Lasers

The argon-ion laser curing light was developed about the same time as the PAC lights were introduced, and they are also claimed to deliver a high irradiance and short exposure times. The term laser stands for light amplification by stimulated emission of radiation. Lasers work by delivering electrical energy to specific atoms within the unit. The electrons become "excited" and move from a low-energy orbit to a higher-energy orbit around the atom's nucleus. When these electrons then return to their normal or "ground" state, they emit photons of light that are all of the same wavelength. The argon-ion laser generates several very intense emission peaks in the blue spectral region and is a viable light source for a high-power curing light [25].

Typical exposure times when using a laser curing light are less than 10 s. However, laser curing lights never became less popular because they are expensive, they are not portable, they have a narrow emission spectrum, and they cannot be battery operated.

4.2.4 Light-Emitting Diode (LED) Technology

The next innovation in dental photocuring was introduced in the early 1990s when blue LED curing lights became available [27, 28]. Using LEDs as the light source has many advantages because the units are solid state, battery operated, and lightweight, and the light they produce does not need to be filtered. The LED emitters are very efficient, and they deliver at least two to three times the luminous output per watt compared to a typical QTH bulb [2]. Also, when used correctly, the LED emitters can provide a long working life of many thousands of hours [1, 2] instead of just 50 or so hours for a QTH bulb [1, 2].

LEDs are semiconductor light sources that have been doped with impurities to create specific electron-excessive (n) and electron-depleted (p) surfaces in two different semiconductor materials [2]. The semiconductor substrate on the n side, or cathode, has an excess of electrons and will rise in potential when sufficient electrical energy is applied. Electrons from the n substrate then pass through and "fall" into "holes" in the electron-deficient medium in the p side, or anode. When an electron meets a "hole" in the p side, it "falls" into a lower energy level and releases energy in the form of a photon of light of a specific wavelength by a process called electroluminescence. The very specific color of the light emitted from the LED corresponds to the energy of the photon that is in turn determined by the composition of the two semiconductors and their resulting "band gap" potential [2]. The semiconductor material in blue LEDs is made of a mix of gallium nitride (GaN) and indium nitride (InN). The emitted light has a relatively narrow bandwidth with a full width half maximum (FWHM) range of only about 25 nm, and this FWHM is much narrower than from QTH lights. By selecting the right proportions of gallium nitride (GaN) and indium nitride (InN), the emission spectrum from "blue" LEDs can be "tuned" to match the specific excitation wavelengths of the photoinitiators used in dental resins.

4.2.5 First-Generation LED Lights

The first generation of dental LED-based light curing units contained a collection of many individual LED "cans" [1] (Fig. 4.4).

The wavelength of the blue light emitted from these early blue LEDs was in the range of maximum absorption of camphorquinone (~470 nm). This made these blue LEDs very efficient at producing the free radicals required to photocure dental resins. Since these early LED lights had a relatively low power output, it was thought that all LED-curing lights generated little or no heat. However, this was due to their low radiant power output rather than to any property of the photons emitted from LED curing lights.

4.2.6 Second-Generation LED Lights

LED chip design has evolved to produce small surface area emitting LED pads, instead of larger discrete LED cans. These LED pads deliver a greater radiant power output, and the number of photons emitted within the absorption range of camphorquinone is now greater than from QTH or PAC lights [1]. However, with this increase in radiant power output, it is necessary to cool the LED chip using large metal heat sinks and/or internal cooling fans. Often, the metal body of these powerful LED-curing lights is used as a heat sink.

Although these "second-generation" curing lights are more powerful than the "first generation" of LED lights, neither the first nor the second generation LED lights deliver much, if any, spectral radiant power below 420 nm (Fig. 4.5). Consequently, they are unable to activate some of the "alternative" photoinitiators, such

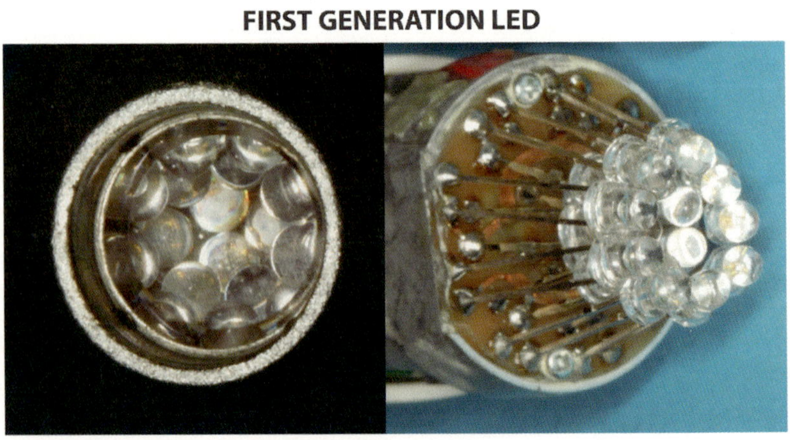

Fig. 4.4 Example of the use of multiple LED cans in a first-generation LED light curing light

as Lucirin TPO®; however, most will activate the recently introduced germanium-based photoinitiator, Ivocerin™, that can be activated by wavelengths of light up to 460 nm [29, 30].

4.2.7 Third-Generation LED Lights: Multi-wave, Multi-peak, and Polywave®

The camphorquinone (CQ) photoinitiator used in the majority of dental resins has a bright yellow color, and this yellow color is problematic when trying to produce very light or translucent shades of restorative resin. As a result, some manufacturers have incorporated co-initiators to boost the effectiveness of CQ so that they could reduce the overall concentration of CQ, while others started using more efficient "alternative" photoinitiators to reduce the concentration of CQ [1]. These "alternative" initiators, such as Lucirin TPO®, impart less of a yellow color than those that contain CQ. However, these alternative photoinitiators are activated by shorter wavelengths of light closer to violet light (at or below 410 nm), and although they can be activated by the broader emission spectrum from QTH curing lights, they are only weakly activated by second-generation LED curing lights that emit little light below 420 nm (Fig. 4.5). To solve the problem caused by the narrow emission spectrum from the blue-only LED units, additional LED emitters were added to the blue LED array. Each additional LED pad produces a different narrow range of wavelengths, and by incorporating several different LED pads into the curing light, a broad spectral range can now be delivered. These curing lights have been called "third-generation" LED curing lights, meaning that they emit light of more than one wavelength range, usually violet and blue (Fig. 4.6). Curing lights of this generation have also been described as "multi-wave" or "multi-peak" dental curing lights, with one manufacturer trademarking the name "Polywave®" to signify this concept within their product line.

The emission spectrum from broad-spectrum LED lights should be able to activate all the photoinitiators currently used in dental resins and bonding agents. Since manufacturers rarely disclose all of the proprietary constituents used in their resins, it is best to assume that if a resin manufacturer produces a broad spectrum LED curing light, then their resins will likely benefit from the use of a broad spectrum LED curing

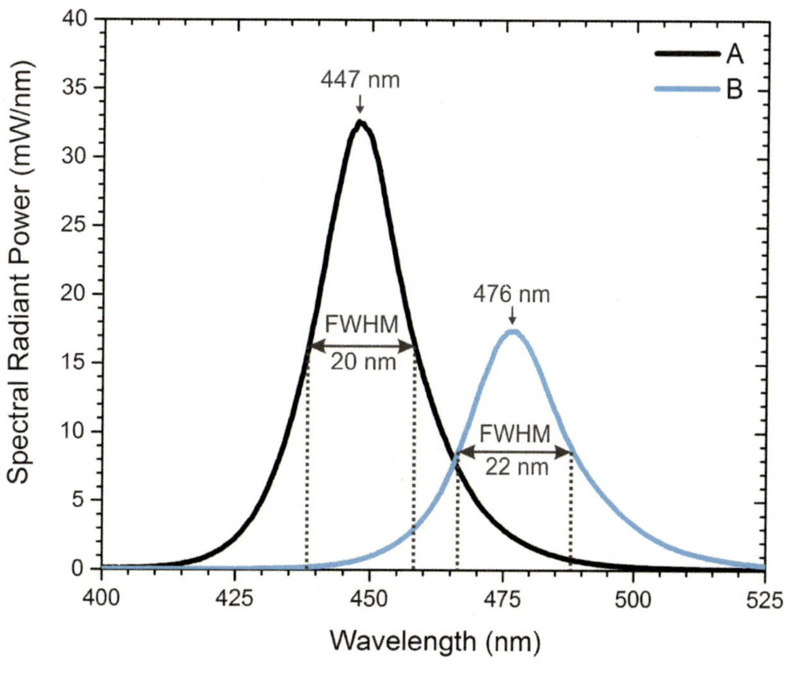

Fig. 4.5 Example of the light output from two different second-generation LED curing lights. Note the peak spectral emission (nm), the limited power output below 420 nm, and the narrow full width at half maximum (FWHM) outputs

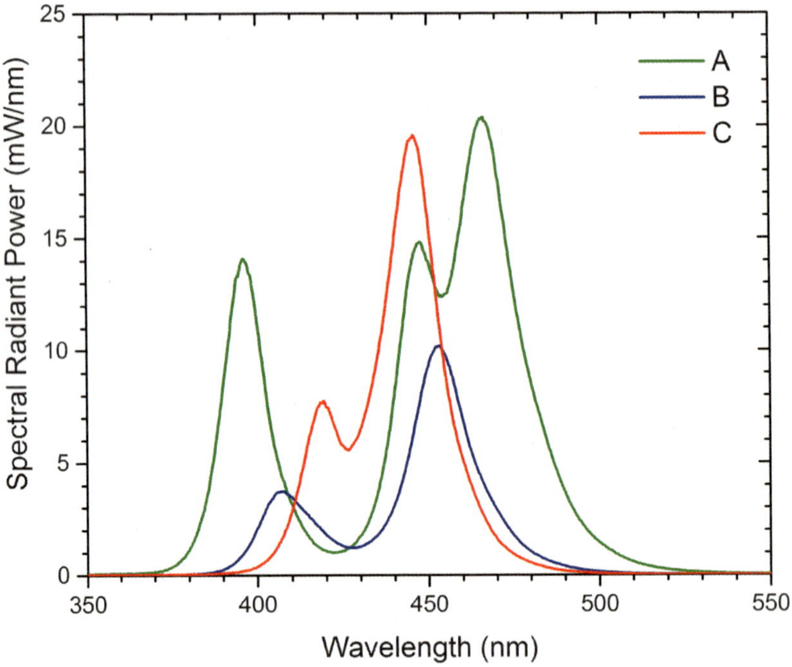

Fig. 4.6 Emission spectra from three broad-spectrum, LED curing lights. Note the emission spectra are all different among these lights and from the second generation lights in Fig. 4.5

light, e.g., Ivoclar Vivadent or Ultradent Products. Conversely, if the manufacturer, e.g., 3M, makes a single peak wavelength curing light only, then their resins are unlikely to require the use of a broad-spectrum polywave® LED curing light.

4.2.8 "Turbo" Light Guides

Conventional, glass-fibered light guides come in a variety of diameters, but usually the proximal entrance and the distal exit apertures of the light guide are the same physical size. In an attempt to increase the irradiance, the proximal entrance to the "turbo" light guide is larger than the exit diameter (Fig. 4.7). Both the entrance and the exit of these light guides contain the same number of fibers, but the fibers at the exit end are smaller than at the entrance. Thus, the same number of photons that enter into the wide entrance to the light guide are emitted over a smaller exit area. Since the same radiant power (number of photons) is now emitted over a smaller area, the radiant exitance, "irradiance" (mW/cm^2), from these turbo light guides is increased [31].

Unfortunately, the irradiance delivered to a resin from these turbo light guides declines rapidly as the distance from the tip increases [21] and at 6 mm away from the tip; these light guides usually deliver less irradiance than a conventional light guide [21]. Some curing lights also include a special boosted output mode, where the voltage to the light source is raised for a short time. However, overdriving the light source to boost the light output shortens its life expectancy, and it also generates more heat.

4.2.9 Exposure Reciprocity

Photopolymerization reaction rates are affected by many factors such as the irradiance received, the concentration of the photoinitiators, the quantum yield for radical generation, the effects of radical recombination/termination, the impact of oxygen inhibition, the resin viscosity, the amount of heat generated, the material thickness, the matching of the resin and filler refractive indices, the filler particle size, and the shade. As a general recommendation, it has been proposed

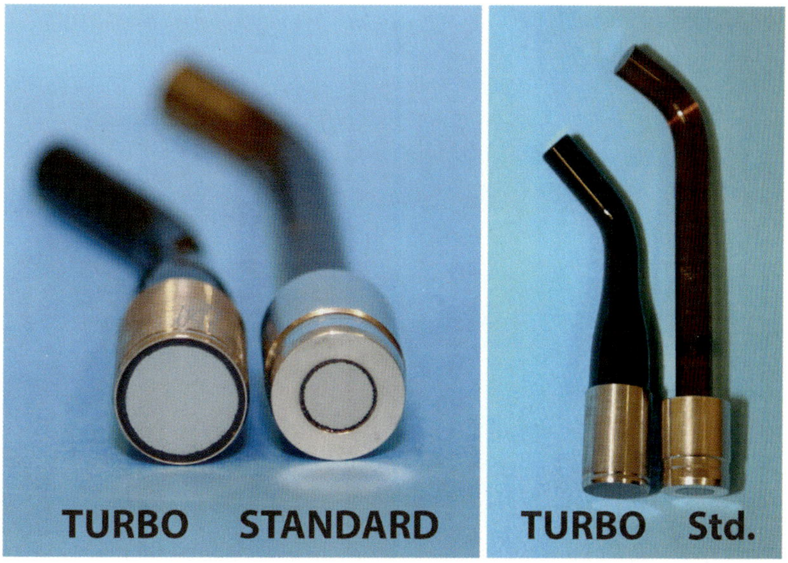

Fig. 4.7 Example of a conventional and a "turbo" light guide where the entrance fiber diameter is larger than the exit fiber diameter. Note how the turbo light guide tapers to a smaller tip

that a QTH curing light delivering an irradiance of 400 mW/cm² should be used for 60 s to adequately polymerize a 1.5–2-mm-thick increment of resin composite [32]. If this irradiance is multiplied by the exposure time, this means that a radiant exposure of 24–36 J/cm² should adequately polymerize most resin composites, recognizing that brand, shade, and opacity of the resin will all affect the exact amount of energy required [33, 34]. Some believe that using a high-intensity curing light is a way to provide timesavings and increase profitability [35]. Behind this is the belief that if the curing light delivers double the irradiance, then you can halve the time spent light curing. However, this is not the case. True reciprocity between the duration of light exposure and the irradiance to achieve the same level of resin polymerization does not exist [36–40]. Instead, it has been calculated that the reaction rate is at best related to the square root of the irradiance [41]. Thus, even under ideal circumstances, reducing the light exposure time from 20 to 5 s will require 16x the irradiance to achieve the same level of polymerization within the resin. Thus, delivering 4000 mW/cm² for 5 s will not achieve the same resin polymerization as 500 mW/cm² delivered for 40 s, despite the fact that in both cases the resin would receive the same 20 J/cm² of radiant exposure. Additionally, it is known that the depth of cure within the resin increases by the logarithm of the radiant exposure, i.e., there is an exponential relationship between depth of cure and the amount of energy delivered, -doubling the radiant exposure received will not double the depth of cure [42]. Thus, it is inadvisable to exceed the resin manufacturer's recommended increment thickness and hope that by using a longer exposure time, the resin will be fully cured.

4.2.10 High-Output Curing Lights and Stress Development During Polymerization

Fast polymerization of dental resin-based composites is thought to adversely affect both the mechanical properties of the polymer network [43, 44] and the physical properties of the resin [45]. With some contemporary dental resins that use CQ photoinitiator systems, rapid photopolymerization produces shorter chain lengths because there is insufficient time for long polymer chains to form before the solid state is reached and no further movement is possible [43]. Also, as long as the system is a liquid, it can physically deform, and little stress is developed. However, beyond the "gel point," the resin becomes a solid, and the polymerization shrinkage deforms the resin thus creating stresses both within the network and at the bonded interfaces. If this gel point is reached very rapidly, as would occur when using a high irradiance, this may result in increased stress [46], increased bond failure, and more gaps between the tooth and restorative material [47, 48].

4.2.11 Soft-Start Exposures

In an attempt to decrease the damaging effects of rapid photopolymerization, a range of different light curing cycles have been proposed. An example is the "soft-start" curing mode, where a low irradiance value is applied to the resin surface for a short time and then, either immediately or over a short period of time, the light output increases to its full operating level for the remainder of the exposure [47, 49, 50]. This technique is intended to allow the partially photopolymerized resin to deform and thus relieve the stresses that are developing within the resin that is cured and rigid. Another method, the pulse-delay, delivers an initial low-level, short-duration exposure, and then the light is turned off. After waiting some 3–5 min, the final exposure is provided at the full light output [47]. It was hoped that the use of such an exposure mode would reduce the rate at which the photopolymerized material reacted, thus allowing movement within the unreacted or partially reacted resin that would then reduce the overall amount of polymerization contraction stress [46, 47, 51–54]. However, it has been reported that using the pulse-delay method results in a lower cross-link density within the photocured resin. This produced polymers that were more susceptible to softening in ethanol [55] and that also stained more readily [56]. Clinically, none of these attempts to control the polymerization shrinkage rate and stress development have been found to provide significantly better performance when compared to a continuous light exposure [1, 57], and in one study restorations photopolymerized with the pulse-delay technique had the highest failure rate after 7 years of service in the mouth [57].

4.2.12 Batteries

Originally, LED curing lights were powered by nickel-cadmium (NiCad) batteries. These batteries can be damaged if they are deeply discharged, or if they are overcharged. Smaller, high-capacity, nickel-metal hydride batteries soon replaced these NiCad batteries [1], but most currently available curing lights now use either lithium-ion batteries or "ultracapacitors." Ultracapacitors can deliver high bursts of power for a short time and are used in at least one LED curing light (Demi Ultra, Kerr Corp., Orange, CA) that can deliver approximately 25, 10-s light exposures before the unit must be recharged. Although ultracapacitors cannot store the same amount of electrical energy as lithium-ion batteries, they can be fully recharged in as little as 40 s and should provide a sufficient number of light exposures to treat one patient.

4.2.13 Curing Light Output Monitoring

Although it has been reported that only 46.8% of dentists use a radiometer regularly to monitor the irradiance [6], it is important that the light output from the curing light be monitored on a regular basis because the light output will decrease for many reasons [25] such as aging and degradation of the light source, the buildup of scale on the fiber-optic light probe after autoclaving [58], breakage or fracture at the light tip [59, 60], or the presence of cured resin on the light tip [59, 61] (Fig. 4.8). In addition, disinfectant sprays can erode the O-rings that stabilize the light guide, and liquids can become baked onto the lens or reflectors inside the housing, thus reducing the light output [62].

Since, dental curing lights have different emission spectra and different light tip diameters, low-cost dental radiometers are often unable to accurately report the irradiance value from a range of curing lights [63–67]. This can lead clinicians to believe that they are delivering sufficient energy to their restorations, when this may not be the case [64]. A new type of dental

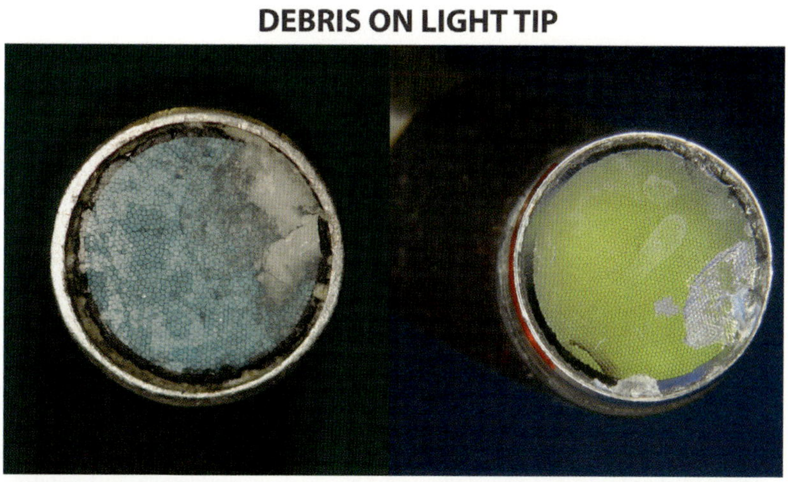

Fig. 4.8 Examples of damaged (**a**) and debris-contaminated (**b**) curing light tips

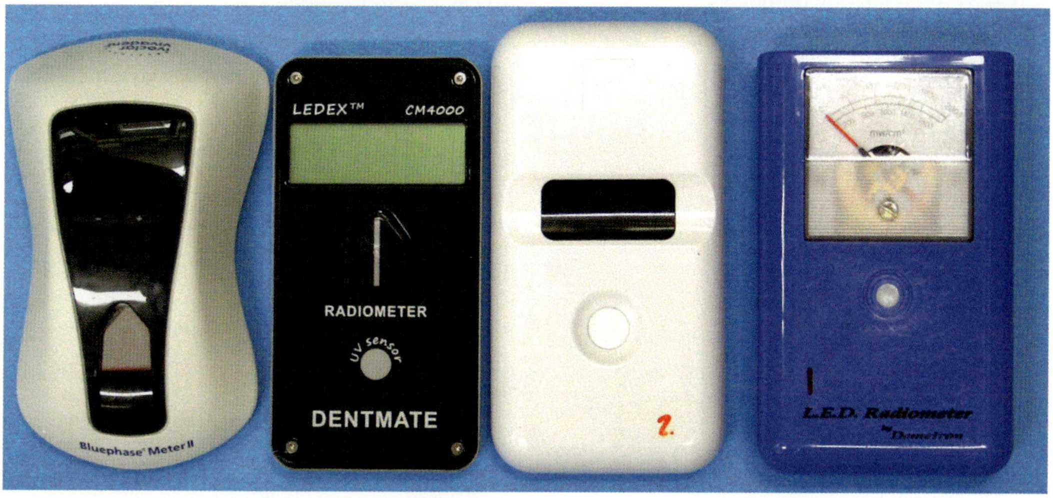

Fig. 4.9 Examples of four commercial dental radiometers. The Bluephase Meter II on the left has a large entrance aperture and currently is the only dental radiometer that is able to measure all the power from a 13-mm diameter light tip

radiometer, the Bluephase Meter II (Ivoclar Vivadent, Amherst, NY, USA), has been introduced that can measure both the radiant power and the irradiance (Fig. 4.9). The meter uses a large sensor that allows it to accurately measure the radiant power from light tips that are up to 13 mm in diameter [68], and if the tip diameter (in mm) is entered into the device, this meter can also calculate the irradiance. When using these radiometers, it is important that the same light guides are used each time the curing light is measured and that the values are recorded for medicolegal reasons.

4.3 Practical Considerations for Light Curing Dental Resins in the Mouth

4.3.1 Temperature Considerations

It is important not to arbitrarily increase the light exposure time in an attempt to assure complete polymerization without understanding the adverse thermal effects this can have on the pulp and oral tissues. Contrary to initial claims, high-power LED curing lights can produce unwanted temperature increases [69–74]. When the light tip is close to soft tissue, or where the remaining tooth structure is thin, there is a risk of thermal damage when the LCU delivers greater than 1200 mW/ cm^2 [75]. It is recommended that when the LCU is used for extended curing times, then the tooth be air-cooled, or the operator should wait at least 2–3 s between every 10 s of light curing [76].

4.3.2 The "Blue Light Hazard"

The dentist has a duty to protect both the patient and their employees from harm [77]. Recently, there has been concern that blue light from high-power curing lights may cause ocular damage [77–81]. This hazard can be prevented by using appropriate eye protection that is provided by the orange-colored shields or glasses (blue light blockers) that are supplied with the curing lights, but these items are not universally used in the dental office [5, 6, 82].

The "blue light hazard" is greatest at 440 nm [83, 84], and this is within the output range from dental LCUs [1, 3] (Fig. 4.10). Blue light is transmitted through the ocular media and absorbed by the retina at the back of the eye. While high levels of blue light can cause immediate and irreversible retinal burning, of greater concern is the chronic exposure to low levels of blue light that may cause accelerated retinal aging and accelerate age-related macular degeneration (ARMD) [84, 85]. Most countries follow international guidelines, such as those from the International Commission on Non-Ionizing Radiation Protection (ICNIRP) and American Conference of Governmental Industrial Hygienists (ACGIH), that limit exposure to all types of hazardous optical radiation [83, 84]. If the operator does not use appropriate eye protection, these limits may be easily reached during a normal workday by dental personnel using high-power curing lights. It has been shown that, after looking at the light for even just the first second of the curing cycle before averting the eyes, it may take as little as seven light exposures to exceed the maximum daily cumulative exposure [79]. It should be noted that the maximum recommended exposure times have been calculated for individuals who have normal photosensitivity. Children, persons who have had cataract surgery, or those who are taking photosensitizing medications have a greater susceptibility for retinal damage. In these circumstances, ocular injury may occur after shorter exposure times [83, 84]. If appropriate eye protection is used when light curing, instead of looking away from the bright blue light on the tooth, the operator can safely watch what they are doing and so can increase the amount of light they deliver to the restoration [86–90] (Fig. 4.11).

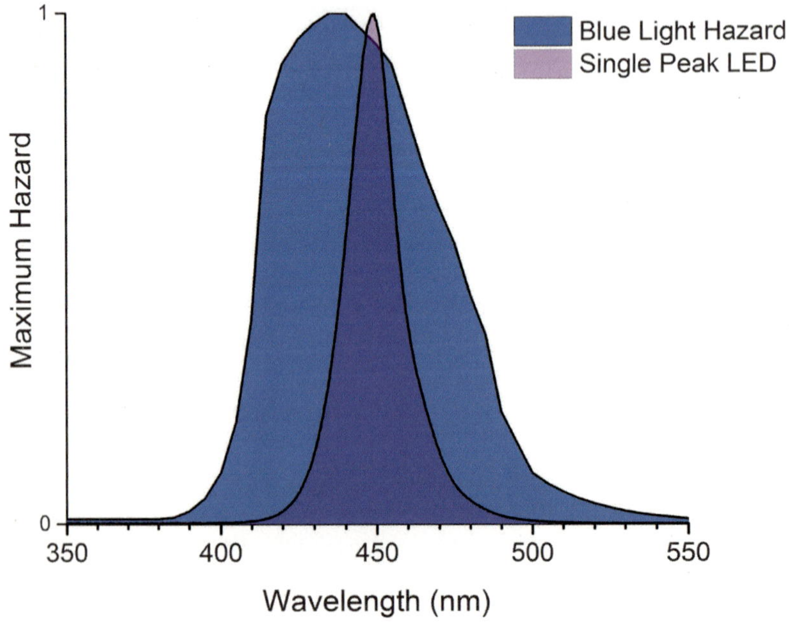

Fig. 4.10 Graphical depiction of the blue light hazard related to the wavelength of light. Superimposition of the emission spectrum from a second-generation LED dental curing light shows that all the blue light delivered from this LED curing light is in the hazardous range

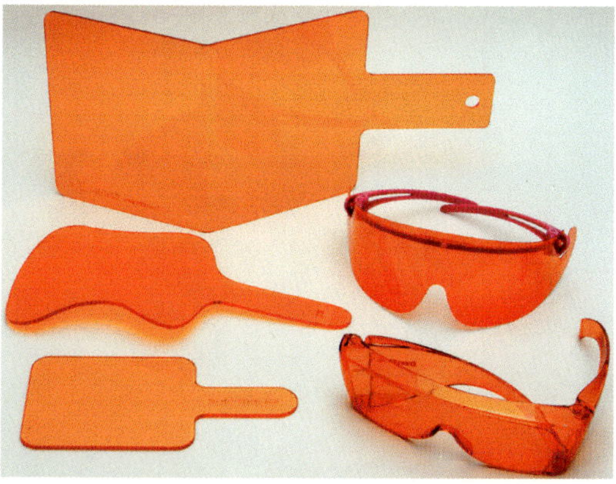

Fig. 4.11 Examples of "blue light" blocking glasses and shields

4.3.3 Light Guide Tip Diameter

The diameter of the light tip has a significant impact on the light coverage and the energy delivered to the restoration [21, 91]. Wide light tips that are 11 or 13 mm in diameter were once popular, but recently, in an attempt to deliver high irradiance values, smaller 6–8-mm diameter light tips have become commonplace. Dentistry is now in the era of bulk filling and bulk curing large resin restorations. With the dimensions of a mandibular molar being approximately 11.0 mm mesiodistally and 10.5 mm buccolingually at the crown [92], the clinician who wishes to reduce the time spent light curing restorations should use a curing light with a light-emitting tip that completely covers the entire surface of the restoration. In the case of a mesial-occlusal-distal restoration in a molar tooth, this means the diameter of the light guide should be at least 11 mm. Otherwise, multiple and overlapping exposures must be delivered so that all areas of the restorative material are covered by the light tip, as seen in Fig. 4.12.

4.3.4 Budget Curing Lights

In today's Internet age, the dental profession can purchase dental equipment, including curing lights, directly online at a lower cost instead of using an approved distributor. While this may seem appealing, many of these "budget curing lights" are unregulated, and some use small diameter (6–7 mm) light guides. Consequently, despite only delivering a low power, they can deliver the same irradiance values as curing lights from major manufacturers that use wider diameter tips. The light beam profiles from these budget lights can also be inferior compared to well-designed curing lights from major manufacturers [14, 19], and the electronics in these budget lights may not compensate for the fall in the output as the battery discharges. Thus, the light output from some of the budget battery-operated curing lights may decline without warning the operator [14]. In addition, some of these budget curing lights may not have been tested for safety or efficacy, and the use of such medical devices on a patient should be regarded as *in vivo* testing on a patient who has not given informed consent [23].

4.3.5 Distance to Target

Curing lights do not act as a point source of light (Fig. 4.13), and depending on the design and the optics of the unit, some deliver well-collimated light beams. Since light may be emitted at different degrees of beam divergence from the tip end of curing lights, the effect of tip distance on the irradiance received at the target is not the same for all lights (Fig. 4.14). The effect of distance from the tip on the decrease in the amount of light received at the target might be assumed to obey the inverse square law; however, because the inverse square law describes a point source of radiation that is emitting 360 degrees in space, much like the Sun, the law does not apply to the partially collimated light from curing lights.

Figure 4.14 displays how increasing the tip-to-target distance can produce very different results from different brands of curing lights. Some curing lights have been reported to deliver only 25%, or even less, of the irradiance measured at the tip at a distance of 8–9 mm from the tip, while others deliver 75% or more [21, 93–97]. Thus, the dentist should know how clinically relevant distances (up to 10 mm) may affect the irra-

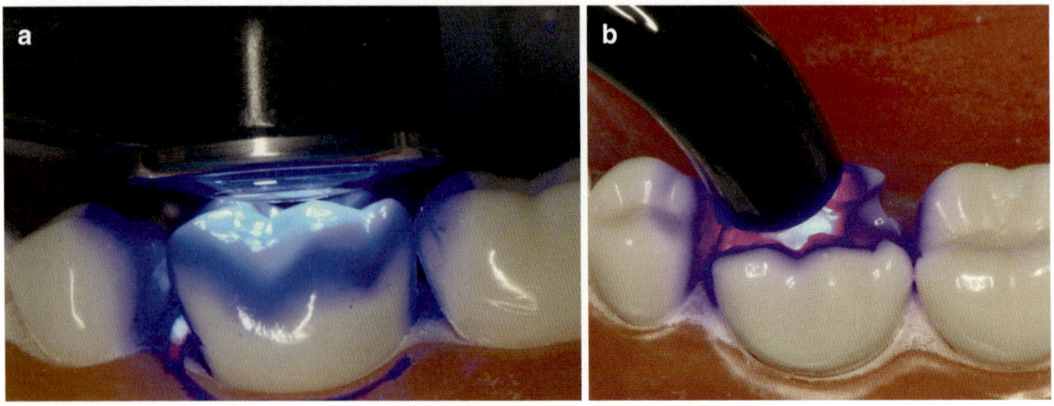

Fig. 4.12 A large diameter light tip (**a**) can cover an entire molar tooth, whereas smaller diameter light tip (**b**) will require multiple exposures to cover an entire molar mesial-occlusal-distal restoration

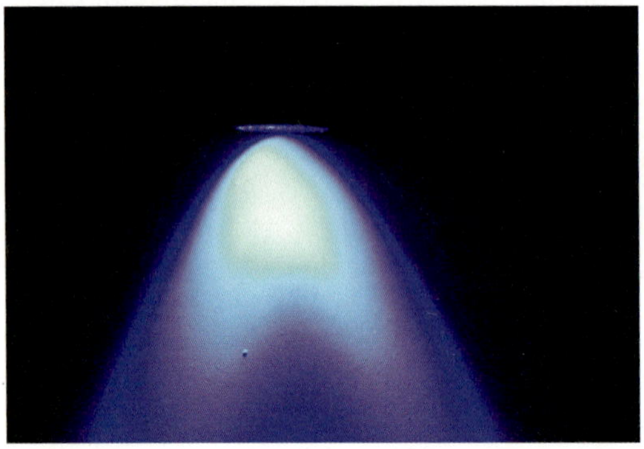

Fig. 4.13 Example of the light beam dispersion from a dental curing light. Note the inhomogeneity in the light beam (brightness)

diance delivered by their curing light to the resin surface (Fig. 4.14).

The light output from the curing light does not just affect the polymerization of the restorative resin, it also affects the bond strength to the tooth. Xu and co-workers investigated the adhesion of composite resin as the distance from the light guide increased [95]. Their investigation was prompted by a number of studies that reported increased microleakage at the gingival margin of restorations when compared to the occlusal enamel margins that were closest to the light. They demonstrated that there was an exponential relationship between the radiant exposure received by the resin and the bond strength to the tooth. They also showed that it was easy to halve the bond strength, just by delivering less energy. They concluded that when curing adhesives in deep proximal boxes with a curing light of 600 mW/cm^2, the exposure time should be increased to 40–60 s to deliver sufficient energy and thus achieve optimal photopolymerization and bonding to the tooth.

4.3.6 Ergonomics and Clinical Access

Access to a restoration is usually not an issue in the laboratory or for the facial surfaces of the anterior teeth. However, curing lights differ in their ability to reach all regions of the mouth, notably the posterior teeth. Figure 4.15 illustrates the excellent ability of a pen style curing light (A) to access the second molar tooth, whereas a curing light with an angled light guide (B) could only access the second molar when the tip was positioned at an angle to the occlusal surface. Such an angle will affect the amount of energy delivered, cause shadows, and ultimately may negatively affect the success of the resin restoration [86, 97] (Fig. 4.16).

4.3.7 Infection Control

Although some fiber-optic light guides can be autoclaved, the curing light itself cannot. Thus, the entire curing light should be covered with a form fitting infection control barrier, and the seam should not impede the light output (Fig. 4.17).

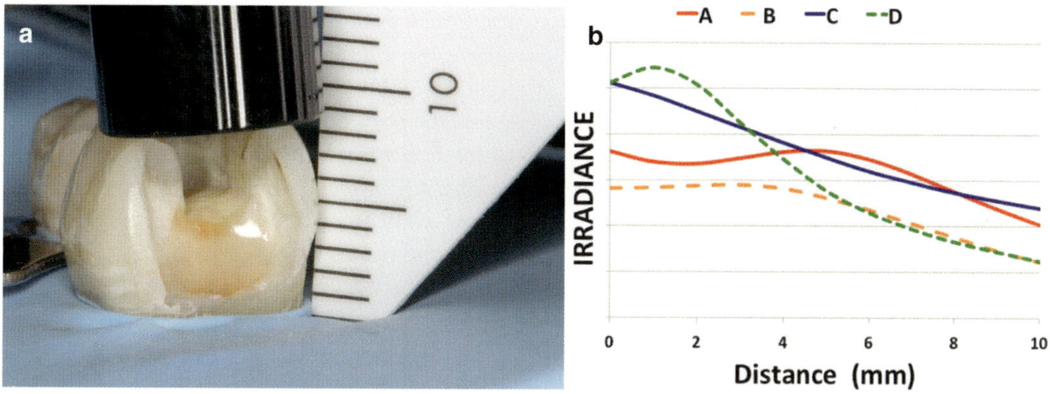

Fig. 4.14 Effect of distance from the light tip on the irradiance. The distance between the light tip and the resin can easily be 6 to 8-mm (**a**). Depending on their design, curing lights can deliver a similar irradiance at the light tip (**C** and **D**), but very different at 6 to 10-mm distances

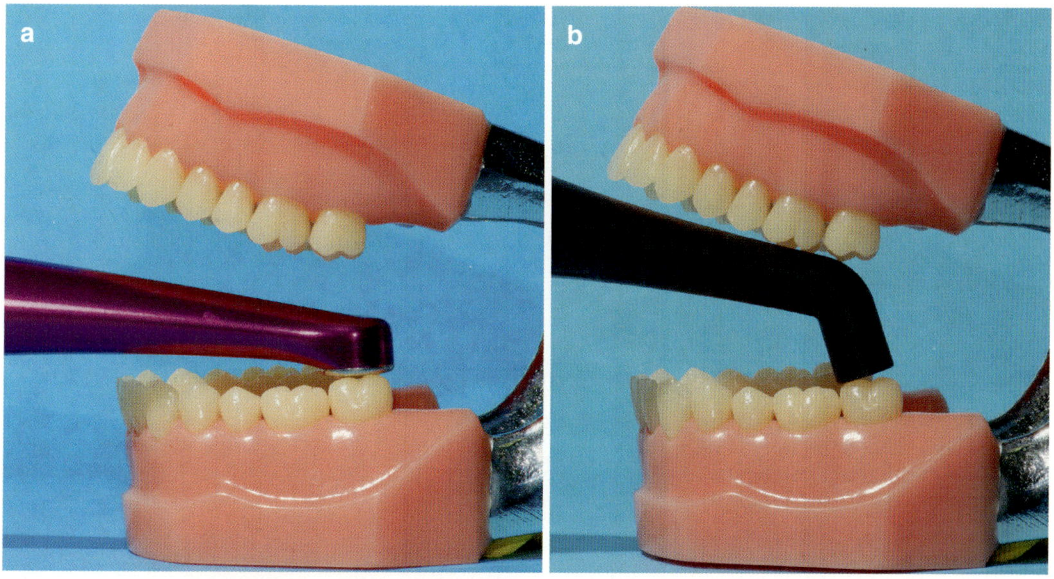

Fig. 4.15 Example of the ability of different dental curing lights to access the mandibular second molar tooth. Light **b** can only access the second molar at an angle whereas light (**a**) has direct access to the tooth

Some commercial barriers can reduce the radiant exitance by up to 40% [15, 98–100]. Latex-based barriers have been reported to cause the greatest reduction in irradiance. This can produce significantly lower resin conversion values [100] unless the exposure time is extended. Consequently, the output from curing lights should be tested with the barrier over the light tip. Clear, plastic food wrap is a highly effective and inexpensive infection control barrier that has minimal effect on light output, but it can appear messy [60, 98, 100].

When using cold sterilizing techniques, only cleaning solutions approved by the light manufacturer should be used because some disinfectant sprays can damage the plastic casing, remove the paint, or damage the rubber O-rings used to stabilize light guides. The disinfectant spray can then leak into the unit and be baked onto the light source or reflectors inside the curing light, thus

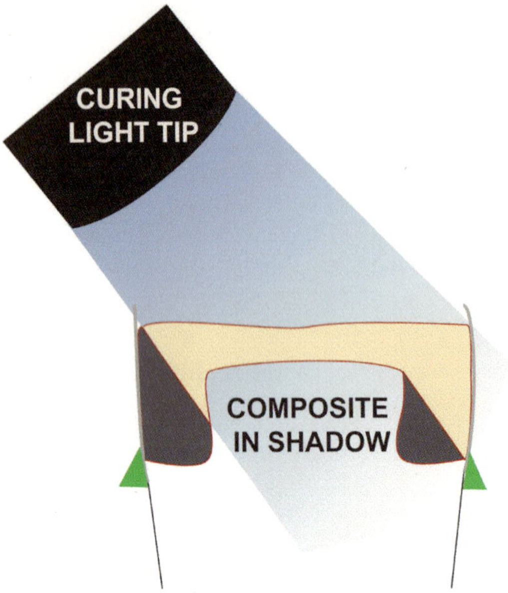

Fig. 4.16 An angled curing light can produce unwanted shadows, as shown by the dark grey shading

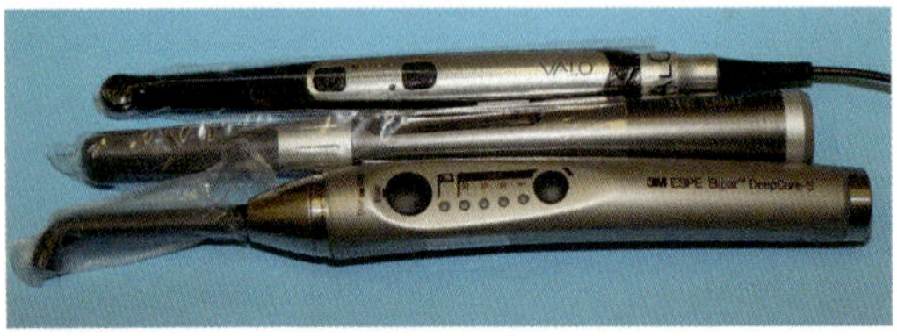

Fig. 4.17 Examples of plastic barriers on the curing light. Unlike the loose fitting barrier over just the tip in the bottom image, the plastic barrier should also cover the control buttons as shown on the other two lights

decreasing the light output [62]. If possible, the light guide should be removed from time to time, and the lens or filter inside the curing light checked to ensure that it and the entrance to the light guide are both clean and undamaged.

4.3.8 Effect of Training

Currently, most of the training provided to dentists, dental students, and dental assistants on how to best use the curing light is inadequate. While there are elaborate descriptions of techniques used for cavity preparation and the use of restorative materials, a critical phase of the procedure is often limited to five words "and then you light cure" [101]. It is common practice not to watch the position of the curing light tip over the restoration when light curing because the light is so bright. Consequently, the light tip sometimes moves away from the resin the operator is trying to photocure. This will negatively affect the amount of energy received and thus the extent of resin polymerization [73, 87, 88, 97, 102].

Operator variability in how much light they deliver can be significantly reduced, and the radiant exposure delivered to restorations can be significantly increased if the user has been trained how to light cure simulated restorations in a dental mannequin (MARC Patient Simulator, BlueLight Analytics, Halifax, Canada) (Fig. 4.18).

Using the simulator, the user is taught how to position the patient to improve light access and how to optimally position the light tip over the restoration throughout the light curing process.

The immediate feedback to the operator on how much irradiance and energy they delivered, together with instructor coaching on how to avoid mistakes, has been shown to be an effective method to teach how to successfully light cure a restoration [86–90].

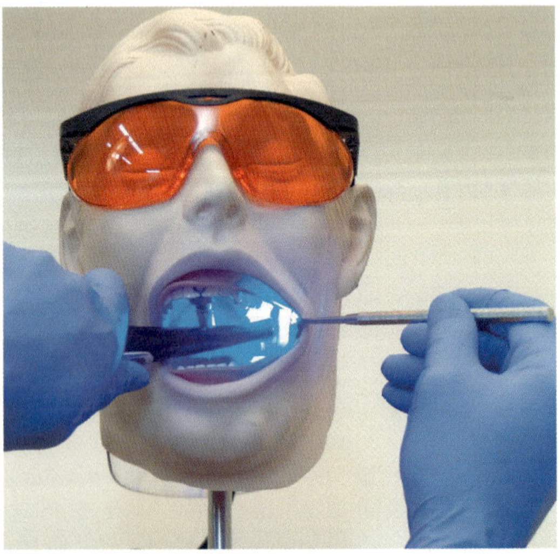

Fig. 4.18 Light curing a simulated restoration using the MARC Patient Simulator

4.3.9 Choosing a Curing Light

When light curing, the clinician should deliver sufficient radiant exposure at the correct wavelengths of light required by the photoinitiator(s) in the resin they are using. Thus, when making a decision about which curing light to purchase, the clinician should ask:

1. What is the radiant power output (watts) from the light?
2. What is the emission spectrum from the curing light? Does the spectral emission from the light match the sensitivity of the resin I use?
3. What is the active tip size, and how much of a typical restoration will receive useful light?
4. Is the light beam homogeneous?
5. What is the effect of distance from the light tip on the irradiance received by my restorations? Does the irradiance drop dramatically as the distance from the tip increases?
6. Does the unit have an ergonomic shape that is comfortable to use, and does it allow full access to all regions of the mouth?
7. Could the light produce an unacceptable temperature rise in the pulp or oral mucosa?
8. How do I disinfect the light?
9. What barriers are available and how do they affect the light output?
10. If it is battery operated, how frequently will it require replacing, and at what cost?
11. Is the curing light approved for use in my country?
12. Who do I contact if I have a problem with the light, or if the patient has a complaint?

4.3.10 Clinical Recommendations When Using a Curing Light

Having chosen a curing light, the following clinical recommendations should help improve how the curing light is used [22].

1. Monitor the performance of curing light, and keep a logbook of the output from the light from the date of purchase. To guide any adjustments in exposure duration, carry out depth of cure scrape tests using different shades of resin that have been light-cured at clinically representative distances and angles.
2. Learn how to use the curing light to maximize the amount of energy delivered to the resin.
3. Maximize the output from the curing light by routinely examining the light tip for damage and remove remnants of previously cured resin. Clean or replace the tip as necessary.
4. Protect the eyes of everyone in the operatory who could be exposed to the bright light from the curing light by using appropriate orange (blue light blocking) safety glasses or shields.
5. When light curing, remember that light travels in a straight line. Place the central axis of the tip of the curing light directly over and normal to the resin surface; the emitting end should be parallel to the resin surface being exposed. Where undercuts that cause shadows are present, move the light tip around and increase the exposure time. Use supplementary buccolingual curing (but beware of overheating).
6. Protect the oral mucosa from the light with gauze and air-cool, or wait several seconds between each light curing cycle when using a powerful curing light that may produce a damaging increase in temperature.

Acknowledgments The author wishes to acknowledge the valuable contributions of Professor F. Rueggeberg when preparing this text and his contributions to dental education.

References

1. Rueggeberg FA. State-of-the-art: dental photocuring – a review. Dent Mater. 2011;27:39–52.
2. Jandt KD, Mills RW. A brief history of LED photopolymerization. Dent Mater. 2013;29:605–17.
3. Price RB, Ferracane JL, Shortall AC. Light-curing units: a review of what we need to know. J Dent Res. 2015;94:1179–86.
4. Santini A, Turner S. General dental practitioners' knowledge of polymerisation of resin-based composite restorations and light curing unit technology. Br Dent J. 2011;211:E13.
5. McCusker N, Bailey C, Robinson S, Patel N, Sandy JR, Ireland AJ. Dental light curing and its effects on color perception. Am J Orthod Dentofac Orthop. 2012;142:355–63.

6. Kopperud SE, Rukke HV, Kopperud HM, Bruzell EM. Light curing procedures - performance, knowledge level and safety awareness among dentists. J Dent. 2017;58:67–73.
7. El-Mowafy O, El-Badrawy W, Lewis DW, Shokati B, Soliman O, Kermalli J, et al. Efficacy of halogen photopolymerization units in private dental offices in Toronto. J Can Dent Assoc. 2005;71:587.
8. Ernst CP, Busemann I, Kern T, Willershausen B. Feldtest zur Lichtemissionsleistung von Polymerisationsgeräten in zahnärztlichen Praxen. Dtsch Zahnarztl Z. 2006;61:466–71.
9. Barghi N, Fischer DE, Pham T. Revisiting the intensity output of curing lights in private dental offices. Compend Contin Educ Dent. 2007;28:380–4. quiz 5-6
10. Hegde V, Jadhav S, Aher GB. A clinical survey of the output intensity of 200 light curing units in dental offices across Maharashtra. J Conserv Dent. 2009;12:105–8.
11. Al Shaafi M, Maawadh A, Al QM. Evaluation of light intensity output of QTH and LED curing devices in various governmental health institutions. Oper Dent. 2011;36:356–61.
12. Hao X, Luo M, Wu J, Zhu S. A survey of power density of light-curing units used in private dental offices in Changchun City, China. Lasers Med Sci. 2015;30:493–7.
13. Maghaireh GA, Alzraikat H, Taha NA. Assessing the irradiance delivered from light-curing units in private dental offices in Jordan. J Am Dent Assoc. 2013;144:922–7.
14. AlShaafi MM, Harlow JE, Price HL, Rueggeberg FA, Labrie D, AlQahtani MQ, et al. Emission characteristics and effect of battery drain in "budget" curing lights. Oper Dent. 2016;41:397–408.
15. Vandewalle KS, Roberts HW, Rueggeberg FA. Power distribution across the face of different light guides and its effect on composite surface microhardness. J Esthet Restor Dent. 2008;20:108–17. discussion 18
16. Price RB, Labrie D, Rueggeberg FA, Felix CM. Irradiance differences in the violet (405 nm) and blue (460 nm) spectral ranges among dental light-curing units. J Esthet Restor Dent. 2010;22:363–77.
17. Michaud PL, Price RB, Labrie D, Rueggeberg FA, Sullivan B. Localised irradiance distribution found in dental light curing units. J Dent. 2014;42:129–39.
18. Price RB, Labrie D, Rueggeberg FA, Sullivan B, Kostylev I, Fahey J. Correlation between the beam profile from a curing light and the microhardness of four resins. Dent Mater. 2014;30:1345–57.
19. Shimokawa CA, Turbino ML, Harlow JE, Price HL, Price RB. Light output from six battery operated dental curing lights. Mater Sci Eng C Mater Biol Appl. 2016;69:1036–42.
20. Yearn JA. Factors affecting cure of visible light activated composites. Int Dent J. 1985;35:218–25.
21. Price RB, Dérand T, Sedarous M, Andreou P, Loney RW. Effect of distance on the power density from two light guides. J Esthet Dent. 2000;12:320–7.
22. Price RB, Shortall AC, Palin WM. Contemporary issues in light curing. Oper Dent. 2014;39:4–14.
23. Shortall AC, Price RB, MacKenzie L, Burke FJ. Guidelines for the selection, use, and maintenance of LED light-curing units - part II. Br Dent J. 2016;221:551–4.
24. Shortall AC, Price RB, MacKenzie L, Burke FJ. Guidelines for the selection, use, and maintenance of LED light-curing units - Part 1. Br Dent J. 2016;221:453–60.
25. Rueggeberg F. Contemporary issues in photocuring. Compend Contin Educ Dent Suppl. 1999:S4–15.
26. Yaman BC, Efes BG, Dorter C, Gomec Y, Erdilek D, Buyukgokcesu S. The effects of halogen and light-emitting diode light curing on the depth of cure and surface microhardness of composite resins. J Conserv Dent. 2011;14:136–9.
27. Fujibayashi K, Shimaru K, Takahashi N, Kohno A. Newly developed curing unit using blue light-emitting diodes. Dent Jpn. 1998;34:49–53.
28. Mills RW, Jandt KD, Ashworth SH. Dental composite depth of cure with halogen and blue light emitting diode technology. Br Dent J. 1999;186:388–91.
29. Moszner N, Fischer UK, Ganster B, Liska R, Rheinberger V. Benzoyl germanium derivatives as novel visible light photoinitiators for dental materials. Dent Mater. 2008;24:901–7.
30. Burtscher P. Ivocerin in comparison to camphorquinone. Ivoclar Vivadent Report, No. 19. July 2013.
31. Curtis JW Jr, Rueggeberg FA, Lee AJ. Curing efficiency of the turbo tip. Gen Dent. 1995;43:428–33.
32. Rueggeberg FA, Caughman WF, Curtis JW Jr. Effect of light intensity and exposure duration on cure of resin composite. Oper Dent. 1994;19:26–32.
33. Fan PL, Schumacher RM, Azzolin K, Geary R, Eichmiller FC. Curing-light intensity and depth of cure of resin-based composites tested according to international standards. J Am Dent Assoc. 2002;133:429–34.
34. Calheiros FC, Daronch M, Rueggeberg FA, Braga RR. Degree of conversion and mechanical properties of a BisGMA:TEGDMA composite as a function of the applied radiant exposure. J Biomed Mater Res B Appl Biomater. 2008;84:503–9.
35. Christensen GJ. Ask Dr. Christensen. Dental Economics. 2009;99. http://www.dentaleconomics.com/articles/print/volume-99/issue-9/departments/ask-dr-christensen/ask-dr-christensen.html.
36. Musanje L, Darvell BW. Polymerization of resin composite restorative materials: exposure reciprocity. Dent Mater. 2003;19:531–41.
37. Leprince JG, Hadis M, Shortall AC, Ferracane JL, Devaux J, Leloup G, et al. Photoinitiator type and applicability of exposure reciprocity law in filled and unfilled photoactive resins. Dent Mater. 2011;27:157–64.
38. Hadis M, Leprince JG, Shortall AC, Devaux J, Leloup G, Palin WM. High irradiance curing and anomalies of exposure reciprocity law in resin-based materials. J Dent. 2011;39:549–57.

39. Wydra JW, Cramer NB, Stansbury JW, Bowman CN. The reciprocity law concerning light dose relationships applied to BisGMA/TEGDMA photopolymers: theoretical analysis and experimental characterization. Dent Mater. 2014;30:605–12.
40. Selig D, Haenel T, Hausnerova B, Moeginger B, Labrie D, Sullivan B, et al. Examining exposure reciprocity in a resin based composite using high irradiance levels and real-time degree of conversion values. Dent Mater. 2015;31:583–93.
41. Kloosterboer JG, Lijten GFCM. Photopolymers exhibiting a large difference between glass transition and curing temperatures. Polymer. 1990;31: 95–101.
42. Cook WD, Standish PM. Cure of resin based restorative materials. II. White light photopolymerized resins. Aust Dent J. 1983;28:307–11.
43. Burdick JA, Lovestead TM, Anseth KS. Kinetic chain lengths in highly cross-linked networks formed by the photoinitiated polymerization of divinyl monomers: a gel permeation chromatography investigation. Biomacromolecules. 2003;4:149–56.
44. Feng L, Carvalho R, Suh BI. Insufficient cure under the condition of high irradiance and short irradiation time. Dent Mater. 2009;25:283–9.
45. Rueggeberg FA, Cole MA, Looney SW, Vickers A, Swift EJ. Comparison of manufacturer-recommended exposure durations with those determined using biaxial flexure strength and scraped composite thickness among a variety of light-curing units. J Esthet Restor Dent. 2009;21:43–61.
46. Taubock TT, Feilzer AJ, Buchalla W, Kleverlaan CJ, Krejci I, Attin T. Effect of modulated photoactivation on polymerization shrinkage behavior of dental restorative resin composites. Eur J Oral Sci. 2014;122:293–302.
47. Kanca J 3rd, Suh BI. Pulse activation: reducing resin-based composite contraction stresses at the enamel cavosurface margins. Am J Dent. 1999;12:107–12.
48. Randolph LD, Palin WM, Watts DC, Genet M, Devaux J, Leloup G, et al. The effect of ultra-fast photopolymerisation of experimental composites on shrinkage stress, network formation and pulpal temperature rise. Dent Mater. 2014;30:1280–9.
49. Suh BI, Feng L, Wang Y, Cripe C, Cincione F, de Rjik W. The effect of the pulse-delay cure technique on residual strain in composites. Compendium. 1999;20:4–12.
50. Feng L, Suh BI. A mechanism on why slower polymerization of a dental composite produces lower contraction stress. J Biomed Mater Res B Appl Biomater. 2006;78:63–9.
51. Bouschlicher MR, Rueggeberg FA. Effect of ramped light intensity on polymerization force and conversion in a photoactivated composite. J Esthet Dent. 2000;12:328–39.
52. Chye CH, Yap AU, Laim YC, Soh MS. Post-gel polymerization shrinkage associated with different light curing regimens. Oper Dent. 2005;30:474–80.
53. Lopes LG, Franco EB, Pereira JC, Mondelli RF. Effect of light-curing units and activation mode on polymerization shrinkage and shrinkage stress of composite resins. J Appl Oral Sci. 2008;16:35–42.
54. Ilie N, Jelen E, Hickel R. Is the soft-start polymerisation concept still relevant for modern curing units? Clin Oral Investig. 2011;15:21–9.
55. Soh MS, Yap AU. Influence of curing modes on crosslink density in polymer structures. J Dent. 2004;32:321–6.
56. Aguiar FH, Oliveira TR, Lima DA, Paulillo LA, Lovadino JR. Effect of light curing modes and ethanol immersion media on the susceptibility of a microhybrid composite resin to staining. J Appl Oral Sci. 2007;15:105–9.
57. van Dijken JW, Pallesen U. A 7-year randomized prospective study of a one-step self-etching adhesive in non-carious cervical lesions. The effect of curing modes and restorative material. J Dent. 2012;40:1060–7.
58. Rueggeberg FA, Caughman WF, Comer RW. The effect of autoclaving on energy transmission through light-curing tips. J Am Dent Assoc. 1996;127:1183–7.
59. Poulos JG, Styner DL. Curing lights: changes in intensity output with use over time. Gen Dent. 1997;45:70–3.
60. McAndrew R, Lynch CD, Pavli M, Bannon A, Milward P. The effect of disposable infection control barriers and physical damage on the power output of light curing units and light curing tips. Br Dent J. 2011;210:E12.
61. Strydom C. Dental curing lights – maintenance of visible light curing units. SADJ. 2002;57:227–33.
62. Strassler HE, Price RB. Understanding light curing, Part II. Delivering predictable and successful restorations. Dent Today. 2014:1–8; quiz 9.
63. Leonard DL, Charlton DG, Hilton TJ. Effect of curing-tip diameter on the accuracy of dental radiometers. Oper Dent. 1999;24:31–7.
64. Roberts HW, Vandewalle KS, Berzins DW, Charlton DG. Accuracy of LED and halogen radiometers using different light sources. J Esthet Restor Dent. 2006;18:214–22. discussion 23-4
65. Price RB, Labrie D, Kazmi S, Fahey J, Felix CM. Intra-and inter-brand accuracy of four dental radiometers. Clin Oral Investig. 2012;16:707–17.
66. Marovic D, Matic S, Kelic K, Klaric E, Rakic M, Tarle Z. Time dependent accuracy of dental radiometers. Acta Clin Croat. 2013;52:173–80.
67. Kameyama A, Haruyama A, Asami M, Takahashi T. Effect of emitted wavelength and light guide type on irradiance discrepancies in hand-held dental curing radiometers. Sci World J. 2013;2013:647941.
68. Shimokawa CA, Harlow JE, Turbino ML, Price RB. Ability of four dental radiometers to measure the light output from nine curing lights. J Dent. 2016;54:48–55.
69. Baroudi K, Silikas N, Watts DC. In vitro pulp chamber temperature rise from irradiation and exotherm of flowable composites. Int J Paediatr Dent. 2009;19:48–54.
70. Atai M, Motevasselian F. Temperature rise and degree of photopolymerization conversion of

nanocomposites and conventional dental composites. Clin Oral Investig. 2009;13:309–16.
71. Leprince J, Devaux J, Mullier T, Vreven J, Leloup G. Pulpal-temperature rise and polymerization efficiency of LED curing lights. Oper Dent. 2010;35:220–30.
72. Matalon S, Slutzky H, Wassersprung N, Goldberg-Slutzky I, Ben-Amar A. Temperature rises beneath resin composite restorations during curing. Am J Dent. 2010;23:223–6.
73. Shortall A, El-Mahy W, Stewardson D, Addison O, Palin W. Initial fracture resistance and curing temperature rise of ten contemporary resin-based composites with increasing radiant exposure. J Dent. 2013;41:455–63.
74. Gomes M, DeVito-Moraes A, Francci C, Moraes R, Pereira T, Froes-Salgado N, et al. Temperature increase at the light guide tip of 15 contemporary LED units and thermal variation at the pulpal floor of cavities: an infrared thermographic analysis. Oper Dent. 2013;38:324–33.
75. Mouhat M, Mercer J, Stangvaltaite L, Örtengren U. Light-curing units used in dentistry: factors associated with heat development—potential risk for patients. Clin Oral Investig. 2017;21:1687–96.
76. Onisor I, Asmussen E, Krejci I. Temperature rise during photo-polymerization for onlay luting. Am J Dent. 2011;24:250–6.
77. Stamatacos C, Harrison JL. The possible ocular hazards of LED dental illumination applications. J Tenn Dent Assoc. 2013;93:25–9. quiz 30-1
78. Bruzell Roll EM, Jacobsen N, Hensten-Pettersen A. Health hazards associated with curing light in the dental clinic. Clin Oral Investig. 2004;8:113–7.
79. Labrie D, Moe J, Price RB, Young ME, Felix CM. Evaluation of ocular hazards from 4 types of curing lights. J Can Dent Assoc. 2011;77:b116.
80. McCusker N, Lee SM, Robinson S, Patel N, Sandy JR, Ireland AJ. Light curing in orthodontics; should we be concerned? Dent Mater. 2013;29:e85–90.
81. Price RB, Labrie D, Bruzell EM, Sliney DH, Strassler HE. The dental curing light: a potential health risk. J Occup Environ Hyg. 2016;13:639–46.
82. Hill EE. Eye safety practices in U.S. dental school restorative clinics, 2006. J Dent Educ. 2006;70:1294–7.
83. American Conference of Governmental Industrial Hygienists (ACGIH): TLVs and BEIs Based on the Documentation for Threshold Limit Values for Chemical Substances and Physical Agents and Biological Exposure Indices. 2015; Cincinnati, OH.
84. International Commission on Non-Ionizing Radiation Protection. Guidelines on limits of exposure to broad-band incoherent optical radiation (0.38 to 3 μm). Health Phys. 1997;73:539–54.
85. Ham WT Jr, Ruffolo JJ Jr, Mueller HA, Clarke AM, Moon ME. Histologic analysis of photochemical lesions produced in rhesus retina by short-wavelength light. Investig Ophthalmol Vis Sci. 1978;17:1029–35.
86. Price RB, McLeod ME, Felix CM. Quantifying light energy delivered to a class I restoration. J Can Dent Assoc. 2010;76:a23.
87. Seth S, Lee CJ, Ayer CD. Effect of instruction on dental students' ability to light-cure a simulated restoration. J Can Dent Assoc. 2012;78:c123.
88. Federlin M, Price R. Improving light-curing instruction in dental school. J Dent Educ. 2013;77:764–72.
89. Mutluay MM, Rueggeberg FA, Price RB. Effect of using proper light-curing techniques on energy delivered to a class 1 restoration. Quintessence Int. 2014;45:549–56.
90. Price RB, Strassler HE, Price HL, Seth S, Lee CJ. The effectiveness of using a patient simulator to teach light-curing skills. J Am Dent Assoc. 2014;145:32–43.
91. Nitta K. Effect of light guide tip diameter of LED-light curing unit on polymerization of light-cured composites. Dent Mater. 2005;21:217–23.
92. Ash MM, Nelson SJ, Ash MM. Dental anatomy, physiology, and occlusion. 8th ed. Philadelphia: W.B. Saunders; 2003.
93. Corciolani G, Vichi A, Davidson CL, Ferrari M. The influence of tip geometry and distance on light-curing efficacy. Oper Dent. 2008;33:325–31.
94. Vandewalle KS, Roberts HW, Andrus JL, Dunn WJ. Effect of light dispersion of LED curing lights on resin composite polymerization. J Esthet Restor Dent. 2005;17:244–54. discussion 54-5
95. Xu X, Sandras DA, Burgess JO. Shear bond strength with increasing light-guide distance from dentin. J Esthet Restor Dent. 2006;18:19–27. discussion 8
96. Price RB, Labrie D, Whalen JM, Felix CM. Effect of distance on irradiance and beam homogeneity from 4 light-emitting diode curing units. J Can Dent Assoc. 2011;77:b9.
97. Konerding KL, Heyder M, Kranz S, Guellmar A, Voelpel A, Watts DC, et al. Study of energy transfer by different light curing units into a class III restoration as a function of tilt angle and distance, using a MARC patient simulator (PS). Dent Mater. 2016;32:676–86.
98. Scott BA, Felix CA, Price RB. Effect of disposable infection control barriers on light output from dental curing lights. J Can Dent Assoc. 2004;70:105–10.
99. Coutinho M, Trevizam NC, Takayassu RN, Leme AA, Soares GP. Distance and protective barrier effects on the composite resin degree of conversion. Contemp Clin Dent. 2013;4:152–5.
100. Sword RJ, Do UN, Chang JH, Rueggeberg FA. Effect of curing light barriers and light types on radiant exposure and composite conversion. J Esthet Restor Dent. 2016;28:29–42.
101. Strassler HE. Successful light curing- not as easy as it looks. Oral Health. 2013;103:18–26.
102. Price RB, Felix CM, Whalen JM. Factors affecting the energy delivered to simulated class I and class V preparations. J Can Dent Assoc. 2010;76:a94.

Degree of Conversion

5

Zrinka Tarle and Matej Par

5.1 Introduction

Composite resins as the most commonly used dental material for a variety of applications have greatly evolved since they were introduced with an aim to fulfill different mechanical, biological, and esthetic requirements [1]. Progress in composite material formulation, such as improved filler morphology and improved existing polymeric matrix, and novel monomer technologies may improve the disadvantages of resin composite materials [2, 3]. Therefore, investigations as well as knowledge and understanding of their properties are the foundations for establishing the clinical use guidelines.

The degree of conversion (DC) can be defined as the extent to which monomers react to form polymers or as the ratio of C=C double bonds that are converted into C–C single bonds [4]. A high degree of composite polymerization is an essential material feature for obtaining optimal physical and mechanical properties and biocompatibility [5–9] and has a crucial impact on the utmost success of a composite restoration. It strongly affects each property of a composite material such as hardness, strength, elastic modulus, water sorption, solubility, color stability, dimensional stability with consequential microleakage, secondary caries, and possible pulpal reactions [3, 6]. Various factors like filler particle size and loading, monomer type and amount, polymerization initiator type and concentration [10, 11], the shade and translucency of the material [7], intensity and wavelength of the light source, and irradiation time [12] can influence the DC of dental composite materials.

It would be ideal to have all of the composite resin monomers converted to polymer during the polymerization reaction. However, the conversion is never complete and reaches a degree of about 50% to 75% for conventional composites [13]; for bulk-fill composite materials, values range from 50% to 81% [14, 15] and for preheated conventional and bulk-fill composites from 67% to 84% [16]; 24 h post-cure values vary from 68% to 86% [17], while for the experimental remineralizing composites based on amorphous calcium phosphate, DC values can reach even up to 87% [18].

In this chapter, factors determining DC, composite properties dependent upon DC, and methods for the evaluation of DC will be described.

Z. Tarle (✉)
Department of Endodontics and Restorative Dentistry, School of Dental Medicine, University of Zagreb, Gunduliceva 5, 10000 Zagreb, Croatia
e-mail: tarle@sfzg.hr

M. Par
Private Dental Practice, Dankovecka 9, Zagreb, Croatia

V. Miletic (ed.), *Dental Composite Materials for Direct Restorations*, http://doi.org/10.1007/978-3-319-60961-4_5

5.2 Factors Determining the Degree of Conversion

The characteristics of dental composite resins result from their perplexed composition which means resin and filler type and amount. Factors determining DC can be classified as intrinsic and extrinsic.

5.2.1 Intrinsic Factors

Intrinsic factors imply composite properties and include resin composition, filler composition, and photoinitiator system [2].

Composite resins consist of the mixtures of various methacrylate monomers which are converted into a cross-linked polymer matrix during the polymerization reaction. Optimal combination of monomers is of exceptional importance in achieving a composite resin with outstanding properties. The DC is primarily determined by the structure and relative ratio of the individual monomers [19, 20]. The most common base monomers in contemporary commercial composites are bisphenol A-glycidyl methacrylate (Bis-GMA, molecular weight: 512 g/mol) and urethane dimethacrylate (UDMA, molecular weight: 471 g/mol). The Bis-GMA monomer is characterized by high molecular weight, rigid structure, and high viscosity. Its main benefits are lower polymerization shrinkage, fast setting, and strong and stiff polymeric networks [19]. However, its high viscosity impairs mobility during polymerization and prevents the polymer from attaining high DC values. For this reason, the Bis-GMA-based resins are admixed with monomers of lower viscosity, e. g., triethyleneglycol dimethacrylate (TEGDMA), urethane dimethacrylate (UDMA), or bisphenol A polyethylene glycol diether dimethacrylate (Bis-EMA) in order to improve the final DC [3]. Comonomers based on Bis-EMA, a monomer of high molecular weight and lower viscosity, usually show higher DC than the Bis-GMA/TEGDMA mixtures [21, 22]. Other monomers with higher molecular weight aimed to reduce shrinkage such as urethane dimethacrylate resin DX511 from Dupont (molecular weight: 895 g/mol) have been developed. On the other hand, dimer acid-based monomers have also relatively high molecular weight, i.e., 673–849 g/mol, and have been shown to have high DC while undergoing lower polymerization shrinkage than Bis-GMA systems [23, 24]. Tricyclodecane (TCD) urethane low viscosity monomers have lower shrinkage and polymerization stress but also high DC compared to others containing conventional dimethacrylates [1, 25].

The DC gradually decreases with increasing thickness of a composite resin layer. Curing light is attenuated by the absorption and scattering as the layer thickness increases and fewer radicals are formed to initiate polymerization [26]. The bulk-fill composite materials have been developed to fulfill challenging request of higher efficiency and enable adequate polymerization up to 4 or 5 mm depth. Optical properties between conventional and bulk-fill composites differ vastly. Bulk-fill composites are generally more translucent in order to ensure sufficient curing of thick increments [27]. Usually, the intensity of the curing light that reaches the bottom of a composite layer is considerably lower than that on the surface. To compensate the polymerization decrease in deeper layers, it is possible to improve the absorption spectrum and the initiator's reactivity, to increase the translucency of the materials and to optimize the LED light source [28, 29]. This approach combines intrinsic factors dealing with photoinitiator system and translucency of composites with extrinsic ones which include polymerization conditions.

In any case, concerning intrinsic factors, photoinitiator which is almost always used is a combination of camphorquinone (CQ) and various types of tertiary amines [30]. However, other photopolymerization systems such as phenylpropanedione (PPD), mono- or bis-acylphosphine oxides (MAPO and BAPO), benzoyl germanium, or benzil [31, 32] have also been introduced. There is a difference among photoinitiators regarding initiation of polymerization—while each converted CQ molecule generates only one free radical, others are able to generate several, e.g., two for MAPO and four for BAPO [33].

Dibenzoyl germanium derivatives are also more light reactive than CQ [34]. While taking into account advantages of some photoinitiators over the CQ system, one should also consider them in relation to comonomer composition and ratio, filler content and size, as well as some extrinsic factors such as light spectrum, irradiance, and irradiation time.

Unavoidable factor in composite resins are fillers responsible for reducing monomer content and consequently for many crucial properties of the material such as strength, resistance to occlusal loads, shrinkage, handling, translucency, opalescence, radiopacity, etc. To increase depth of cure, it is necessary to increase the translucency of composites by decreasing the filler content and increasing filler size in an effort to ensure that more photons penetrate into deeper layers [28]. The amount of scattered and absorbed light influences the light transmittance through a composite material. Large filler-matrix interface area causes a considerable light scattering because of differences in the refractive indices between filler particles and resin matrix [14], while similar refractive indices of the components of composites have been shown to improve translucency in experimental materials.

5.2.2 Extrinsic Factors

5.2.2.1 Light Sources and Curing Conditions

Preferred curing mode of composite resins is photopolymerization, and complete understanding of the photopolymerization process is essential for achieving optimal properties of the material. Light curing has greatly revolutionized dentistry and is required in almost any clinical procedure. Technology behind light sources in dentistry changed from UV curing (wavelength about 365 nm) to a visible light curing (wavelength about 470 nm) that was introduced in 1976.

Quartz-tungsten-halogen lights were the main light source for photopolymerization for decades. During that time, a wide range of adaptations and improvements were made such as bulb power increase, output values increased from average to extreme, the adaptation of curing gun, and introduction of different curing modes [28]. The spectral emission of conventional curing lights includes wavelengths that induce heating of the resin and tooth during curing. Despite their popularity, conventional halogen light-curing units have serious drawbacks, such as a limited effective lifetime (40–100 h), reflector and filter degradation over time due to high operating temperatures, and the significant amount of heat produced during curing. Many halogen units have been shown to not reach the minimum power output specified by the manufacturers [35]. The most frequently used photoinitiator in resin composites, CQ, is sensitive to light in the blue region of the visible spectrum, with an absorption peak at 470 nm. Therefore, every light source with adequate irradiance in this region can be used as a curing unit. To overcome the problems of halogen technology, alternative light sources have been suggested, such as argon laser [36], pulsed laser [37, 38], plasma light [39, 40], and blue superbright light-emitting diodes (LEDs) [8, 9].

Today, LEDs are the light source of choice due to much higher efficiency compared to previous technologies. Their emission in the blue part of the spectrum is attained by using indium gallium nitride and matches the maximal absorption of the most frequently used photoinitiator CQ [28]. The first generation of LEDs (commercial) was introduced in the beginning of the new millennium. Their typical design was a combination of multiple, individual LED from 7 to 64 LEDs [28]. These units have a narrow spectral distribution range and are much more energy efficient (30% compared to 4% of halogen lights is used into light) and can be battery-powered. This LED generation demonstrated an irradiance of 150–350 mW/cm^2 [41]. Photoactivated composites can be successfully cured with lower irradiance while maintaining high final DC and minimizing shrinkage stress [8]. Second generation of LEDs implies 1 W chips into curing lights generating 140 mW/cm^2 output and 5 W chip generating 600 mW/cm^2 output which means great increase in output in the similar wavelength range [28].

Third generations of LEDs were developed in order to enable polymerization of restorative materials using different photoinitiators. They feature high irradiance at multiple wavelengths as well as appropriate shape and dimension of the light guide to closely approach every area in the mouth.

There are many curing factors influencing DC such as the "total energy" concept, meaning that the radiant energy is the product of irradiance and exposure time (which means the higher the irradiance, the shorter the exposure time), temperature buildup during light-curing procedures, maintenance of curing units, as well as measurements of the power density [41].

The photopolymerization method has a profound influence on DC and shrinkage stress [42]. High-intensity lights provide higher DC values, but they also produce higher contraction stress. A slower curing process that allows composite flow may act for stress relaxation during polymerization [43]. The aim of optimal photopolymerization is to enable, for as long as possible, the pre-gel phase and to decrease the rate of polymeric chain growth, allowing more plastic deformation to occur and preventing the buildup of interfacial stresses [13]. For this purpose, modified photo curing protocols with variable intensities throughout the cure cycle were devised [44, 45].

5.2.2.2 Pre-heating of Composites

Increased curing temperature favors radical and monomer mobility which in turn results with a higher DC [16, 46]. This affects both physical and mechanical polymer properties as well as the biocompatibility of pre-heated composites. Raising the cure temperature reduces viscosity and enhances molecular mobility and collision frequency of reactive species. On the other hand, it postpones diffusion-controlled propagation, which then increases the final limiting conversion [46]. Pre-heating composites before photo curing decreases their viscosity, enhances marginal adaptation, and reduces microleakage [16]. However, increased degree conversion of pre-heated composite resins leads to higher shrinkage and possibly greater polymerization shrinkage stress [47].

The effect of temperature on the DC depends on the photoinitiator system. In the study of Tauböck et al. [16], the only bulk-fill composite material showing higher DC upon pre-heating contains an additional germanium-based photoinitiator besides CQ/amine system [34]. Unlike the aforementioned report [47], this study showed that composite resin pre-heating can reduce polymerization shrinkage forces of bulk-fill and conventional composite resins, whereas the DC remains the same or increases [16].

5.2.2.3 Post-cure Reaction

Post-cure polymerization is a direct result of the nature of multifunctional methacrylate polymerization reaction. A considerable increase in viscosity and a decrease of reactive species mobility are caused by the initial rapid reaction [18, 48]. Free radicals and unreacted monomers remain trapped within the matrix shortly after the start of illumination. The reaction has the potential to continue at a slow rate [49] and can be continued for as long as there are free radicals available and reactants which are sufficiently mobile [50].

Post-cure reaction was found to be more extensive in materials with an initially lower DC. In cases of highly polymerized materials, reactive sites are immobilized in the polymer network, while in samples with an initially lower DC, a higher amount of unreacted radicals allows increased mobility to make contact with other reactive species. According to Burtscher [49], even a small increase in the extent of DC toward the end of polymerization process can greatly influence the density of cross-linking and optimize the properties of composite resins. From the clinical standpoint, the post-cure DC increase (Fig. 5.1) implies that final mechanical properties and biocompatibility of a composite are not attained immediately after curing but rather developed gradually over the post-cure period. In the study of Par et al. [17], the highest post-cure increase was achieved in materials with patented modified UDMA as well as proprietary monomers analogous to Bis-GMA and Procrylat resin. It is possible that these modified monomers acted to alter polymerization kinetics and retard the conversion of monomers [51].

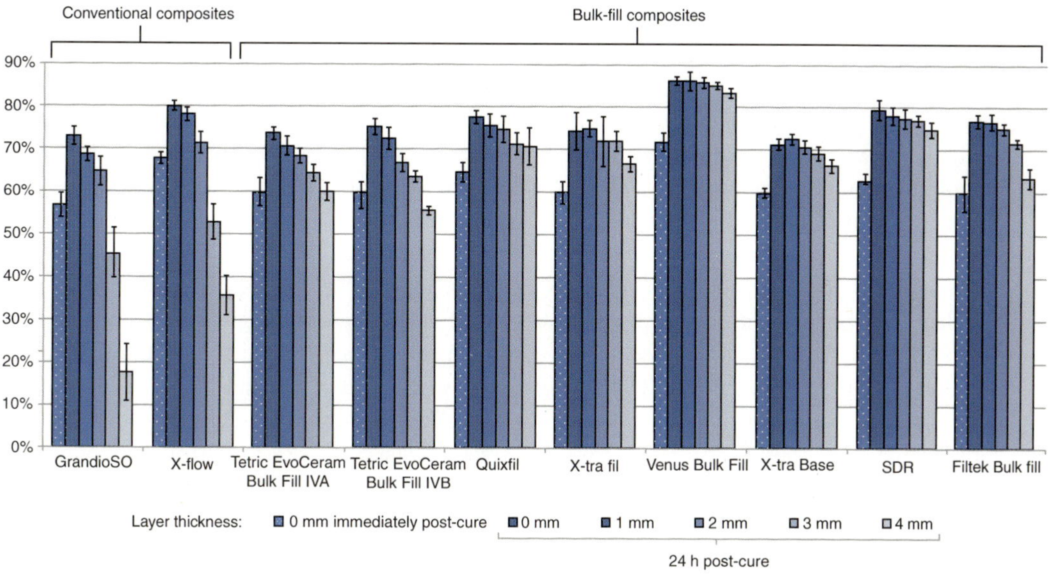

Fig. 5.1 Degree of conversion of some commercial composites measured immediately after light curing and 24 h post-cure. Error bars denote ±1 standard deviation. Reprinted with permission from [17]

5.3 Composite Properties Dependent on the Degree of Conversion

The DC is a fundamental attribute of a cured composite since it affects virtually all other material properties [2]. Most of these properties are important for the clinical success of the restoration, either in short or long term [52]. Although the composition of contemporary composites is fine-tuned to attain optimal DC and the related properties if properly handled and light-cured [15, 53, 54], poor DC due to unfavorable curing conditions or operators' insufficient understanding of the curing procedure may affect critical material properties and increase the risk of clinical failure [55]. The influence of the DC on various composite properties is described below.

5.3.1 Mechanical Properties

Higher DC implies that more double bonds were consumed for the formation of an infinite polymeric network and that lower amount of unreacted monomer is left to plasticize the network structure [56]. Both of these factors improve mechanical properties, such as strength, elastic modulus, hardness, and glass transition temperature [56–60]. However, the well-known correlation between the DC and mechanical properties is valid only for a given composite formulation since mechanical properties do not depend solely on the DC but also on multiple other factors, most prominently filler load and resin composition [19, 61, 62]. While the filler load and particle geometry are primary determinants of mechanical properties, monomer composition determines the mobility of reactive medium during polymerization, consequently influencing the final DC and polymer structure. In this regard, varying the monomer composition could increase the final DC by virtue of increasing the resin mobility, but this does not necessarily improve material properties [14, 63]. For example, increasing the ratio of the diluent monomer TEGDMA in a Bis-GMA/TEGDMA copolymer improves the DC but renders the composite very brittle [19, 64]. Conversely, increasing the ratio of Bis-GMA may not reduce strength or hardness despite the decline in final DC [56, 57]. This exemplifies that the molecular architecture of monomers is an important determinant of mechanical properties—excessively increasing DC at the cost of the ratio of high molecular weight monomers impairs final mechanical properties of the cured resin. Thus, tailoring a composite with optimal DC and mechanical properties implies attaining a delicate balance between the stiffer "base" monomers and the DC-improving diluent monomers [19].

The kinetics of polymerization reaction, which is for a given composite determined by light-curing conditions, governs the final polymeric structure and the relative amount of cycles, linear chains, and cross-links [65]. Additionally, the polymeric network is substantially heterogeneous, containing high-DC microgel regions, regions of lower DC and unreacted monomer pools [66]. The heterogeneity is DC dependent and increases at higher conversions [67]. These complex structural features are not described by the DC [68, 69] and can only be assessed indirectly through measurements of material softening, glass transition temperature, or dielectric properties [58, 70, 71]. Thus, although the mechanical properties on macro- and microscale might appear constant and correlate well with the DC, a considerable heterogeneity always exists on the fundamental scale. The DC is simply the average measure of consumed double bonds which provides information on neither structural heterogeneity nor cross-linking density [72, 73]. Even within a given material, the final polymeric structure is highly dependent on light-curing conditions [74, 75], and the same DC values may not necessarily suggest identical polymer architecture and mechanical properties [45, 76]. Besides, small changes in the DC at late stages of polymerization can have a considerable effect on mechanical properties, as they mostly contribute to cross-linking [71], resulting in an exponential improvement in mechanical properties [77]. All of these facts indicate that although the DC correlates well with mechanical properties on the clinically relevant scale, it does not provide a complete description of subtle differences in network structure on the molecular level.

5.3.2 Polymerization Shrinkage and Shrinkage Stress

The polymerization reaction of methacrylates is inseparably linked to volumetric shrinkage, due to the conversion of intermolecular distances among separate monomer molecules of 0.3–0.4 nm into the distance of covalent bonds of about 0.15 nm [19]. As described previously, the amount of shrinkage is linearly related to the DC [78]. While a high DC is desirable to ensure optimal composite properties, it is accompanied with high volumetric shrinkage, contributing to the interfacial stress [79]. Attaining high DC and preserving marginal integrity are therefore conflicted aims, and this issue persists throughout the history of dental composites [80].

Unlike volumetric shrinkage, shrinkage stress developed under constrained conditions shows a highly nonlinear dependence on the DC. Shrinkage stress is a function of volumetric shrinkage and elastic modulus, both of which rise simultaneously during polymerization and are directly dependent on the DC [81]. Whereas low levels of the DC either allow viscous flow (prior to gelation) or high compliance due to low elastic modulus (prior to vitrification), at later stages of polymerization, the stress buildup increases rapidly [82]. After the vitrification point, the material is characterized by high elastic modulus, and small increases DC can have a huge impact on the shrinkage stress [83].

A popular approach for mitigating shrinkage stress in a clinical setting is by using modulated curing protocols, so-called soft start or pulse delay curing [44, 45]. The former combines a period of low irradiance followed by a high irradiance, whereas the latter introduces a time delay between two expositions. Both approaches are intended to allow more viscous flow to diminish the shrinkage stress buildup as well as to change the relative amount of linear chains and cross-links [44, 75]. Some authors argued that the observed benefits in terms of reduced shrinkage stress are not due to delayed gelation or vitrification but due to inferior DC or network microstructural differences resulting from the modulated curing protocols [60, 84]. It is important to note that some of the modulated protocols may impair material properties without being reflected on the DC [45]. The previously discussed subtle structural differences arising from different curing conditions may be the reason for the conflicting literature reports on the stress-decreasing efficiency of modulated curing protocols [2, 60, 83, 85, 86]. The material dependence of the effect of different curing protocols is another possible explanation for the inconsistent literature evidence about their benefits [87].

5.3.3 Biocompatibility

Various components are released in an aqueous environment from a cured composite material: monomers, components of the photoinitiator system, and various degradation products [88, 89]. As the most abundant mobile species present within the cured composite, residual monomer has traditionally been attributed the majority of the toxic effect, but other compounds may elute in comparable or even higher amounts [89] and exert a toxic effect [90]. The final DC of contemporary dental composites ranges from about 50% to 80%, suggesting that 20–50% of double bonds remained unreacted [21]. However, not all of these bonds can be eluted, since most of them are embedded in the polymeric network as pendant double bonds [91]. It is estimated that only 5–10% of the total amount of unreacted double bonds is capable of being eluted from the cured composite, amounting to approximately 2 wt% of the resin component [88]. The inverse relationship between the DC and the amount of eluted monomers is well documented in the literature [91–93]. Higher DC not only leaves less free monomer available for leaching out of the cured composite but also implies a denser network which reduces water diffusivity [94], thus hindering the release of monomer and other leachable species. The inverse relationship between the DC and biocompatibility is particularly relevant for the class of "bulk-fill" composites, whose application in thick layers may lead to the higher release of potentially toxic compounds [92]. An additional concern regarding bulk-fill composites is due to manufacturer's recommendations of very short curing times which may be insufficient to attain optimal DC throughout thick layers [15, 95]. It should be noted that despite an established correlation, the DC is not a single determinant of the amount of available leachable species, since different architectures of polymer network as a function of curing conditions may lead to different amounts of leachable molecules within a single material at similar DC values [75, 91].

In addition to the release of potentially toxic components, biocompatibility issues related to low DC arise from the propensity of unreacted monomers to promote bacterial colonization [96]. Furthermore, some products of composite degradation can influence biofilm formation and survival of *S. mutans* on restoration surfaces [97]. This is particularly relevant to the development of secondary caries at the proximal cavity floor [98], which has the highest risk of remaining undercured in a clinical situation, especially when the "bulk-fill" technique is used. The risk of secondary caries at this site is additionally heightened by faster degradation of poorly cured composite [99].

5.3.4 Water Sorption, Solubility, Degradation, and Color Stability

The amount of water absorbed by a composite is mainly determined by the filler ratio and hydrophilicity of the resin [94, 100]. Although the polymeric matrix is insoluble, it can be penetrated and expanded by water molecules which show affinity to certain functional groups or bonds contained within the network, e.g., hydroxyl groups and ester or ether bonds [101]. By affecting the network density, the DC determines the amount and diffusivity of absorbed water [94]. Additionally, DC also determines the amount of unreacted monomer, which can leach out of the polymerized material. Thus, both water sorption and solubility show a good correlation with the DC for a given composite [102].

All composite components undergo a degradation process when exposed to oral environment; polymeric network is cleaved by hydrolysis and enzymatic breakdown, siloxane bonds at the filler/matrix interface are hydrolyzed, and components of filler particles are solubilized and eroded [88, 103, 104]. Since all of these reactions occur in an aqueous medium, the DC-dependent mobility and amount of water within the polymeric network determine the extent and rate of degradation [94]. Additionally, DC affects the amount of unreacted monomer which by its elution forms porosities within the material, allowing more water sorption and facilitating degradation [101]. Color stability is jeopardized by material degradation and uptake of pigment particles from oral environment, both of which depend on porosity and water sorption [105, 106]. Exposition to water diminishes mechanical properties by plasticization and swelling of the matrix [107]. These effects are more pronounced in the case of low DC and lead to increased abrasive wear [108].

As is the case with other DC-dependent properties, the correlation of water sorption, solubility, and degradation with the DC does not hold for comparison across different composites due to the influence of multiple other factors. Additionally, the same material with similar DC values attained under various curing conditions can show different water sorption and susceptibility to degradation [45], once again highlighting the fact that DC by itself is insufficient for a complete characterization of the network structure, as it is considerably influenced by structural complexities that cannot be described with a simple proportion of converted double bonds [65, 76, 109].

5.4 Methods for the DC Evaluation

5.4.1 Vibrational Spectroscopies: Infrared and Raman

5.4.1.1 Theoretical Background

Every molecule is characterized by a specific set of energetic states that are determined by its atomic arrangement. The collection of energetic transitions between these states gives rise to the pattern that is unique for a certain chemical compound. Probing the sample by means of vibrational spectroscopies gives a spectrum in which the transitions between vibrational states are represented by spectral bands. The position of the band within the spectrum is determined by transition energy between vibrational states and is commonly expressed in wavenumbers (cm^{-1}). By assigning the specific vibrational band to a certain functional group or bond within the molecule, vibrational spectroscopies can provide both qualitative and quantitative information [110]. The translation of spectroscopic data into absolute concentration values requires the usage of calibration curves, which relate the concentration of a particular species with the intensity of its respective vibrational band. Alternatively, the ratio of concentrations can be calculated without using calibration curves; instead the spectra can be normalized by using the internal standard, i.e., the vibrational band whose intensity remains constant [111]. In the case of dental composites, this means using a band which undergoes no change throughout the polymerization. Thus, the DC calculations do not require calibration curves, as only the relative amount of the double bonds consumed during polymerization is evaluated [112, 113]. Since the double C=C bonds are contained within different monomers, the underlying assumption is that their infrared absorptivity and Raman scattering intensity are independent on the molecular structure of the monomer. This assumption holds for infrared absorptivity, while the Raman scattering intensity of the C=C bonds may differ among different monomers [114]. However, this difference is neglected when evaluating the DC by means of Raman spectroscopy, since the spectra of polymerized and unpolymerized material used for the calculation have qualitatively the same monomer composition [114].

The physical phenomena behind the infrared and Raman spectroscopy are different; however, both methods are equally used for the DC measurements and give similar results [29, 115]. The choice of the method probably depends on the convenience for a particular experimental design and availability of the instrumentation. Overall, infrared spectroscopy is considered more traditional method for DC measurements and is more frequently used [15, 16, 53, 68, 116].

5.4.1.2 Infrared Spectroscopy

Infrared spectroscopy is based on absorption of photons with energy equal to the energy difference between molecular vibrational energy states. The infrared spectrometer operates by illuminating the sample with infrared beam and recording the radiation that is transmitted through or reflected from the sample. The remaining radiation carries information on how much of the incident radiation was absorbed for a particular wavelength and is used to produce the vibrational infrared spectrum. Most of the contemporary infrared spectrometers are based on an interferometer and use Fourier transform to convert an interferogram into a spectrum, thus the term Fourier-transform infrared (FTIR) spectroscopy [117].

Infrared spectroscopy can be performed in different regions of the infrared spectrum, which are named after their relative position to the visible light as near-infrared (14,000–4000 cm^{-1}), mid-infrared (4000–400 cm^{-1}), and far-infrared (400–4 cm^{-1}) [117]. The DC of dental composites is commonly measured in the mid-infrared region by quantifying the change in the intensity of the vibrational band at 1640 cm^{-1} that corresponds to the stretching vibration of aliphatic C=C bonds in methacrylate molecules [112]. Assuming the proportionality of the aliphatic C=C bonds concentration to the corresponding vibrational band intensity, information on the amount of converted bonds can be extracted by comparing the band intensity in polymerized and unpolymerized material [114]. As an internal standard, the band at 1610 cm^{-1} representing the aromatic C=C absorption is commonly used. The availability of this vibrational band depends on the presence of methacrylate monomers containing an aromatic core, such as Bis-GMA and Bis-EMA. In composites based on aliphatic monomers, e.g., UDMA, the vibrational band at 1610 cm^{-1} is absent, and other alternative reference bands are used [53, 118].

For spectrum processing, various methods of baseline subtraction and band deconvolution can be performed [119–121]. The linear relationship between the aliphatic C=C concentration and the corresponding band intensity is highly dependent on the baseline selection. Different baselines may cause considerable variations in the final DC results, reaching up to 20% [120]. Further issue related to the baseline position is the change in intensity of the nearby C=O band at 1715 cm^{-1} due to the conjugation of C=O group with C=C bonds consumed during polymerization [64, 122]. Thus, some authors recommended using band height instead of the band area, since the former is less affected by the baseline change [115]. Another procedure that may affect the DC values is the decomposition procedure (peak fitting) that is performed to resolve partially overlapping bands at 1610 and 1640 cm^{-1} [119]. However, it was shown that accurate DC calculations can also be performed using original, unfitted spectra [120]; thus, some authors find the fitting procedure unnecessary [115]. In any case, the variations in spectra processing do affect the final results to a various degree [115, 120, 123], and this fact should be considered when comparing DC values among different studies. Unfortunately, the detailed information about spectra processing is rarely reported in research papers.

Vibrational band intensities are used to calculate the DC by the equation [124]:

$$\mathrm{DC} = 1 - \frac{\left(\dfrac{I_{\mathrm{C=C}}}{I_{\mathrm{reference}}}\right)_{\mathrm{polymerized}}}{\left(\dfrac{I_{\mathrm{C=C}}}{I_{\mathrm{reference}}}\right)_{\mathrm{unpolymerized}}} \tag{5.1}$$

where $I_{C=C}$ and $I_{reference}$ represent the band intensity of aliphatic C=C stretching (1640 cm^{-1}) and the intensity of the reference band (Fig. 5.2). In this equation, the expression contained within the fraction essentially represents the ratio of the aliphatic C=C bonds remaining after polymerization, while subtracting this value from unity gives the percentage of the consumed double bonds, which is the definition of DC [112].

Sample preparation for infrared measurements varies according to the mode of collecting the spectra. The most classical technique for recording in transmission mode involves grinding the tested material, mixing it with potassium bromide (KBr) powder, and pressing the mixture into a thin pellet [16]. The pellet contains only a small concentration of the sample (0.3–1% by weight), dispersed in the KBr matrix which is

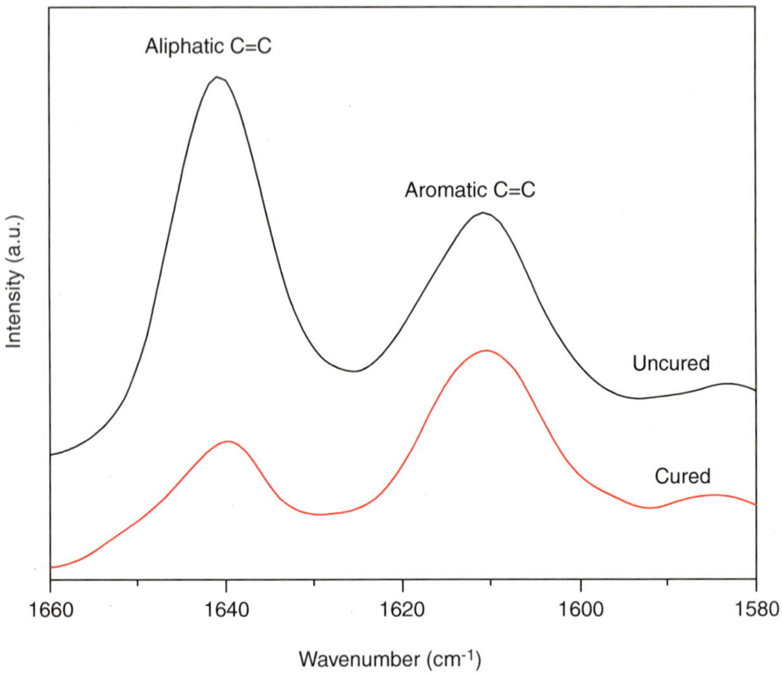

Fig. 5.2 The part of the infrared spectrum used for the DC evaluation. The spectra of uncured and cured sample are normalized to the reference band at 1610 cm^{-1}, and the change in intensity of the band at 1640 cm^{-1} is used to calculate the DC

transparent for infrared radiation. The pellet is then illuminated with an infrared beam, and the transmitted radiation is registered by a detector (Fig. 5.3). Main shortcomings of this approach are its destructiveness and elaborate sample preparation. Alternatively, infrared spectrum can be recorded in transmittance mode by pressing a composite into a sufficiently thin film [124] or in reflectance modes—attenuated total reflectance (ATR) and diffuse and specular reflectance. ATR mode is gaining popularity due to its convenience [125], whereas other reflectance modes are practically possible but not widely employed. In the ATR mode, the sample is positioned in a tight contact with the crystal of high refractive index, e.g., zinc selenide, diamond, or germanium. By directing the infrared beam at a certain angle onto the crystal, light is totally reflected from the border between the crystal and the sample. During the process of total reflection, infrared light penetrates the sample, while the absorption occurs at the crystal surface in contact with the sample. After multiple internal reflections, attenuated beam exiting the crystal is guided to the detector [117]. The major advantage of ATR is that it requires no additional sample preparation besides applying the uncured composite paste or clamping the polymerized composite sample onto the crystal (Fig. 5.4). ATR mode also allows evaluation of polymerization kinetics through the real-time DC measurements during the light curing with high data acquisition rate [126, 127].

The caution must be exercised when recording the spectra in the mid-infrared region, since the vibrational bands of interest (1640 and 1610 cm^{-1}) are located within the absorption spectrum of water [117]. Therefore, the samples must be dry, and the air humidity in the sample compartment must be kept constant; otherwise, water vibrational bands may interfere with the DC measurement. The effect of water can be eliminated by purging the sample compartment with inert gas (e.g., nitrogen) or by switching to the near-infrared region in which the vibrational bands used for DC evaluation are not affected by the presence of water [111]. Measuring the DC in near-infrared region provides some additional advantages. Due to lower absorptivity in the near-infrared region, much higher path-lengths are allowed (up to 4 mm), enabling measurements through the bulk of the samples without any previous preparation [128]. If the sample

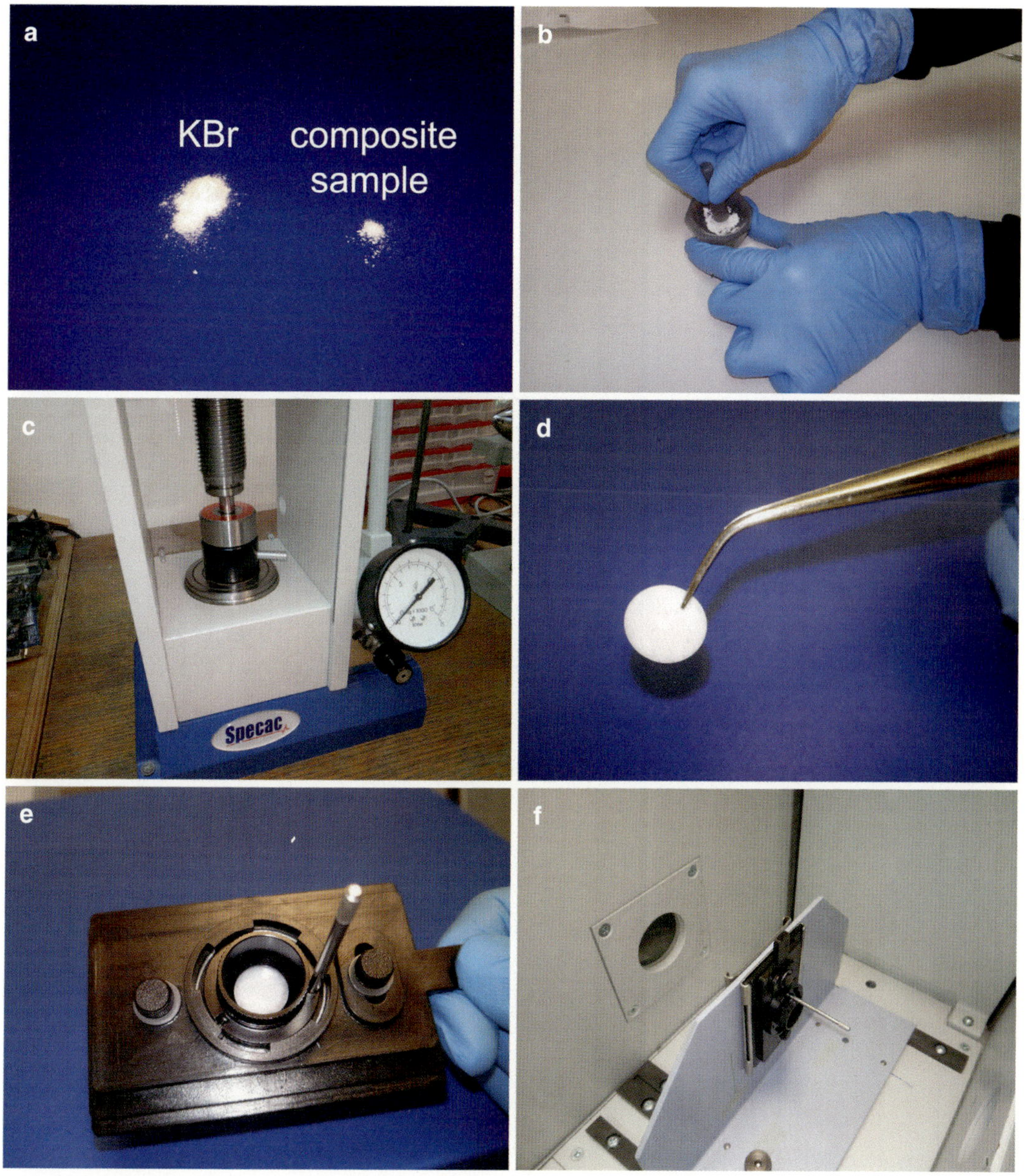

Fig. 5.3 Sample preparation for infrared spectroscopy in transmission mode. A small amount of composite sample (**a**) is ground with potassium bromide into powder (**b**), pressed into a pellet (**c**, **d**) which is mounted into a holder (**e**), and positioned inside the sample compartment of (**f**) an infrared spectrometer

geometry is precisely determined, using near-infrared eliminates the need for the internal standard, and only the intensity of the =C-H_2 vibration band at 6165 cm^{-1} is assessed for the DC calculation [128, 129]. Despite these benefits, the near-infrared region is much less often used for DC measurements than the mid-infrared.

5.4.1.3 Raman Spectroscopy

Raman spectroscopy probes molecular vibrations by means of inelastic Raman scattering. Unlike the elastic (Rayleigh) scattering, inelastic scattering is characterized by different energies of incident and scattered photons. Raman scattering is induced by exciting a molecule to a virtual energy

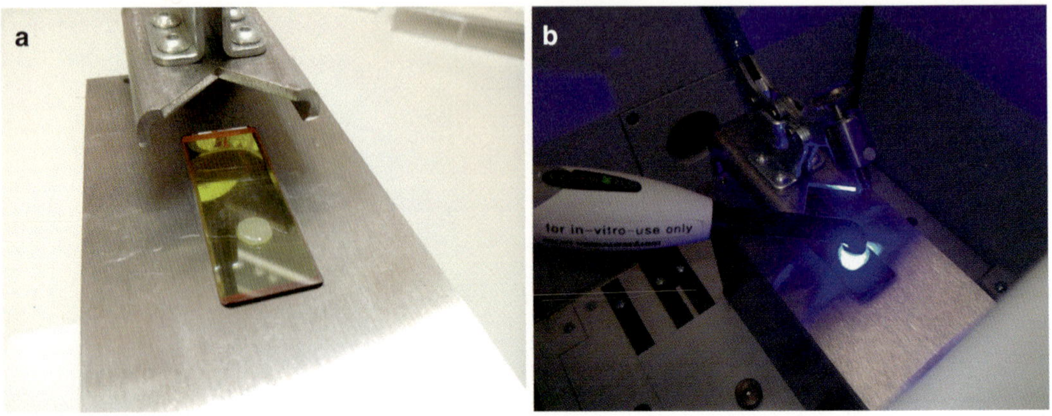

Fig. 5.4 Attenuated total reflectance (ATR) accessory of the infrared spectrometer and experimental setup for real-time measurements. Uncured composite is applied in the direct contact with zinc selenide crystal of the ATR accessory (**a**). The light-curing unit tip is positioned immediately above the composite sample, allowing spectra recording and light curing to be performed simultaneously (**b**)

state and its subsequent relaxation to an energy state that is either higher or lower than the original state. If the molecule undergoes an excitation from ground energy state and then relaxes to one of the higher energy states, the energy of scattered photon is lower than that of the incident photon (Stokes Raman scattering). Inversely, the excitation from one of the excited vibrational energy states and then relaxation to the ground energy state result with the scattered photon having higher energy than the incident photon (anti-Stokes Raman scattering, Fig. 5.5). In both cases, the energy difference represents the Raman shift and corresponds to the characteristic vibrational energy transition of a molecule [110].

In a Raman spectrometer, the scattering effect is induced by illuminating the sample with monochromatic laser radiation in the ultraviolet, visible, or near-infrared region. The light scattered on the sample is collected with a lens, and the elastically scattered photons (Rayleigh) are filtered out. These photons have the same energy as the incident photons emitted by a laser and carry no information on vibrational spectrum of the molecule. Only the small portion of photons which were inelastically scattered (about 1 in 10 million) is led to the detector for the reconstruction of the Raman spectrum [130]. Various Raman spectrometers offer a wide range of excitation laser wavelengths. Since the Raman scattering intensity is proportional to the negative fourth power of the excitation wavelength, shorter wavelengths are beneficial due to higher signal intensity. However, shorter wavelengths induce more unwanted fluorescence which interferes with the signal in the spectral region of interest. This can be overcome by using the excitation laser of longer wavelength (near-infrared), since its energy is insufficient to excite the energetic transitions responsible for fluorescence [114]. Such infrared lasers are usually a part of the hybrid FTIR/FT-Raman instruments that share the same optics and hardware for both techniques. The drawback of near-infrared excitation is lower intensity of Raman scattering and the need to use higher laser power or longer acquisition times in order to improve the signal [18]. Another important consideration regarding the selection of excitation wavelength is to avoid its overlapping with the absorption spectrum of the photoinitiator system [131], in order to avoid any additional photocuring during the measurement.

Raman and infrared spectroscopy are complementary techniques, as each vibrational transition may be active in infrared, Raman, or both. Generally, infrared spectroscopy is more sensitive for polar bonds, yielding strong vibrational bands with high signal-to-noise ratio, whereas Raman is more appropriate for examining nonpolar bonds. The vibrational bands pertaining to

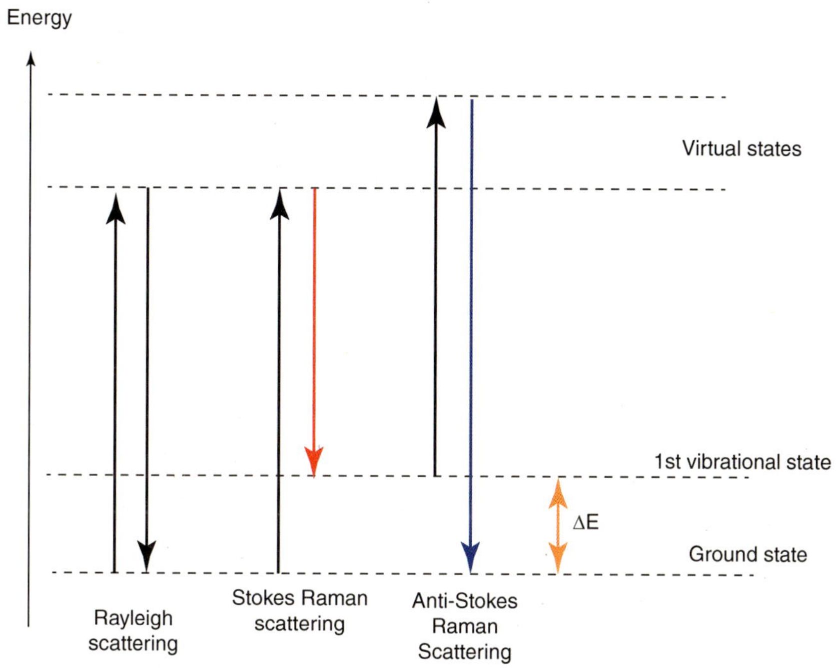

Fig. 5.5 A schematic representation of elastic (Rayleigh) and inelastic (Raman) scattering. Inelastically scattered photons have either lower (Stokes) or higher (anti-Stokes) energy than the incident photons. This energy difference (ΔE) represents Raman shift

aliphatic C=C and aromatic C=C used for the DC assessment are well detectable in both Raman and FTIR; thus, both methods can be used interchangeably. The Raman spectrum is processed by baseline subtraction and deconvolution similarly to the infrared spectrum, and the same equation (Eq. 5.1) is used for the DC calculation. As in the case of the infrared spectroscopy, the parameters of spectra processing that influence the final DC results [115] are often reported with insufficient parameters, affecting the inter-study comparability of DC values.

Raman can be advantageous over the infrared spectroscopy due to much simpler sample preparation. The uncured or cured composite is mounted on the sample holder "as is" and aligned with the laser beam (Fig. 5.6), eliminating the need for laborious preparation of KBr pellets or using the accessories for various reflectance modes in the case of infrared spectroscopy [17]. The measurements can be done in situ, on samples of any geometry and without damaging the samples. Another advantage of Raman spectroscopy is its insensitivity to water, which eliminates the need to control the environmental humidity and allows measurements on wet samples. Raman spectrometer can be coupled with a microscope to enable focusing of the laser beam onto small areas of the sample (micro-Raman) for assessing the local DC (Fig. 5.7). A set of such local measurements can be used to create a DC map and investigate the DC as a function of the position within the sample [132].

There are several drawbacks regarding the use of Raman for DC measurements. Due to the low intensity of Raman scattering, longer acquisition times are needed to obtain a good signal-to-noise ratio compared to the infrared measurements. This prevents real-time DC monitoring and may also present a problem if measurements are performed before the slowly developing DC has stabilized [133]. Thus, Raman is more suitable for assessing the DC in what can be considered a static system, which usually means 24 h after light curing [134]. Another concern regarding Raman spectroscopy may be localized

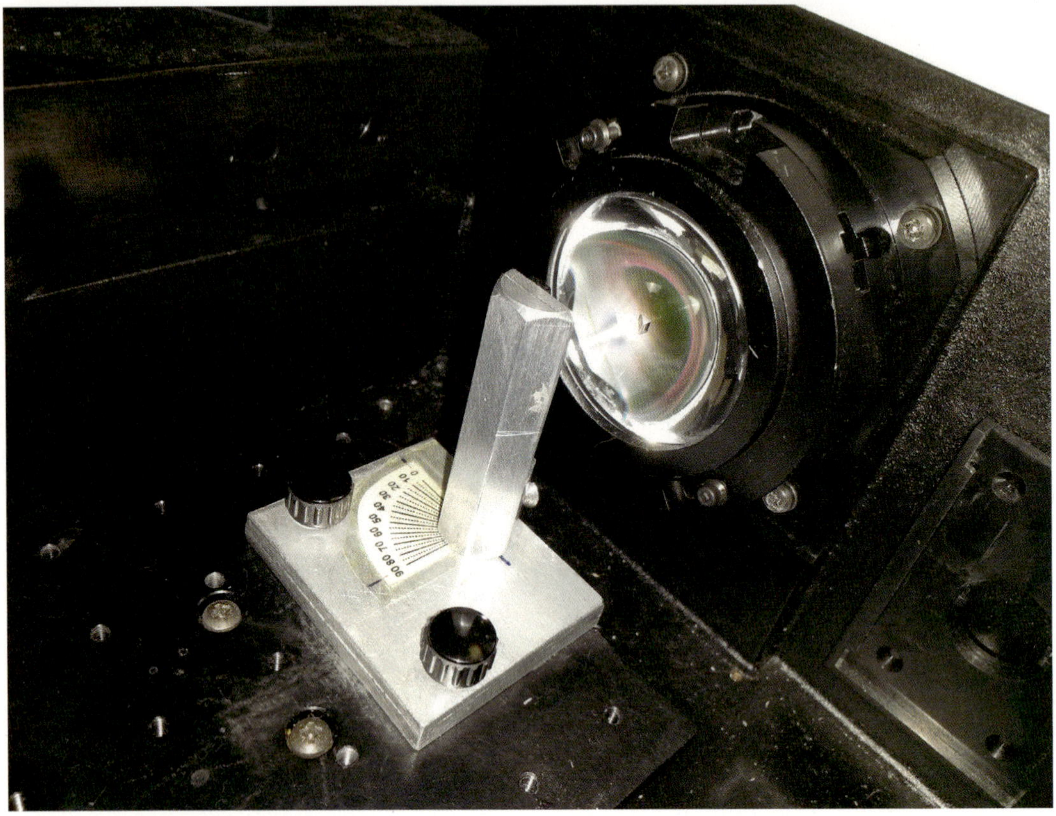

Fig. 5.6 Sample compartment of a FT-Raman spectrometer. The sample in its original state is mounted on the universal holder and aligned with the excitation laser beam. The lens collects scattered photons, which are subsequently filtered and led to the detector

temperature increase at the spot excited with laser beam, which may increase the mobility of unreacted monomers and free radicals, thus furthering the polymerization. The concerns about detrimental effect of heating by excitation laser were expressed for biological samples [135], but there are no reports of the laser heating effect on the DC of dental composites.

5.4.1.4 Limitations of the Spectroscopic Techniques

The inherent shortcoming of infrared and Raman spectroscopy is their inability to differentiate between the aliphatic C=C bonds that originate from methacrylate monomers from these contained within the silane molecules. The double bonds in silane molecules undergo conversion in the same way as the monomeric double bonds, but they show lower reactivity, especially if located in deeper parts of the silane layer [136]. The amount of silane varies greatly among composites due to differences in the filler load and particle size [54]. Both these factors determine the effective particle surface area that needs to be covered with silane. For instance, in experimental composites with low filler load (40–50 wt%) and a small amount of nano-sized particles, up to 4.4% of the total number of C=C bonds were contained within silane molecules [18]. Commercial composites contain much higher filler loads, and the contribution of the silane to the total filler load ranging from 2.8% to 9.0% [137] is not negligible. In light of these facts, the net conversion of C=C bonds from methacrylate monomers is generally somewhat higher than the spectroscopically determined DC, which takes into account both monomeric and silane C=C bonds.

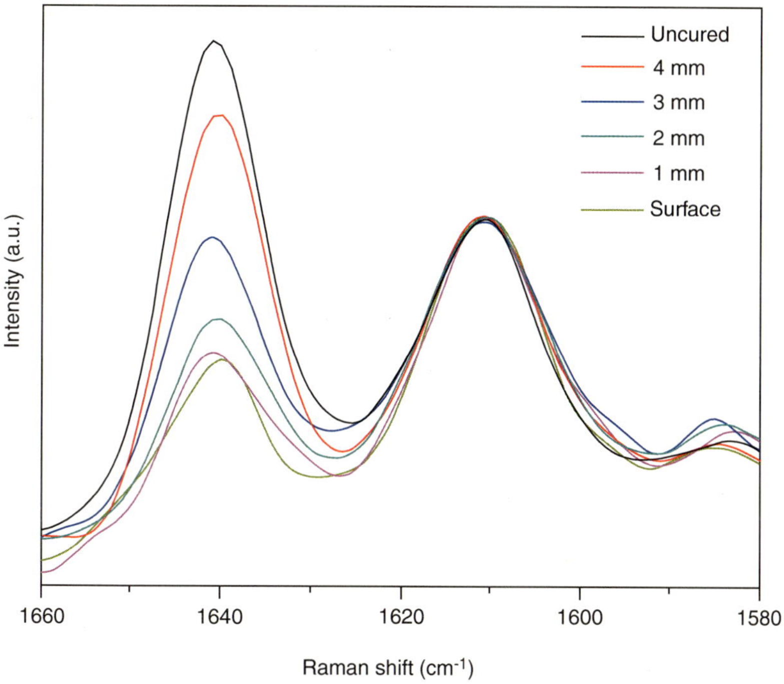

Fig. 5.7 Raman spectrum of the uncured composite (*black*) and spectra collected from various depths of the cured sample. The sample of a conventional composite was light cured from one side, and measurements were done at increasing distance ("depth") from the cured surface. All spectra are normalized to the reference band at 1610 cm^{-1} so that intensities of the band at 1640 cm^{-1} can be directly compared. Lower intensities of the band at 1640 cm^{-1} indicate higher consumption of aliphatic C=C double bonds at the surface and nearby depths (1 and 2 mm), whereas DC considerably declines as the measurement depth increases further, approaching that of the uncured material

A major issue regarding laboratory investigations of DC is its sensitivity to experimental conditions that are often not sufficiently controlled. The DC is commonly investigated as a function of material, layer thickness, and curing protocol [15]; however, some important factors are either ignored or beyond the control of investigators. For example, mold size and reflectivity play an important role in the reflection of curing light from mold borders [138, 139]. Furthermore, the mold material determines its thermal capacitance and conductivity, thus affecting the heat dissipation from the specimen. The amount of the material contained in the specimen influences the amount of released heat and temperature rise, which has an impact on polymerization kinetics and final DC values [140]. Additionally, environmental temperature and storage conditions affect the polymerization kinetics both during and after light curing [133]. The aforementioned differences in spectra processing further contribute to the variability of the DC results. All of these facts must be considered when comparing DC results obtained from different experimental setups. Currently no standardized method for the DC evaluation exists, but developing one in the future would highly improve the interlaboratory comparability of results [141].

5.4.2 Indirect Methods for the DC Evaluation

In addition to the spectroscopic techniques which are considered "direct" methods for the DC evaluation, the extent of conversion can be assessed indirectly by several methods that measure various other properties which change along with the DC. Due to the complex influence of multiple factors that are either unknown or difficult to assess, some of these properties are useful only as approximate indicators of the polymerization progress, and most of them are impossible to translate into absolute DC values. Among the indirect methods, microhardness testing is by far the most frequently used but also often criticized. Together with another classical (and disputed) method, the ISO 4049 depth of cure, microhardness is classically used to evaluate the efficiency of curing at depth. These and other less conventional methods for indirect DC assessment are briefly described below.

5.4.2.1 Microhardness

Microhardness measurements are performed by impressing a diamond indenter of a specific geometry into the composite surface. The surface of indentation is measured and together with a known force of indentation used to calculate the microhardness value [142]. In practical terms, microhardness represents the resistance of a material to plastic deformation and wear by abrasion. Due to a good correlation between microhardness and DC [69, 77], this method has a long history of use for indirectly measuring the efficiency of cure [73] (Fig. 5.8). The correlation is valid only when the DC and microhardness values are compared for samples of various conversions within a single composite formulation and does not hold for different composites as both properties are independently influenced by other factors [143]. Microhardness shows an exponential dependence on DC [77, 144] since it is considerably influenced by cross-linking which is scarce in the early stage of the polymerization and increases as the polymerization progresses [48]. Thus, the sensitivity of microhardness measurements increases at higher conversions, allowing the detection of small changes in the DC [77].

5.4.2.2 The Depth of Cure (DoC) Concept

Since the curing light is attenuated while passing through a composite material due to light scattering and absorption, there is a gradual decline in the DC through the composite layer (Fig. 5.1) [17]. The DoC concept is intended to detect the distance from the composite surface at which the DC heterogeneity becomes clinically unacceptable. Thus, the DoC is defined as the maximum thickness of a composite material that can be adequately cured in a single layer [69]. The term "adequately" has raised much dispute rendering the DoC concept itself rather controversial. Basically, the cure is defined as adequate if microhardness values are higher than 80% of the maximum value which is often, but not always, obtained at the surface [15]. Although originally devised for microhardness, the similar principle of identifying the depth with 80% of the maxi-

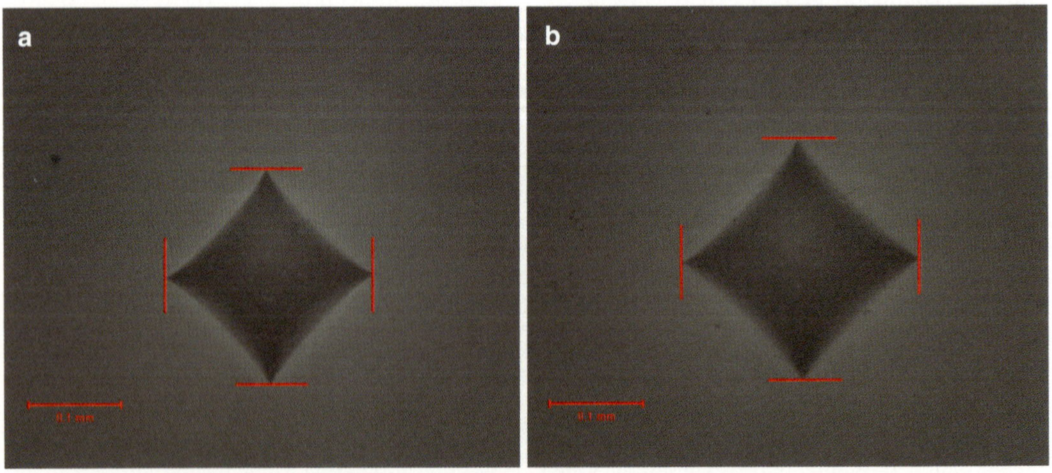

Fig. 5.8 Micrograph of indentations made on the top (**a**) and bottom (**b**) of a 6-mm-thick specimen of a bulk-fill composite. Greater surface area of the bottom indentation (**b**) reflects DC decline due to the curing light attenuation at depth

mum value has also been applied to the DC [145]. Alternatively, the 90% of the maximum DC value is sometimes considered as the "adequate cure" [132], since it was estimated that 80% reduction in hardness corresponds to 90% reduction in DC [146]. A major issue with the DoC concept is that the postulated cutoff values (whether microhardness or DC) are selected completely arbitrarily with neither physical meaning nor any measurable change in composite properties occurring at the threshold value [147]. The gradual decline in all composite properties with depth is inevitable, but there is no clear rationale for setting either the 80% or 90% cutoff value for any of the measured properties. Despite the controversy and lack of physical foundation, the DoC concept continues to be used to assess curing efficiency, and 80% of the maximum microhardness value is routinely quoted as adequate [15, 145, 146, 148]. An alternative definition of the DoC, as the depth of transition from glassy to rubbery state, has been proposed [69]. Despite being more physically justified, this approach is not commonly used as a criterion for the DoC.

5.4.2.3 ISO 4049 Depth of Cure

The simplest method to evaluate light-curing efficiency as a function of depth is devised by the International Organization for Standardization (ISO) and known as the ISO 4049 DoC. Briefly, a cylindrical composite specimen is prepared in a stainless-steel mold with the diameter of 4 mm. Both apertures of the mold are covered with Mylar strips, and the composite is cured through the upper aperture. Immediately after light curing, the specimen is removed from the mold, and the uncured material is removed with a plastic spatula. The height of the remaining cylinder is measured with a micrometer and divided by two. The obtained value is regarded as the maximum thickness of the composite increment that can be cured in a single exposition, i.e., the DoC [149].

Unlike other DoC testing methods, the ISO 4049 DoC requires no sophisticated instrumentation. It is intended for a quick and cost-effective screening of the relative performance of various combinations of composite materials and curing conditions, without claiming any correlation with mechanical properties or clinical performance [138]. There is much criticism of the ISO 4049 DoC, arising from the lack of either physical or clinical rationale for the procedure and calculation performed, poor correlation with values obtained by other DoC methods [69], sensitivity on the operator technique, and dependence on the mold characteristics [138, 139]. Despite criticism, the ISO 4049 DoC test fulfills the basic requirement of a standard testing method, which is to be as simple and as reproducible as possible [150] and is currently mandatory for determining maximum layer thickness and recommended curing times for all commercial composites [139].

5.4.2.4 Other Indirect Indicators of Conversion

Differential scanning calorimetry [151] and *differential thermal analysis* [152] measure the enthalpy of the polymerization reaction and make use of the known amount of heat released for a mole of the methacrylate functional group converted (approximately 55 kJ/mol) to calculate the DC [153]. By measuring the heat flow in real time, information on polymerization kinetics can be obtained [154].

Polymerization shrinkage can be used to indirectly evaluate the DC in a similar manner. Since each mole of converted double bonds contributes to a particular amount of polymerization shrinkage of approximately 20 cm^3/mol [155], shrinkage data can be translated into DC [156].

Softening in ethanol and *glass transition temperature* are indirect measures of cross-linking density, since more cross-linked polymeric networks are less prone to hardness deterioration in a solvent and undergo glass transition at higher temperatures [58, 70]. Although the cross-linking density increases along with the DC, it must not be considered a simple function of the DC since cross-linking is independently affected by curing conditions which influence the rates of initiation and termination and thus control the number of active growth centers [2].

Light transmittance undergoes a gradual change as the DC increases, due to the changes in resin refractive index and consumption of photoinitiator [157]. Although the clear relationship with DC cannot be determined due to the convolution of many simultaneously occurring processes, monitoring the light transmittance in real time is a simple method that can provide some insight into polymerization kinetics [126, 158].

Impedance spectroscopy operates by measuring electrical properties of the sample over the range of alternating current frequencies. Since the formation of polymeric network occurring during polymerization is reflected as the change in electrical conductivity, the latter can be used for real-time monitoring of the polymerization kinetics [159, 160].

References

1. Ilie N, Hickel R. Resin composite restorative materials. Aust Dent J. 2011;56(Suppl 1):59–66.
2. Leprince JG, Palin WM, Hadis MA, Devaux J, Leloup G. Progress in dimethacrylate-based dental composite technology and curing efficiency. Dent Mater. 2013;29(2):139–56.
3. Ferracane JL. Resin composite—state of the art. Dent Mater. 2011;27(1):29–38.
4. Yoshida K, Greener EH. Effects of two amine reducing agents on the degree of conversion and physical properties of an unfilled light-cured resin. Dent Mater. 1993;9(4):246–51.
5. Calheiros FC, Daronch M, Rueggeberg FA, Braga RR. Degree of conversion and mechanical properties of a BisGMA:TEGDMA composite as a function of the applied radiant exposure. J Biomed Mater Res B Appl Biomater. 2008;84(2):503–9.
6. Krifka S, Seidenader C, Hiller KA, Schmalz G, Schweikl H. Oxidative stress and cytotoxicity generated by dental composites in human pulp cells. Clin Oral Investig. 2012;16(1):215–24.
7. Tarle Z, Meniga A, Ristic M, Sutalo J, Pichler G, Davidson CL. The effect of the photopolymerization method on the quality of composite resin samples. J Oral Rehabil. 1998;25(6):436–42.
8. Knezević A, Tarle Z, Meniga A, Sutalo J, Pichler G, Ristić M. Degree of conversion and temperature rise during polymerization of composite resin samples with blue diodes. J Oral Rehabil. 2001;28(6):586–91.
9. Tarle Z, Meniga A, Knezević A, Sutalo J, Ristić M, Pichler G. Composite conversion and temperature rise using a conventional, plasma arc, and an experimental blue LED curing unit. J Oral Rehabil. 2002;29(7):662–7.
10. Miletic V, Santini A. Optimizing the concentration of 2,4,6-trimethylbenzoyldiphenylphosphine oxide initiator in composite resins in relation to monomer conversion. Dent Mater J. 2012;31(5):717–23.
11. Turssi CP, Ferracane JL, Vogel K. Filler features and their effects on wear and degree of conversion of particulate dental resin composites. Biomaterials. 2005;26(24):4932–7.
12. Uctasli S, Tezvergil A, Lassila LV, Vallittu PK. The degree of conversion of fiber-reinforced composites polymerized using different light-curing sources. Dent Mater. 2005;21(5):469–75.
13. Tarle Z, Knezevic A, Demoli N, Meniga A, Sutaloa J, Unterbrink G, Ristic M, Pichler G. Comparison of composite curing parameters: effects of light source and curing mode on conversion, temperature rise and polymerization shrinkage. Oper Dent. 2006;31(2):219–26.
14. Czasch P, Ilie N. In vitro comparison of mechanical properties and degree of cure of bulk fill composites. Clin Oral Investig. 2012;17(1):227–35.
15. Tarle Z, Attin T, Marovic D, Andermatt L, Ristic M, Taubock TT. Influence of irradiation time on subsurface degree of conversion and microhardness of high-viscosity bulk-fill resin composites. Clin Oral Investig. 2015;19(4):831–40.
16. Taubock TT, Tarle Z, Marovic D, Attin T. Preheating of high-viscosity bulk-fill resin composites: effects on shrinkage force and monomer conversion. J Dent. 2015;43(11):1358–64.
17. Par M, Gamulin O, Marovic D, Klaric E, Tarle Z. Raman spectroscopic assessment of degree of conversion of bulk-fill resin composites—changes at 24 hours post cure. Oper Dent. 2015;40(3):E92–101.
18. Par M, Gamulin O, Marovic D, Skenderovic H, Klaric E, Tarle Z. Conversion and temperature rise of remineralizing composites reinforced with inert fillers. J Dent. 2016;48:26–33.
19. Peutzfeldt A. Resin composites in dentistry: the monomer systems. Eur J Oral Sci. 1997;105(2):97–116.
20. Amirouche-Korichi A, Mouzali M, Watts DC. Effects of monomer ratios and highly radiopaque fillers on degree of conversion and shrinkage-strain of dental resin composites. Dent Mater. 2009;25(11):1411–8.
21. Stansbury JW. Dimethacrylate network formation and polymer property evolution as determined by the selection of monomers and curing conditions. Dent Mater. 2012;28(1):13–22.
22. Skrtic D, Antonucci JM. Effect of chemical structure and composition of the resin phase on vinyl conversion of amorphous calcium phosphate-filled composites. Polym Int. 2007;56(4):497–505.
23. Lu H, Trujillo-Lemon M, Ge J, Stansbury JW. Dental resins based on dimer acid dimethacrylates: a route to high conversion with low polymerization shrinkage. Compend Contin Educ Dent. 2010;31(Special Issue 2):1–4.
24. Bracho-Troconis C, Trujillo-Lemon M, Boulden J, Wong N, Wall K, Esquibel K. Characterization of N'Durance: a nanohybrid composite based on new nano-dimer technology. Compend Contin Educ Dent. 2010;31(Special Issue 2):5–9.

25. Kurokawa R, Finger WJ, Hoffmann M, Endo T, Kanehira M, Komatsu M, Manabe A. Interactions of self-etch adhesives with resin composites. J Dent. 2007;35(12):923–9.
26. Lee SK, Kim TW, Son SA, Park JK, Kim JH, Kim HI, Kwon YH. Influence of light-curing units on the polymerization of low-shrinkage composite resins. Dent Mater J. 2013;32(5):688–94.
27. Bucuta S, Ilie N. Light transmittance and micromechanical properties of bulk fill vs. conventional resin based composites. Clin Oral Investig. 2014;18(8):1991–2000.
28. Rueggeberg FA. State-of-the-art: dental photocuring—a review. Dent Mater. 2011;27(1):39–52.
29. Leloup G, Holvoet PE, Bebelman S, Devaux J. Raman scattering determination of the depth of cure of light-activated composites: influence of different clinically relevant parameters. J Oral Rehabil. 2002;29(6):510–5.
30. Jakubiak J, Allonas X, Fouassier JP, Sionkowska A, Andrzejewska E, Linden LÅ, Rabek JF. Camphorquinone–amines photoinitiating systems for the initiation of free radical polymerization. Polymer. 2003;44(18):5219–26.
31. Neshchadin D, Rosspeintner A, Griesser M, Lang B, Mosquera-Vazquez S, Vauthey E, Gorelik V, Liska R, Hametner C, Ganster B, Saf R, Moszner N, Gescheidt G. Acylgermanes: photoinitiators and sources for Ge-centered radicals. Insights into their reactivity. J Am Chem Soc. 2013;135(46):17314–21.
32. Leprince JG, Hadis M, Shortall AC, Ferracane JL, Devaux J, Leloup G, Palin WM. Photoinitiator type and applicability of exposure reciprocity law in filled and unfilled photoactive resins. Dent Mater. 2011;27(2):157–64.
33. Neumann MG, Schmitt CC, Ferreira GC, Correa IC. The initiating radical yields and the efficiency of polymerization for various dental photoinitiators excited by different light curing units. Dent Mater. 2006;22(6):576–84.
34. Moszner N, Fischer UK, Ganster B, Liska R, Rheinberger V. Benzoyl germanium derivatives as novel visible light photoinitiators for dental materials. Dent Mater. 2008;24(7):901–7.
35. Jandt KD, Mills RW, Blackwell GB, Ashworth SH. Depth of cure and compressive strength of dental composites cured with blue light emitting diodes (LEDs). Dent Mater. 2000;16(1):41–7.
36. Pradhan RD, Melikechi N, Eichmiller F. The effect of irradiation wavelength bandwidth and spot size on the scraping depth and temperature rise in composite exposed to an argon laser or a conventional quartz–tungsten–halogen source. Dent Mater. 2002;18(3):221–6.
37. Tarle Z, Meniga A, Ristic M, Sutalo J, Pichler G. Polymerization of composites using pulsed laser. Eur J Oral Sci. 1995;103(6):394–8.
38. Meniga A, Tarle Z, Ristic M, Sutalo J, Pichler G. Pulsed blue laser curing of hybrid composite resins. Biomaterials. 1997;18(20):1349–54.
39. Park SH, Krejci I, Lutz F. Microhardness of resin composites polymerized by plasma arc or conventional visible light curing. Oper Dent. 2002;27(1):30–7.
40. Knezević A, Tarle Z, Meniga A, Sutalo J, Pichler G, Ristić M. Photopolymerization of composite resins with plasma light. J Oral Rehabil. 2002;29(8):782–6.
41. Burtscher P. Visible light curing of composite resins—report. Research and development Ivoclar Vivadent AG, Schaan, Liechtenstein 18; 2007. p. 29–32.
42. Silikas N, Eliades G, Watts DC. Light intensity effects on resin-composite degree of conversion and shrinkage strain. Dent Mater. 2000;16(4):292–6.
43. Yap AU, Seneviratne C. Influence of light energy density on effectiveness of composite cure. Oper Dent. 2001;26(5):460–6.
44. Ilie N, Jelen E, Hickel R. Is the soft-start polymerisation concept still relevant for modern curing units? Clin Oral Investig. 2011;15(1):21–9.
45. Asmussen E, Peutzfeldt A. Influence of pulse-delay curing on softening of polymer structures. J Dent Res. 2001;80(6):1570–3.
46. Daronch M, Rueggeberg FA, De Goes MF, Giudici R. Polymerization kinetics of pre-heated composite. J Dent Res. 2006;85(1):38–43.
47. Lohbauer U, Zinelis S, Rahiotis C, Petschelt A, Eliades G. The effect of resin composite pre-heating on monomer conversion and polymerization shrinkage. Dent Mater. 2009;25(4):514–9.
48. Andrzejewska E. Photopolymerization kinetics of multifunctional monomers. Prog Polym Sci. 2001;26:605–65.
49. Burtscher P. Stability of radicals in cured composite materials. Dent Mater. 1993;9(4):218–21.
50. Leprince J, Lamblin G, Truffier-Boutry D, Demoustier-Champagne S, Devaux J, Mestdagh M, Leloup G. Kinetic study of free radicals trapped in dental resins stored in different environments. Acta Biomater. 2009;5(7):2518–24.
51. Par M, Lapas-Barisic M, Gamulin O, Panduric V, Spanovic N, Tarle Z. Long term degree of conversion of two bulk-fill composites. Acta Stomatol Croat. 2016;50(4):292–300.
52. Opdam NJ, van de Sande FH, Bronkhorst E, Cenci MS, Bottenberg P, Pallesen U, Gaengler P, Lindberg A, Huysmans MC, van Dijken JW. Longevity of posterior composite restorations: a systematic review and meta-analysis. J Dent Res. 2014;93(10):943–9.
53. Alshali RZ, Silikas N, Satterthwaite JD. Degree of conversion of bulk-fill compared to conventional resin-composites at two time intervals. Dent Mater. 2013;29(9):e213–7.
54. Ilie N, Hickel R. Investigations on mechanical behaviour of dental composites. Clin Oral Investig. 2009;13(4):427–38.
55. Price RB, Ferracane JL, Shortall AC. Light-curing units: a review of what we need to know. J Dent Res. 2015;94(9):1179–86.

56. Ferracane JL, Greener EH. The effect of resin formulation on the degree of conversion and mechanical properties of dental restorative resins. J Biomed Mater Res. 1986;20(1):121–31.
57. Asmussen E. Restorative resins: hardness and strength vs. quantity of remaining double bonds. Scand J Dent Res. 1982;90(6):484–9.
58. Lovell LG, Lu H, Elliott JE, Stansbury JW, Bowman CN. The effect of cure rate on the mechanical properties of dental resins. Dent Mater. 2001;17(6):504–11.
59. Lovell LG, Newman SM, Donaldson MM, Bowman CN. The effect of light intensity on double bond conversion and flexural strength of a model, unfilled dental resin. Dent Mater. 2003;19(6):458–65.
60. Dewaele M, Asmussen E, Peutzfeldt A, Munksgaard EC, Benetti AR, Finne G, Leloup G, Devaux J. Influence of curing protocol on selected properties of light-curing polymers: degree of conversion, volume contraction, elastic modulus, and glass transition temperature. Dent Mater. 2009;25(12):1576–84.
61. Chung KH, Greener EH. Correlation between degree of conversion, filler concentration and mechanical properties of posterior composite resins. J Oral Rehabil. 1990;17(5):487–94.
62. Leprince JG, Palin WM, Vanacker J, Sabbagh J, Devaux J, Leloup G. Physico-mechanical characteristics of commercially available bulk-fill composites. J Dent. 2014;42(8):993–1000.
63. Musanje L, Ferracane JL. Effects of resin formulation and nanofiller surface treatment on the properties of experimental hybrid resin composite. Biomaterials. 2004;25(18):4065–71.
64. Sideridou I, Tserki V, Papanastasiou G. Effect of chemical structure on degree of conversion in light-cured dimethacrylate-based dental resins. Biomaterials. 2002;23(8):1819–29.
65. Hadis M, Leprince JG, Shortall AC, Devaux J, Leloup G, Palin WM. High irradiance curing and anomalies of exposure reciprocity law in resin-based materials. J Dent. 2011;39(8):549–57.
66. Bowman CN, Kloxin CJ. Toward an enhanced understanding and implementation of photopolymerization reactions. AIChE J. 2008;54(11):2775–95.
67. Kannurpatti AR, Anseth JW, Bowman CN. A study of the evolution of mechanical properties and structural heterogeneity of polymer networks formed by photopolymerizations of multifunctional (meth) acrylates. Polymer. 1998;39(12):2507–13.
68. Frauscher KE, Ilie N. Degree of conversion of nano-hybrid resin-based composites with novel and conventional matrix formulation. Clin Oral Investig. 2013;17(2):635–42.
69. Leprince JG, Leveque P, Nysten B, Gallez B, Devaux J, Leloup G. New insight into the "depth of cure" of dimethacrylate-based dental composites. Dent Mater. 2012;28(5):512–20.
70. Schneider LF, Moraes RR, Cavalcante LM, Sinhoreti MA, Correr-Sobrinho L, Consani S. Cross-link density evaluation through softening tests: effect of ethanol concentration. Dent Mater. 2008;24(2):199–203.
71. Lovell LG, Berchtold KA, Elliott JE, Lu H, Bowman CN. Understanding the kinetics and network formation of dimethacrylate dental resins. Polym Adv Technol. 2001;12:335–45.
72. Soh MS, Yap AU. Influence of curing modes on crosslink density in polymer structures. J Dent. 2004;32(4):321–6.
73. Ferracane JL. Correlation between hardness and degree of conversion during the setting reaction of unfilled dental restorative resins. Dent Mater. 1985;1(1):11–4.
74. Peutzfeldt A, Asmussen E. Resin composite properties and energy density of light cure. J Dent Res. 2005;84(7):659–62.
75. Ilie N, Obermaier J, Durner J. Effect of modulated irradiation time on the degree of conversion and the amount of elutable substances from nano-hybrid resin-based composites. Clin Oral Investig. 2014;18(1):97–106.
76. Barszczewska-Rybarek IM. Structure-property relationships in dimethacrylate networks based on Bis-GMA, UDMA and TEGDMA. Dent Mater. 2009;25(9):1082–9.
77. Rueggeberg FA, Craig RG. Correlation of parameters used to estimate monomer conversion in a light-cured composite. J Dent Res. 1988;67(6):932–7.
78. Rueggeberg F, Tamareselvy K. Resin cure determination by polymerization shrinkage. Dent Mater. 1995;11(4):265–8.
79. Braga RR, Ferracane JL. Contraction stress related to degree of conversion and reaction kinetics. J Dent Res. 2002;81(2):114–8.
80. Ferracane JL. Buonocore Lecture. Placing dental composites—a stressful experience. Oper Dent. 2008;33(3):247–57.
81. Schneider LF, Cavalcante LM, Silikas N. Shrinkage stresses generated during resin-composite applications: a review. J Dent Biomech. 2010;2010:131630.
82. Braga RR, Ballester RY, Ferracane JL. Factors involved in the development of polymerization shrinkage stress in resin-composites: a systematic review. Dent Mater. 2005;21(10):962–70.
83. Stansbury JW, Trujillo-Lemon M, Lu H, Ding X, Lin Y, Ge J. Conversion-dependent shrinkage stress and strain in dental resins and composites. Dent Mater. 2005;21(1):56–67.
84. Asmussen E, Peutzfeldt A. Two-step curing: influence on conversion and softening of a dental polymer. Dent Mater. 2003;19(6):466–70.
85. Feng L, Suh BI. A mechanism on why slower polymerization of a dental composite produces lower contraction stress. J Biomed Mater Res B Appl Biomater. 2006;78(1):63–9.
86. Cunha LG, Alonso RC, Pfeifer CS, Correr-Sobrinho L, Ferracane JL, Sinhoreti MA. Modulated photo-activation methods: influence on contraction stress, degree of conversion and push-out bond strength of composite restoratives. J Dent. 2007;35(4):318–24.
87. Hofmann N, Denner W, Hugo B, Klaiber B. The influence of plasma arc vs. halogen standard or

soft-start irradiation on polymerization shrinkage kinetics of polymer matrix composites. J Dent. 2003;31(6):383–93.
88. Ferracane JL. Elution of leachable components from composites. J Oral Rehabil. 1994;21(4):441–52.
89. Van Landuyt KL, Nawrot T, Geebelen B, De Munck J, Snauwaert J, Yoshihara K, Scheers H, Godderis L, Hoet P, Van Meerbeek B. How much do resin-based dental materials release? A meta-analytical approach. Dent Mater. 2011;27(8):723–47.
90. Nomura Y, Teshima W, Kawahara T, Tanaka N, Ishibashi H, Okazaki M, Arizono K. Genotoxicity of dental resin polymerization initiators in vitro. J Mater Sci Mater Med. 2006;17(1):29–32.
91. Durner J, Obermaier J, Draenert M, Ilie N. Correlation of the degree of conversion with the amount of elutable substances in nano-hybrid dental composites. Dent Mater. 2012;28(11):1146–53.
92. Pongprueksa P, De Munck J, Duca RC, Poels K, Covaci A, Hoet P, Godderis L, Van Meerbeek B, Van Landuyt KL. Monomer elution in relation to degree of conversion for different types of composite. J Dent. 2015;43(12):1448–55.
93. Randolph LD, Palin WM, Bebelman S, Devaux J, Gallez B, Leloup G, Leprince JG. Ultra-fast light-curing resin composite with increased conversion and reduced monomer elution. Dent Mater. 2014;30(5):594–604.
94. Martin N, Jedynakiewicz N. Measurement of water sorption in dental composites. Biomaterials. 1998;19(1–3):77–83.
95. Rueggeberg FA, Cole MA, Looney SW, Vickers A, Swift EJ. Comparison of manufacturer-recommended exposure durations with those determined using biaxial flexure strength and scraped composite thickness among a variety of light-curing units. J Esthet Restor Dent. 2009;21(1):43–61.
96. Brambilla E, Gagliani M, Ionescu A, Fadini L, Garcia-Godoy F. The influence of light-curing time on the bacterial colonization of resin composite surfaces. Dent Mater. 2009;25(9):1067–72.
97. Khalichi P, Singh J, Cvitkovitch DG, Santerre JP. The influence of triethylene glycol derived from dental composite resins on the regulation of *Streptococcus mutans* gene expression. Biomaterials. 2009;30(4):452–9.
98. Mjor IA. Clinical diagnosis of recurrent caries. J Am Dent Assoc. 2005;136(10):1426–33.
99. da Silva EM, Almeida GS, Poskus LT, Guimarães JG. Relationship between the degree of conversion, solubility and salivary sorption of a hybrid and a nanofilled resin composite. J Appl Oral Sci. 2008;16(2):161–6.
100. Yiu CK, King NM, Carrilho MR, Sauro S, Rueggeberg FA, Prati C, Carvalho RM, Pashley DH, Tay FR. Effect of resin hydrophilicity and temperature on water sorption of dental adhesive resins. Biomaterials. 2006;27(9):1695–703.
101. Ferracane JL. Hygroscopic and hydrolytic effects in dental polymer networks. Dent Mater. 2006;22(3):211–22.
102. Pearson GJ, Longman CM. Water sorption and solubility of resin-based materials following inadequate polymerization by a visible-light curing system. J Oral Rehabil. 1989;16(1):57–61.
103. Drummond JL. Degradation, fatigue, and failure of resin dental composite materials. J Dent Res. 2008;87(8):710–9.
104. Soares LE, Nahorny S, Martin AA. FT-Raman spectroscopy study of organic matrix degradation in nanofilled resin composite. Microsc Microanal. 2013;19(2):327–34.
105. Dietschi D, Campanile G, Holz J, Meyer JM. Comparison of the color stability of ten new-generation composites: an in vitro study. Dent Mater. 1994;10(6):353–62.
106. Asmussen E. Factors affecting the color stability of restorative resins. Acta Odontol Scand. 1983;41(1):11–8.
107. Ferracane JL, Berge HX, Condon JR. In vitro aging of dental composites in water—effect of degree of conversion, filler volume, and filler/matrix coupling. J Biomed Mater Res. 1998;42(3):465–72.
108. Ruyter IE. Methacrylate-based polymeric dental materials: conversion and related properties. Summary and review. Acta Odontol Scand. 1982;40(5):359–76.
109. Sideridou ID, Achilias DS. Elution study of unreacted Bis-GMA, TEGDMA, UDMA, and Bis-EMA from light-cured dental resins and resin composites using HPLC. J Biomed Mater Res B Appl Biomater. 2005;74(1):617–26.
110. Chalmers JM, Griffiths PR, editors. Handbook of vibrational spectroscopy. Chichester: Wiley; 2001.
111. Moraes LG, Rocha RS, Menegazzo LM, de Araújo EB, Yukimito K, Moraes JC. Infrared spectroscopy: a tool for determination of the degree of conversion in dental composites. J Appl Oral Sci. 2008;16(2):145–9.
112. Ruyter IE, Svendsen SA. Remaining methacrylate groups in composite restorative materials. Acta Odontol Scand. 1978;36(2):75–82.
113. Ruyter IE, Oysaed H. Conversion in different depths of ultraviolet and visible light activated composite materials. Acta Odontol Scand. 1982;40(3):179–92.
114. Shin WS, Li XF, Schwartz B, Wunder SL, Baran GR. Determination of the degree of cure of dental resins using Raman and FT-Raman spectroscopy. Dent Mater. 1993;9(5):317–24.
115. Pianelli C, Devaux J, Bebelman S, Leloup G. The micro-Raman spectroscopy, a useful tool to determine the degree of conversion of light-activated composite resins. J Biomed Mater Res. 1999;48(5):675–81.
116. Al-Ahdal K, Ilie N, Silikas N, Watts DC. Polymerization kinetics and impact of post polymerization on the degree of conversion of bulk-fill resin-composite at clinically relevant depth. Dent Mater. 2015;31(10):1207–13.
117. Smith BC. Fundamentals of Fourier transform infrared spectroscopy. 2nd ed. Boca Raton, FL: CRC Press, Taylor & Francis Group; 2011.

118. Marovic D, Taubock TT, Attin T, Panduric V, Tarle Z. Monomer conversion and shrinkage force kinetics of low-viscosity bulk-fill resin composites. Acta Odontol Scand. 2015;73(6):474–80.
119. Acquaviva PA, Cerutti F, Adami G, Gagliani M, Ferrari M, Gherlone E, Cerutti A. Degree of conversion of three composite materials employed in the adhesive cementation of indirect restorations: a micro-Raman analysis. J Dent. 2009;37(8):610–5.
120. Rueggeberg FA, Hashinger DT, Fairhurst CW. Calibration of FTIR conversion analysis of contemporary dental resin composites. Dent Mater. 1990;6(4):241–9.
121. Nomoto R, Asada M, McCabe JF, Hirano S. Light exposure required for optimum conversion of light activated resin systems. Dent Mater. 2006;22(12):1135–42.
122. De Santis A. Photo-polymerisation effects on the carbonyl CO bands of composite resins measured by micro-Raman spectroscopy. Polymer. 2005;46(14):5001–4.
123. Ilie N, Hickel R. Can CQ be completely replaced by alternative initiators in dental adhesives? Dent Mater J. 2008;27(2):221–8.
124. Ferracane JL, Greener EH. Fourier transform infrared analysis of degree of polymerization in unfilled resins—methods comparison. J Dent Res. 1984;63(8):1093–5.
125. Ilie N, Fleming GJ. In vitro comparison of polymerisation kinetics and the micro-mechanical properties of low and high viscosity giomers and RBC materials. J Dent. 2015;43(7):814–22.
126. Ilie N, Durner J. Polymerization kinetic calculations in dental composites: a method comparison analysis. Clin Oral Investig. 2014;18(6):1587–96.
127. Scherzer T, Decker U. Real-time FTIR–ATR spectroscopy to study the kinetics of ultrafast photopolymerization reactions induced by monochromatic UV light. Vib Spectrosc. 1999;19(2):385–98.
128. Stansbury JW, Dickens SH. Determination of double bond conversion in dental resins by near infrared spectroscopy. Dent Mater. 2001;17(1):71–9.
129. Trujillo M, Newman SM, Stansbury JW. Use of near-IR to monitor the influence of external heating on dental composite photopolymerization. Dent Mater. 2004;20(8):766–77.
130. Lewis IR, Edwards HGM, editors. Handbook of Raman spectroscopy. New York: CRC Press, Taylor & Francis Group; 2001.
131. Stansbury JW. Curing dental resins and composites by photopolymerization. J Esthet Dent. 2000;12(6):300–8.
132. Li X, Pongprueksa P, Van Meerbeek B, De Munck J. Curing profile of bulk-fill resin-based composites. J Dent. 2015;43(6):664–72.
133. Par M, Gamulin O, Marovic D, Klaric E, Tarle Z. Effect of temperature on post-cure polymerization of bulk-fill composites. J Dent. 2014;42(10):1255–60.
134. Pilo R, Cardash HS. Post-irradiation polymerization of different anterior and posterior visible light-activated resin composites. Dent Mater. 1992;8(5):299–304.
135. Marigheto NA, Kemsley EK, Potter J, Belton PS, Wilson RH. Effects of sample heating in FT-Raman spectra of biological materials. Spectrochim Acta A Mol Biomol Spectrosc. 1996;52(12):1571–9.
136. Halvorson RH, Erickson RL, Davidson CL. The effect of filler and silane content on conversion of resin-based composite. Dent Mater. 2003;19(4):327–33.
137. Sabbagh J, Ryelandt L, Bachérius L, Biebuyck JJ, Vreven J, Lambrechts P, Leloup G. Characterization of the inorganic fraction of resin composites. J Oral Rehabil. 2004;31(11):1090–101.
138. Price RB, Rueggeberg FA, Harlow J, Sullivan B. Effect of mold type, diameter, and uncured composite removal method on depth of cure. Clin Oral Investig. 2016;20(7):1699–707.
139. Erickson RL, Barkmeier WW. Curing characteristics of a composite. Part 2: the effect of curing configuration on depth and distribution of cure. Dent Mater. 2014;30(6):e134–45.
140. Price RB, Whalen JM, Price TB, Felix CM, Fahey J. The effect of specimen temperature on the polymerization of a resin-composite. Dent Mater. 2011;27(10):983–9.
141. Sakaguchi RL. Review of the current status and challenges for dental posterior restorative composites: clinical, chemistry, and physical behavior considerations. Summary of discussion from the Portland Composites Symposium (POCOS) June 17–19, 2004, Oregon Health and Science University, Portland, Oregon. Dent Mater. 2005;21(1):3–6.
142. Watts DC, Amer OM, Combe EC. Surface hardness development in light-cured composites. Dent Mater. 1987;3(5):265–9.
143. Marovic D, Panduric V, Tarle Z, Ristic M, Sariri K, Demoli N, Klaric E, Jankovic B, Prskalo K. Degree of conversion and microhardness of dental composite resin materials. J Mol Struct. 2013;1044:299–302.
144. Erickson RL, Barkmeier WW, Halvorson RH. Curing characteristics of a composite – part 1: cure depth relationship to conversion, hardness and radiant exposure. Dent Mater. 2014;30(6):e125–33.
145. Bouschlicher MR, Rueggeberg FA, Wilson BM. Correlation of bottom-to-top surface microhardness and conversion ratios for a variety of resin composite compositions. Oper Dent. 2004;29(6):698–704.
146. Miletic V, Pongprueksa P, De Munck J, Brooks NR, Van Meerbeek B. Curing characteristics of flowable and sculptable bulk-fill composites. Clin Oral Investig. 2016;21:1201–12.
147. Musanje L, Darvell BW. Curing-light attenuation in filled-resin restorative materials. Dent Mater. 2006;22(9):804–17.

148. Ilie N, Stark K. Effect of different curing protocols on the mechanical properties of low-viscosity bulk-fill composites. Clin Oral Investig. 2015;19(2):271–9.
149. International Standard 4049. Polymer-based restorative materials. Geneva: ISO; 2009.
150. Della Bona A, Wozniak WT, Watts DC. International dental standards—order out of chaos? Dent Mater. 2011;27(7):619–21.
151. Antonucci JM, Toth EE. Extent of polymerization of dental resins by differential scanning calorimetry. J Dent Res. 1983;62(2):121–5.
152. Imazato S, McCabe JF, Tarumi H, Ehara A, Ebisu S. Degree of conversion of composites measured by DTA and FTIR. Dent Mater. 2001;17(2):178–83.
153. Miyazaki K, Horibe T. Polymerization of multifunctional methacrylates and acrylates. J Biomed Mater Res. 1988;22(11):1011–22.
154. Rosentritt M, Shortall AC, Palin WM. Dynamic monitoring of curing photoactive resins: a methods comparison. Dent Mater. 2010;26(6):565–70.
155. Dewaele M, Truffier-Boutry D, Devaux J, Leloup G. Volume contraction in photocured dental resins: the shrinkage-conversion relationship revisited. Dent Mater. 2006;22(4):359–65.
156. Venhoven BA, de Gee AJ, Davidson CL. Polymerization contraction and conversion of light-curing BisGMA-based methacrylate resins. Biomaterials. 1993;14(11):871–5.
157. Howard B, Wilson ND, Newman SM, Pfeifer CS, Stansbury JW. Relationships between conversion, temperature and optical properties during composite photopolymerization. Acta Biomater. 2010;6(6):2053–9.
158. Par M, Marovic D, Skenderovic H, Gamulin O, Klaric E, Tarle Z. Light transmittance and polymerization kinetics of amorphous calcium phosphate composites. Clin Oral Investig. 2016;21:1173–82.
159. Steinhaus J, Hausnerova B, Haenel T, Grossgarten M, Moginger B. Curing kinetics of visible light curing dental resin composites investigated by dielectric analysis (DEA). Dent Mater. 2014;30(3):372–80.
160. Par M, Santic A, Gamulin O, Marovic D, Mogus-Milankovic A, Tarle Z. Impedance changes during setting of amorphous calcium phosphate composites. Dent Mater. 2016;32(11):1312–21.

Part III

Classification and New Formulations

6 Developing a More Appropriate Classification System for Modern Resin-Based Composite Technologies

Luc D. Randolph, William M. Palin, and Julian G. Leprince

6.1 Current Terminology

A classification for dental resin composites should be appropriately represented and relevant and assist dental practitioners, serving as a simple guide to material selection. A classification should also facilitate material identification for manufacturers. Innovations which bring significant changes in terms of material application should lead to an update. Conversely, a strong classification should resist the introduction of superfluous terms for trivial novelties.

The properties and requirements of composites are numerous (see Chap. 2, Fig. 6.1). Currently there exist several perceived "classes" or labels of commercial dental resin composites, by application or material viscosity, "anterior/posterior" or "universal" and "flowable/packable," or by filler morphology—hybrid, micro- or nanohybrid, "nanofill," etc. Further modern labels include "low-shrink" or "bulk-fill" and have been heavily marketed by manufacturers aiming to attract the attention of practitioners. All these terms and labels refer to some extent to which aspect of a composite a manufacturer focused on (Fig. 6.1). Some labels are logical: an "anterior" resin composite should mimic the optical properties of enamel/dentin and allow for excellent sculpting. These properties are immediately perceivable and can be checked by dental practitioners. Other labels, such as "bulk-fill" or "low-shrink," describe physical properties that cannot be perceived. These resin composites do not necessarily outperform conventional "hybrids" in terms of curing depths [1] or shrinkage stress [2, 3], which is nevertheless intended

L.D. Randolph (✉)
Advanced Drug Delivery and Biomaterials, Louvain Drug Research Institute, Université Catholique de Louvain, Brussels, Belgium

Institute of Condensed Matter and Nanosciences, Bio- and Soft-Matter, Université Catholique de Louvain, Louvain-la-Neuve, Belgium
e-mail: luc.randolph@uclouvain.be

W.M. Palin
College of Medical and Dental Sciences, Institute of Clinical Sciences, Birmingham Dental School and Hospital, University of Birmingham, 5 Mill Pool Way, Birmingham, UK

J.G. Leprince
Advanced Drug Delivery and Biomaterials, Louvain Drug Research Institute, Université Catholique de Louvain, Brussels, Belgium

Institute of Condensed Matter and Nanosciences, Bio- and Soft-Matter, Université Catholique de Louvain, Louvain-la-Neuve, Belgium

School of Dentistry and Stomatology, Cliniques universitaires St Luc, Université Catholique de Louvain, Brussels, Belgium

V. Miletic (ed.), *Dental Composite Materials for Direct Restorations*, http://doi.org/10.1007/978-3-319-60961-4_6

Physical (intrinsic)	Physical (observable)	Application
Filler size "Micro", "Nano","Fine", "Ultra-fine"	**Handling** "Flowable"/"packable"	**Restoration type** "Anterior"/"Posterior" "Universal"
Filler size distribution "Hybrid", "Nano-hybrid"		**Technique** "Direct"/"Indirect" "Bulk-fill"
Filler type / resin mod. "Ormocer"		
Polymerization shrinkage "Low-shrink"		**Type** "Aesthetic"

Fig. 6.1 Characteristics and properties (*black*), terms, and labels (in *blue*) used to describe past and current dental composites

through the labels. Performance cannot hence be predicted by labels. Additionally, since it is perceived that pastes may not conform to the line angles and corners of a cavity, many dental practitioners might adopt the use of a "flowable" resin composite base layer. However, clinically, the advantage of such strategy has been rejected [4]. Clearly, the current terminology, with its numerous terms and apparent loose appropriation of labels, does not help in classifying resin composites.

6.2 Current Classification Based on Filler Size Distribution

Generally, the filler content of commercial dental resin composites is high (>50 vol%) [5, 6]. As dental composites become ever more versatile, the need for more reliable materials is paramount for load-bearing restorations. From a mechanical standpoint, a resin composite should replace dentin by appropriately transferring masticatory stresses, homogeneously throughout a restoration and with minimal deformation. Glass filler particles which display elastic moduli of 50 GPa and above serve as fillers and mostly contribute to the rigidity of dental composites. As noted previously, resin composites can be described by several intrinsic characteristics pertaining to the fillers, including the filler size distribution, geometry, and composition.

Historically, dental resin composites have usually been classified according to the filler size distribution and size regimes. Traditionally, glass particles, with an average size in the range of 20–50 μm, were used. The advances in grinding yielded "fine" and "ultra-fine" composites (Fig. 6.2), with smaller fillers. With the evolution of production methods, "microfilled" composites appeared in the 1970s; however, and by definition, such materials contained nanoparticles (<100 nm). Most materials produced thereafter became "hybrids," incorporating both, so-called nano- and micron-sized particles. The terminology and size distribution of hybrids have further broadened. Today, broad classification methods are in no way informative of material performance and often falsely applied [5]. In particular the distinction between "micro- "and "nanohybrids" is unclear (Fig. 6.2), as the latter may include greater amounts of nanoparticles and prepolymerized fillers. Here again, the terminology fails to inform and allow prediction of material performance.

A practitioner can only "see" the color or "feel" the handling of a resin composite. Interestingly, the viscosity and firmness are closely related to intrinsic characteristics, such as the resin composition or filler content. Since the current classification based on filler size distribution is too broad, using handling would hence appear as a sensible candidate. Consequently, the flowable/packable distinction will now be reviewed.

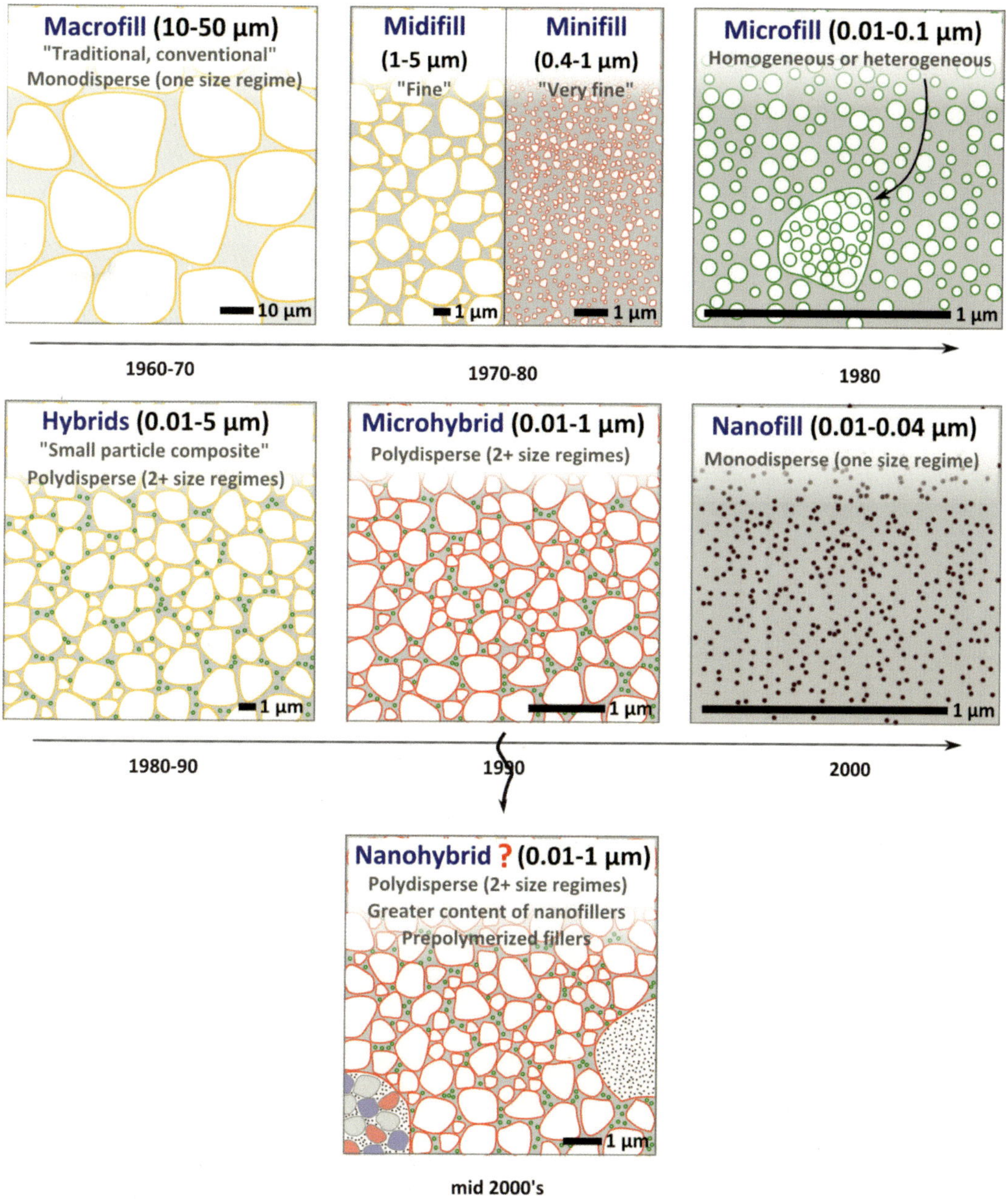

Fig. 6.2 Evolution of particle size and classification of dental composites. Modern materials are labeled "nanohybrids," a loosely defined term which at the very least indicates the use of nano- and micron-sized particles

6.3 A Classification Based on Handling Properties

The handling of resin composites is one of the two properties observable by practitioners without access to scientific equipment—the other being color and more specifically its hue. The handling can be detailed as both the viscosity and *thixotropy*, which refers to the time-dependent decrease in viscosity when shear stress is increased, i.e., as the resin composite is applied (via ultrasonic excitation or otherwise) through a

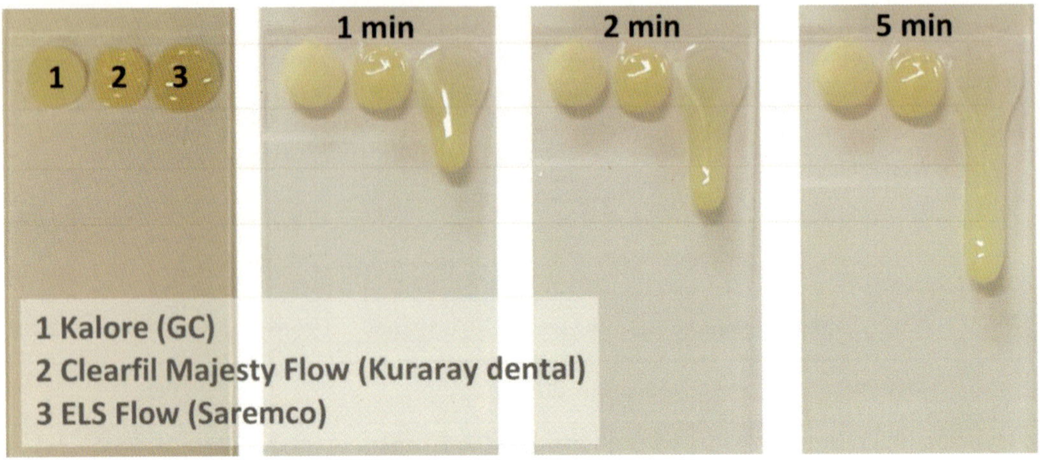

Fig. 6.3 Flowability of three different commercial composites, one aesthetic with a paste consistency (*1*) and two "flowables" (*2* and *3*). Note the downward displacement with time. The step between the *dotted lines* is 1 cm

compule, the resin composite "flows." When the shear stress is removed, the material regains initial viscosity. Dental practitioners may welcome a pseudoplastic resin composite but most importantly a sculptable material.

The viscosity of a dental composite is mainly influenced by two characteristics: the resin composition and the silanization of fillers. The filler content also plays a role, but to a lesser extent in highly filled materials. Thixotropy, a property, can be obtained with the addition of nano-sized filler particulates. Already one can see that a binary classification based on the *flowable*/*packable* distinction in fact relies on several characteristics. While a practitioner would potentially choose a *flowable* for its fluidity compared to a *packable*, a choice among different *flowables* would still have to be made. As exemplified in Fig. 6.3, two commercial "flow" composites display very different viscosities. The mechanical properties and water sorption of such materials also differ [5], along with their intrinsic characteristics. For example, the filler contents of material 2 and 3 are 59 and 28 vol%, respectively (manufacturer's data), and display flexural moduli of 6.7 and 3.7 GPa, a 50% difference.

Overall a classification based on the handling of resin composites provides little discriminatory power and limited information to practitioners. No single characteristic correlates with the observable viscosity and fulfills the requirements of the basis for classification.

Clearly, the key concern of any classification system is less of observable traits but rather the characteristics associated with intrinsic material properties, which vary considerably over a wide range of commercial resin composites. In order to discuss the relevance of a classification, the basis for organizing materials should now be defined. Such basis should be:

- *Intrinsic*, i.e., be specific to a component without which a composite would not perform the same
- *Global*, i.e., general and applicable to all composites
- *Informative*, i.e., have identifiable key characteristic(s) that significantly affect material performance
- *Explicit*, i.e., not conceptual properties but obvious to the practitioners

The best candidates are characteristics that govern major properties of composites (Fig. 6.4). For example, at first glimpse, the color of dental composites could constitute the basis for a classification. The color however does not inform in any way on how a composite behaves, whether chemically or physically. One may reconsider the filler size distribution in light of Fig. 6.4, in

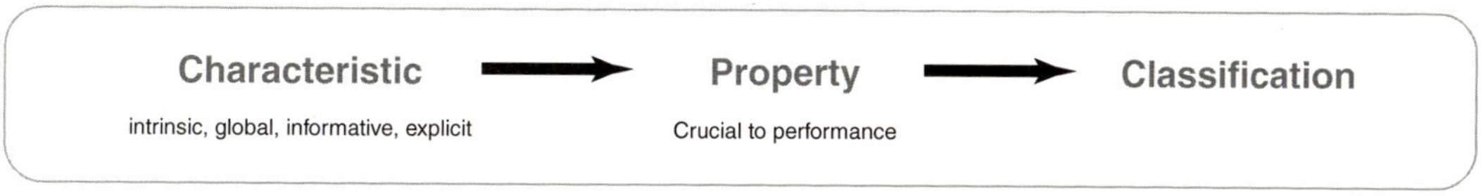

Fig. 6.4 Scheme summarizing the steps coming ahead of setting up a classification

particular since it is related to polishability and gloss retention. An alternative classification to the current one (Fig. 6.2) may be suggested.

6.4 An Alternative Classification Based on Filler Size Distribution

In order to obtain high *polishability*, particle size distribution must allow for an efficient removal of matter: after bulk reduction, the surface of a resin composite is polished using abrasive tools to remove traces of defects created during reduction and to progressively decrease surface roughness. To do so, tools coated with hard particles (alumina, silicon carbide, diamond) of decreasing sizes are applied to the surface. Conceptually, one may picture roughness as the distance between peaks and valleys. The smaller the filler particles of resin composites are, the smoother the surface can be since the minimum peak-to-valley distance will be lower [7]. Further, a decrease in surface roughness is related to an increase in gloss [8], i.e., of specular reflection versus diffuse reflection. "Specular" refers to a reflection for which light cone is narrow, making a surface appear shiny and reflective as with metals. "Diffuse" refers to reflection emitted in a wide range of directions, making a surface appear matte. Consequently for resin composites, which must display a high level of gloss, smaller particle size distributions are also of interest. Highly filled materials do require multimodal size distributions to maximize packing. However, by optimizing these distributions, the minimization of the upper limit of the size range would lead to an increased surface aspect during polishing and surface gloss. This is supported by the high surface roughness, observed in "macrofills," that is resin composites based on particles larger than 10 μm, even after careful polishing compared to nanohybrids and nanofills which conversely display excellent polishability [9]. After investigating a representative series of modern resin composites, a classification could hence be designed associating levels of surface roughness clinically achievable using current finishing and polishing tools to filler size distributions.

In order to obtain high *gloss retention*, a resin composite must display a high resistance to wear during the lifetime of a restoration. As stated above, gloss depends on the amount of specular light reflected. Gloss retention, that is, the preservation of a glossy surface aspect during the lifetime of a restoration, is directly related to the resistance to wear [10]. Further, increased resistance to wear is associated to increased filler contents, and this is experimentally observed in "microfills" ([11], 0.04 μm filler size). Further, "microhybrids" (≤1 μm) with multimodal distributions perform as well as "microfills" (0.1 μm) and better than fine-particle (1 or 1.5 μm) resin composites with regards to wear resistance [12]. It should be noted that surface degradation in the oral cavity is complex and dependent on extrinsic factors such as physical/chemical (temperature, pH, moisture, etc.), mechanical (masticatory load), and abrasive media (food bolus, size of abrasive particles, etc.). However, inherent material properties also play an important role, and material selection could again rely on size distribution. A classification could be designed similarly to that suggested based on surface roughness but using gloss retention as the property of interest. Materials already on the market designed with stress absorbing structures (clusters) and displaying high elastic moduli should perform better in terms of gloss retention [13]. Further, the use of prepolymerized fillers which contain submicron particles [5] would also be advantageous to obtain a high gloss and conserve it over time.

6.5 Suggestions for New Informative Classifications

Filler characteristics clearly offer a strong base for designing a classification. Some suggestions were made previously regarding the use of filler size distribution. However, there are additional characteristics that fit the requirements and framework shown in Fig. 6.4. More specifically, three characteristics that are intrinsic to materials and which could directly guide a practitioner when selecting a composite can be identified:

- The filler volume content.
- The thixotropy.
- The matting of the surface when handling.

6.5.1 Filler Volume Content

According to the rule of mixtures (ROM), filler volume content is directly related to the elastic modulus of each phase of a composite, although this is a nonlinear relationship, since the mechanical properties of fillers are significantly different from that of the resin. Estimations of the elastic modulus have been made in the past, with upper and lower theoretical bounds [14, 15]. A simplified, phenomenological model was designed taking into account the difference between elastic moduli of the fillers and resin:

$$E = E_r \left(E_r / E_f\right)^{1-\left(1-V_f\right)^{\beta}}$$

where E and V_f are the elastic modulus and the filler content by volume. β is a constant dependent on Poisson's ratios of each phase (v_f and v_r) [15]:

$$\beta = \frac{2\left[\left(1-v_f^2\right)/\left(1-v_r^2\right)\right]^{1.7}}{\ln\left(E_f / E_r\right)}$$

While the form of this phenomenological model is of great interest to predict the mechanical performance of commercial materials, in a daily practice, the practitioner should simply remember to select a material with the higher filler volume content. Such choice would be most suitable for load-bearing restorations. When overlapping this model to a dataset of a series of "anterior," "posterior," "microhybrid," and "nanohybrid" commercial resin composites, one can observe a good fit (Fig. 6.5). Some exceptions exist, in particular for composites based on the Ormocer technology or incorporating prepolymerized fillers. In such cases, the filler content comprises particles (inorganic-organic macromolecules/aggregates or resin-rich particles, respectively) that may not significantly contribute to the mechanical reinforcement of the material. Nevertheless, with a classification based on the filler volume content, an informed practitioner would then refer to the literature to determine the "inorganic filler volume content" for materials available. This amount refers to the particles made of glass and ceramic which were quantified during a volumetric test, for example, based on Archimedes' principle. Filler particles should display a much higher elastic moduli than the resin and solely play a role of matrix stiffener. This classification is simple and universal. Categories would be determined based on filler contents, attributing thresholds according to manufacturing limitations or, for example, by observing the thixotropic/matting of a range of materials (see below) as a function of the inorganic filler volume content.

6.5.2 Thixotropy and Surface Matting

In order to facilitate composite placement and sculpting, practitioners may welcome some amount of thixotropy. The appreciation of this behavior is purely subjective as some may prefer "packable" materials that can be pressed and resist sculpting. Nevertheless, in material selection, one should try a pellet of composite and manipulate it with a flat instrument, a spatula, for example. If stressed the material becomes easier to handle, and the composite displays thixotropy. On the contrary, if the surface becomes matte, the composite is "shear thickening", i.e., the viscosity increases with the shear rate. This behavior could be indicative of issues with particle size distribution (particle stacking) and resin compo-

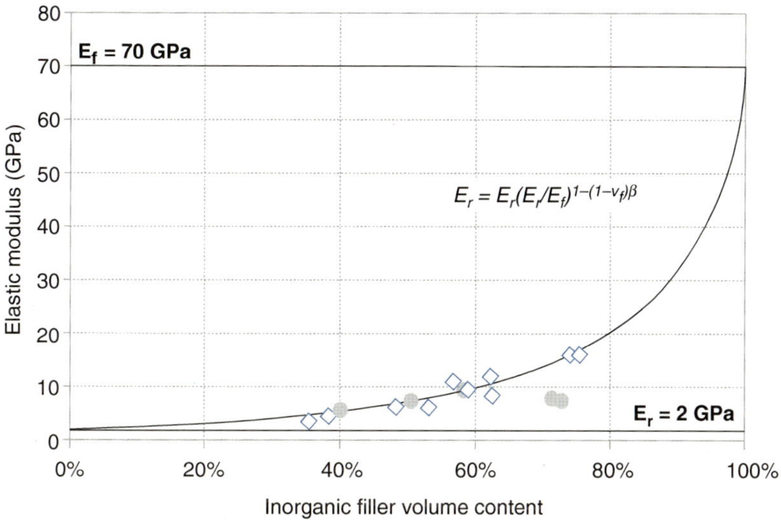

Fig. 6.5 Correlation between the elastic modulus and filler volume content based on the model from [15]. The elastic moduli of resin and fillers E_r and E_f were chosen as 2 and 70 GPa, respectively. Poisson's ratios for the resin and filler phase were chosen as 0.33 and 0.15, respectively. The overlapped data was extracted from [5]

sition (particle wetting and flow). Compared to the current packable/flowable distinction, a classification using the matte/shiny one, which again specifically informs on the composition and quality would be more informative, although the concepts underlying the distinction may not be easily grasped by practitioners.

In summary, current resin-based dental composites for direct restorations differ from each other based on various characteristics. Such characteristics may (e.g., filler volume content) or may not (e.g., particle size) be predictive of the materials' properties. It is the opinion of the authors of the present chapter that a classification should not be purely descriptive but as much as possible informative and predictive of such properties, in order to facilitate the material selection by practitioners in the clinics. Although probably imperfect, the suggested new avenues for classification have the advantage of directly informing on some aspects of the clinical behavior of a restoration and, as such, are worth keeping in mind. As it is, the current "hybrid" classification does not inform on material properties, and commercial labels are misleading. Hence, great care should be taken when interpreting marketing information, regardless of which "kind" of composite appeals most.

Acknowledgments L.D. Randolph is a FRIA (F.R.S--FNRS) scholar.

References

1. Bucuta S, Ilie N. Light transmittance and micromechanical properties of bulk fill vs. conventional resin based composites. Clin Oral investig. 2014;18:1991–2000.
2. Yamasaki LC, De Vito Moraes AG, Barros M, Lewis S, Francci C, Stansbury JW, et al. Polymerization development of "low-shrink" resin composites: reaction kinetics, polymerization stress and quality of network. Dent Mater. 2013;29:e169–79.
3. Jang JH, Park SH, Hwang IN. Polymerization shrinkage and depth of cure of bulk-fill resin composites and highly filled flowable resin. Oper Dent. 2015;40:172–80.
4. van Dijken JW, Pallesen U. Clinical performance of a hybrid resin composite with and without an intermediate layer of flowable resin composite: a 7-year evaluation. Dent Mater. 2011;27:150–6.
5. Randolph LD, Palin WM, Leloup G, Leprince JG. Filler characteristics of modern dental resin composites and their influence on physico-mechanical properties. Dent Mater. 2016;32:1586–99.
6. Adabo GL, Dos Santos Cruz CA, Fonseca RG, LsG V. The volumetric fraction of inorganic particles and the flexural strength of composites for posterior teeth. J Dent. 2003;31:353–9.
7. Marghalani HY. Effect of filler particles on surface roughness of experimental composite series. J Appl Oral Sci. 2010;18:59–67.

8. Kakaboura A, Fragouli M, Rahiotis C, Silikas N. Evaluation of surface characteristics of dental composites using profilometry, scanning electron, atomic force microscopy and gloss-meter. J Mater Sci Mater Med. 2007;18:155–63.
9. Costa JD, Ferracane J, Paravina RD, Mazur RF, Roeder L. The effect of different polishing systems on surface roughness and gloss of various resin composites. J Esthet Restor Dent. 2007;19:214–24.
10. Lee Y-K, Lu H, Oguri M, Powers JM. Changes in gloss after simulated generalized wear of composite resins. J Prosthet Dent. 2005;94:370–6.
11. Lim B-S, Ferracane JL, Condon JR, Adey JD. Effect of filler fraction and filler surface treatment on wear of microfilled composites. Dent Mater. 2002;18:1–11.
12. Turssi CP, Ferracane JL, Vogel K. Filler features and their effects on wear and degree of conversion of particulate dental resin composites. Biomaterials. 2005;26:4932–7.
13. Heintze SD, Zellweger G, Zappini G. The relationship between physical parameters and wear of dental composites. Wear. 2007;263:1138–46.
14. Hashin Z, Shtrikman S. A variational approach to the theory of the elastic behaviour of multiphase materials. J Mech Phys Solids. 1963;11:127–40.
15. Chantler PM, Hu X, Boyd NM. An extension of a phenomenological model for dental composites. Dent Mater. 1999;15:144–9.

Low-Shrinkage Composites

7

Vesna Miletic

7.1 Introduction

Polymerization shrinkage is an inherent property of methacrylate-based composites. In uncured composite, monomers are at intermolecular van der Waals distances and come closer as polymerization progresses to form covalent intramolecular bonds within the polymer. The result of this process is deformation or strain of the polymer also known as "polymerization shrinkage."

In general, shrinkage of sculptable dental composites is between 2 and 4% [1], whereas flowable composites shrink considerably more, between 3.5 and 6.5% [2–4]. Higher shrinkage of flowable composites is associated with the lower filler and greater resin fraction in the mixture. Shrinkage vectors are directed toward the inner parts of the material and are influenced by adhesion to cavity walls [4, 5] as well as cavity geometry and C-factor [6, 7].

The adhesive system that bonds composite to the cavity walls places a considerable constraint on the composite as the pulling action of the adhesive is directly opposite to the shrinkage vector of the composite resin. During polymerization, composite has the ability to flow within the growing polymer compensating for the adhesive restriction and composite shrinkage. However, this only happens up to a certain point, known as the "gel point" when material flow is no longer possible. Further polymerization of the polymer with increased stiffness results in stresses along the restoration-cavity wall.

Shrinkage stresses are higher in materials with high elastic modulus, i.e., rigid materials [8] as well as those with faster polymerization rate and greater post-gel shrinkage [9, 10]. Shrinkage stress of most dental composites was reported to be in the range of 1.5–15 MPa [1, 11–13], with few exceptions exhibiting higher stresses such as Filtek Z100 (3M ESPE) whose polymerization stress was shown to exceed 20 MPa [1]. An inverse linear fit was found between shrinkage and stress indicating that composites with lower volumetric shrinkage are likely to be associated with higher shrinkage stress. Tensile modulus was also shown to inversely correlate to shrinkage and directly to shrinkage stress [1].

It is assumed that shrinkage stress exceeding the compliance of the adhesive system would lead to microcracks and gaps along the restoration-tooth interface or within the tooth or composite restoration. Compromised marginal adaptation is likely one of the important factors contributing to secondary caries [14] which has been identified as the primary reason for restoration failure [15]. A recent review by Ferracane and Hilton [14] summarizes in vitro and in vivo evidence in an attempt to reveal whether or not

V. Miletic
DentalNet Research Group, School of Dental Medicine, University of Belgrade, Belgrade, Serbia
e-mail: vesna.miletic@stomf.bg.ac.rs

V. Miletic (ed.), *Dental Composite Materials for Direct Restorations*,
http://doi.org/10.1007/978-3-319-60961-4_7

shrinkage stress is clinically meaningful. In vitro evidence suggesting negative effects of shrinkage stress on marginal adaptation was not corroborated by clinical studies with "circumstantial evidence" for this link at best. However, shrinkage stress was concluded to be clinically meaningful in light of its perceived influence on the recommended clinical procedures involving bonding, composite placement, and curing protocols [14].

In a review by Braga and Ferracane [16], three strategies for the reduction of shrinkage stress were outlined: (1) nonbonded fillers would enable the flow of monomers and interaction between resin matrix and fillers without constraint; (2) increased concentration of inhibitors from 0.05 to 1 wt% would reduce polymerization rate and extend the pregel phase; and (3) high-density polyethylene spheres would reduce elastic modulus or volumetric shrinkage.

In addition, developments regarding low-shrinkage monomers, though in experimental phases, were mentioned as the promising pathways: (1) addition of spiro orthocarbonates to dimethacrylate and epoxy resins, (2) esterified multi-methacrylate oligomers, (3) cycloaliphatic epoxy resins (oxiranes), and (4) combined siloxanes and oxiranes (siloranes).

Oxiranes and siloranes seemed especially promising for dental use based on high-strength polymerization uninhibited by atmospheric oxygen and ring-opening cationic polymerization which reduces shrinkage compared to BisGMA [16].

7.2 Low-Shrinkage Strategies in Commercial Composites

Table 7.1 summarizes information on low-shrinkage composites that were or still are available on the market. The materials were labeled 'low-shrinkage' either by the manufacturers or researchers. Two main strategies for reduced shrinkage may be identified in commercial low-shrinkage composites: (1) high filler content (>80 wt%) and (2) modified resin matrix.

7.2.1 High Filler Content

Because shrinkage is the result of resin polymerization, the idea behind high filler content is that by increasing the amount of filler, the reduced amount of resin would shrink less in a given volume of composite. In commercial low-shrinkage composites, the filler content varies between 84 wt% (Premise; Kerr) and 92 wt% (Clearfil Majesty Posterior; Kuraray). Variations in particle size allow optimized particle distribution and high density contributing to reduced shrinkage and maintained handling properties of such composites. Commercial low-shrinkage composites contain a combination of micro- (1–1.5 μm) or sub-micro-sized (~0.5 μm) glass or glass-ceramic particles and amorphous silica nano-sized particles (40 nm). They may also contain larger prepolymerized fillers (~10 μm) of already polymerized composite milled to form organic-inorganic filler particles.

7.2.2 Modified Resin Matrix

7.2.2.1 Replacement of TEGDMA with BisEMA

Due to the high viscosity of BisGMA, diluent monomers of lower molecular weight, such as TEGDMA, are added to the resin mixture to optimize viscosity and allow filler inclusion. Flexible TEGDMA contributes to the increased degree of conversion of a BisGMA-TEGDMA mixture compared to the bulky and rigid BisGMA monomer alone. TEGDMA also increases polymerization shrinkage of its respective composite due to its higher number of reactive species per volume unit [17].

One strategy to reduce polymerization shrinkage in dental composites is to reduce or completely replace diluent monomers of low molecular weight. TEGDMA is commonly replaced by monomers of higher molecular weight, such as UDMA and especially BisEMA (often referred to as ethoxylated BisGMA). Lower viscosity of BisEMA may be attributed to the absence of hydrogen bonding due to the lack of hydroxyl groups. In Extra Low Shrinkage

Table 7.1 Low-shrinkage composites

Material	Manufacturer/type	Low-shrink strategy	Composition[a]	Dedicated adhesive
Filtek P90/Filtek Silorane	3M ESPE/microhybrid	Silorane chemistry; ring-opening polymerization	Resin: Silorane resin (23 wt%) Initiating system: CQ, iodonium salt, electron donor (0.9 wt%) Fillers: quartz (0.1–1 μm) + yttrium fluoride fillers (76 wt%) Other: Stabilizers (0.13%), pigments (0.005%)	YES. P90/silorane system adhesive
Extra low shrinkage (ELS)	Saremco/microhybrid	Lack of TEGDMA, inclusion of BisEMA	Resin: BisGMA, BisEMA (26%) Fillers: Ba-Al-B-Si glass filler (avg. 0.7 μm, range 50 nm–3 μm) (73% wt%) Other: Initiator, inhibitor, stabilizer, pigments (<1%)	NO
Kalore	GC/microhybrid	High-molecular-weight cross-linker (DX-511 monomer), high filler content	Resin: UDMA, DX-511 comonomer, dimethacrylate (18%) Fillers: Fluoroaluminosilicate glass, prepolymerized filler, SiO_2 (82 wt%) Other: Initiators, inhibitors, stabilizers, pigments (<1%)	NO
Venus Diamond	Heraeus Kulzer/nanohybrid	High-molecular-weight cross-linker (urethane- and tricyclodecane-based monomer), high filler content	Resin: TCD-DI-HEA, UDMA (<20%) Fillers: Barium aluminum fluoride glass, highly discrete nanoparticles (80–82 wt%) Other: Rheology modifier, initiator system, stabilizers, pigments	NO
N'Durance	Septodont/nanohybrid	High-molecular-weight cross-linker (dimer acid dimethacrylate), lack of TEGDMA, inclusion of BisEMA, high filler content	Resin: Dimer dicarbamate dimethacrylate, BisEMA (EBPADMA), UDMA, hexanediol dimethacrylate (19%) Fillers: Ytterbium fluoride (avg. 40 nm) + silica nanofillers (10 nm), and barium glass fillers (avg. 0.5 μm) + TiO_2 (80 wt%) Other: Camphorquinone, tert. amine, inhibitors, stabilizers, pigments (<1%)	NO
Clearfil Majesty Posterior	Kuraray/nanohybrid	High filler content	Resin: BisGMA, TEGDMA, hydrophobic aromatic dimethacrylate (<7%) Fillers: Alumina and silica nanofiller (20 nm) + glass-ceramic filler (1.5 μm) (92 wt%) Other: CQ, accelerators, pigments (<1%)	NO

(continued)

Table 7.1 (continued)

Material	Manufacturer/type	Low-shrink strategy	Composition[a]	Dedicated adhesive
Grandio	Voco/nanohybrid	High filler content	Resin: BisGMA, TEGDMA, UDMA (~12 wt%) Fillers: Glass-ceramic filler, silica nanofiller (87 wt%) Other: initiators, pigments, amines, additives (<1 wt%)	NO
Premise	Kerr/nanofilled	High filler content, trimodal filler distribution	Resin: BisEMA, TEGDMA (~15%) Fillers: Ba-Al-B-Si glass, Ba glass fillers (avg. 0.4 μm), prepolymerized fillers, silica nanofillers (40 nm) (84 wt%) Other: Camphorquinone, tert. amine, inhibitors, stabilizers, pigments (<1%)	NO
AElite LS posterior	Bisco/microhybrid	High filler content	Resin: BisGMA, BisEMA, TEGDMA (~11%) Fillers: Glass frit + amorphous silica (88 wt%) Other: Initiators, stabilizers, inhibitors, pigments (<1%)	NO
Inten-S	Ivoclar Vivadent/hybrid	High filler content, modified resin matrix[b]	Resin: Dimethacrylates (17.5 wt%) Filler: Barium glass + ytterbium trifluoride (41.9 wt%), copolymer filler (40 wt%) Other: Stabilizers and catalysts (0.3 wt%), additives (0.3 wt%), pigments (<0.1 wt%)	NO
Reflexions XLS dentin	Bisco/nanohybrid	High filler content	Yamamoto et al. [60] Resin: BisEMA (~12 wt%) Fillers: Glass + amorphous silica (88 wt%)	NO

[a]According to manufacturer's technical data

[b]Reduced/omitted high-shrinkage monomer (as stated by the manufacturer)

BisGMA bisphenol A diglycidylmethacrylate, *TEGDMA* triethylene glycol dimethacrylate, *UDMA* urethane dimethacrylate, *BisEMA (EBPADMA)*, ethoxylated bisphenol-A dimethacrylate, *CQ* camphorquinone

(ELS) composite (Saremco) TEGDMA is completely substituted by BisEMA and appears to be the only manufacturer's strategy to reduce shrinkage as the filler content of this microhybrid composite is not increased (73 wt%). BisEMA is often used in other low-shrinkage composites to partially replace TEGDMA (Table 7.1).

7.2.2.2 Silorane Chemistry and Filtek Silorane

For 40 years, no monomers other than methacrylates were used in dental composites. In 2005 Weinmann et al. [18] compared the properties of a silorane-based experimental composite to methacrylate-based composites. Based on two known strategies for the reduction of polymerization shrinkage, i.e., reduction of reactive sites per volume unit and the use of different resins, silorane monomer was developed for dental use. It consists of a siloxane backbone and four cycloaliphatic oxirane moieties (Fig. 7.1). Cationic polymerization is initiated through interaction of camphorquinone, iodonium salt, and an electron donor resulting in reactive acidic cationic species which open the epoxy group of the oxirane ring creating a carbocation. Further reaction with oxirane moieties results in the formation of highly cross-linked polymer network.

Polymerization shrinkage of siloranes, compensated by oxirane ring-opening, was shown to be substantially lower than that of methacrylate polymer formed via free radical polymerization. Another important finding was slower shrinkage progression by silorane than methacrylate-based composites leading to the hypothesis that shrinkage stress would also be lower, though it was not calculated by Weinmann et al. [18].

Following this report, attempts were intensified to achieve an optimal material composition based on silorane chemistry for dental use. There were several reports on experimental silorane- and oxirane-based materials [12, 19–22]. Compared to microhybrid composites, those early silorane-based formulations had lower wear

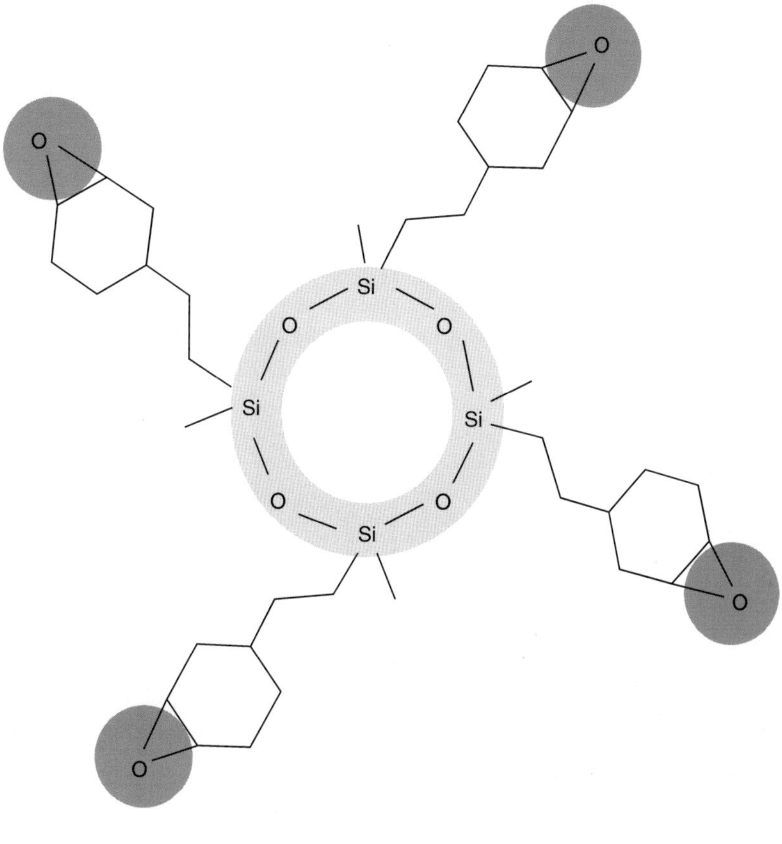

Fig. 7.1 Silorane molecule consisting of a siloxane (*light gray*) backbone and oxirane (*dark gray*) moieties

resistance, higher surface fatigue [20], and lower degree of conversion but similar or improved hardness [21]. Smaller cuspal deflection was inconsistent with the observed microleakage around MOD restorations [21].

Siloranes were found to be more stable in aqueous media than oxiranes [19]. Along with a previous report by Schweikl et al. [23] pointing to a lower mutagenic potential of siloranes than oxiranes, these findings suggested that siloranes were more biologically acceptable than oxiranes.

Experimental silorane-based composite Hermes (3M ESPE) showed similar microleakage around Class I restorations compared to hybrid and nanofilled control composites [22]. Mean shrinkage stress of 3.5 MPa found for Hermes was lower than 4.8 MPa of a nanofilled composite (Filtek Supreme, 3M ESPE) [12]. Curing time of 20 s with high-intensity light-curing units (1200 mW/cm^2) was recommended as the upper light limit that allows stress rate control [12].

Incorporating previous knowledge on silorane chemistry and properties of experimental materials, Filtek Silorane (3M ESPE) was launched on the market in 2007 and advertised as the first commercial composite with polymerization shrinkage below 1% and 2 MPa shrinkage stress [24]. A composite with different name (Filtek P90, 3M ESPE) but the same material composition as Filtek Silorane was also marketed. Both Filtek Silorane and Filtek P90 appear in the scientific literature, but the reported properties essentially refer to the same material. Resin matrix of Filtek Silorane consists of 23 wt% silorane resin and 76 wt% quartz and ytterbium fluoride fillers, according to the manufacturer's data. A study by Leprince et al. [25] found similar filler mass fraction using thermogravimetric analysis (about 75%) to the one claimed by the manufacturer. An SEM analysis showed that filler particles were irregularly shaped and 0.1–1 μm in size. The inability to produce quartz fillers by a sol-gel process was suggested as the likely reason for irregular particle shape in Filtek Silorane [25].

A number of studies investigated various properties of Filtek Silorane, especially shrinkage and stress [26–30] but also other physico-mechanical [25, 28, 30–34], esthetic [35], and biological properties [36, 37] as well as and marginal adaptation [38–43]. A few studies also investigated the effects of curing on cuspal deflection [44–46]. Several clinical trials were also reported [47–55].

7.2.2.3 High-Molecular Weight Monomers

TCD-DI-HEA of Venus Diamond (Fig. 7.2) contains the rigid central part of the monomer (tricyclodecane) which is said to reduce monomer vibrations in the uncured material allowing closer distances between TCD-DI-HEA monomers. This so-called higher packing density of the cross-linking monomers results in smaller changes in distances during polymerization, thereby, reducing polymerization shrinkage. Urethane groups increase reactivity and result in high monomer-to-polymer conversion. It was previously shown that degree of conversion is generally related to good mechanical properties and low leachability of dental composites [30, 56–59]. Side arms are said to be responsible for lower shrinkage stress due to increased flexibility, which was confirmed by previous studies [26, 60].

DX-511 of Kalore (Fig. 7.3) is a very long monomer, twice the molecular weight of UDMA and nearly twice the molecular weight of BisGMA. The number of reactive sites per volume unit, responsible for reduced shrinkage, is even smaller in DX-511 than in TCD-DI-HEA. Similarly to TCD-DI-HEA, DX-511 contains a rigid core which is claimed to maintain monomer shape and prevent deformation of the long chain. Furthermore, flexible side arms and urethane groups increase the reactivity and ensure the formation of a 3D polymer network.

Dimer acid dimethacrylate of N'Durance (Fig. 7.4) is a dimer acid derivative monomer which also contains a core including an aromatic moiety, urethane groups, and two side arms. It is stated that this high-molecular-weight monomer is responsible for high conversion, low shrinkage, and increased hydrophobicity.

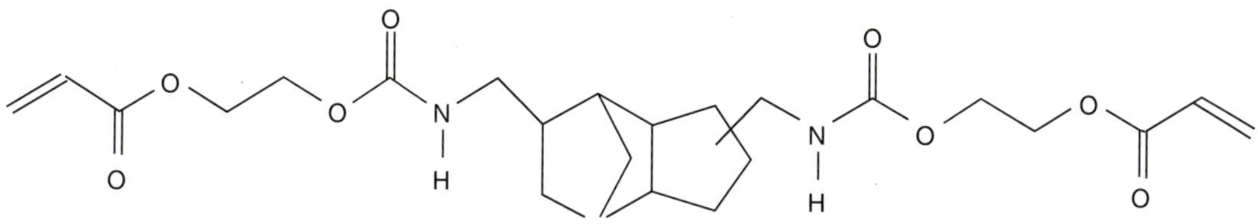

Fig. 7.2 TCD-DI-HEA, a cross-linking low-shrinkage monomer in Venus Diamond (Heraeus Kulzer)

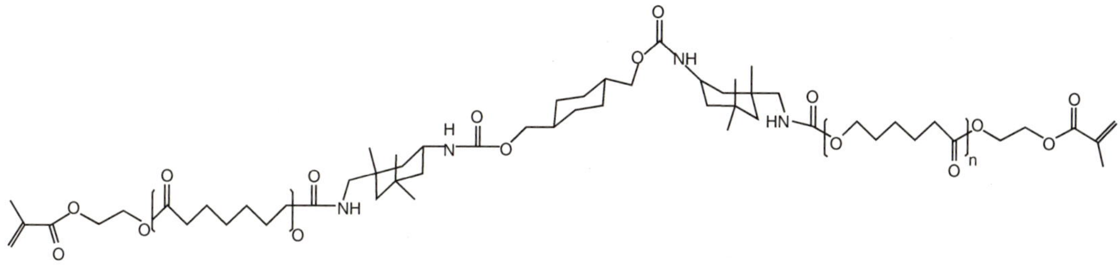

Fig. 7.3 DX-511, a cross-linking low-shrinkage monomer in Kalore (GC)

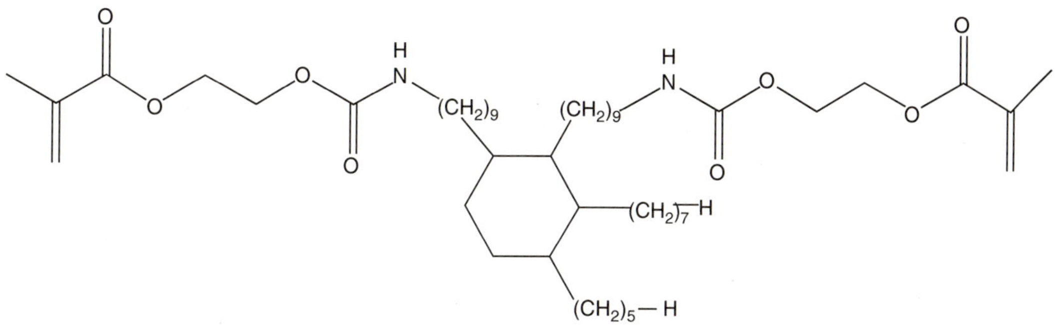

Fig. 7.4 DDCDMA, a cross-linking monomer in N'Durance

7.3 Properties of Commercial Low-Shrinkage Composites

7.3.1 Monomer Conversion

Monomer conversion in low-shrinkage composites varies much to the same extent as in any other group or class of composite materials. Moreover, the degree of conversion of low-shrinkage composites is generally in the same range as other composites. Only individual differences between materials were reported. For example, Premise showed about 10% higher degree of conversion than Grandio (61–74% and 55–63%, respectively) for a number of curing conditions and curing lights [61, 62], whereas Venus Diamond and AElite LS Posterior were in the range of 58–65%, hence comparable to Grandio [62]. A study by Yamasaki et al. [30] reported higher degree of conversion for N'Durance than Filtek Silorane and Kalore. Boaro et al. [34] found similar or higher degree of conversion for low-shrinkage composites (N'Durance, AElite LS Posterior) compared to the microfilled Heliomolar, microhybrid Filtek Z250, and nanofilled Filtek Supreme but lower than microhybrid Point 4.

The degree of conversion of Filtek Silorane has been a challenge due to its unique monomer chemistry. Two studies found unexpectedly low degrees of conversion (30–40%) for Filtek

Silorane [30, 34]. Conversely, a degree of conversion in the range of 70–83% was found for Filtek Silorane in another study [62]. Currently, Fourier transform infrared spectroscopy (FTIR) or micro-Raman spectroscopy are the two methods used to determine monomer conversion in dental composites. In methacrylate-based composites, the ratio of aliphatic (1640 cm^{-1}) and aromatic C=C bonds (1610 cm^{-1}) [63] or aliphatic to vinyl group (6155 cm^{-1}) [34] in cured and uncured materials is commonly used to calculate the degree of conversion. With its different monomer chemistry, Filtek Silorane presents a certain difficulty in identifying the appropriate peaks associated with oxirane-opening rings and internal standard groups that remain unchanged during polymerization. About 20% difference in the degree of conversion was reported when two different peak areas associated with epoxy groups (4156 and 4071 cm^{-1}) were used for calculation [30]. Comparing epoxy C-O-C rings at 883 cm^{-1} with the reference CH bond at 1257 cm^{-1} resulted in up to 50% higher conversion [62]. It may be assumed that certain differences would exist between studies but not as high as 20% or 50% given the fact that it is customary to set up an experiment to produce the highest degree of conversion for relevant curing conditions. Differences in monomer conversion observed for Filtek Silorane seem more related to the choice of peaks in FTIR/Raman spectra than to the material or experimental setup, pointing out the need to determine a more appropriate method to calculate the degree of conversion of Filtek Silorane.

7.3.2 Polymerization Shrinkage and Shrinkage Stress

Lower shrinkage was reported for early materials from this group, Inten-S and AElite LS Posterior, compared to microhybrid composites [64]. However, shrinkage stress was similar or higher than microfilled and microhybrid controls with consequently greater microleakage around Class V restorations [65]. Later studies reported inconsistent findings on AElite LS Posterior, ranging from lower shrinkage and/or shrinkage stress compared to microfilled, microhybrid, and nanofilled control composites [10, 66, 67] to no better than the control composites [27].

Lower shrinkage (1.3–1.5%) was found for Filtek Silorane than other low-shrinkage composites Premise, Clearfil Majesty Posterior [39], N'Durance [34], AElite LS Posterior [34, 67], and ELS [34, 39]. Filtek Silorane also exhibited lower shrinkage (~1.5%) than various other composites: compomer Dyract Extra (Dentsply), giomer Beautifil II (Shofu), microhybrid Esthet-X (Dentsply), Filtek Z250 (3M ESPE) [31, 34], Point 4 (Kerr), microfilled Heliomolar (Ivoclar Vivadent) [34, 67], nano-ceramic Ceram-X (Dentsply) [39], and nanofilled Filtek Supreme (3M ESPE) [31, 34], which were all in the range of 2.2–3.2% [31]. Linear axial shrinkage of Filtek Silorane (~1%) was also lower than that of Filtek Z250 (2.3%) [44]. Other low-shrinkage composites Kalore (1.8%) and Venus Diamond (1.7%) had lower shrinkage than Filtek Z250 (2.0%) despite a different measurement technique, micro-computed tomography [68].

Li et al. [69] introduced a noncontact technique, digital image correlation, based on a single camera, for shrinkage strain measurements and used Premise as a model composite. By measuring local shrinkage fields across material depth, they found that the maximum volumetric shrinkage of 1.5% occurred 1 mm below the irradiated surface. This finding was explained by reduced monomer conversion at the surface due to the presence of an oxygen inhibition layer.

Regarding shrinkage stress, Venus Diamond showed lower values than Filtek Silorane using two measurement techniques, strain-stress analyzer and universal testing machine [26]. Venus Diamond and Filtek Silorane had lower shrinkage than AElite LS Poster, ELS, and N'Durance with values for all ranging between 1.4% (Venus) and 2.4% (N'Durance). However, shrinkage stress showed different pattern (ELS < Venus Diamond < AElite LS Posterior < Filtek

Silorane < N'Durance) with values ranging from 2.7 MPa (ELS) to 4.6 MPa (N'Durance). The tested low-shrinkage composites did not present improvements compared to microfilled, nanofiller, and microhybrid control composites (Durafill, Heliomolar, Filtek Supreme, Filtek Z250, and Point 4) [27]. Venus Diamond consistently showed lower shrinkage stress (0.6–2.5 MPa) than other low-shrinkage composites Kalore (2.7–4.7 MPa) and Reflexions (3.3–6.9 MPa) as well as the microfilled Heliomolar (4–6 MPa) though shrinkage followed a different trend: Reflexions (1.8%) < Kalore (2%) < Heliomolar (2.3%) < Venus Diamond (2.5%) [60].

One study where a similar trend was observed between shrinkage and shrinkage stress was by Yamasaki et al. [30] who reported shrinkage in the order of Filtek P90 (1.7%) < Kalore (1.9%) < N'Durance (2.2%) and shrinkage stress Filtek P90 (2.6 MPa) < Kalore (2.7 MPa) < N'Durance (3.6 MPa). High shrinkage stress of N'Durance was explained by high monomer conversion (45%) after material vitrification [30]. On the other hand, lower shrinkage and conversion beyond the vitrification point are likely reasons for lower shrinkage stress of Kalore and Filtek P90 [30].

Monomer conversion beyond the gel point leads to post-gel shrinkage. Shrinkage stress was found to correlate with post-gel shrinkage but not total shrinkage [27, 46]. Mathematical modeling confirmed that shrinkage stress is related to post-gel shrinkage, but also to elastic modulus and a number of increments during placement [10]. Total shrinkage may be related to the shrinkage rate at the beginning of polymerization [29]. Filtek Silorane and Kalore showed lower shrinkage rate over the first 5 s of light curing than the control microhybrid, giomer, and nanofilled composites resulting in generally lower total shrinkage [29].

A study by Watts and Alnazzawi [70] found that shrinkage-stress rate was dependent on temperature, this being more pronounced in methacrylate-based composites than low-shrinkage composites based on high-molecular-weight monomers (Kalore and Venus Diamond). Generally higher final stress was found for methacrylate-based composites but not Kalore and Venus Diamond which showed stress compensation ability [70]. Conflicting findings were reported by Jongsma and Kleverlaan [71] in that higher final shrinkage and shrinkage stress occurred in Venus Diamond and Premise as well as microhybrid controls at elevated temperatures (37 and 44 °C) than room temperature (23 °C). The highest shrinkage and stress leap occurred between 23 and 30 °C. Therefore, a balance is required between the beneficial increase in monomer conversion and adverse increase in shrinkage stress by preheating composites in clinical practice. There is no conclusive evidence that preheating material has a positive clinical effect on composite restorations.

One of the first bulk-fill composites on the market, SDR (Dentsply), exhibited significantly lower shrinkage stress of 1.1 MPa than Filtek Silorane (3.6 MPa) [28]. The flowable nature of SDR and stress-relieving sites within the growing polymer were associated with reduced shrinkage stress.

7.3.3 Mechanical Properties

Higher flexural strength and modulus of Filtek Silorane than Kalore and N'Durance were associated with its highest cross-link density [30]. In another study, higher flexural strength and modulus of Filtek Silorane than the microfilled Heliomolar were associated with the filler composition [67]. Despite virtually the same percentage of fillers in Filtek Silorane (76 wt%) and Heliomolar (77 wt%), the former contains predominantly quartz particles which are harder than prepolymerized and amorphous silica particles in the latter. Similar flexural strength and modulus were found for low-shrinkage and microhybrid, microfilled, and nanofilled control composites [34]. Kalore exhibited lower and Venus Diamond similar flexural strength and modulus compared to the microhybrid Filtek Z250 [68]. Flexible high-molecular-weight monomer DX-511 and prepolymerized fillers seem to compromise mechanical properties of Kalore. Also lower flexural modulus, found for Filtek Silorane and AElite LS Posterior compared to Filtek Z250, was accounted for lower shrinkage stress of the low-shrinkage composites than Filtek Z250 [41].

A battery of physical tests were used to compare Filtek Silorane with various methacrylate-based composites: giomer Beautifil II, compomer Dyract Extra, microhybrid Filtek Z250 and Esthet-X [31], ormocer Admira, nanohybrid Tetric EvoCeram, Synergy D6 and Grandio [25], and nanofilled Filtek Supreme [25, 31]. Compressive strength [31] and dynamic modulus of elasticity [25] of Filtek Silorane were inferior to other composites, while other properties (diametral flexural strength, flexural strength and modulus, fracture toughness, and hardness) were similar to most control composites. Knoop hardness was higher than that of compomer [31]. Knoop and Vickers hardness showed moderate values for Filtek Silorane, no worse than most control composites [25, 31]. Mixed performance of Filtek Silorane was very difficult to explain due to differences in resin composition, filler type, size, and fraction. Lower compressive strength and dynamic modulus of elasticity suggest that Filtek Silorane may not be recommended for areas of high occlusal load.

Grandio, another low-shrinkage composite, showed higher hardness, elastic moduli than most control composites and similar flexural strength [25]. Such good mechanical properties are certainly due to high filler content of Grandio (87 wt%). High elastic modulus of Grandio may be associated with its relatively high shrinkage stress [72, 73], thus, restraining the use of Grandio in cavities with low C-factor.

Two studies compared the performance of low-shrinkage composites Filtek P90/Silorane [32] and Venus Diamond [74] to the microhybrid control Filtek Z250. As expected, fracture resistance of restored teeth deteriorated with cavity extension and/or cusp weakening. Filtek P90 (Silorane) performed comparable to Filtek Z250 in terms of fracture resistance and fracture pattern of restored teeth [32]. Conversely, Venus Diamond resulted in better fracture resistance, marginal integrity, and smaller cusp deformation than Filtek Z250 in restored premolars [74]. These similarities between Venus Diamond and Filtek Z250 could be associated with comparable flexural strength and modulus [68].

7.3.4 Sorption and Solubility

Low-shrinkage composites generally have lower sorption than control microhybrid, microfilled, and nanofilled composites. However, the results for solubility were somewhat inconsistent [34]. Conflicting data for low-shrinkage composite were reported in another study [33]. Filtek Silorane had lower water sorption and solubility than the microfilled Heliomolar and nanohybrid Tetric EvoCeram [33]. Increased hydrophobicity of resin in low-shrinkage composites based on either silorane, high-molecular weight monomers or BisEMA are likely reasons for low affinity to water and low sorption and solubility of low-shrinkage composites.

7.3.5 Elution

Kopperud et al. [37] followed elution from Filtek Silorane in water and ethanol for 72 h and found 4 silorane monomers and iodonium salt but no camphorquinone eluates in ethanol. No elution was detected in water. Quantification of eluates was impossible because monomers were not available as reference materials [37].

Similarly, initiator camphorquinone, inhibitor BHT, and UV stabilizer benzophenone were found to elute in methanol but not in water from ELS. As high as 950 μmol/L of benzophenone was detected while the amounts of camphorquinone and BHT were much lower, about 6 μmol/L and 10 μmol/L, respectively [75]. These findings are not surprising as greater elution from dental composites was found in ethanol than water in previous studies [76, 77]. This is due to the organic nature of the solvent and hydrophobic nature of dental composites which result in greater ethanol than water uptake by composite materials and subsequent dissolution [78].

7.3.6 Esthetic Properties

Esthetic properties of low-shrinkage composite were reported in only a few studies. Similar color changes were reported for Filtek Silorane and the control microhybrid Filtek Z250, ormocer Admira, and nanofilled Filtek Supreme following storage in colored beverages (red wine, coffee, cola, tea) and water. The greatest color changes were induced by red wine [35]. Color change of AElite LS Posterior induced by mouthwashes was found to be among those for other composites, nanoceramic Ceram-X, and nanofilled Filtek Supreme. Though the values were within the clinically acceptable range, Listerin mouthwash induced the greatest color change in AElite LS Posterior [79]. More important are color changes that occur in composites during polymerization as these values were found to exceed the clinically acceptable range for a number of materials including the low-shrinkage Premise [80].

7.4 Clinical Considerations

7.4.1 Marginal Adaptation

Generally low-shrinkage composites benefit from the "layering" placement technique. Favorable effect of the "layering" techniques on bond strength to dentin was found for N'Durance, Kalore, and Filtek Silorane [42]. However, an increase in C-factor adversely affected bonding of Filtek Silorane especially if it is placed in "bulk" [40]. This finding was associated with challenging adaptation of stiff Filtek Silorane to the cavity walls. In addition to the "layering" technique, curing a flowable liner if one is used beneath Filtek Silorane was also recommended [40]. Increased C-factor affected bond strength to dentin of Filtek Silorane and AElite LS Posterior to a smaller extent than that of the microhybrid Filtek Z250. This result was associated with lower shrinkage stress of low-shrinkage composites than the microhybrid control [41].

The best marginal adaptation and highest bond strength to dentin for Filtek Silorane is obtained using its dedicated adhesive system [42]. This did not hold for other methacrylate-based low-shrinkage composites, as it was shown that adhesive systems and composite from the same manufacturer do not necessarily result in the highest bond strength to dentin [81]. For example, Premise showed the best results with two-step self-etch adhesive Clearfil SE Bond (Kuraray) and worst with two-step etch-rinse adhesive from the same manufacturer (Optibond Solo Plus; Kerr) [81].

Low-shrinkage Filtek Silorane and AElite LS Posterior exerted smaller cuspal deformation than the nanofilled Filtek Supreme (3M ESPE) which was associated with lower post-gel shrinkage, smaller number of increments and lower elastic modulus [10, 45]. An optimal balance of post-gel shrinkage and elastic modulus were suggested reasons for lower cuspal deformation reported for Filtek Silorane and Kalore but not for Premise and Reflexions compared to the control Filtek Supreme composite [46].

7.4.2 Filtek Silorane Adhesive System

As the composition of Filtek Silorane is radically different than that of methacrylate-based composites, a new adhesive system was developed for adequate bonding to tooth tissues. Siloxane moiety is responsible for hydrophobicity of the silorane monomer, lower water sorption, and solubility of Filtek Silorane than methacrylate-based composites [33]. The designated adhesive system must overcome the greater hydrophilic-to-hydrophobic "conversion" between tooth substrate, particularly dentin, and silorane-based restorations. Silorane adhesive is designed as a two-step self-etch system: hydrophilic primer is based on a mixture of acidic methacrylate monomers that partially demineralize enamel and dentin as the first step. Hydrophobic bond contains hydrophobic dimethacrylates tailored for interaction with the primer on one side and oxirane groups of silorane on the other. Silorane adhesive system differs from other two-step self-etch adhesives in that primer and bond are cured separately.

Given the fact that primer and bond are cured separately, it is seems more relevant to compare the hybrid layer of Silorane adhesive to one-step than two-step self-etch systems. Santini and Miletic [82] reported thinner hybrid layer of Silorane adhesive compared to etch-and-rinse adhesives but similar or thicker than one-step self-etch adhesives. Resin tags were 2–3 μm thick and somewhat funnel shaped but without any significant lateral branching (Fig. 7.5) [82]. As would be expected, Filtek Silorane was compatible only with its adhesive system; the use of phosphoric acid etching did not significantly improve bond strength to dentin but increased silver nanoleakage within the hybrid layer [83].

7.4.3 Clinical Trials

As shown in the previous section, Filtek Silorane has been the most frequently tested low-shrinkage composite in laboratory studies. In line with this is the researchers' inclination to test Filtek Silorane more often than other low-shrinkage composite materials in clinical trials. Only a few studies compared clinical performance of other low-shrinkage composites.

The early commercial low-shrinkage composite Inten-S was compared by Van Dijken and Lindberg to a microhybrid composite Point 4 (Kerr) over 5 and 15 years of clinical service [84, 85]. They found no significant differences between of the two composites in Class II cavities. Secondary caries was identified as the main reason for restoration failure after 5 years [84], while secondary caries and material fracture were the main reasons for restoration failure after 15 years [85].

Kramer et al. [86] evaluated Grandio and the control Tetric Ceram after 10 years of placement in Class II cavities. Marginal adaptation deteriorated continuously over the years resulting in progressive marginal discoloration in both tested composites. The main reasons for composite degradation were enamel cracks and material chipping. Grandio deteriorated more than the control in terms of surface roughness and color match indicating compromised esthetic properties.

Schmidt el al [52, 53]. compared Filtek Silorane to a nanoceramic composite, Ceram-X (Dentsply) in Class II restorations after 1 and 5 years. Ceram-X showed significantly better occlusal and gingival marginal adaptation after 1 year of clinical service, but no difference was found after 5 years. Furthermore, no significant differences were found between other modified USPHS criteria, namely, hypersensitivity, proximal contact, anatomic form, fracture, and secondary caries, and both composites were concluded to be acceptable for Class II cavities.

Filtek Silorane and Ceram-X were also compared by another group, Yaman et al. [55] in Class V restorations. A 3-year follow-up showed comparable performance by both composites.

Baracco et al. [47, 48] compared Filtek Silorane to a microhybrid composite, Filtek Z250 (3M ESPE) in Class I and II restorations after 2 and 5 years of clinical service using modified USPHS criteria. At follow-up periods, no significant difference was found between Filtek Silorane and Z250 combined with an etch-and-rinse adhesive. Z250 placed following a self-etch adhesive showed considerable marginal discoloration and was inferior to the former two groups.

Walter et al. [54] compared Filtek Silorane to a nanohybrid composite, Tetric EvoCeram (Ivoclar Vivadent) in Class II restorations after 3 years. More elaborate FDI criteria were used, but no differences were found between the two composites. It was interesting to note that among the esthetic criteria, the ones with lowest scores were color stability and translucency; fracture and retention were mostly compromised in the functional group and periodontal response in the biological group of the evaluated criteria.

Burke et al. [49] followed Filtek Silorane as Class I and II restorative 2 years after placement in a UK practice-based research network. Overall satisfactory clinical performance was concluded.

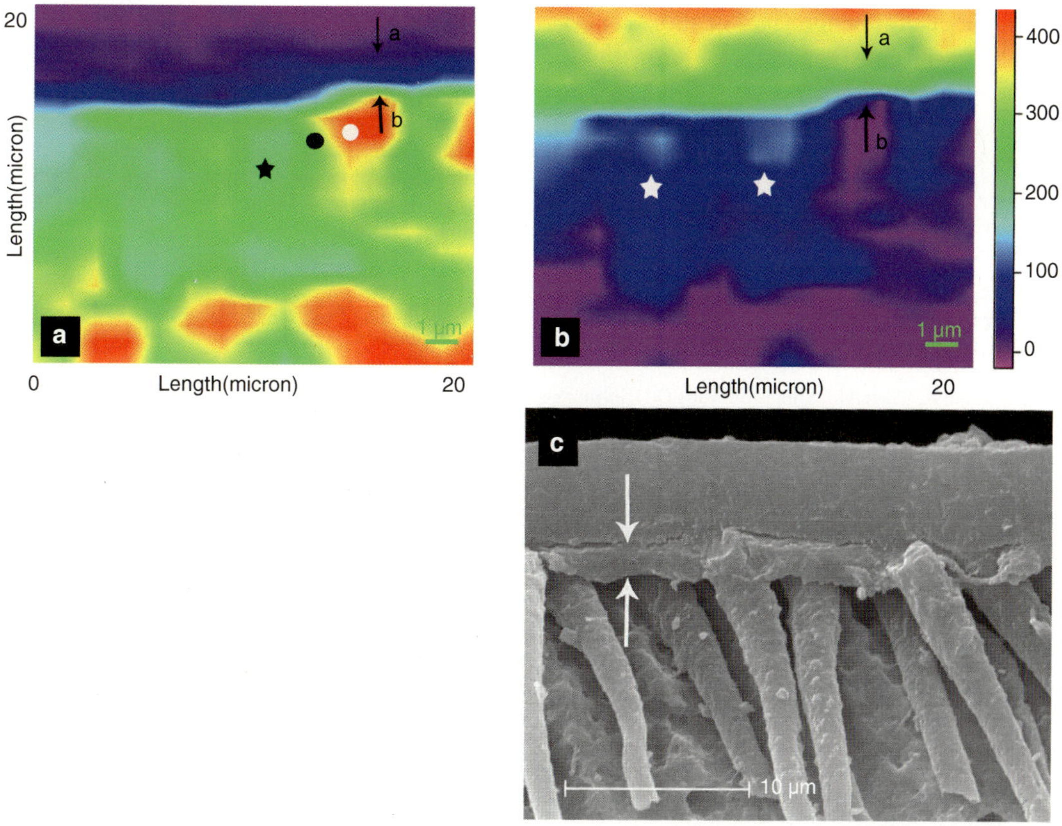

Fig. 7.5 Silorane adhesive-dentin interface visualized using micro-Raman spectroscopy and SEM. (**a**) A 2D map of dentin containing different intensity of spectral features ranging from the least intense area corresponding to demineralized dentin (point "a," *black arrow*) to maximum intensity area corresponding to unaffected dentin (point "b," *black arrow*). The *black star* indicates a dentinal tubule, the *black circle* peritubular dentin, and the *white circle* intertubular dentin. (**b**) Identical specimen area and the range of intensity of spectral features associated with Silorane adhesive starting from maximum intensity at the adhesive layer (point "a," *black arrow*) to the minimum intensity at the bottom of the hybrid layer (point "b," *black arrow*). The *white star* indicates a resin tag. The color scale shows intensity (arbitrary units). The area between points "a" and "b" corresponds to the hybrid layer. (**c**) An SEM micrograph of the same specimen used for micro-Raman spectroscopic analysis. The hybrid layer is indicated by *white arrows*. Reprinted from [82] with permission

However, the evaluated criteria did show signs of deterioration, especially marginal discoloration which was rated optimal in 77% of cases.

Popoff et al. [50, 51] followed the outcome of restoration repair using Filtek P90 and P60 (3M ESPE) after 1 and 2 years. Modified USPHS criteria were used, but no significant differences were observed between the two composites. Significantly worse marginal adaptation was found for Filtek P90 at 2 years compared to the baseline.

The reviewed clinical trials suggest that Filtek Silorane is as acceptable posterior restorative as other hybrid composites with no improvement in any of the clinically relevant esthetic, functional, or biological category. Marginal adaptation seems the most compromised aspect of Filtek Silorane restorations in clinical conditions.

In conclusion, low-shrinkage composites are a rather variable "class" of materials, both in composition and performance. Though shrinkage of some low-shrinkage composites does appear lower than conventional hybrid composites, other properties do not present any improvements. Mixed and inconsistent properties confirm the heterogeneity of this "class" of composites which does not allow the practitioner any predictability as to the clinical performance of these composites. Clinical trials confirm that low-shrinkage composites fail to improve clinical practice to a significant level and at best perform as good as conventional hybrid composites.

References

1. Kleverlaan CJ, Feilzer AJ. Polymerization shrinkage and contraction stress of dental resin composites. Dent Mater. 2005;21:1150–7.
2. Baroudi K, Saleh AM, Silikas N, Watts DC. Shrinkage behaviour of flowable resin-composites related to conversion and filler-fraction. J Dent. 2007;35:651–5.
3. Garcia D, Yaman P, Dennison J, Neiva G. Polymerization shrinkage and depth of cure of bulk fill flowable composite resins. Oper Dent. 2014;39:441–8.
4. Takemura Y, Hanaoka K, Kawamata R, Sakurai T, Teranaka T. Three-dimensional X-ray micro-computed tomography analysis of polymerization shrinkage vectors in flowable composite. Dent Mater J. 2014;33:476–83.
5. Hirata R, Clozza E, Giannini M, Farrokhmanesh E, Janal M, Tovar N, et al. Shrinkage assessment of low shrinkage composites using micro-computed tomography. J Biomed Mater Res B Appl Biomater. 2015;103:798–806.
6. Chuang SF, Chang CH, Chen TY. Spatially resolved assessments of composite shrinkage in MOD restorations using a digital-image-correlation technique. Dent Mater. 2011;27:134–43.
7. Van Ende A, Van de Casteele E, Depypere M, De Munck J, Li X, Maes F, et al. 3D volumetric displacement and strain analysis of composite polymerization. Dent Mater. 2015;31:453–61.
8. Davidson CL, Feilzer AJ. Polymerization shrinkage and polymerization shrinkage stress in polymer-based restoratives. J Dent. 1997;25:435–40.
9. Feilzer AJ, Dauvillier BS. Effect of TEGDMA/BisGMA ratio on stress development and viscoelastic properties of experimental two-paste composites. J Dent Res. 2003;82:824–8.
10. Bicalho AA, Valdivia AD, Barreto BC, Tantbirojn D, Versluis A, Soares CJ. Incremental filling technique and composite material--part II: shrinkage and shrinkage stresses. Oper Dent. 2014;39:E83–92.
11. Kim RJ, Kim YJ, Choi NS, Lee IB. Polymerization shrinkage, modulus, and shrinkage stress related to tooth-restoration interfacial debonding in bulk-fill composites. J Dent. 2015;43:430–9.
12. Ilie N, Jelen E, Clementino-Luedemann T, Hickel R. Low-shrinkage composite for dental application. Dent Mater J. 2007;26:149–55.
13. Al Sunbul H, Silikas N, Watts DC. Polymerization shrinkage kinetics and shrinkage-stress in dental resin-composites. Dent Mater. 2016;32:998–1006.
14. Ferracane JL, Hilton TJ. Polymerization stress–is it clinically meaningful? Dent Mater. 2016;32:1–10.
15. Opdam NJ, Bronkhorst EM, Roeters JM, Loomans BA. A retrospective clinical study on longevity of posterior composite and amalgam restorations. Dent Mater. 2007;23:2–8.
16. Braga RR, Ferracane JL. Alternatives in polymerization contraction stress management. Crit Rev Oral Biol Med. 2004;15:176–84.
17. Peutzfeldt A. Resin composites in dentistry: the monomer systems. Eur J Oral Sci. 1997;105:97–116.
18. Weinmann W, Thalacker C, Guggenberger R. Siloranes in dental composites. Dent Mater. 2005;21:68–74.
19. Eick JD, Smith RE, Pinzino CS, Kostoryz EL. Stability of silorane dental monomers in aqueous systems. J Dent. 2006;34:405–10.
20. Palin WM, Fleming GJ, Burke FJ, Marquis PM, Pintado MR, Randall RC, et al. The frictional coefficients and associated wear resistance of novel low-shrink resin-based composites. Dent Mater. 2005;21:1111–8.
21. Palin WM, Fleming GJ, Nathwani H, Burke FJ, Randall RC. In vitro cuspal deflection and microleakage of maxillary premolars restored with novel low-shrink dental composites. Dent Mater. 2005;21:324–35.
22. Yamazaki PC, Bedran-Russo AK, Pereira PN, Wsift EJ Jr. Microleakage evaluation of a new low-shrinkage composite restorative material. Oper Dent. 2006;31:670–6.
23. Schweikl H, Schmalz G, Weinmann W. The induction of gene mutations and micronuclei by oxiranes and siloranes in mammalian cells in vitro. J Dent Res. 2004;83:17–21.
24. 3M ESPE. Filtek(TM) Silorane, Low shrink posterior restorative; Silorane adhesive system, Self-Etch Primer & Bond, 2007.
25. Leprince J, Palin WM, Mullier T, Devaux J, Vreven J, Leloup G. Investigating filler morphology and mechanical properties of new low-shrinkage resin composite types. J Oral Rehabil. 2010;37:364–76.
26. Marchesi G, Breschi L, Antoniolli F, Di Lenarda R, Ferracane J, Cadenaro M. Contraction stress of low-shrinkage composite materials assessed with different testing systems. Dent Mater. 2010;26:947–53.
27. Boaro LC, Goncalves F, Guimaraes TC, Ferracane JL, Versluis A, Braga RR. Polymerization stress, shrinkage and elastic modulus of current low-shrinkage restorative composites. Dent Mater. 2010;26:1144–50.
28. Ilie N, Hickel R. Investigations on a methacrylate-based flowable composite based on the SDR technology. Dent Mater. 2011;27:348–55.
29. Naoum SJ, Ellakwa A, Morgan L, White K, Martin FE, Lee IB. Polymerization profile analysis of resin composite dental restorative materials in real time. J Dent. 2012;40:64–70.
30. Yamasaki LC, De Vito Moraes AG, Barros M, Lewis S, Francci C, Stansbury JW, et al. Polymerization development of "low-shrink" resin composites: reac-

tion kinetics, polymerization stress and quality of network. Dent Mater. 2013;29:e169–79.
31. Lien W, Vandewalle KS. Physical properties of a new silorane-based restorative system. Dent Mater. 2010;26:337–44.
32. Taha NA, Maghaireh GA, Bagheri R, Abu HA. Fracture strength of root filled premolar teeth restored with silorane and methacrylate-based resin composite. J Dent. 2015;43:735–41.
33. Giannini M, Di Francescantonio M, Pacheco RR, Cidreira Boaro LC, Braga RR. Characterization of water sorption, solubility, and roughness of silorane- and methacrylate-based composite resins. Oper Dent. 2014;39:264–72.
34. Boaro LC, Goncalves F, Guimaraes TC, Ferracane JL, Pfeifer CS, Braga RR. Sorption, solubility, shrinkage and mechanical properties of "low-shrinkage" commercial resin composites. Dent Mater. 2013;29:398–404.
35. Barutcigil C, Yildiz M. Intrinsic and extrinsic discoloration of dimethacrylate and silorane based composites. J Dent. 2012;40(Suppl 1):e57–63.
36. Buergers R, Schneider-Brachert W, Hahnel S, Rosentritt M, Handel G. Streptococcal adhesion to novel low-shrink silorane-based restorative. Dent Mater. 2009;25:269–75.
37. Kopperud HM, Schmidt M, Kleven IS. Elution of substances from a silorane-based dental composite. Eur J Oral Sci. 2010;118:100–2.
38. Bagis YH, Baltacioglu IH, Kahyaogullari S. Comparing microleakage and the layering methods of silorane-based resin composite in wide class II MOD cavities. Oper Dent. 2009;34:578–85.
39. Papadogiannis D, Kakaboura A, Palaghias G, Eliades G. Setting characteristics and cavity adaptation of low-shrinking resin composites. Dent Mater. 2009;25:1509–16.
40. Van Ende A, De Munck J, Mine A, Lambrechts P, Van Meerbeek B. Does a low-shrinking composite induce less stress at the adhesive interface? Dent Mater. 2010;26:215–22.
41. El-Sahn NA, El-Kassas DW, El-Damanhoury HM, Fahmy OM, Gomaa H, Platt JA. Effect of C-factor on microtensile bond strengths of low-shrinkage composites. Oper Dent. 2011;36:281–92.
42. Van Ende A, Mine A, De Munck J, Poitevin A, Van Meerbeek B. Bonding of low-shrinking composites in high C-factor cavities. J Dent. 2012;40:295–303.
43. Juloski J, Carrabba M, Aragoneses JM, Forner L, Vichi A, Ferrari M. Microleakage of class II restorations and microtensile bond strength to dentin of low-shrinkage composites. Am J Dent. 2013;26:271–7.
44. Kwon Y, Ferracane J, Lee IB. Effect of layering methods, composite type, and flowable liner on the polymerization shrinkage stress of light cured composites. Dent Mater. 2012;28:801–9.
45. Bicalho AA, Pereira RD, Zanatta RF, Franco SD, Tantbirojn D, Versluis A, et al. Incremental filling technique and composite material–part I: cuspal deformation, bond strength, and physical properties. Oper Dent. 2014;39:E71–82.
46. Tantbirojn D, Pfeifer CS, Braga RR, Versluis A. Do low-shrink composites reduce polymerization shrinkage effects? J Dent Res. 2011;90:596–601.
47. Baracco B, Fuentes MV, Ceballos L. Five-year clinical performance of a silorane- vs a methacrylate-based composite combined with two different adhesive approaches. Clin Oral Investig. 2016; 20:991–1001.
48. Baracco B, Perdigao J, Cabrera E, Ceballos L. Two-year clinical performance of a low-shrinkage composite in posterior restorations. Oper Dent. 2013;38:591–600.
49. Burke FJ, Crisp RJ, James A, Mackenzie L, Pal A, Sands P, et al. Two year clinical evaluation of a low-shrink resin composite material in UK general dental practices. Dent Mater. 2011;27:622–30.
50. Popoff DA, de Magalhaes CS, de Freitas OW, Soares LA, de Almeida Santa Rosa TT, Ferreira RC, et al. Two-year clinical performance of dimethacrylate based composite restorations repaired with a silorane-based composite. J Adhes Dent. 2014;16:575–83.
51. Popoff DA, Santa Rosa TT, Ferreira RC, Magalhaes CS, Moreira AN, Mjor IA. Repair of dimethacrylate-based composite restorations by a silorane-based composite: a one-year randomized clinical trial. Oper Dent. 2012;37:E1–10.
52. Schmidt M, Dige I, Kirkevang LL, Vaeth M, Horsted-Bindslev P. Five-year evaluation of a low-shrinkage Silorane resin composite material: a randomized clinical trial. Clin Oral Investig. 2015;19:245–51.
53. Schmidt M, Kirkevang LL, Horsted-Bindslev P, Poulsen S. Marginal adaptation of a low-shrinkage silorane-based composite: 1-year randomized clinical trial. Clin Oral Investig. 2011;15:291–5.
54. Walter R, Boushell LW, Heymann HO, Ritter AV, Sturdevant JR, Wilder AD Jr, et al. Three-year clinical evaluation of a silorane composite resin. J Esthet Restor Dent. 2014;26:179–90.
55. Yaman BC, Dogruer I, Gumustas B, Efes BG. Three-year randomized clinical evaluation of a low-shrinkage silorane-based resin composite in non-carious cervical lesions. Clin Oral Investig. 2014;18:1071–9.
56. Santini A, Miletic V, Swift MD, Bradley M. Degree of conversion and microhardness of TPO-containing resin-based composites cured by polywave and monowave LED units. J Dent. 2012;40:577–84.
57. Miletic V, Pongprueksa P, De Munck J, Brooks NR, Van Meerbeek B. Curing characteristics of flowable and sculptable bulk-fill composites. Clin Oral Investig. 2016;21(4):1201–12.
58. Czasch P, Ilie N. In vitro comparison of mechanical properties and degree of cure of a self-adhesive and four novel flowable composites. J Adhes Dent. 2013;15:229–36.
59. Pongprueksa P, De Munck J, Duca RC, Poels K, Covaci A, Hoet P, et al. Monomer elution in relation to degree of conversion for different types of composite. J Dent. 2015;43:1448–55.

60. Yamamoto T, Kubota Y, Momoi Y, Ferracane JL. Polymerization stresses in low-shrinkage dental resin composites measured by crack analysis. Dent Mater. 2012;28:e143–9.
61. Hadis M, Leprince JG, Shortall AC, Devaux J, Leloup G, Palin WM. High irradiance curing and anomalies of exposure reciprocity law in resin-based materials. J Dent. 2011;39:549–57.
62. Lee SK, Kim TW, Son SA, Park JK, Kim JH, Kim HI, et al. Influence of light-curing units on the polymerization of low-shrinkage composite resins. Dent Mater J. 2013;32:688–94.
63. Miletic VJ, Santini A. Remaining unreacted methacrylate groups in resin-based composite with respect to sample preparation and storing conditions using micro-Raman spectroscopy. J Biomed Mater Res B Appl Biomater. 2008;87:468–74.
64. Yap AU, Soh MS. Post-gel polymerization contraction of "low shrinkage" composite restoratives. Oper Dent. 2004;29:182–7.
65. Calheiros FC, Sadek FT, Braga RR, Cardoso PE. Polymerization contraction stress of low-shrinkage composites and its correlation with microleakage in class V restorations. J Dent. 2004;32:407–12.
66. Cadenaro M, Biasotto M, Scuor N, Breschi L, Davidson CL, Di Lenarda R. Assessment of polymerization contraction stress of three composite resins. Dent Mater. 2008;24:681–5.
67. Arrais CA, Oliveira MT, Mettenburg D, Rueggeberg FA, Giannini M. Silorane- and high filled-based "low-shrinkage" resin composites: shrinkage, flexural strength and modulus. Braz Oral Res. 2013;27:97–102.
68. de Oliveira DC, Rovaris K, Hass V, Souza-Junior EJ, Haiter-Neto F, Sinhoreti MA. Effect of low shrinkage monomers on physicochemical properties of dental resin composites. Braz Dent J. 2015;26:272–6.
69. Li J, Fok ASL, Satterthwaite J, Watts DC. Measurement of the full-field polymerization shrinkage and depth of cure of dental composites using digital image correlation. Dent Mater. 2009;25:582–8.
70. Watts DC, Alnazzawi A. Temperature-dependent polymerization shrinkage stress kinetics of resin-composites. Dent Mater. 2014;30:654–60.
71. Jongsma LA, Kleverlaan CJ. Influence of temperature on volumetric shrinkage and contraction stress of dental composites. Dent Mater. 2015;31:721–5.
72. Pereira RA, Araujo PA, Castaneda-Espinosa JC, Mondelli RF. Comparative analysis of the shrinkage stress of composite resins. J Appl Oral Sci. 2008;16:30–4.
73. Pick B, Pelka M, Belli R, Braga RR, Lohbauer U. Tailoring of physical properties in highly filled experimental nanohybrid resin composites. Dent Mater. 2011;27:664–9.
74. Barreto Bde C, Van Meerbeek B, Van Ende A, Sousa SJ, Silva GR, Soares PV, et al. Biomechanical behavior of extensively restored premolars: cusp deformation, marginal integrity, and fracture resistance. J Adhes Dent. 2015;17:213–8.
75. Hogg C, Maier M, Dettinger-Maier K, He X, Rothmund L, Kehe K, et al. Effect of various light curing times on the elution of composite components. Clin Oral Investig. 2015;20(8):2113–21.
76. Manojlovic D, Radisic M, Lausevic M, Zivkovic S, Miletic V. Mathematical modeling of cross-linking monomer elution from resin-based dental composites. J Biomed Mater Res B Appl Biomater. 2013;101:61–7.
77. Tabatabaei MH, Sadrai S, Bassir SH, Veisy N, Dehghan S. Effect of food stimulated liquids and thermocycling on the monomer elution from a nanofilled composite. Open Dent J. 2013;7:62–7.
78. Zhang Y, Xu J. Effect of immersion in various media on the sorption, solubility, elution of unreacted monomers, and flexural properties of two model dental composite compositions. J Mater Sci Mater Med. 2008;19:2477–83.
79. Celik C, Yuzugullu B, Erkut S, Yamanel K. Effects of mouth rinses on color stability of resin composites. Eur J Dent. 2008;2:247–53.
80. Celik EU, Aladag A, Turkun LS, Yilmaz G. Color changes of dental resin composites before and after polymerization and storage in water. J Esthet Restor Dent. 2011;23:179–88.
81. Thomsen KB, Peutzfeldt A. Resin composites: strength of the bond to dentin versus mechanical properties. Clin Oral Investig. 2007;11:45–9.
82. Santini A, Miletic V. Comparison of the hybrid layer formed by Silorane adhesive, one-step self-etch and etch and rinse systems using confocal micro-Raman spectroscopy and SEM. J Dent. 2008;36:683–91.
83. Duarte S Jr, Phark JH, Varjao FM, Sadan A. Nanoleakage, ultramorphological characteristics, and microtensile bond strengths of a new low-shrinkage composite to dentin after artificial aging. Dent Mater. 2009;25:589–600.
84. van Dijken JW, Lindberg A. Clinical effectiveness of a low-shrinkage resin composite: a five-year evaluation. J Adhes Dent. 2009;11:143–8.
85. van Dijken JW, Lindberg A. A 15-year randomized controlled study of a reduced shrinkage stress resin composite. Dent Mater. 2015;31:1150–8.
86. Kramer N, Reinelt C, Frankenberger R. Ten-year clinical performance of posterior resin composite restorations. J Adhes Dent. 2015;17:433–41.

Bulk-Fill Composites

8

Annelies Van Ende

The indications to use composites as a minimally invasive restorative in the posterior region have increased considerably in the latest years. While not so long ago, composites were considered unsuitable to restore extensive lesions in the posterior, load-bearing area, new clinical evidence shows favorable outcomes for cusp-replacing restorations in posterior composites [1]. These findings are especially important in light of the phasedown of the use of amalgam [2], which calls for new treatment alternatives in these clinical situations. With the increasing use of composites in extreme indications, convenience and simplicity of these materials have become increasingly important.

Classically, a restoration is placed in increments that are cured separately. The limited depth of cure of conventional composites, usually no more than 2 or 2.5 mm, has precluded the use of thicker layers. Another reason to opt for an incremental technique is to reduce the polymerization shrinkage stress [3–5], although this argument has also been contradicted [6–8]. Low-shrinkage composites were developed to manage shrinkage-induced stress, but layering was still required due to the limited depth of cure [9].

A. Van Ende
TP Van Ende, Kinrooi, Belgium
e-mail: annelies.vanende@gmail.com

Bulk-filling, as opposed to the incremental technique, obviously offers attractive benefits, since the latter can be very time-consuming, especially in large cavities. Moreover, the risk of including voids or gaps between the consecutive layers can be avoided. However, several criteria should be met before a composite is truly eligible for bulk-filling. The restorative must be able to be polymerized at the full depth of the restoration. Shrinkage stress should be reduced to a minimum. Meanwhile, the handling properties should enable the placement of composite without the inclusion of air and voids. Finally, the composite must have sufficient resistance to fracture and wear to endure the occlusal forces in the posterior region.

8.1 Classification and Composition

Although bulk-fill is a rather recent term for composites that can be placed without the necessity of using an incremental technique, the concept is not new; composites with similar properties already existed on the market before the introduction of this terminology with the launch of SDR posterior flowable base (Dentsply; Surefil SDR flow in America). The depth of cure of Quixfil (Dentsply), a high-viscosity posterior restorative from the same company, is also claimed to be 4 mm. Moreover, some light-cured core buildup materials (e.g., Clearfil Photo Core,

V. Miletic (ed.), *Dental Composite Materials for Direct Restorations*,
http://doi.org/10.1007/978-3-319-60961-4_8

Kuraray) are also claimed to be suitable for bulk placement with a depth of cure beyond 4 mm.

Usually, bulk-fill composites are divided in high-viscosity [10] and flowable [11] composites. The flowable composites usually require an additional capping layer, while the high-viscosity composites do not [12, 13].

An outsider in this classification is SonicFill 2 (Kerr) (the successor of SonicFill, Kerr), which has a high viscosity that decreases considerably when the material is sonicated [14] and thus does not strictly belong to either of the groups.

It has been pointed out in the scientific literature that differences between individual composites are more distinct than differences between bulk-fill and conventional composites [15].

Hence, it is not surprising that their chemical composition is not particularly different from other conventional composites. Some composites have unique constituents. Tetric EvoCeram Bulk Fill (Ivoclar Vivadent) contains a patented germanium-based photoinitiator, called Ivocerin [16], which has a higher potency than the traditional photoinitiator camphorquinone, albeit at lower peak wavelength. A patented urethane-based methacrylate resin incorporating a photoactive group is included in SDR (Dentsply) to alter the radical polymerization process [17].

8.2 Clinical Evidence

Since bulk-fill composites are a rather new class, no long-term studies are available at the moment. Some results on the medium term have been published by Manhart et al. [18] on Quixfill and by Van Dijken et al. [19] on SDR. Those studies show that in a period of up to 5 years, those two bulk-fill composites do not perform significantly different from conventional composite restorations in the posterior, load-bearing area. However, this does not mean that those results can be extrapolated to other bulk-fill materials, as their properties vary widely. No randomized controlled clinical trials exist for any of the high-viscosity composites. More controlled clinical trials that exclusively focus on extensive (comprising a wide isthmus or replacing at least one cusp), deep restorations are necessary to elucidate whether they are truly suitable for these indications. The currently available evidence is clearly not substantial enough to make definitive conclusions.

8.3 Laboratory Properties

When a considerable volume of composite is placed in load-bearing areas, good mechanical properties are required. Extensive studies have been conducted comparing the flexural strength of several flowable and high-viscosity bulk-fill composites [13, 20–22]. Overall, the high-viscosity bulk-fill composites have better mechanical properties such as flexural strength and fracture toughness than their flowable counterparts; however, variations between the individual products are so large that it would be ill-considered to make general conclusions. When looking at the individual products, we find that some flowable bulk-fill composites consistently show better strength than some of the high-viscosity bulk-fill composites [13, 20–22]. On the other hand, wear resistance will be less relevant for the flowable bulk-fill composites, since the manufacturers instruct to cap them with a conventional composite [12, 13, 15].

Another thought that deserves consideration is that the finally constituted polymer network of the composite and its properties are not entirely homogeneous. What mostly seems to distinguish bulk-fill composites from other conventional composites is the claim that their depth of cure is increased to 4 mm or beyond. In the literature, there are large variations in the measured depth of cure of bulk-fill composites [21, 23–34], which can easily be explained by the differences in setup. Besides the fact that the depth of cure is not only dependent of the restorative but also on the used light source, irradiation parameters, and the timing of the measurements, there is no consensus on how an acceptable depth of cure should be established. Several methods have been used, such as microhardness measurements and degree of conversion. However, maximum hardness and degree of conversion that can be obtained are dependent on the composition of the composites and, even so, do not reflect the quality of the polymer network *per se* [35, 36]. Hence, it becomes rather difficult to claim an absolute depth as the depth of cure. Nevertheless, some observations can be made. Irradiance of composites will inevitably drop with decreasing depth because of attenuation due to absorption, scattering, and reflection [35]. Hence, the better light at wavelengths absorbed by the used initiators (camphorquinone has a peak absorbance around 468 nm [37] and the germanium-based Ivocerin around 408 nm [32], respectively) can pass (lower attenuation coefficient); the closer the quality of the cured resin will be in the deeper layers. Indeed, it has been confirmed that bulk-fill materials are more translucent [28, 38–40] than conventional composites. The flowable bulk-fill composites tend to be more translucent than the high-viscosity composites. As a result, they also tend to cure faster [33]. This increased translucency might result in esthetical compromises, although the more translucent flowable variants are masked by their capping layer. Another observation is that short curing times might not be sufficient to reach optimum levels of conversion in deeper layers, which once again confirms that the "exposure reciprocity law" is not absolute [41–43]. Shorter exposure to a higher irradiance renders inferior mechanical properties in depth when compared to a longer exposure to lower irradiance [10, 11, 32].

While the volumetric shrinkage of the high-viscosity bulk-fill composites is comparable with that of conventional posterior composites, with reported values around 2%, shrinkage of the flowable bulk-fill composites tends to be somewhat higher, around 3% [25, 44].

8.4 Adaptation, Shrinkage Stress, and Handling

Ideally, a restoration should seal the cavity outline perfectly without the occurrence of gaps. There are two main causes for the occurrence of gaps and voids in a restoration that are caused by the restorative rather than the adhesive: air inclusion during insertion due to the handling properties [45] and gaps arising due to shrinkage of the material [25, 46]. Unlike amalgam, composites are not condensable materials. Handling is quite subjective and has not been widely studied in the literature. The viscosity of the bulk-fill materials is similar to conventional high-viscosity and flowable composites for both classes, respectively. However, it has been reported that it is difficult to achieve intimate adaptation with high-viscosity composites [45, 47], while with flowable composites, it is more difficult to achieve a tight proximal contact with the adjacent tooth [48].

In the ongoing research regarding shrinkage stress of bulk-fill composites, despite a multitude of publications [21, 49–51], results remain largely contradicting and inconclusive. One of the main reasons is that shrinkage stress is not a material property but depends largely on the compliance and the configuration of the cavity [52] as well as the development of the properties over time [53]. Most studies report lower shrinkage stress with bulk-fill composites when compared to conventional composites [21, 49, 54, 55], but differences found between the flowable and high-viscosity bulk-fill composites vary largely. Moreover, apart from some conflicting reports on cuspal strain [12, 56–58], the stress measurements do not take the application technique (single increment vs. multiple increments) into account.

Conclusion

While the mechanical properties of bulk-fill composites vary largely between the individual products, they are, in general, comparable to conventional composites. The main distinctive feature of bulk-fill composites is increased translucency and consequently increased depth of cure. In the short term, the use of bulk-fill composites renders clinical results that are comparable with conventional composite placement. However, since few products have been tested in clinical trials, it is too early to draw general conclusions.

References

1. Fennis WM, Kuijs RH, Roeters FJ, Creugers NH, Kreulen CM. Randomized control trial of composite cuspal restorations: five-year results. J Dent Res. 2014;93:36–41. doi:10.1177/0022034513510946.
2. Lynch CD, Wilson NHF. Managing the phase-down of amalgam: part II. Implications for practising arrangements and lessons from Norway. Br Dent J. 2013;215:159–62. doi:10.1038/sj.bdj.2013.788.
3. Lee MR, Cho BH, Son HH, Um CM, Lee IB. Influence of cavity dimension and restoration methods on the cusp deflection of premolars in composite restoration. Dent Mater. 2007;23:288–95. doi:10.1016/j.dental.2006.01.025.
4. Park J, Chang J, Ferracane J, Lee IB. How should composite be layered to reduce shrinkage stress: incremental or bulk filling? Dent Mater. 2008;24:1501–5. doi:10.1016/j.dental.2008.03.013.
5. Kwon Y, Ferracane J, Lee IB. Effect of layering methods, composite type, and flowable liner on the polymerization shrinkage stress of light cured composites. Dent Mater. 2012;28:801–9. doi:10.1016/j.dental.2012.04.028.
6. Bicalho AA, Pereira RD, Zanatta RF. Incremental filling technique and composite material–part I: cuspal deformation, bond strength, and physical properties. Oper Dent. 2014;39(2):E71–82. doi:10.2341/12-441-L.
7. Bicalho AA, Valdivia AC, Barreto B de CF, Tantbirojn D, Versluis A, Soares JC. Incremental filling technique and composite material–part II: shrinkage and shrinkage stresses. Oper Dent. 2014;39:E83–92. doi:10.2341/12-442-L.
8. Soares CJ, Bicalho AA, Tantbirojn D, Versluis A. Polymerization shrinkage stresses in a premolar restored with different composite resins and different incremental techniques. J Adhes Dent. 2013;15:341–50. doi:10.3290/j.jad.a29012.
9. Goracci C, Cadenaro M, Fontanive L, Giangrosso G, Juloski J, Vichi A, et al. Polymerization efficiency and flexural strength of low-stress restorative composites. Dent Mater. 2014;30:688–94. doi:10.1016/j.dental.2014.03.006.
10. Ilie N, Stark K. Curing behaviour of high-viscosity bulk-fill composites. J Dent. 2014;42:977–85. doi:10.1016/j.jdent.2014.05.012.
11. Ilie N, Stark K. Effect of different curing protocols on the mechanical properties of low-viscosity bulk-fill composites. Clin Oral Investig. 2015;19:271–9. doi:10.1007/s00784-014-1262-x.
12. Tomaszewska IM, Kearns JO, Ilie N, Fleming GJP. Bulk fill restoratives: to cap or not to cap–that is the question? J Dent. 2015;43:309–16. doi:10.1016/j.jdent.2015.01.010.
13. Ilie N, Bucuta S, Draenert M. Bulk-fill resin-based composites: an in vitro assessment of their mechanical performance. Oper Dent. 2013;38:618–25. doi:10.2341/12-395-L.
14. Ching K. Deep and fast: Kerr's SonicFill bulk fill composite. HDA Now. 2012:24–5.
15. Engelhardt F, Hahnel S, Preis V, Rosentritt M. Comparison of flowable bulk-fill and flowable resin-based composites: an in vitro analysis. Clin Oral Investig. 2016;20(8):2123–30. doi:10.1007/s00784-015-1700-4.
16. Mahn E. Changing the paradigm of composite placement: Tetric EvoCeram Bulk Fill. Ivoclar Vivadent n.d.;Special Ed:1–24.
17. Ilie N, Hickel R. Investigations on a methacrylate-based flowable composite based on the SDR™ technology. Dent Mater. 2011;27:348–55. doi:10.1016/j.dental.2010.11.014.
18. Manhart J, Chen H-Y, Hickel R. Clinical evaluation of the posterior composite Quixfil in class I and II cavities: 4-year follow-up of a randomized controlled trial. J Adhes Dent. 2010;12:237–43. doi:10.3290/j.jad.a17551.
19. van Dijken JWV, Pallesen U. Posterior bulk-filled resin composite restorations: a 5-year randomized controlled clinical study. J Dent. 2016;51:29–35. doi:10.1016/j.jdent.2016.05.008.
20. Garoushi S, Säilynoja E, Vallittu PK, Lassila L. Physical properties and depth of cure of a new short fiber reinforced composite. Dent Mater. 2013;29:835–41. doi:10.1016/j.dental.2013.04.016.
21. El-Damanhoury H, Platt J. Polymerization shrinkage stress kinetics and related properties of bulk-fill resin composites. Oper Dent. 2013;39:374–82. doi:10.2341/13-017-L.
22. Leprince JG, Palin WM, Vanacker J, Sabbagh J, Devaux J, Leloup G. Physico-mechanical characteristics of commercially available bulk-fill composites. J Dent. 2014;42:993–1000. doi:10.1016/j.jdent.2014.05.009.
23. Flury S, Hayoz S, Peutzfeldt A, Hüsler J, Lussi A. Depth of cure of resin composites: is the ISO 4049 method suitable for bulk fill materials? Dent Mater. 2012;28:521–8. doi:10.1016/j.dental.2012.02.002.
24. Finan L, Palin WM, Moskwa N, McGinley EL, Fleming GJP. The influence of irradiation potential on the degree of conversion and mechanical properties of two bulk-fill flowable RBC base materials. Dent Mater. 2013;29:906–12. doi:10.1016/j.dental.2013.05.008.
25. Benetti AR, Havndrup-Pedersen C, Honoré D, Pedersen M, Pallesen U. Bulk-fill resin composites: polymerization contraction, depth of cure, and gap formation. Oper Dent. 2014;40(2):190–200. doi:10.2341/13-324-L.
26. Par M, Gamulin O, Marovic D, Klaric E, Tarle Z. Effect of temperature on post-cure polymerization of bulk-fill composites. J Dent. 2014;42:1255–60. doi:10.1016/j.jdent.2014.08.004.
27. Alrahlah A, Silikas N, Watts DC. Post-cure depth of cure of bulk fill dental resin-composites. Dent Mater. 2014;30:149–54. doi:10.1016/j.dental.2013.10.011.
28. Bucuta S, Ilie N. Light transmittance and micro-mechanical properties of bulk fill vs. conventional resin

based composites. Clin Oral Investig. 2014;18:1991–2000. doi:10.1007/s00784-013-1177-y.
29. Tarle Z, Attin T, Marovic D, Andermatt L, Ristic M, Tauböck TT. Influence of irradiation time on subsurface degree of conversion and microhardness of high-viscosity bulk-fill resin composites. Clin Oral Investig. 2014;19(4):831–40. doi:10.1007/s00784-014-1302-6.
30. Garcia D, Yaman P, Dennison J, Neiva G. Polymerization shrinkage and depth of cure of bulk fill flowable composite resins. Oper Dent. 2014;39:441–8. doi:10.2341/12-484-L.
31. Awad D, Stawarczyk B, Liebermann A, Ilie N. Translucency of esthetic dental restorative CAD/CAM materials and composite resins with respect to thickness and surface roughness. J Prosthet Dent. 2015;113(6):534–40. doi:10.1016/j.prosdent.2014.12.003.
32. Zorzin J, Maier E, Harre S, Fey T, Belli R, Lohbauer U, et al. Bulk-fill resin composites: polymerization properties and extended light curing. Dent Mater. 2015;31:293–301. doi:10.1016/j.dental.2014.12.010.
33. Miletic V, Pongprueksa P, de Munck J, Brooks NR, van Meerbeek B. Curing characteristics of flowable and sculptable bulk-fill composites. Clin Oral Investig. 2016;21(4):1201–12. doi:10.1007/s00784-016-1894-0.
34. Yap AUJ, Pandya M, Toh WS. Depth of cure of contemporary bulk-fill resin-based composites. Dent Mater J. 2016;35:503–10. doi:10.4012/dmj.2015-402.
35. Musanje L, Darvell BW. Curing-light attenuation in filled-resin restorative materials. Dent Mater. 2006;22:804–17. doi:10.1016/j.dental.2005.11.009.
36. Leprince JG, Leveque P, Nysten B, Gallez B, Devaux J, Leloup G. New insight into the "depth of cure" of dimethacrylate-based dental composites. Dent Mater. 2012;28:512–20. doi:10.1016/j.dental.2011.12.004.
37. Van Landuyt KL, Snauwaert J, De Munck J, Peumans M, Yoshida Y, Poitevin A, et al. Systematic review of the chemical composition of contemporary dental adhesives. Biomaterials. 2007;28:3757–85. doi:10.1016/j.biomaterials.2007.04.044.
38. Son SA, Park JK, Seo DG, Ko CC, Kwon YH. How light attenuation and filler content affect the microhardness and polymerization shrinkage and translucency of bulk-fill composites? Clin Oral Investig. 2016;21(2):559–65. doi:10.1007/s00784-016-1920-2.
39. Lassila LVJ, Nagas E, Vallittu PK, Garoushi S. Translucency of flowable bulk-filling composites of various thicknesses. Chin J Dent Res. 2012;15:31–5.
40. Li X, Pongprueksa P, Van Meerbeek B, De Munck J. Curing profile of bulk-fill resin-based composites. J Dent. 2015;43(6):664–72. doi:10.1016/j.jdent.2015.01.002.
41. Musanje L, Darvell BW. Polymerization of resin composite restorative materials: exposure reciprocity. Dent Mater. 2003;19:531–41. doi:10.1016/S0109-5641(02)00101-X.
42. Feng L, Carvalho R, Suh BI. Insufficient cure under the condition of high irradiance and short irradiation time. Dent Mater. 2009;25:283–9. doi:10.1016/j.dental.2008.07.007.
43. Leprince JG, Palin WM, Hadis MA, Devaux J, Leloup G. Progress in dimethacrylate-based dental composite technology and curing efficiency. Dent Mater. 2013;29:139–56. doi:10.1016/j.dental.2012.11.005.
44. Yu P, Yap A, Wang X, Yu P, Yap AUJ, Wang X-Y. Degree of conversion and polymerization shrinkage of bulk- fill resin-based composites. Oper Dent. 2017;42(1):82–9. doi:10.2341/16-027-L.
45. Agarwal R, Hiremath H, Agarwal J, Garg A. Evaluation of cervical marginal and internal adaptation using newer bulk fill composites: an in vitro study. J Conserv Dent. 2015;18:56–61. doi:10.4103/0972-0707.148897.
46. Feng L, Suh BI, Shortall AC. Formation of gaps at the filler-resin interface induced by polymerization contraction stress: gaps at the interface. Dent Mater. 2010;26:719–29. doi:10.1016/j.dental.2010.03.004.
47. Scotti N, Alovisi C, Comba A, Ventura G, Pasqualini D, Grignolo F, et al. Evaluation of composite adaptation to pulpal chamber floor using optical coherence tomography. J Endod. 2015;42:160–3. doi:10.1016/j.joen.2015.10.006.
48. Loomans BA, Opdam NJ, Roeters JF, Bronkhorst EM, Plasschaert AJ. Influence of composite resin consistency and placement technique on proximal contact tightness of class II restorations. J Adhes Dent. 2006;8:305–10.
49. Rullmann I, Schattenberg A, Marx M, Willershausen B, Ernst C-P. Photoelastic determination of polymerization shrinkage stress in low-shrinkage resin composites. Schweiz Monatsschr Zahnmed. 2012;122:294–9.
50. Kim RJ-Y, Kim Y-J, Choi N-S, Lee I-B. Polymerization shrinkage, modulus, and shrinkage stress related to tooth-restoration interfacial debonding in bulk-fill composites. J Dent. 2015;43(4):430–9. doi:10.1016/j.jdent.2015.02.002.
51. Kalliecharan D, Germscheid W, Price RB, Stansbury J, Labrie D. Shrinkage stress kinetics of bulk fill resin-based composites at tooth temperature and long time. Dent Mater. 2016;32:1322–31. doi:10.1016/j.dental.2016.07.015.
52. Fok AS-L. Shrinkage stress development in dental composites–an analytical treatment. Dent Mater. 2013;29:1108–15. doi:10.1016/j.dental.2013.08.198.
53. Abu-elenain DA, Lewis SH, Stansbury JW. Property evolution during vitrification of dimethacrylate photopolymer networks. Dent Mater. 2013;29:1173–81. doi:10.1016/j.dental.2013.09.002.
54. Kim HJ, Park SH. Measurement of the internal adaptation of resin composites using micro-CT and its correlation with polymerization shrinkage. Oper Dent. 2014;39:E57–70. doi:10.2341/12-378-L.
55. Jang J-H, Park S-H, Hwang I-N. Polymerization shrinkage and depth of cure of bulk-fill resin composites and highly filled flowable resin. Oper Dent. 2015;40:172–80. doi:10.2341/13-307-L.

56. Campodonico C, Tantbirojn D, Olin P, Versluis A. Cuspal deflection and depth of cure in resin-based composite restorations filled by using bulk, incremental and transtooth-illumination techniques. J Am Dent Assoc. 2011;142:1176–82.
57. Moorthy A, Hogg CH, Dowling AH, Grufferty BF, Benetti AR, Fleming GJP. Cuspal deflection and microleakage in premolar teeth restored with bulk-fill flowable resin-based composite base materials. J Dent. 2012;40:500–5. doi:10.1016/j.jdent.2012.02.015.
58. Francis AV, Braxton AD, Ahmad W, Tantbirojn D, Simon J, Versluis A. Cuspal flexure and extent of cure of a bulk-fill flowable base composite. Oper Dent. 2015;40(5):515–23. doi:10.2341/14-235-L.

9 Fiber-Reinforced Composites

Sufyan Garoushi

9.1 Introduction

Nowadays particulate filler composite resin (PFC) enables the dentist to cover a much larger spectrum of indications than few years ago. The ability to bond PFC to tooth enamel and dentin makes it a desired material to use. Among other things, this is due to substantial improvements in the physical parameters of PFC, in particular their enhanced wear resistance, strength, and color stability. However, the development of fiber-reinforced composite (FRC) has given the practitioner the first real opportunity to create reliable composite structures. The parameter which has been developed to its maximum potential within classic composites is flexural strength and fracture toughness. FRCs have highly favorable mechanical properties, and their strength to weight ratios are superior even to those of most alloys [1]. When compared to metal alloys, FRCs offer many other advantages as well including non-corrosiveness, translucency, good bonding properties, and repair facility. Additionally, FRCs give alternatives for chairside and laboratory fabrication. Therefore, it is not surprising that FRCs have potential for use in many applications in dentistry [1]. The use of FRCs in dental applications has been discussed in the literature since the early 1960s. However, it took almost 30 years before dental FRCs were applied in clinical use.

FRCs are structural materials that have at least two distinct constituents. The reinforcing component provides strength and stiffness, while the surrounding matrix supports the reinforcement and provides workability (Fig. 9.1). The polymer matrix also protects the fibers from the effects of mechanical damage and moisture [1].

FRCs can be categorized according to the reinforcement and polymer matrices used. The most commonly used fibers are glass fibers of various kinds. Also carbon/graphite, aramid, boron, and metal fibers are used for various

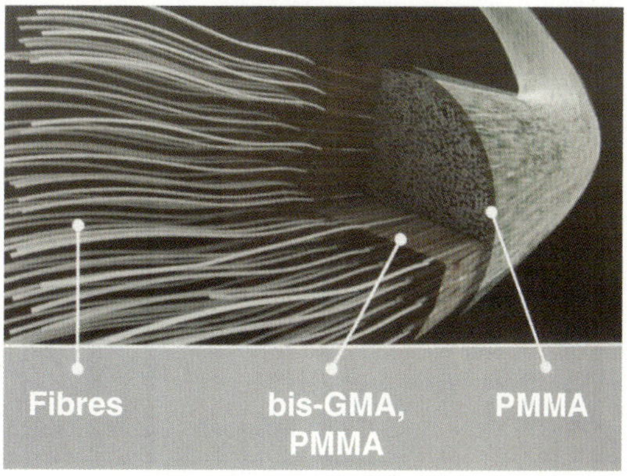

Fig. 9.1 Unidirectional semi-interpenetrating polymer network (semi-IPN) resin-impregnated fiber-reinforced composite

S. Garoushi
Department of Biomaterials Science and Turku Clinical Biomaterials Center–TCBC, Institute of Dentistry, University of Turku, Turku, Finland
e-mail: sufgar@utu.fi

V. Miletic (ed.), *Dental Composite Materials for Direct Restorations*,
http://doi.org/10.1007/978-3-319-60961-4_9

purposes [2]. FRCs can also be divided into groups based on fiber length and orientation. Long fibers containing FRCs are called continuous FRCs, but there are also discontinuous short FRCs. The three main structural types of FRC products presently available are continuous unidirectional, bidirectional fibers (weaves), and multidirectional discontinuous.

The mechanical advantages provided by FRCs are their flexural strength, fatigue strength, elastic modulus, and bond strength (of fiber substructure to veneering composites and resin luting cements). Additionally, FRCs are metal-free and esthetic and allow a minimally invasive treatment technique even with direct treatment technique. However, until recently, FRCs have not been widely accepted clinically although they successfully reinforce long-term restorations such as crowns and bridges [3–6]. The first issue limiting wide acceptance was the sensitive technique of using FRC, and the second was the mechanical properties that were well below theoretical calculations and expectations. This was due to the low fiber content in the definite appliance as well as due to the inadequate impregnation of the fibers with the resins, which were often highly viscous [7]. In order to establish an improved technique, some manufacturers produce industrial resin-impregnated FRC materials. Moreover, one manufacturer (StickTech, member of GC group, Turku, Finland) established and used polymethyl methacrylate (PMMA)-dimethacrylate (BisGMA)-based semi-interpenetrating polymer network (semi-IPN) [8]. Semi-IPN (Fig. 9.1) allowed the surface of the FRC structure to be reactivated in order to have a durable bond when cementing laboratory-manufactured restorations to abutments, cementing root canal posts, layering veneering composite on FRC substructure, or repairing FRC restorations. In addition, the handling properties of FRC were improved [1].

9.2 Structure and Properties of FRC

In order to achieve a good reinforcing outcome with fiber reinforcements, all the strength-related factors of FRCs should be thoroughly taken into account. Several factors influence the mechanical properties of FRC.

9.2.1 Reinforcing Fibers Used in FRC

Glass fibers (GF) are the most commonly used reinforcing fibers in both dental and industrial applications. They have high tensile strength combined with low extensibility. Their transparent appearance makes them well suited for dental applications with high cosmetic demands. Glass fibers are formed by heating the raw materials (sand, kaolin, limestone, and colemanite) in an oven at a temperature of 1600 °C. The liquid glass mass is then drawn into 10–24 μm fibers. According to the chemical composition of the glass mass, glass fibers are classified into A-, C-, D-, E-, R-, and S-glass types, with difference in mechanical and chemical resistance properties. E-glass is the main type used in reinforced plastic. E-glass has a calcium-alumino-borosilicate composition. It has good tensile and compressive strength and stiffness and a relatively low cost. R- and S-glasses are sometimes also used in dental applications, such as root canal posts. Their chemical composition is different from E-glass, giving them slightly higher tensile strength and modulus.

Aramid fibers (AF) are created from aromatic polyamide fibers, more commonly known as Kevlar® fibers. These fibers have high strength and low density, with anisotropic tensile strength as fibers. They are resistant to chemicals and thermally stable and have high mechanical stability and high glass transition temperature. Aramid fibers have been used to reinforce the denture base polymers with and without silane treatment [9]. However, the yellow color of the fibers, lack of bonding between fibers and resin, and poor polishing surface limit their use in dental applications.

Carbon fibers (CF) or carbon/graphite fibers are the most common high strength and high modulus of elasticity reinforcing fibers. They exhibit high strength in both tension and compression. In contrast, their impact strength is lower than that of glass or aramid FRC [10].

The first article on carbon fiber reinforcement of denture base polymer was published in the 1970s [11], and after that numerous authors have reported the use of CF in reinforcing denture base polymers. Carbon fiber reinforcements have not met wide clinical acceptance because of their difficult handling characteristics and black color resulting in poor esthetics [12]. However, carbon FRCs were used as root canal posts [13].

Ultra-high molecular weight (UHMW)-polyethylene fibers are one of the most durable reinforcing fibers available. They are made of aligned polymer chains, have low modulus and density, and present good impact resistance [10]. They are white in color and thus it is possible to use them in dental applications. Several authors have investigated the reinforcing effect of polyethylene fibers on dental polymers [14, 15]. Their clinical use is limited because of poor bonding the fibers to dental resin and potential problems related to increased adhesion of oral microbes to FRC [16].

9.2.2 Fiber Orientation

Fiber orientation (direction) influences the mechanical and thermal properties of FRC [17]. Continuous unidirectional fibers give strength, stiffness, and anisotropic mechanical strength to the composite in the direction of the fibers, and thus, they are suitable for applications in which the direction of the highest stress is known. The reinforcing efficiency (Krenchel's factor) of unidirectional fibers is theoretically 100% which means that reinforcing properties can be obtained in one direction [10]. Continuous bidirectional (woven) fibers have reinforcing fibers in two directions, so they have a reinforcing effect equally in two directions [10]. The theoretical reinforcing efficiency of such fibers is 50% or 25% (Fig. 9.2).

Woven fibers add toughness to the polymer and act as a crack stopper. They are especially suitable in cases where the direction of the load is unknown or there is no space for unidirectional fibers. Woven reinforcement has been shown to increase the strain at fracture for polymers [1]. Properties of woven fiber-reinforced composites are called orthotropic, in contrast to the anisotropic properties of unidirectional FRC.

If the fibers are orientated randomly as in chopped short FRC, the mechanical properties are the same in all directions. Composites that have randomly oriented fibers are isotropic in their mechanical and thermal properties; in other words, the strength of the FRC is not

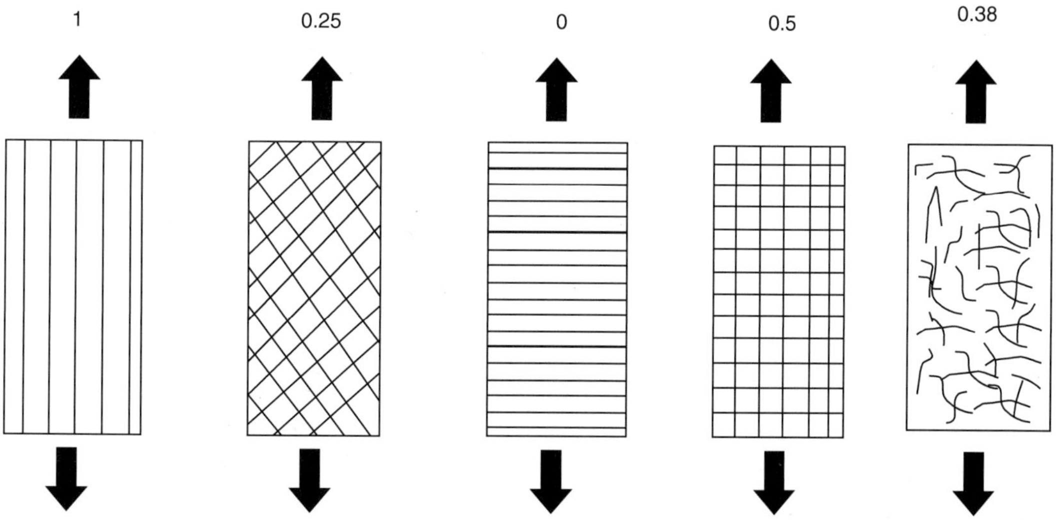

Fig. 9.2 Reinforcing efficiency (Krenchel's factor) (*left–right*) unidirectional fibers in the direction of the load (0°), bidirectional fibers 45°/45° to the load, unidirectional fibers 90° to the direction of the load, bidirectional fibers 0°/90° in the direction of the load, and short random fibers. Values above the figure describe the reinforcing efficiency

related to the direction of the fracture force [18]. The theoretical reinforcing efficiency of such fibers is 20% in three dimensions, whereas in two dimensions orientation gives 38% reinforcing efficiency (Fig. 9.2) [10].

9.2.3 Impregnation and Adhesion of Fibers

Fibers should be well impregnated (embedded) within the polymer matrix, in order to have adequate adhesion of fibers to the polymer matrix. To gain good impregnation of fibers with resin matrix of high viscosity, i.e., multiphasic denture base resins, preimpregnation of the fibers with porous PMMA was introduced many years ago. Other impregnation methods utilize the use of light-curing dimethacrylate monomers or monomer-polymer systems that form a semi-IPN matrix for the FRC [8]. Adequate adhesion of the fibers to the polymer matrix is one of the important requirements for composite strength [1]. The chemical bond between the polymer and the fibers should ideally be of a covalent nature. Proper adhesion makes it possible to transfer stress from the polymer matrix to the reinforcing fibers. Adhesion requires accurate impregnation of the fibers with the matrix, and ideally, all the fibers should be embedded in the polymer matrix. Silane coupling agents have been used effectively to expand the adhesion between polymers and glass fibers, in addition to other dental substrates [19]. The function of silane coupling agents is rooted in the formation of siloxane bridges and hydrogen bonds on the glass surface.

9.2.4 Fiber Placement and Quantity

The fiber quantity of FRC itself and relative quantity in FRC device affect the strength and load-bearing capacity of the system. Research has been conducted regarding the effect of varying the amount of fiber reinforcement in dental FRC. The results show that as the fiber quantity increases in the definite appliance, the mechanical properties become more like the fibrous elements. When fibers are positioned in the direction of highest stress, partial fiber reinforcement can be sufficient to hinder the formulation of a fracture line [20]. The fibers should be placed on the tension side of the device during mastication and perpendicular to the possible fracture line.

Fiber concentration is regularly reported with the unit of fiber content by weight. The weight fraction of the fibers can be changed to the volume fraction when the density of the polymer and the fiber is known. The fiber quantity in FRC-reinforced device or in FRC follows the basic principle of the rule of mixtures, asserting that as a constituent amount increases, the performance of the device or composite shifts toward the behavior of the constitute [21]. This can be achieved if factors such as impregnation and adhesion of fibers with polymer matrix are optimized. Moreover, the theoretically expected modulus of FRC was calculated using the rule of mixtures in terms of stiffness [22]:

$$E_e = E_f V_f + E_m V_m$$

where E_e = expected elastic modulus of the composite, E_f = elastic modulus of fiber, V_f = volume fraction of fiber, E_m = elastic modulus of matrix, and V_m = volume fraction of matrix.

9.2.5 Interfacial Adhesion of FRC and Resin Composites

All modern PFC and FRC restorations are based on effective adhesive procedures using dental adhesives. Dental adhesive systems are complex mixtures containing hydrophilic and hydrophobic monomers, solvents (including water), sometimes fillers, and polymerization initiators and co-initiators. Their challenge is firstly to completely penetrate a hydrophilic etched tooth surface (enamel or dentin) to obtain an acceptable mechanical retention and secondly to achieve a strong bond through the reaction of copolymerization (oxygen-inhibited layer) with the hydrophobic matrix of composites or luting resins. This process can be performed clinically in different ways according to the presentation of the adhesive system. Enamel adhesion through the acid etching has been shown to be effective, whereas the development of dentin adhesion techniques is in constant progress [23].

In addition to the importance of resin adhesion to the tooth, adhesion of adhesives to indirectly made restorations is also of importance. The composition of the polymer matrix and fiber orientation has the major role in bonding ability and durability of PFC to the FRC or resin luting cement. It has been concluded that preimpregnation of the fibers with the light-polymerizable dimethacrylate resin system containing linear polymer phases is of importance to optimize the interfacial adhesion of FRC to PFCs. However, preimpregnation can be based on using any monomer resin (e.g., dimethacrylate, trimethacrylate, or dendrimer), but using a combination of dimethacrylate monomer resin and linear polymer, which forms semi-IPN polymer network after being polymerized, offers better bonding site for PFC [1, 8]. The FRC with a semi-IPN resin matrix can be adhered with resin composites by means of interdiffusion bonding. Two different kinds of semi-IPNs are available for dental use; one requires manual further impregnation by resin, and the other is fully preimpregnated by the manufacturer.

The bond strength of chairside-fabricated FRC to the tooth surface is as good as PFC [24]. Some recent studies have shown that especially HEMA-containing adhesive resins or MMA monomer in combination with some dimethacrylate monomer systems could promote the diffusion of the adhesive resin and dissolve the linear polymer phases of the FRC on the bonding surface, to form interdiffusion bonding. In addition, FRC layer at the adhesive interface can change the path of crack propagation at the interface, which limits the cohesive fracture of the tooth structure [24].

Previous studies have shown good adhesion between FRC with different orientations and PFC [24, 25]. On the other hand, short randomly oriented FRC with a rough surface (microretention) and a higher fraction of polymer matrix can ease the penetration of the monomers inside the materials, thus offering a better bonding site for the tooth substrate and PFC [26].

Another alternative for bonding of PFC to FRC is to use oxygen-inhibited layer on the FRC surfaces [26]. The PFC reacts during free-radical polymerization with the oxygen-inhibited layer and provides a reliable bond. It needs to be noted that an oxygen-inhibited layer can only be used in the veneering stage of FRC substructures or frameworks, not in the bonding of an indirectly made restoration or in repairs of old restorations.

There have also been some attempts to use tribochemical silica coating of FRC surface in order to improve bonding of PFC through silane coupling agents [27].

9.3 Applications of FRCs in Dentistry

FRCs are currently commonly used in several fields of dentistry. In addition to prosthodontic and restorative dentistry, applications of FRCs extend to periodontal, orthodontic, and surgical fields in the form of various splints.

9.3.1 Prosthodontic Application

The recurrent fractures of removable dentures can be eliminated by the use of FRC as a reinforcement [28]. The impact strength of maxillary complete denture can be increased by a factor greater than two when reinforced with bidirectional FRC [29]. However, as in the cases of any other applications for fiber reinforcement, the positioning of fiber is of importance in order to achieve an efficient reinforcing effect [28]. FRC can also be used as framework in overdenture or implant-supported prosthesis. Combining FRCs with light-polymerizable dimethacrylate resins and particulate filler composite systems enables the use of fibers in fixed prosthodontics and other adhesively luted restorations. FRC-based resin-bonded restorations are claimed to have certain benefits over conventional materials. Lower elastic modulus of FRC in comparison with cast metal alloy helps to diminish interfacial stresses between the tooth and the resin-bonded fixed partial denture (FPD). Fixed restorations using adhesive technique can be fabricated using either a direct or indirect technique. With the indirect technique, the restorations are manufactured by a dental technician and adhesively luted in place with a luting resin cement [30, 31], whereas in the direct technique, preimpregnated FRCs are used by the dentist as a chairside approach for teeth replacements [32–34]. Surface-retained, inlay, onlay, and full-cover crown-retained devices can be used. According to the clinical need, hybrid-type fixed prosthesis can be prepared by integrating various retainer types into the same prosthetic device.

Based on current clinical results, it is reasonable to expect FRC-FPD to attain a longevity of 5–10 years [3–6]. However, it has been emphasized that FRC prosthesis with a veneering composite offers an alternative, not necessarily a substitute for conventional prosthetic devices. Computer-aided design/computer-aided manufacturing (CAD/CAM) processes of FRC blocks made of short random fiber-oriented FRCs in polyamide matrix (nylon) are also available for FRC framework fabrication.

9.3.2 Endodontic Application

FRCs are also increasingly used as root canal posts in restoring severely damage endodontically treated teeth. FRC endodontic posts have been introduced to be used instead of metal alloys and ceramics. It was found that prefabricated FRC posts showed lower flexural properties than an individually polymerized material [13, 35, 36]. However the mechanical properties depend on the composition, structure, and diameter of endodontic posts. The individually polymerized FRC material showed almost the same degree of conversion after light polymerization as monomer resin without fibers. The individually formed FRC post material with a semi-IPN polymer matrix bonded better to composite resin luting cement than the prefabricated posts with a cross-linked polymer matrix [35]. There is less risk to loss of retention due to higher bond strength values of IPN posts than prefabricated FRC posts [36]. FRC post's strength and elastic modulus depend on the type of stresses they are subjected to. Tensile, shear, flexural, or compressive stresses lead to different values of elastic modulus or maximum strength for the same composite material. Furthermore these values depend also on the angle between the fiber and the load direction. In addition, an individually formed FRC post offers a possibility to build the post and the bridge framework out of the same material in order to achieve maximum attachment in special cases and reduces the risk of root fracture, because of its isoelasticity with dentin [35, 36].

Recently, there has been scientific debate and published data regarding the failure and the risk of using the prefabricated (solid) fiber posts in the way conventional metal posts have been used. They were reported different failure modes of the fiber post-core-crown restorations; however, in all situations, damage is associated with the stress caused by occlusion and force of mastication and resistance of the restored tooth to withstand fatigue stresses for years. These failures can be explained by the insufficient bonding of fiber post to root canal dentin, and post system is not able to carry the load and consequently diminishes the tensile stress at the crown margin. Many studies showed a significant increase in the fracture resistance of restored teeth when the fiber posts were adapted closely to the canal walls [37–39]. Through the use of an individually formed post technique, it is possible to fill the large and irregular root cavities more efficiently than with a single, prefabricated centrally positioned post. Because of the IPN matrix structure, the individually made fiber posts have good bonding with cement and direct composite core\restorations enabling reliable surface-retained applications. Moreover, with an individually made fiber post, the amount of luting cement can be minimized, thus reducing the residual shrinkage of the cement and resulting in a better adaptation of the fiber post [39].

9.3.3 Tooth Filling and Core-Buildup Application

Attempts have been made to reinforce posterior composite restorations by using FRC as substructure with different orientations in order to enhance composite strength and toughness. This bilayered composite structure is a type of restoration which includes both FRC and PFC (Fig. 9.3). Several studies showed that FRC substructure supports the PFC surface layer and serves as a crack prevention layer [33, 40–43]. FRC substructure's thickness has prior importance, as it influences the failure mode and the crack-arresting mechanism. Furthermore, the type of the FRC substructure and the thickness of the veneering composite play also a significant role [44]. In addition to these laboratory studies, there are also clinical reports on the use of various bilayered restorations exhibited promising results [45–47].

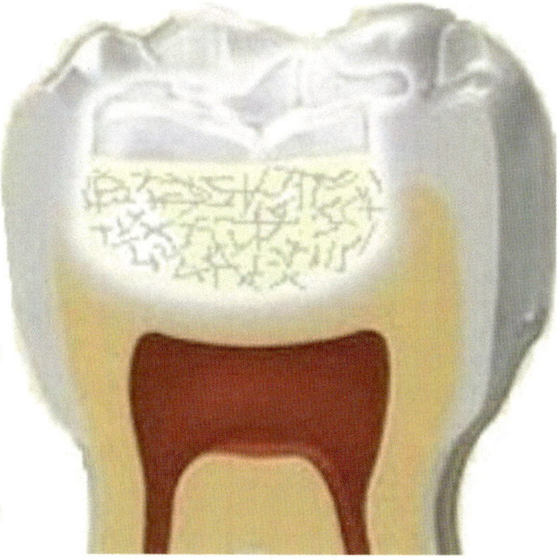

Fig. 9.3 Schematic representation of bilayered posterior composite restoration: lost dentin is replaced by tough short FRC and covered by surface layer of PFC

In order to simplify the clinical technique of using FRC inside cavities, recently in 2013, discontinuous or short FRC resin (everX Posterior) has been introduced as a dental restorative composite resin [47, 48]. The composite resin is intended to be used as bulk base filling material in high stress-bearing areas especially in large cavities of vital and non-vital posterior teeth (Fig. 9.3). It consists of a combination of a resin matrix, randomly orientated E-glass fibers, and inorganic particulate fillers. The resin matrix contains BisGMA, TEGDMA, and PMMA forming a semi-IPN which provides good bonding properties and improves toughness of the polymer matrix. The in vitro studies showed improvements in the load-bearing capacity and fracture toughness of short FRC resin in comparison with conventional PFC resin [18, 48, 49]. The short FRC resin showed significantly higher fracture toughness (2.4 $MPa{\cdot}m^{0.5}$), flexural strength (124 MPa), and flexural modulus (12,6 GPa) than all other comparative composite materials [48, 49]. The reinforcing effect of the fiber fillers is based on stress transfer from the polymer matrix to fibers but also on the behavior of individual short fibers as crack stoppers (Fig. 9.4). Random fiber orientation and lowered cross-linking density of the polymer matrix by the semi-IPN structure likely had a significant role in mechanical properties.

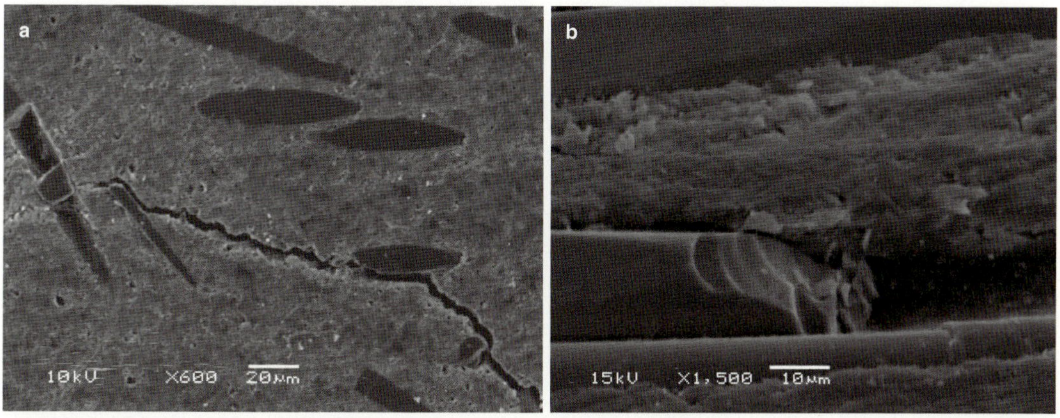

Fig. 9.4 SEM photomicrographs at different magnifications of fracture surfaces of a short FRC composite showing fiber-arrested crack propagation (**a**) and a fractured individual glass fiber (**b**)

Curing depth was found to be 4.6 mm which was similar to other bulk fill composites and higher than conventional hybrid PFC [48]. They also showed lower percentage of shrinkage strain (0.17%) compared to other tested composites [48]. The short FRC resin has also exhibited control of the polymerization shrinkage stress by fiber orientation, and thus marginal microleakage was reduced compared with conventional PFC resins [43, 50]. On the basis of the promising published data, it is suggested that short FRC resin could be used to fulfill the requirements for ideal posterior composite restorations. It is intended to be used as bulk substructure material which will be covered by a layer of PFC resin (1–2 mm). It is difficult to predict clinical long-term performance from only laboratory experiments. One-year clinical report showed good clinical performance of this novel material combination of bulk short FRC substructure and surface layer of PFC in high stress-bearing areas [47].

9.3.4 Periodontal Splint Application

Because of brittleness and natural rigidity of conventional composite resins, the composites as splints with metal wires are prone to failure. To overcome this clinical limitation, preimpregnated unidirectional FRC has allowed clinicians to replace metal wires. FRC periodontal splints are thin and simple in design and have the potential for excellent bonding and durability [32]. Different types of commercial FRC splints are available for the purpose of conservative splinting. These fiber-reinforced splints have sufficient mechanical strength and satisfactory esthetics, do not disturb the occlusion, and allow maintaining proper oral hygiene [32, 51, 52].

There are also some clinical reports of using FRCs as bonded retainers after orthodontic therapy and space maintainers for short-term space maintenance [51, 52].

Conclusions

This chapter describes briefly FRC that can be used in dentistry. It is concluded that FRC materials offer a combination of strength and toughness that is comparable to dental tissues. The specific mechanical and physical strength and specific modulus of these FRC materials may be markedly superior to those of existing resin-based composites and metallic materials.

Within the limitations of the clinical trials available to review, FRC is a promising material giving clinicians alternative treatment options. They suggest reasonable success for FRC restorations including endodontic posts, fixed partial dentures, and posterior composite restorations. However, multiyear clinical studies are still needed to determine the value and usefulness of FRC restorations as long-term tooth structure replacement.

References

1. Vallittu PK. High-aspect ratio fillers: fiber-reinforced composites and their anisotropic properties. Dent Mater. 2015;31:1–7.
2. Edwards KL. An overview of the technology of fiber-reinforced plastics for design purposes. Mater Des. 1998;19:1–10.
3. Vallittu PK. Survival rates of resin-bonded, glass fiber-reinforced composite fixed partial dentures with a mean follow-up of 42-months: a pilot study. J Prosthet Dent. 2004;91:241–7.
4. Gohring TN, Roos M. Inlay-fixed partial dentures adhesively and reinforced by glass fiber: clinical and scanning electron microscopy analysis after five years. Eur J Oral Sci. 2005;113:60–9.
5. Spinas E, Aresu M, Canargiu F. Prosthetic rehabilitation interventions in adolescents with fixed bridges: a 5-year observational study. Eur J Paediatr Dent. 2013;14:59–62.
6. van Heumen CC, van Dijken JW, Tanner J, Pikaar R, Lassila LV, Creugers NH, Vallittu PK, Kreulen CM. Five-year survival of 3-unit fiber-reinforced composite fixed partial dentures in the anterior area. Dent Mater. 2009;25:820–7.
7. Vallittu PK. Some aspects of the tensile strength of unidirectional glass fiber-polymethyl methacrylate composite used in dentures. J Oral Rehabil. 1998;25:100–5.
8. Lastumäki TM, Lassila LV, Vallittu PK. The semi-interpenetrating polymer network matrix of fiber-reinforced composite and its effect on the surface adhesive properties. J Mater Sci Mater Med. 2003;14:803–9.
9. Mullarky R. Aramid fiber reinforcement of acrylic appliances. J Clin Orthod. 1985;19:655–8.
10. Murphy J. Reinforced plastics handbook. 2nd ed. Oxford: Elsevier Advanced Technology; 1998. p. 265.

11. Schreiber C. Polymethylmethacrylate reinforced with carbon fibers. Br Dent J. 1971;130:29–30.
12. Bowman AJ, Manley TR. The elimination of breakages in upper denture by reinforcement with carbon fiber. Br Dent J. 1984;156:87–9.
13. Lassila LV, Tanner J, Bell AM, Narva K, Vallittu PK. Flexural properties of fiber reinforced root canal posts. Dent Mater. 2004;20:29–36.
14. Vallittu PK. Ultra-high-modulus polyethylene ribbon as reinforcement for denture polymethyl methacrylate: a short communication. Dent Mater. 1997;13:381–2.
15. Gutteridge D. Reinforcement of poly (methyl methacrylate) with ultra- high- modulus polymethylene fibers. J Dent. 1992;20:50–4.
16. Tanner J, Carlén A, Söderling E, Vallittu PK. Adsorption of parotid saliva proteins and adhesion of Streptococcus Mutans ATCC 21752 to dental fiber-reinforced composites. J Biomed Mater Res B Appl Biomater. 2003;66:391–8.
17. Dyer SR, Lassila LV, Jokinen M, Vallittu PK. Effect of fiber position and orientation on fracture load of fiber-reinforced composite. Dent Mater. 2004;20:947–55.
18. Garoushi S, Vallittu PK, Lassila LV. Short glass fiber reinforced restorative composite resin with semi-inter penetrating polymer network matrix. Dent Mater. 2007;23:1356–62.
19. Vallittu PK. Comparison of two different silane compounds used for improving adhesion between fibers and acrylic denture base material. J Oral Rehabil. 1993;20:533–9.
20. Vallittu PK. Curing of silane coupling agent and its effect on the transverse strength of autopolymerizing polymethylmethacrylate glass fiber composite. J Oral Rehabil. 1997;24:124–30.
21. Herakovich C. Mechanics of fibrous composites. New York: Wiley and Sons Publ. Co; 1998.
22. Goldberg AJ, Burstone CJ. The use of continuous fiber reinforcement in dentistry. Dent Mater. 1992;8:197–202.
23. Cocco AR, Rosa WL, Silva AF, Lund RG, Piva E. A systematic review about antibacterial monomers used in dental adhesive systems: current status and further prospects. Dent Mater. 2015;31:1345–62.
24. Tezvergil A, Lassila LV, Vallittu PK. The shear bond strength of bidirectional and random- oriented fiber-reinforced composite to tooth structure. J Dent. 2005;33:509–16.
25. Kallio TT, Lastumäki TM, Vallittu PK. Bonding of restorative and veneering composite resin to some polymeric composites. Dent Mater. 2001;17:80–6.
26. Keski-Nikkola MS, Lassila LV, Vallittu PK. An *in vitro* investigation of bond strength of veneering composite resin to glass fiber veil reinforced composite. Eur J Prosthodont Restor Dent. 2004;12:80–6.
27. Rosentritt M, Behr M, Kolbeck C, Handel G. *In vitro* repair of three-unit fiber-reinforced composite FPDs. Int J Prosthodont. 2001;14:344–9.
28. Narva KK, Vallittu PK, Helenius H, Yli-Urpo A. Clinical survey of acrylic resin removable denture repairs with glass-fiber reinforcement. Int J Prosthodont. 2001;14:219–24.
29. Kim SH, Watts DC. The effect of reinforcement with woven E-glass fibers on the impact strength of complete dentures fabricated with high-impact acrylic resin. J Prosthet Dent. 2004;91:274–80.
30. Freilich M, Duncan J, Meiers J, Goldberg A. Preimpregnated fiber-reinforced prostheses. Part I. Basic rationale and complete-coverage and intracoronal fixed partial denture designs. Quintessence Int. 1998;29:689–96.
31. Ahlstrand W, Finger W. Direct and indirect fiber-reinforced fixed partial dentures: case reports. Restor Dent. 2002;33:359–65.
32. Meiers J, Duncan J, Freilich M, Goldberg A. Preimpregnated fiber reinforced prosthesis. Part II. Direct applications: splint and fixed partial dentures. Quintessence Int. 1998;29:761–8.
33. Garoushi S, Vallittu PK, Lassila LVJ. Use of isotropic short fiber reinforced composite with semi-interpenetrating polymer network matrix in fixed partial dentures. J Dent. 2007;35:403–8.
34. Garoushi S, Lassila LVJ, Vallittu PK. Direct composite resin restoration of an anterior tooth: effect of fiber-reinforced composite substructure. Eur J Prosthodont Restor Dent. 2007;15:61–6.
35. Bell AM, Lassila LV, Kangasniemi I, Vallittu PK. Bonding of fiber-reinforced composite post to root canal dentin. J Dent. 2005;33:533–9.
36. Hatta M, Shinya A, Vallittu PK, Shinya A, Lassila LV. High volume individual fiber post versus low volume fiber post: the fracture load of the restored tooth. J Prosthodont Res. 2011;55:146–53.
37. Fráter M, Forster A, Jantyik Á, Braunitzer G, Nagy K, Grandini S. In vitro fracture resistance of premolar teeth restored with fiber-reinforced composite posts using a single or a multi-post technique. Aust Endod J. 2017;43(1):16–22. [Epub ahead of print]
38. Le Bell-Rönnlöf AM, Lassila LV, Kangasniemi I, Vallittu PK. Load-bearing capacity of human incisor restored with various fiber-reinforced composite posts. Dent Mater. 2011;27:107–15.
39. Vallittu PK. Are we misusing fiber posts? Guest editorial. Dent Mater. 2016;32:125–6.
40. Garoushi S, Lassila LVJ, Tezvergil A, Vallittu PK. Static and fatigue compression test for particulate filler composite resin with fiber-reinforced composite substructure. Dent Mater. 2007;23:17–23.
41. Garoushi S, Vallittu PK, Lassila L. Fracture resistance of short, randomly oriented, glass fiber-reinforced composite premolar crowns. Acta Biomater. 2007;3:779–84.
42. Garoushi S, Vallittu PK, Lassila L. Direct restoration of severely damaged incisors using short fiber-reinforced composite resin. J Dent. 2007;35:731–6.
43. Garoushi SK, Hatem M, Lassila L, Vallittu PK. The effect of short fiber composite base on microleakage and load-bearing capacity of posterior restorations. Acta Biomater Odontol Scand. 2015;1:6–12.

44. Garoushi S, Lassila L, Tezvergil A, Vallittu PK. Load bearing capacity of fiber-reinforced and particulate filler composite resin combination. J Dent. 2006;34:179–84.
45. Rocca GT, Rizcalla M, Kjejci I. Fiber-reinforced resin coating for endocrown preparations: a technical report. Oper Dent. 2013;38:242–8.
46. Garoushi S, Shinya A, Shinya A, Vallittu PK. Fiber-reinforced onlay composite resin restoration: a case report. J Contemp Dent Pract. 2009;10:104–10.
47. Garoushi S, Tanner J, Vallittu PK, Lassila L. Preliminary clinical evaluation of short fiber-reinforced composite resin in posterior teeth: 12-months report. Open Dent J. 2012;6:41–5.
48. Garoushi S, Sailynoja E, Vallittu PK, Lassila L. Physical properties and depth of cure of a new short fiber reinforced composite. Dent Mater. 2013;29:835–41.
49. Bijelic-Donova J, Garoushi S, Vallittu PK, Lassila L. Mechanical properties, fracture resistance, and fatigue limits of short fiber reinforced dental composite resin. J Prosthet Dent. 2016;115:95–102.
50. Garoushi S, Vallittu PK, Watts DC, Lassila LV. Polymerization shrinkage of experimental short glass fiber-reinforced composite with semi-inter penetrating polymer network matrix. Dent Mater. 2008;24:211–5.
51. Garoushi S, Lassila LVJ, Vallittu P. Fiber-reinforced composite in clinical dentistry. Chin J Dent Res. 2008;11:101–8.
52. Khan AS, Azam MT, Khan M, Mian SA, Ur Rehman I. An update on glass fiber dental restorative composites: a systematic review. Mater Sci Eng C Mater Biol Appl. 2015;47:26–39.

Self-Adhering Composites

10

Paulo H.P. D'Alpino, Nádia da Rocha Svizero, and Marcela Carrilho

10.1 Introduction

Tissue loss in the craniofacial region is frequently derived from disease, trauma, and/or congenital anomalies, mostly causing physiologic and psychological consequences for their bearers. As a result, tissue reconstruction to an esthetic and functional state emerges as a high interest medical topic, evolving through the research, clinical experience, and collaboration between these two backgrounds. A myriad of studies can be found in the literature describing novel approaches to the production of biocompatible and structurally bioactive materials that can be applied to replace or repair craniofacial tissues, targeting clinical efficiency and effectiveness [1].

As other medical fields are dependent on biomaterials and bioengineering upgrading, adhesive dentistry greatly evolved over the past decade. A consistent part of this progression is directly endorsed by a better comprehension of dental substrates' bonding principles/limitations and a remarkable advancement in the dental adhesive systems' chemistry, composition, and technology [2, 3]. From the pioneer systems in the 1970s that yielded weak or none bond especially to dentin, to contemporary functional systems that can establish intimate bond to dentin, resin-based adhesives have advanced nothing more than enormously. Convolutions of human dental tissues, however, have not been simple to decode, and the understanding on interaction and molecular interplay between dental tissues and biomaterials is still being depicted, which will keep in turn fomenting new advances in biomaterials/tissue engineering for next years.

The trend of using exclusively chemical-set, multiple component bonding/restorative systems has been moving away toward the use of dual-set, reduced bonding step adhesive systems that are easier to apply. Low-shrinkage, bulk-fill, and self-adhesive resin-based materials are among the newest commercially available restorative materials that have been developed exactly following the appeal of reducing the time at which chairside treatments occur by means of restorative procedure simplification [4–8]. In general, clinicians tend to assume that dental adhesive materials have already been optimized regarding any possible situation that is likely to be clinically found and that subsequent attempts in optimizing speed and efficiency can be eventually reached without

P.H.P. D'Alpino (✉) • M. Carrilho
Biomaterials in Dentistry/Biotechnology and Innovation in Health Programs, Universidade Anhanguera de São Paulo (UNIAN-SP), São Paulo, SP, Brazil
e-mail: paulodalpino@yahoo.com

N. da R. Svizero
Operative Dentistry Department, Hospital for Rehabilitation of Craniofacial Anomalies, Universidade de São Paulo (USP), São Paulo, SP, Brazil

V. Miletic (ed.), *Dental Composite Materials for Direct Restorations*,
http://doi.org/10.1007/978-3-319-60961-4_10

significant trade-offs in the quality or durability of resin-dentin bonds [9]. Thus, the development of new adhesive materials has been also driven by clinician-consumer's requirements for effectively placing their restorations with guarantee economy, in time and cost.

Simplification of clinical adhesive procedures in dentistry appears as one of the major driving forces propelling the current research and development efforts at the dental material industry [10]. In this way, modern materials are packaged in different formats and application facilities. Also, thanks to new formulations, products are launched to fit into fewer bottles. Clinicians may now quickly apply restorative materials with less clinical steps to fill the preparations. With the advent of self-adhering restorative materials, they were somehow down to absolutely no bottles. In other words: a single-step restoration gathers etchant, primer, adhesive, and restorative material.

Although representing a radical change on how direct dental restorations can be nowadays made, dental materials' manufactures have once again speeded up to launch their products based on this new restorative approach that completely suppress the preparation of tooth substrates to be restored. Obviously and over again in scientific evidencing terms, all these materials are, at this point, relatively brand new, and a few or no clinical studies about their performance are therefore available. Even though no long-term evaluations exist to demonstrate the effectiveness of these products, it may be useful to contextualize them with regard to the other materials they derive from and, at the same time, are claimed to be prone to replace and speculate on changes that this emerging class of restorative material can impose for the future of adhesive dentistry; both aspects are mainly addressed in this chapter.

10.2 A Timeline of the Development and Advances of Self-Adhering Direct Restorative Materials

The bonding mechanism of resin-based adhesive systems to enamel and dentin is essentially based on a series of physical-chemical principles that do not change significantly from when this class of material was first launched in the sunrise of the 1970s. Morphophysiological aspects that impair optimal adhesion to challenging bonding substrates such as carious-affected and sclerotic dentin remain, for instance, practically unchanged over the past decades. Because adhesive systems, in realistic terms, need to be universal and capable to couple resin composites with any hard dental structure under extremely limited conditions (i.e., time, temperature, atmospheric pressure, level of hydration), the major and most effective mechanism of interaction between them has been relying on an exchange process, in which minerals removed from dental hard tissues are replaced by resin monomers that upon in situ polymerization become micromechanically interlocked in the created porosities of dental substrates [10, 11]. When this mechanism, widely known as dental hard tissue "hybridization," was described by Nakabayashi et al. [12] for the first time, it provided essential insights into the rationale of resin bonding to dentin, which significantly impacted the course of adhesive dentistry and development of restorative materials in subsequent years.

The biophysical concept of "etch-and-rinse" dental adhesives of keeping unsupported acid-etched dentin matrices in fully extended state to be better infiltrated with resin monomers (i.e., etch-and-rinse approach) and the reintroduction of acidic self-etching primers from earlier prototypes to bond resin to smear layer-covered dentin (i.e., self-etch approach) are the two strategies currently defining how clinicians can repair dental structures when using dental restorative composites. Although these two methods present different ways of dealing with tooth tissues, they essentially interact with dental structures through such resin-diffusion, hybridizing process previously mentioned. It is well true that the quality of the hybrid layer strongly depends on its nanostructure and the reactants formed by the monomer-tooth reaction, but in concert with optimized management of resin composites' polymerization shrinkage stress, these two bonding approaches have contributed to enhance laboratorial and clinical predictability in the bonding of polymeric restorative materials to hard dental tissues, even if considering bias effects due to high product dependency in the outcomes [13–15].

There is a general consensus that non-carious cervical lesions (NCCLs) provide the best and most challenging configuration to test the clinical effectiveness of dental adhesives because they normally require that bonding procedures be performed on both enamel and dentin with none or minimal macroretention resources [16]. Recent published randomized controlled clinical trials showing a favorable performance of self-etch adhesives on NCCLs' restorations at clinically relevant terms (varying between 6 and 13 years) [17–19] steadily embody the aspirations of clinicians and manufactures toward dental bonding procedure simplification.

Unlike etch-and-rinse adhesives, self-etch adhesives do not require a separate etching step, as they contain acidic monomers that simultaneously prepare and interact with dental substrates [20]. Consequently, this approach is not only more user-friendly (shorter application time, fewer steps), but also has been considered less technique sensitive (no wet bonding) and less aggressive, causing less postoperative sensitivity experienced by patients when compared to etch-and-rinse adhesives [21–23]. These characteristics are in accordance with the adhesion decalcification (AD) concept [24]. According to the AD concept, molecules that contain functional carboxyl groups either adhere to or decalcify hydroxyapatite tissues. In the process that involves an adhesion to hydroxyapatite, molecules will remain attached to the hydroxyapatite surface depending on the solubility of the calcium salt in the acidic solution containing functional monomers [11]. In this way, the lower the solubility of the calcium salt on its own acidic solution, the more intense and stable are the molecular adhesion of the acidic functional monomers to hydroxyapatite [13]. In other words, this concept wherein acidic functional monomers favor a bonded restoration to adhere to the tooth tissues more than their ability to decalcify it somehow represents the core idea behind the development of self-adhering restorative materials. This adhesion approach also induces secondary reactions, characterized as chemical bonding, between acidic functional monomers incorporated in the formulation with the hydroxyapatite [25]. Thus, in this adhesion strategy, there is a synergism between micromechanical retention and chemical interactions between monomer acidic groups and hydroxyapatite [13, 26]. In Fig. 10.1, a timeline is depicted highlighting important findings and concepts toward the development and advances which led to the launching of self-adhering restoratives.

The acid-functionalized monomers currently utilized for most self-etch adhesives to promote demineralization and bonding to the tooth hard tissues are still predominantly (meth)acrylate monomers with either carboxylic acid groups, as with 4-methacryloxyethyl trimellitic anhydride (4-META), 4-methacryloxyethyl trimellitic acid (4-MET), and pyromellitic glycerol dimethacrylate (PMGDM), or phosphoric acid groups, as with 2-methacryloxyethyl phenyl hydrogen phosphate (Phenyl-P), 10-methacryloxydecyl dihydrogen phosphate (10-MDP), bis(2-methacryloxyethyl) acid phosphate (BMP), and dipentaerythritol penta-acrylate monophosphate (Penta-P) [27]. The morphological features of the adhesive-tooth interface produced by self-etch adhesives depend to a great extent on the manner in which their functional monomers interact with the dental substrate [28]. Thus, the actual bonding performance attained by self-etch adhesives varies a great deal, depending on the actual composition and, more specifically, on the actual functional monomer included in the adhesive formulation.

Among these monomers so far tested for their chemical bonding potential to dental apatites, 10-MDP has shown to be more proficient regarding other phosphoric acid-derived monomers, like Phenyl-P and 4-MET [13, 29], and the phosphonate-derived ones HAEPA (carboxy-2-[4-(dihydroxyphosphoryl)-2-oxabutyl]acrylic acid), EAEPA (ethyl 2-[4-(dihydroxyphosphoryl)-2-oxabutyl]acrylate), and MAEPA (2,4,6-trimethylphenyl 2-[4-(dihydroxyphosphoryl)-2-oxabutyl] acrylate) [26, 30]. 10-MDP was reported to form aqueous insoluble salt complex with calcium of tooth apatites with a higher stability to dissolution when compared with the calcium complexes

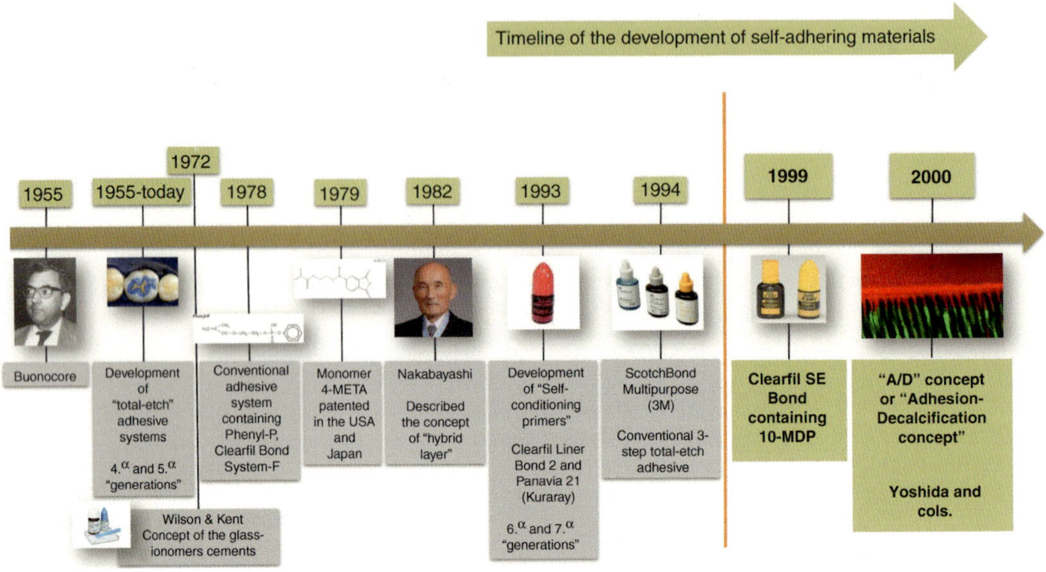

Fig. 10.1 This timeline of major events lays out the most important points in history that guided the developments and advances of self-adhering direct restorative materials. Two events can be considered the keystone for dental material industry toward the development of self-adhesive restoratives: in 1999, the Japanese Company Kuraray launched a 10-MDP-based, two-step self-adhesive system Clearfil SE Bond, considered the gold standard in several important scientific studies; in 2000, Yoshida and coworkers published this important study describing the AD concept that represented the scientific foundation for the understanding of bonding approach of this category of materials

formed with apatite when using 4-MET and Phenyl-P [13, 26, 31, 32]. An important detail to mention is that primary chemical interaction of 10-MDP with dental apatite was shown to occur within a clinically realistic time of 20 s [32]. This represents an extra bonding mechanism for 10-MDP-based adhesives and has been related with improvements in the biodegradation resistance of adhesive interfaces made with dental systems containing this monomer [31, 33–35].

Recently, the so-called multimode or universal adhesives were launched and named in this way due to their versatile clinical indications. *Universal adhesives* are considered one-step self-etching adhesives that can be applied in self-etching mode, etch-and-rinse mode, or selective-etch mode, depending on the clinical procedure [36–38]. This characteristic allows clinicians to decide which adhesive strategy to use for each specific clinical situation [39]. However, studies have been published in the literature considering that these universal adhesives have shown significantly inferior results in terms of bonding ability to the dental tissues, even when applied in self-etching mode [38, 40–43]. *Scotchbond Universal Adhesive* (3M ESPE), launched in 2011, was claimed to be the first universal adhesive [44]. Currently, among other marketed universal adhesives are *All-Bond Universal* (Bisco) and *Prime&Bond Elect* (Dentsply Caulk).

The popularity of self-etch adhesives in today's dental practice was the cornerstone for dental material industry to develop the *self-adhesive resin cements*. *Self-adhesive resin cements* are hybrid materials that blend characteristics of self-etching adhesives, resin restorative composites, and, in some cases, dental cements [45]. Specific compositions for commercial materials can be found in the manufacturer's brochures and have been published in some articles [45–48]. *Self-adhesive resin cements* represent a category of restorative materials created when 3M ESPE *RelyX™ Unicem Aplicap* was commercially available in 2002. This manufacturer claimed that its low pH immediately after mixing (pH 1) would permit this material to act in a similar manner to self-etching adhesive primers to produce a bond with dentin, and, because of this, they do not require technique-sensitive steps, such as acid etching, priming, or bonding [25].

Self-adhesive resin cements are hybrid, dual-curing, two-part materials that require hand mixing, capsule trituration, or delivery by an automixing dispenser. One component basically contains traditional methacrylate monomers that are commonly used in most of restorative resin-based composites and/or dental cements (i.e., Bis-GMA, UDMA, TEGDMA, GDMA, HEMA, and others), while the other component is comprised of acid-functionalized monomers already utilized in current self-etch dental adhesives (i.e., Phenyl-P, PMGDM, 4-META, Penta-P, BMP, MDP) or especially designed to this class of material, such as the neutral monomers based on bisacrylamide structures [27]. If on one side self-adhesive resin cements resemble self-etch adhesives and flowable resin composites due to the presence of methacrylate monomers (functionalized and/or structuring), on the other side they exhibit a polyacid matrix structure that approximates them to polyalkenoate-based materials, like glass ionomer cements (GICs) and resin-modified glass ionomer cements (RMGICs). The polyacid matrix of self-adhesive resin cements is formed, thanks to the low concentrations of fillers consisting mainly of ion-leachable particles, such as barium fluoroaluminosilicate glass, strontium calcium aluminosilicate glass, quartz, colloidal silica, and ytterbium fluoride glass. When in contact with hydrated dental substrates, the acid-functionalized monomers are ionized, acidifying the medium, which triggers an acid-base reaction between the glass fillers and dental substrates that, in sequence, neutralizes the monomer ionization and accordingly creates a polyacid matrix [27].

Actually, self-adhesive resin cements are conceptually similar to an almost extinct class of biomaterial, the compomers, which came available in the market in the end of the 1990s and never gained expressive recognition from researchers or clinicians since these materials seemed not to combine the advantages of resin composites and GICs as idealized in manufactures' prospects, materials they were supposed to derive from, such as capacity to bond hard dental tissues and release fluoride ions [46, 47, 49, 50]. A quite difference between compomers and self-adhesive resin cements is the presence of acidic monomers in the latter. Besides increasing the chances of establishing a chemical bonding with dental substrates via calcium apatite chelation as occurring when using GICs, the likely leaching of fluoride ions from soluble glass fillers of some self-etch resin cements could represent an advantage against occasional caries challenging, even though this should be yet clinically demonstrated [27].

Self-adhesive resin cements are used as luting agents, claimed by the manufacturers to adhere to dental hard tissues and indirect restorations (i.e., inlays, onlays, crowns, and posts) without the requirements of separate adhesive or etchant. The varied types of restorative materials currently applied in a daily based practice were shown as being compatible with self-adhesive resin cements, which include milled or pressed ceramics, full gold crowns, and also porcelain-fused-to-metal restoration, thereby enhancing the array of clinical possibilities wherein these cements can be applied [51]. Yet, quite few results comparing the self-adhesive resin cements and other conventional resin cements are available in the literature, but an in vivo study that evaluated over a 12-month period indirect composite resin restorations cemented with self-adhesive resin cements showed that these materials exhibited a clinical performance that did not differ significantly from that observed for conventional resin cements [52]. However, it can be speculated that under longer periods of evaluation, the dual-bonding mechanism (micromechanical and chemical interaction) could represent an important advantage of self-adhesive cements in terms of bonding stability when compared to other resin cements that essentially bond to the tooth structures simply by micromechanical interactions [53].

Concerns generally related with the low viscosity of resin-based materials, such as reduction in material's elastic modulus, higher volume shrinkage, and, in consequence, elevated shrinkage stress [54–57], potentially limit the use of self-adhesive resin cements in direct restorative

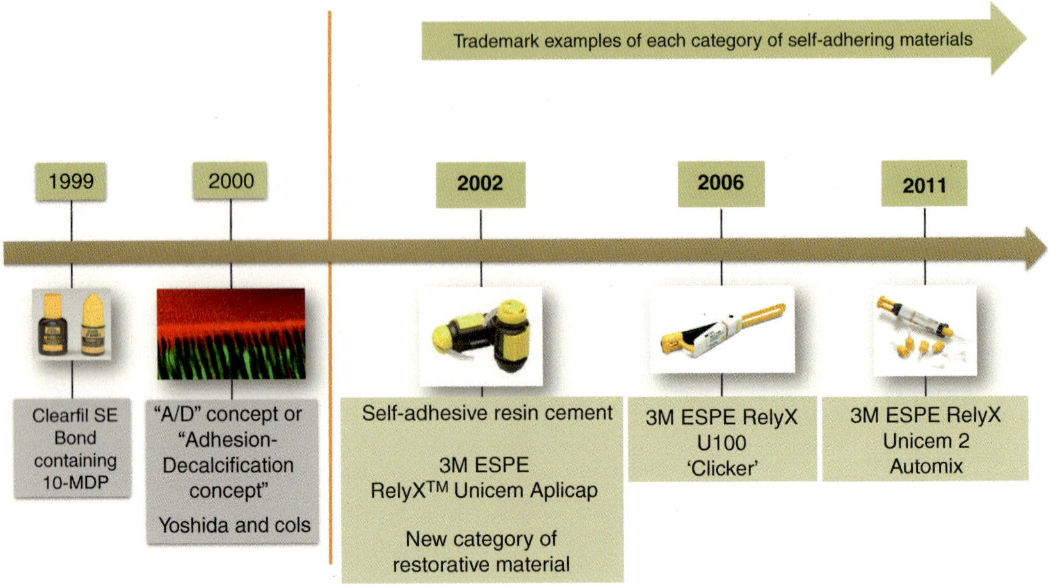

Fig. 10.2 This timeline lays out the development of 3M ESPE self-adhesive resin cement products after the first generation of self-adhesive universal resin cement RelyX™ Unicem, market in 2002; the manufacturer launched RelyX™ U200 in 2011, which represents the last generation of self-adhesive resin cement after the second-generation RelyX™ U100 using the delivery system "Clicker" (launched in 2006). According to the manufacturer, RelyX™ U200 contains an additional monomer and a viscosity modifier in order to optimize its rheological properties. In addition, following the market trend, RelyX™ U200 is also offered with an automix delivery system

procedures. It can be suggested, for instance, an increased bond strength when fiber posts were cemented with self-adhesive resin cements is possible due to the differences in the viscosities when delivering the resin cements and after the setting reactions [58]. Following the market trend and also attentive to scientific findings, dental manufacturers are marketing their products to be delivered using standardized automix tips (Fig. 10.2). This provides a more comfortable handling, time saving, and choices of tips for varied clinical applications, which includes a tip to deliver the cement directly into the root canal.

Commercial products currently available on the market are *Bifix SE* (Voco GmbH), *MaxCem Elite* (Kerr), *G-Cem* (CG), *Clearfil SA Luting* (Kuraray), *SmartCem2* (Dentsply Caulk), *BeautiCem SA* (Shofu), and *Multilink Speed* (Ivoclar Vivadent), among others.

Self-adhesive resin cements thus naturally led to the advent of a new category of self-adhesive materials: the *self-adhesive flowable resin (restorative) composites*. This evolving techology also allowed this category of restorative to adhesively and chemically bond to the tooth tissues in direct restorative procedures, with no need of a separate adhesive step [59], promising to reinforce the paradigm's shift on how resin-based direct restorations will probably be done in the near future.

10.3 Self-Adhering Restorative Materials' Identity: Components and Interaction with Tooth Substrates

Likewise, for self-etch adhesives and self-adhesive resin cements, as previously seen in this chapter, the advent of self-adhering restorative materials (self-adhesive resin composites) is also in part owed to the development of the chemistry of acidic functional groups. Acidic functional monomers were initially added to self-etching adhesives as ligand components allowing a chemical interaction with the hydroxyapatite found in dental hard tissues [60]. This was particularly true when functional monomers, 10-MDP, 4-MET, and Phenyl-P, were added to this category of adhesives [57]. As previously mentioned, among the acidic functional monomers contained in self-etching adhesive systems, 10-MDP was found to be the monomer that "readily and intensively" adheres to apatite [13], and again this has been used to justify the favorable performance of 10-MDP-containing adhesives in many laboratory and clinical studies [33, 34].

It has been described varied possible adsorption and reaction mechanisms of 10-MDP with dental hydroxyapatite via adsorption onto Ca^{2+} sites, reaction with PO_4^{3-} groups of apatite, and/or by substitution of OH^- or PO_4^{3-} groups of the apatite matrix [13, 61]. Other studies have also sustained that the bonding mechanism of 10-MDP-based self-etching adhesives strongly resembles that of obtained when using resin-modified glass ionomers [11, 62] since it only superficially interacts with the dental hard tissues, hardly dissolving the apatite that remains in a non-authentic submicron hybrid layer [60].

Although it would be expected that the chemical bonding contributed to the majority of the bond strength, there may be a consensus that the role of acidic functional groups as chemical ligands to the interfacial area is more related with the stability of the chemical bonding and the adhesives themselves rather than to the bond strengths of the interface [63]. Previous studies demonstrated the bond strength to dentin when a 10-MDP-based two-step self-etch adhesive yields reliable results in terms of bonding effectiveness and durability when compared to other commercially available self-etch adhesives, in both in vitro and in vivo studies [64–66]. Until 2011, Kuraray Company owned MDP patent for 10 years and since then have been incorporated into numerous bonding and luting products, such as primers, adhesives, and resin composites.

Another common component present in self-adhering restorative materials is the monomer Phenyl-P, which is thought to ionically bond to calcium at the apatite surface after severely decalcification of apatite crystals around collagen fibrils. Thanks to its functional group, phosphate (PO_4^3) and hydroxide (OH) ions would be extracted from apatite surface by hydronium ions (H_3O^+), and the interfacial area produced by the Phenyl-P-based adhesive was claimed to have most of the apatite dissolved and the collagen fibril exposed up to a depth of about 1 μm. In this way, the interfacial area is considered less stable due to the presence of unprotected collagen fibrils and the absence of the original apatite crystals [29, 31].

Finally, another monomer usually found in self-adhering restorative formulations, 4-MET, has been described to exhibit a weak chemical bonding potential in comparison with 10-MDP [13], leading to the formation of a submicron hybrid layer with apatite that protects the remaining collagen fibrils. The hybrid layer produced by a 4-MET-based adhesive was demonstrated to exhibit a relatively superficial interaction with dentin, with shallow demineralization and collagen exposure [29, 31], which explains the degradation resistance of the interfacial bond, extending the longevity in comparison to that of a Phenyl-P-based adhesive [31].

Since self-adhering restorative materials evolved from self-adhesive resin cements, they similarly have components that are present in glass ionomer cements. GICs can be considered a type of mild self-etch adhesives as they have an auto-adhesive capability with no need of hard dental tissue pretreatment [20]. The mechanism on how GICs interact with hard dental tissues remains for years under fully obscurity [67], but it is actually regarded to involve a wetting of the hard tissues by the glass ionomer cement and consequent formation of ionic bonds at the intimacy of dentin and enamel tissues, even in the presence of a smear layer [68]. Their ability to adhere to the dental tissues seems to depend initially on the limited demineralization of both enamel and dentin, with consequent infiltration and micromechanical interaction, and on the chemical interaction with the calcium ions between apatite and the polyalkenoic acid, a polymer containing numerous carboxyl functional groups. This allows an ionic bonding, occurring between carboxyl groups of the polyalkenoic acid and calcium of partially remaining apatite crystals [20, 69]. In addition, the acidic feature of GICs' setting reaction also selectively induces dental apatite dissolution, exposing a microporous collagen network [69].

There are six essential constituents found in GICs: polymeric water-soluble acid, basic (ion-leachable) glasses, water [70], silica, alumina, and calcium fluoride [71]. The setting reaction is an acid-base reaction between polymeric carboxylic acid and basic fluoroaluminosilicate glass and requires an aqueous medium in order for the ions to be leached from the glass and to react with the polyacid moiety [71]. Water is the solvent for the polymeric acid allowing the polymer to act as an acid by promoting proton release, the medium in which the setting reaction takes place and, ultimately, represents a component of the set cement [70]. These materials are commonly presented as an aqueous solution of polymeric acid and a finely divided glass powder, which are mixed by an appropriate method to form a viscous paste that sets rapidly [72]. The application of the fresh cement paste allows proper wetting of the tooth surface to take place. However, alternative formulations are commercially found which range from both the acid and the glass being present in the powder, and pure water being added to cause setting, to formulations in which some of the acid is blended with the glass powder and the rest is present in a dilute solution in water [72]. Glass ionomers set within 2–3 min from mixing by an acid-base reaction after which water becomes incorporated into the cement [72]. The displacement of calcium ions with the phosphate ions allows the electron neutrality [73].

The combination of ion-leachable glass particles (like in glass ionomers) and the presence of acidic-functionalized monomers (like in self-etch systems and self-adhesive resin cements) is also found in self-adhering restorative materials and is thought to be advantageous in terms of bond durability [26, 31]. The basic difference between the chemistry when self-etch adhesives and glass ionomers cements are compared is that the former contain functional monomers with usually only one or two functional chemical groups with affinity with apatite crystals [20]. Thus, individual monomers of self-etching adhesives are converted into a polymer linked to dental apatite after polymerization. Conversely, GICs present numerous functional acidic groups attached to the polyalkenoic acid polymer backbone that covalently links to calcium ions at different and remote sites [20].

It has been also pointed out that the glass ionomer "concept" was combined with functionalized monomers to form self-adhesive resin cements, and more recently self-adhering restorative materials, in order to neutralize the initial low pH, which thereby rapidly increases from 1 to 6 when these acidic monomers are ionized in the presence of water [48]. It has been previously demonstrated that the acidic monomers added to methacrylates seem to impair the rate and extent of polymerization because of the deactivating action of the acidic groups on free radicals [74, 75], chemically interfering with the amine initiator [76]. Since additional glass ionomer-type reaction occurs at the same time as the free radical polymerization, particularly in 3M products [77], harmful effects on these materials' final conversion could be compensated with a polyacid matrix formation. It is important to bear in mind therefore that there is a dynamic process wherein the demineralization/monomer permeation process and polymerization kinetics coexist in these materials [78]. This additional glass ionomer-type reaction occurring at the same time as the free radical polymerization also contributes to the overall properties and thus to the potential clinical success of these restorative products [78]. When phosphoric ester groups and methacrylate-functionalized polyalkenoic acid polymers are put together, they allow the inorganic smear layer to be dissolved and the intertubular dentin to be demineralized. This interaction approach gave these materials the ability to bond to dentin in the presence of a variety of moisture levels. In this way, likely in self-adhesive resin cements, they in theory should simultaneously penetrate the demineralized dentin to form the hybrid layer and flow into the dentin tubules, creating resin tags [79, 80].

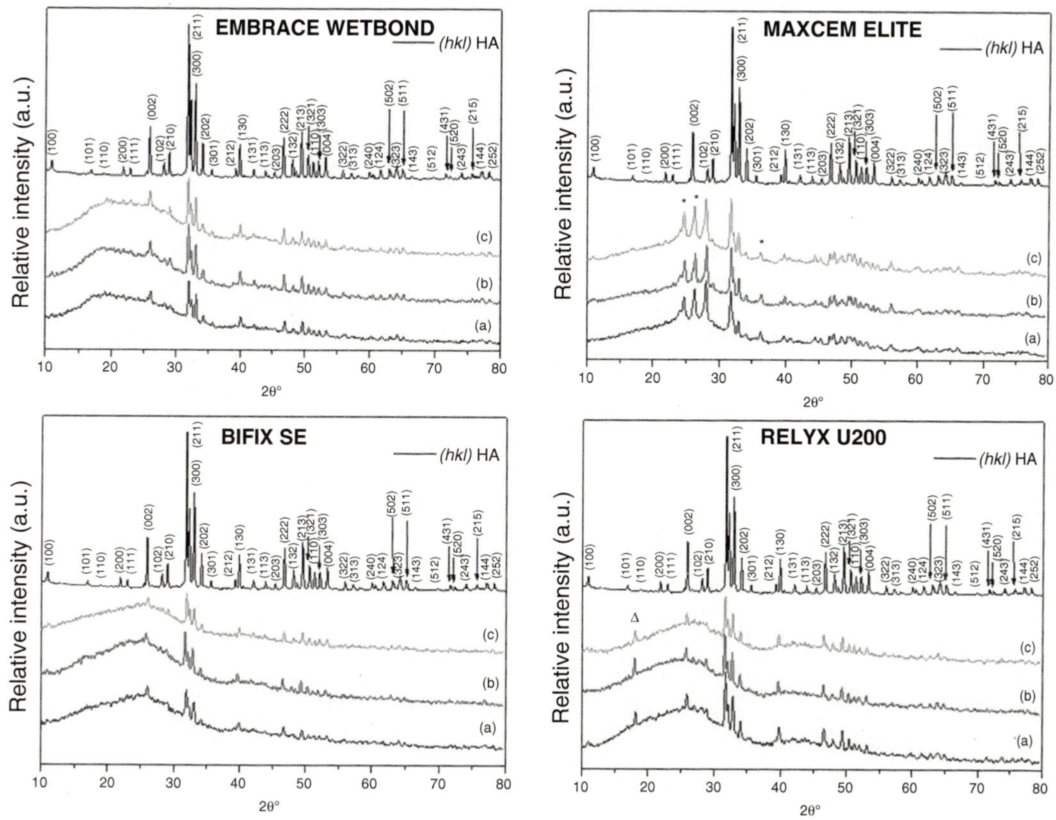

Fig. 10.3 Twenty-four-hour X-ray diffraction patterns of the self-adhesive resin cements: (*a*) immediate photoactivation; (*b*) delayed photoactivation; (*c*) chemical activation. *Asterisks* crystalline peaks of ytterbium fluoride. *Delta* means unidentified crystalline peak at $2\theta = 17.9°$ (from D'Alpino et al. 2015 [78])

The panels in Fig. 10.3 display the changes in the crystalline peaks of pure hydroxyapatite after mixing with different commercial self-adhesive resin cements evaluated with X-ray diffraction. According to the authors [78], changes in crystallinity of hydroxyapatite are representative of the ability of self-adhesive resin cements to superficially demineralize and permeate the tooth tissues. The acidic monomers incorporated in these materials are claimed to incorporate the smear layers, but not sufficiently strong to form an authentic hybrid layer along the resin-tooth interface (Fig. 10.4) [81]. In spite of this, it was also proven that the adhesion strategy of self-adhesive cements relies not only on micromechanical retention but also on chemical interactions between monomer acidic groups and hydroxyapatite [82].

10.4 Self-Adhering Flowable Composites: A Prelude of Self-Adhering Composites for Restoration

The flowable resin composite *Embrace WetBond Class V* (from Pulpdent), marketed since 2002, can be considered a sort of prototype of *self-adhering flowable composites*. Manufacturers however used to recommend etching, and the application of an adhesive system was considered optional. Its chemistry involves di-, tri-, and multifunctional acrylate monomers that are hydrophilic and actually require some moisture to be activated [83]. More recently, in the same way of self-adhesive resin cements, functional monomers were added to flowable composites to

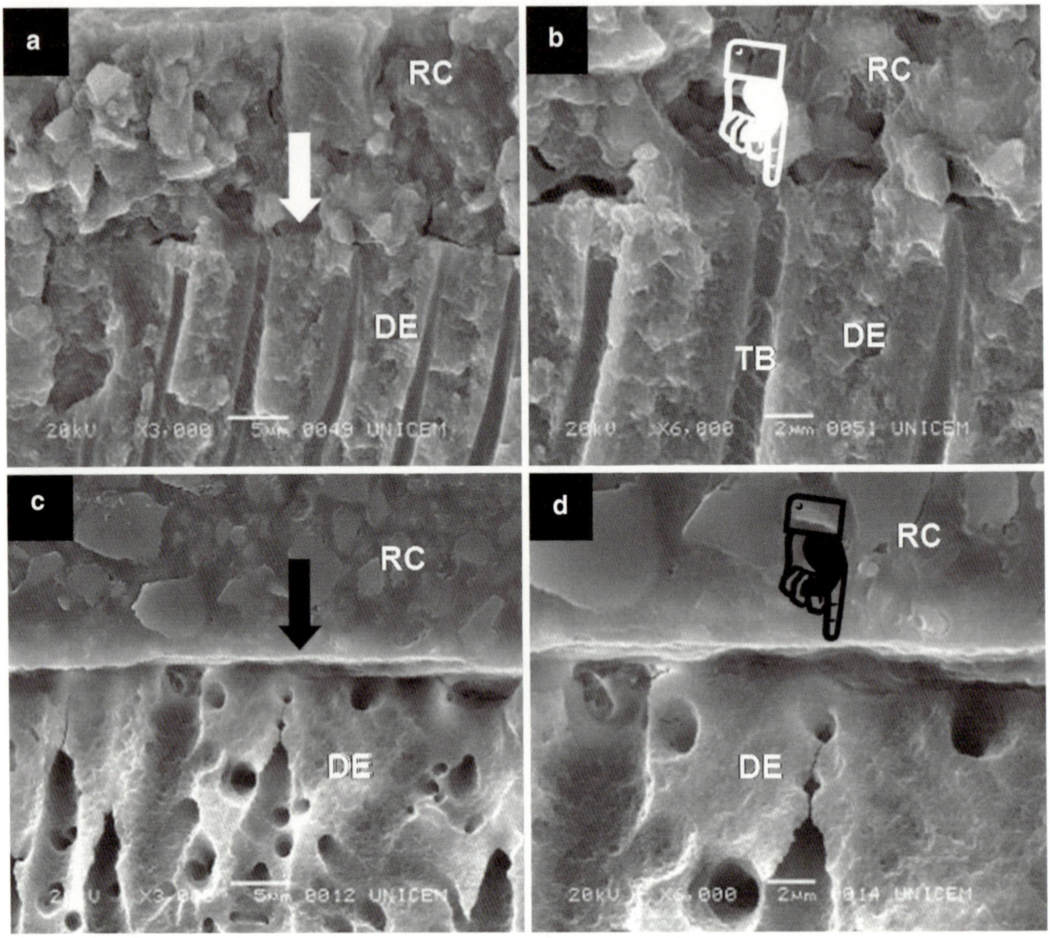

Fig. 10.4 SEM photomicrograph of the self-adhesive resin cement RelyX Unicem (3M ESPE) bonded to dentin. (**a**) (3000×) and (**b**) (6000×) (fractured specimens) exhibit an intimate contact of the resin cement with the dentin tissue (*white arrow*); dentin tubules (TB) with no resin infiltration (*white hand*) were noticed. In (**c**) and (**d**) (conventionally processed specimens), images show a non-authentic hybrid layer (*black arrow*) and also the interaction between the resin cement and the dentin (*black hand*). *RC* resin cement, *DE* dentin (from Vaz et al. 2012 [81])

serve as adhesion promoters and provide bonding to mineralized dental tissues through chemical reaction with apatite [84] with no additional etching, rinsing, or air blowing, apart from light curing which is actually recommended [85].

Flowable composites were initially developed in the 1990s as an important advance in restorative dental materials to repair class V lesions [67]. Flowable composites can be considered low-viscosity resin composites obtained from formulations with 20–25% lower filler loading in comparison to that of conventional composites, providing excellent handling and reduced working time [86, 87]. In fact, the low viscosity of flowable composites can be obtained either by decreasing the percentage of fillers or modifying the resin monomers, for instance, by adding diluents, that is, resin monomers with molecular weight relatively lower in comparison to conventional methacrylates [88]. This lower viscosity of flowables allowed these materials to be placed using injection syringes, easily dispensing with very small-gauge needles, thus limiting its stickiness and making them ideal for use in small preparations [89]. The first generation of flowables was used only as liners due to their low elastic modulus, increased elasticity, and wettability [90]. Compared with the interfacial area formed by a bonding agent and a resin composite, flowable liners are considered to present fewer voids at the interface, as these materials are able to better wet the cavity floor due to their flowability, when a thin layer of a flowable composite is applied, improving the marginal adaptation and sealing [91]. The second-generation flowables developed since 2000 promised increased mechanical properties and were proposed for use in bulk conservative restorations [92].

On the other hand, as already mentioned, common trade-offs caused by the relatively lower filler loading or higher amount of diluents in resin composites are greater degree of polymerization shrinkage and lower mechanical properties compared to other hybrid composites [54–57, 93]. In order to minimize consequences induced by the shrinkage stress of composite material at the interface tooth-composite, several practical steps have been proposed [94]. Because of their low modulus of elasticity, flowable composites have been indicated for lining class V restorations as stress-absorbing intermediate layers. Actually, as liners and base, flowable composites have demonstrated significantly positive effects [95], especially in time-consuming clinical cases in which atypical preparation designs present undercuts or angulations [96]. In these cases, using a flowable composite as a liner can help the dentist to deal with clinical issues where the access and visibility are more difficult, building the preparation out before the application of the resin composite [96]. Conversely, clinicians should be aware about the clinical consequences of shrinkage properties found in flowable composites, as these materials can sometimes shrink up to twice as much as condensable composites [96]. This can result in stress at the adhesive layer with a consequent mechanical failure at the composite/tooth interface, de-bonding, microleakage, secondary caries, and remnant enamel fractures [97, 98].

Flowable composites are offered in a full range of Vita shades to be applied in association with other restoratives [99]. Today, other clinical indications for these materials besides lining include temporary crown repair, veneer cementation, pit-and-fissure sealing, porcelain repair, and small core buildup [89]. In reality flowable composites have been indicated to numerous other applications as well depicted by *Baroudi* and *Rodrigues* [89]. Characteristics of flowable composites may include radiopacity, various viscosities for superior flowability or packing, fluoride release, and also high polishability [92]. Their consistency extended to other categories of resin-based materials, such as ormocers (organically modified ceramics) and compomers. In addition, a wide range of flowable composites with different percentages of fillers (50–70 wt%) are available, being classified as low, medium, and high viscosity.

Flowable composites are now widely used for clinicians and considered an important material in restorative and cosmetic dentistry. Following the same characteristics, self-adhering flowable composites were recently launched. *Fusio Liquid Dentin Dental Flowable Composite* (named *Dyad Flow* in Latin America) from Pentron, launched in May 2009, was marketed for small class I, III, and V restorations, as base liners for larger restorations and as a pit-and-fissure sealant, available in a variety of Vita shades. *Vertise Flow* was then released by Kerr in January 2010, and according to the manufacturer, it is indicated for small class I and class II restorations, as liner for large class I and class II restorations and as pit-and-fissure sealant, and for porcelain repair. This flowable composite is also available in varied shades. Both flowable composites present different chemistry based on traditional methacrylate systems, but their formulations incorporate acidic monomers typically found in dentin bonding agents: *Vertise Flow* contains GPDM (glycerol phosphate dimethacrylate), same of added to Kerr's adhesives (OptiBond), whereas *Fusio Liquid Dentin* is a 4-META-based flowable composite. Since then, the use of self-adhesive flowable resin composites in restorative dentistry increased as these materials are easy to handle and manipulate, the application is quite simple and easy, and there is no need of a previous acid etching [87]. Figure 10.5 presents the timeline and the commercial packaging of the first self-adhering flowable composites launched.

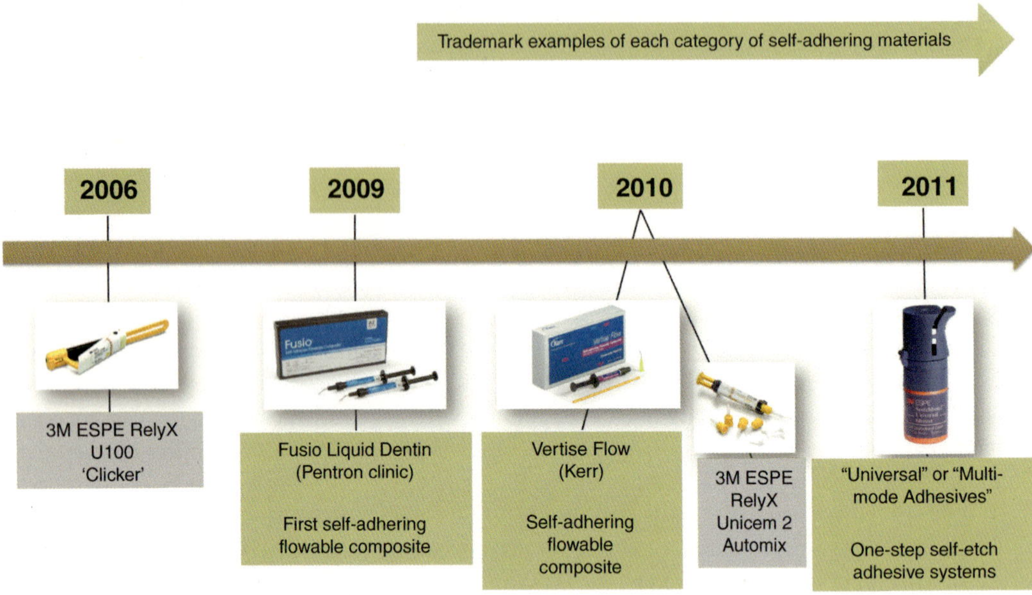

Fig. 10.5 This timeline exemplifies some trademarks of the so-called self-adhering flowable composites. Thanks to their lower viscosity, both *Fusio Liquid Dentin* (launched in 2009) and *Vertise Flow* (launched in 2010) are available in small syringes that allow these commercial materials to be easily dispensed with very small-gauge needles, thus limiting its stickiness and making them ideal for use in small preparations

For being the first materials on the market, the great majority of published studies evaluated these two commercial self-adhering flowable composites. Differences in bonding effectiveness between these two self-adhering flowable composites are determined among other factors, by their actual composition and also by the functional monomer contained in the material formulation. As previously described, *Fusio Liquid Dentin* contains the functional monomer 4-MET that has been attributed with chemical bonding potential to hydroxyapatite and tooth tissue, known to be significantly less strong than that of obtained with 10-MDP [13]. The functional monomer used in *Vertise Flow* according to Kerr's technical profile is GPDM. This phosphate functional group is supposed to be able to chemically bond with the calcium ions of the dental hard tissues. It has been also claimed that the prepolymerized fillers present in the formulation also minimize the shrinkage and enhance properties [100]. However, it has been reported that the functional acidic monomer GPDM present a 2-µm-deep hydroxyapatite-free hybrid layer, indicating that this monomer most likely etches the dentin surface, indicative of an absence of chemical bonding to hydroxyapatite [59]. These results corroborate with another study in which the interfacial dentinal area obtained with *Vertise Flow* exhibited open dentinal tubules and also an exposed collagen network, similar to that of observed when a total-etch adhesive system is applied to dentin [85]. It has been pointed out that, as the functional acidic monomers are not able to deeply penetrate the tooth structures, the self-adhesiveness, which is represented by an effective chemical bonding, would be achieved whether the flowable composites presented a relative viscosity [59].

Apart from differences in terms of formulation, the rheological properties of these two self-adhering flowable composites are also claimed to be completely distinct. *Fusio Liquid Dentin* has been described to be significantly more fluid than *Vertise Flow*. Reasons that explain such difference rely on the filler content that is found to be lower for *Fusio Liquid Dentin* (65 wt%) in comparison with *Vertise Flow* (70 wt%) [59]. Although there may be a practical limit in terms of filler packing for considering these materials as *flowable composites*, this difference pointed out by the authors requires a more accurate analysis considering that other dissimilarities, i.e., in terms of particle sizes, should be also evaluated. *Fusio Liquid Dentin* was also described to present better handling properties, to be less sticky to application instruments, and to exhibit a better wetting of the dental hard tissues [59]. The authors believe that the easier handling may have contributed in part to the improved bonding effectiveness of *Fusio Liquid Dentin* in comparison to that of found for *Vertise Flow* [59]. In another study, *Fusio Liquid Dentin* was also found to present higher bond strength than that of observed for *Vertise Flow* [85].

In spite of these features, these materials have in common the fact that they are friendly-user materials, with easy application: when applied in small class I and II preparations, wash and dry the preparation, brush on *Vertise Flow*, photoactivate it, and apply another layer if necessary. For *Fusio Liquid Dentin*, the manufacturer recommends slight enamel roughening before application, and the material is then applied, agitated, contoured with an explorer, and finally photoactivated. Other self-adhering flowable composites have been launched with the similar indications and easy application.

Despite self-adhering flowable composites, manufactures assure these materials have an ample indication; their use should be pursued with care at least up to when the outcomes can prove their clinical advantages over conventional resin materials [101]. A previous study evaluated the microleakage of self-adhesive flowable composites in comparison with a conventional flowable composite that is regularly associated with an etch-and-rinse adhesive [102]. It was found that *Vertise Flow* presented lower levels of microleakage regarding that of *Fusio Liquid Dentin* [102]. The authors concluded that a previous etching with phosphoric acid may reduce the microleakage for *Fusio Liquid Dentin* in both enamel and dentin, whereas this pretreatment was valid for *Vertise Flow* only at the enamel margin. Both self-adhering flowable composites presented higher microleakage when compared with that of conventional flowable composite.

Although still scarcely, *self-adhering flowable composites* have been also clinically evaluated. In a randomized, controlled, single-center, split-mouth clinical trial, a self-adhesive flowable composite (*Fusio Liquid Dentin*) was evaluated when applied in non-carious cervical lesions [103]. The results were compared with that obtained when using a nanohybrid composite associated with a three-step etch-and-rinse adhesive system [103]. It was found that 27 out of 40 restorations filled with *self-adhering flowable composite* were clinically unacceptable after only 6 months in service (success rate of only 33%). The authors attributed this low success rate to failure in retention against 100% of success rate for the restorations in which the combination of nanohybrid composite and total-etch adhesive was applied. In another study, the bond strength of a self-adhering flowable resin composite (*Vertise Flow*) to dentin in primary molars was evaluated [104]. The results were compared with two ionomer-based cements and one flowable resin composite combined with different adhesive systems. The authors reported similar bond strength means in comparison with those obtained with glass ionomer cements. They also found that the association of this flowable composite with adhesive systems resulted in higher bond strength means when compared with all of the experimental groups. It was pointed out that the incorporation of more operative steps reduces the advantages of this group of materials as it would involve a more complex handling scenario [104].

In general, flowable composites are considered to have well-adapted bonded interfacial morphology [105]. That is why this low modulus restoratives have been indicated for using as stress-absorbing liner materials [106]. Considering that self-adhering flowable composites are currently recommended as liners and that their low viscosity favors an increased interfacial adaptation, these materials should be also considered as low elastic modulus liners, hence being capable to reduce the cusp deformation and gap formation by absorbing polymerization shrinkage stress. Up to now, no studies were found in the literature in this respect.

10.5 Biocompatibility of Self-Adhering Materials

The polymerization reaction in methacrylate-based resins is radical mediated [107]. Ideally, polymer networks should be stable and insoluble and also chemically and thermally stable [108]. However, most of the monomers used in dental resin materials can absorb water and chemicals from the environment, hence releasing by-products to its surroundings [109]. Concern has been expressed regarding a clinically relevant analysis of the biocompatibility of self-adhering materials considering that components are released during their clinical application [78, 110–113]. Polymers formed after the application and photoactivation of dental restoratives are subject to both hygroscopic and hydrolytic effects, influencing the mechanical properties, the dimensional stability, and the biocompatibility [109]. Numerous by-product components are lixiviated from polymerized methacrylate-based resins, varying in nature and amount [78]. Monomer release studies are generally investigated using different solvents such as water, saliva, and other organic solvents [114]. Biological concerns have been also reported as a variety of chemical and physical processes due to the sorption and solubility processes are claimed to produce deleterious effects on the polymeric structure and function of the materials [109].

Another issue is the fact that self-adhering materials are frequently applied to newly exposed dentin, especially when the preparation design exposes a great amount of dentinal tubules, particularly in total crown preparations [78]. Considering the application of self-adhering restorative materials, in contact with the dentinal tubules, monomers and their components lixiviated by the bonded interface might not be totally avoided of reaching the pulp through dentinal fluid flow transport, thus potentially getting in contact with odontoblasts and other pulp cells. Accordingly, all sorts of cell reactions might occur, varying from a slight inflammatory reaction that can lead to necrotic cell death and also noninflammatory apoptotic cell death [115].

The major concern regarding the biocompatibility of self-adhering restoratives relies on their resultant thin and characteristic interfacial layer. The acidic monomers present in the self-adhesive cements were considered not strong enough to etch through smear layers to form an authentic hybrid layer along the interface [81]. Furthermore a thin interfacial layer is formed also because these cements' initial acidity, derived from ionization of its functionalized monomers, is quickly neutralized either due to the polymerization process or because monomers react with alkaline fillers [48]. The smear layer formed after preparation procedures is modified and incorporated into the interfacial area when cementing with self-adhesive resin cements. In consequence, a very fine "hybrid-like layer" is produced with the absence of resin tags [79]. It can be speculated that the interfacial area can be degraded by the presence of the dentinal fluid that easily dissolves the remaining smear plugs and contacting the thin non-authentic hybrid layer [111–113]. In this way, monomers and other oligomers can be initially lixiviated toward the pulp via dentinal tubules and afterward their degradation products.

In a previous study [116], the morphological characteristics of fillers found in self-adhesive resin cements were evaluated using different methods. In one of these methods, an elemental analysis of the fillers was conducted using X-ray spectroscopy analysis and micromorphology under SEM. Based on their findings, the authors found differences in the nature and chemistry of inorganic fractions in the commercial self-adhesive cements tested that seem to influence their clinical performance. It was also found fluorineions in one of the cements tested (G-Cem) and the chemical element chromium in another one (RelyX U200) (Fig. 10.6). The latter one is known for its cytotoxicity, to cause immunologic problems, and also for being mutagenic in certain species [117].

Garcia and coworkers evaluated the cytotoxicity of components released from different resin cements to odontoblastic-like cells and human dental pulp cells [118]. In that study, the authors exposed these cells to the products released from resin-modified glass ionomer cement,

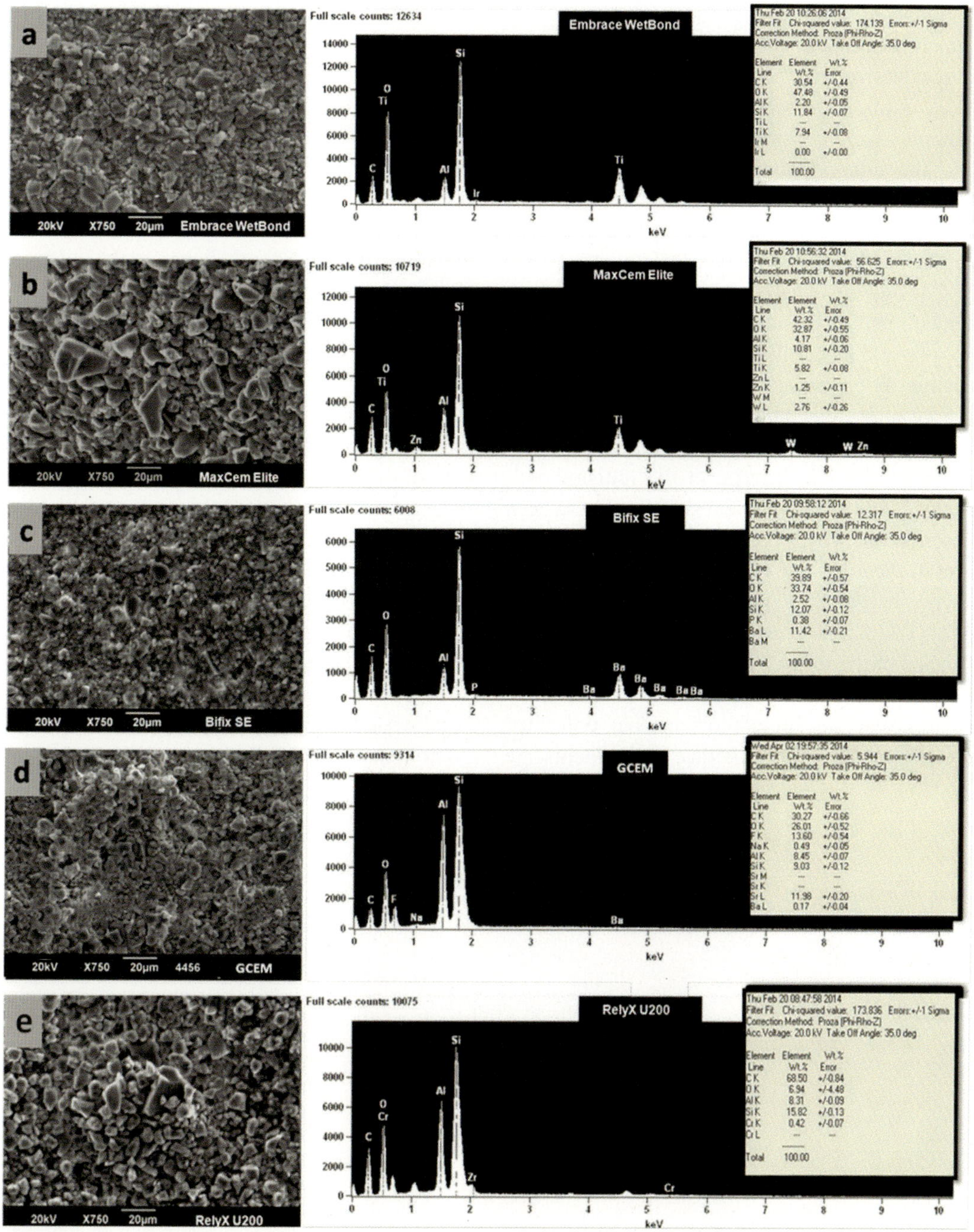

Fig. 10.6 Representative SEM/EDS analyses of the inorganic phase of self-adhesive resin cements are illustrated. The EDS analysis detected strong signals of Si and relatively high amounts of Al in all of the cements investigated. Significant amount of Ti is also observed for Embrace WetBond and MaxCem Elite. Other chemical elements were detected in different amounts, showing the complexity of the composition of the inorganic phase of the self-adhesive resin cements; among them, it can be highlighted the identification of F in the composition of G-Cem taking in account its anticariogenic activity, and Cr in RelyX U200 due to its mutagenic potential (**a**) Embrace WetBond (Pulpdent); (**b**) MaxCem Elite (Kerr); (**c**) Bifix SE (Voco); (**d**) G.Cem (GC); (**e**) RelyX U200 (3M ESPE), (from D'Alpino et al. 2016 [116])

self-adhesive resin cement, and conventional resin cement associated with a conventional etch-and-rinse adhesive system. The results were compared to a control, untreated group. None of the tested materials were considered cytotoxic. In spite of this, the authors pointed out the cytotoxicity of the resin cements is considered material dependent and that the different application protocols to dentin may interfere with their cytotoxicity [118].

Considering that the self-adhesive resin cements present distinctive formulations, low initial pH, and the ability to interact with hydroxyapatite, as previously described, these cements can be also either photoactivated or chemically activated. In both cases, reactive free radicals are generated by cleavage of the initiator molecules [119]. Varied clinical situations have been described in which the polymerization completion in the areas not reached by the curing light energy occurs through chemical reaction [120, 121]. Taking into account that only a certain percentage of the monomers convert into polymers, and the fact that these materials are dual-cured restoratives, the amount of residual unreacted monomers may vary whether the cements are either photoactivated or chemically activated. In a previous study, the cell viability of odontoblastic-like cells was evaluated after exposure to disks of self-adhesive resin cements activated according to the manufacturer's instructions [122]. In this study, odontoblastic-like cells were used in an in vitro model to investigate the cytotoxic effects of five commercial self-adhesive cements containing different acidic functional monomers. The results were compared to that of a control group of unexposed cells. It was found that the results were material dependent (Fig. 10.7). In other words, the composition of the different cements influenced on the cell viability after exposure. Some of them were rather cytotoxic. In spite of these problems described above, the use of resin cements in self-etch approach, in which the restorative procedure involves less technique-sensitive steps, has been claimed to allow a less hostile environment that leads to a "minimum" postoperative sensitivity [51].

Flowable composites have been also reported to produce higher levels of toxicity compared to conventional materials [89]. This increased cytotoxicity was attributed to the addition of

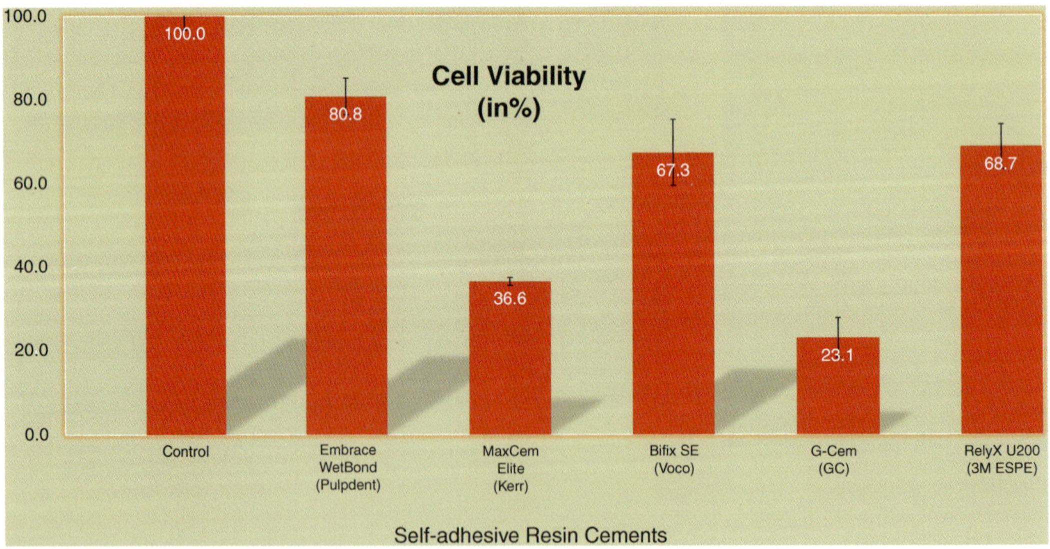

Fig. 10.7 Representative results of a study which evaluated the cytotoxic effect of self-adhesive resin cements containing different acidic functional monomers [122]. In this study, specimens of five commercial cements were immersed in a culture medium in which odontoblast-like cells were previously seeded. Control group consisted of unexposed cells. Cell viability significantly decreased after exposure to the self-adhesive cements, indicating that the tested materials seem to cause varied cytotoxicity when in contact with their lixiviated by-products. Cement G-Cem (GC) was found to cause the highest cytotoxicity

higher percentages of resin diluents considering necessary for conferring these materials' higher flowability [123]. Moreover, their lower filler packing might also be responsible for an increase in materials' temperature during the polymerization set reaction [124]. Accordingly, a significant rise in the temperature in the exothermic setting reaction might also contribute to cause pulpal damage, especially when flowable composites are applied in deep preparations [124]. While being crucial, no studies evaluating the cytotoxicity of self-adhering composites are available so far in the literature, and further in vivo and in vitro studies are fundamental to evaluate the self-adhering restorative material performance.

10.6 Bioactive Restoratives

Today, an important research topic in dentistry is the possibility of the development of restoratives that are "active" rather than "inert" material. This evolving technology is not new as numerous categories of materials release fluorides, such as GICs, RMGICs, and fluoride-containing resin composites/adhesives. The main difference in these advanced materials may allow the remineralization promoted by a slow releasing of calcium and phosphate ions from materials. The varied concentrations of certain ions onto the fluid that baths dental hard tissues would allow the precipitation of new calcium-phosphate mineral on these tissues' surface [125, 126]. Recently, a new category of restorative materials called ACTIVA Bioactive, launched in 2014, claims to combine the benefits of composites and glass ionomers while eliminating the disadvantages associated with those materials (Fig. 10.8). This material, described as being an "enhanced resin-modified glass ionomer restorative material" [127, 128], promises release and recharge calcium, phosphate, and fluoride ions with the surrounding teeth. These topics related to bioactivity of restorative materials are discussed in Chap. 18.

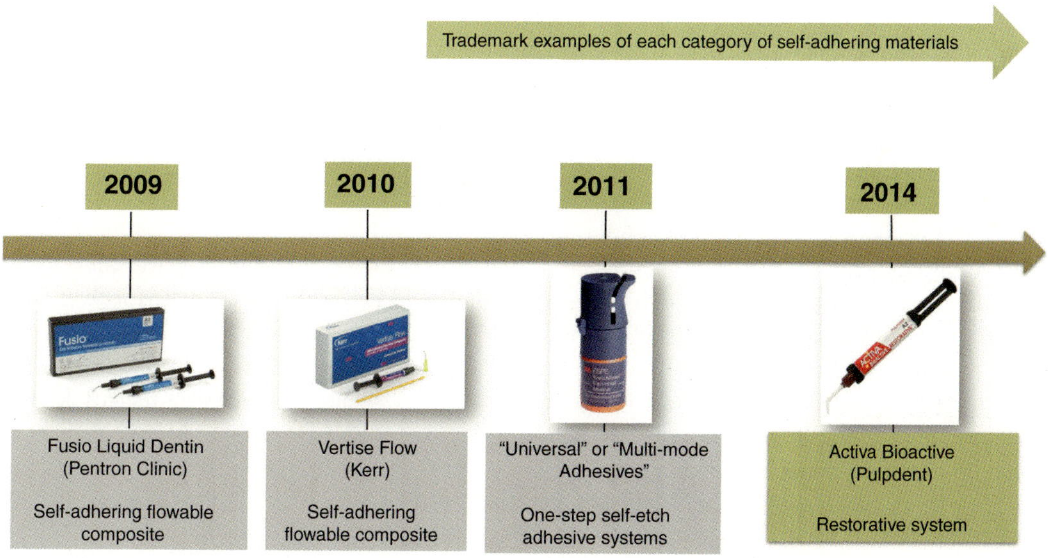

Fig. 10.8 This timeline presents a trademark example of a restorative material with bioactive properties (*ACTIVA Bioactive—Pulpdent*), launched in 2014. It is part of a restorative system, named *ACTIVA Products*, that contains other restoratives with similar formulations and different viscosities (flowable, luting cements, etc.), allowing the application in varied clinical indications

10.7 Self-Adhering Resin Composites: Now and Future

Taking into account the variability of commercial *self-adhering flowable composites* in terms of viscosity, this characteristic allows this group of restoratives to be indicated in different clinical situations, which make them to be considered as an "entry point" for *universal self-adhering composites* [27]. Nowadays, the development of *self-adhering composites* is certainly the main focus of the dental industry. Considering the commercial success and the qualified clinical effectiveness of the flowable composites, the next step is certainly the search of commercial self-adhering composites. As previously discussed, the flowable composite *Embrace WetBond Class V* (from Pulpdent) can be considered the earliest self-adhesive resin composite, launched in 2002. According to the manufacturer's instructions, both etching and the application of an adhesive system were considered optional. The advantages of this restorative material were reported to be wet bonding, tooth integrating, better retention, superior marginal seal, smooth margins, less technique sensitive, and increased fluoride release [129].

Up to now, there are no distinctive *self-adhering resin composites* on the market containing acidic functional monomers with similar indications of conventional resin composites. General indications of current resin composites include fillings requiring high mechanical clinical performance (class IV cavities with occlusal function, large class I, combination or complex class II, class VI). The most suitable composite is that with the higher inorganic load [130]. In this case, more viscous resin composites are indicated. With the advent of high-viscosity bulk-fill materials attempted to simplify and expedite the restoration process, being adequately polymerized in thick layers up to 4 or even 5 mm [131]. This group of materials is claimed to be shaded, sculptable, and, thanks to their higher filler content, present improved strength and wear resistance [132]. Due to differences in rheological properties and application techniques, bulk-fill resin composites can be further classified in low-viscosity (flowable) and high-viscosity (sculptable) material ones [131].

Clinicians that once have demanded for an easier, efficient placement technique to fill posterior composite restorations that rivaled that for amalgam [132] may now claim for an even faster way to complete their bonded restorations. An ideal self-adhering composite would be a well-adapted, chemically and micromechanically bonded material to the confines of the preparation, linking the remaining cusps and extending the fatigue life of the tooth, especially when remaining structure is weak. In this way, these authors propose the development of a *high-viscosity, self-adhering bulk-fill composite*. In spite of their high viscosity, this category of restorative should be able to effectively diffuse and decalcify the underlying enamel and dentin, allowing a better monomer dentinal interaction with the dental tissues, reacting with hydroxyapatite, and enhancing the sealing potential for the prevention of nanoleakage, and possibly extended bonding longevity. Another desired characteristic is that this new category should be biocompatible with respect to the biological interactions between the resin components and the various tissues.

10.8 Final Considerations

Traditionally materials used in dentistry were designed to be passive, that is, not to interplay with body tissues and fluids. Thus, those materials would be positively evaluated if they were able to keep their integrity without interacting with the oral environment. This state of affairs has been gradually modified over the last decade. Modern restorative materials are now thought to be necessarily functional. They are supposed to play specific roles (i.e., to prevent tissue demineralization, to allow remineralization, to chemically react, to be bactericide), undergo decisive changes, and to be responsive materials. It could be bet that the most sophisticated class of restorative materials in the imaginable future will be that which emulate biological systems, through defined, controllable pathways that yield predictable clinical outcomes [133]. The benefit for the patient and the quality of dental therapy will undergo a significant improvement by the time such materials are developed and introduced.

Regardless of how direct restorative materials will be really in the near future, a characteristic they will probably share with their current predecessors is the simpler/easier way of being placed onto dental tissues. The advantage of establishing a stable and durable hybridization with hard dental tissues in a user-friendly manner is undoubtedly a tendency to be pursued for modern restorative materials. The present overview of self-adhering direct restorative materials suggests that these materials are expected to perform similarly (or maybe better than) to their antecessors, that is, the self-etching adhesive systems in association with resin composites and/or the self-adhesive resin cements. Clinical evaluations concerning the overall effectiveness of these materials are only short term so that they do not permit yet to draw conclusions at long-term basis. Although further in vivo and in vitro studies must yet attest their safety and efficacy in dental practice, some of the contemporary direct restorative materials already represent a quite promise for the repair and replacement of dental tissues, and this highlights the significant advances in dental material field to date.

References

1. Ferracane JL, Giannobile WV. Novel biomaterials and technologies for the dental, oral, and craniofacial structures. J Dent Res. 2014;93:1185–6.
2. Beck F, Lettner S, Graf A, Bitriol B, Dumitrescu N, Bauer P, et al. Survival of direct resin restorations in posterior teeth within a 19-year period (1996–2015): a meta-analysis of prospective studies. Dent Mater. 2015;31:958–85.
3. Kramer N, Reinelt C, Frankenberger R. Ten-year clinical performance of posterior resin composite restorations. J Adhes Dent. 2015;17:433–41.
4. Yazici AR, Ustunkol I, Ozgunaltay G, Dayangac B. Three-year clinical evaluation of different restorative resins in class I restorations. Oper Dent. 2014;39:248–55.
5. D'Alpino PH, Bechtold J, dos Santos PJ, Alonso RC, Di Hipolito V, Silikas N, et al. Methacrylate- and silorane-based composite restorations: hardness, depth of cure and interfacial gap formation as a function of the energy dose. Dent Mater. 2011;27:1162–9.
6. Han L, Okamoto A, Fukushima M, Okiji T. Evaluation of physical properties and surface degradation of self-adhesive resin cements. Dent Mater J. 2007;26:906–14.
7. Poss SD. Utilization of a new self-adhering flowable composite resin. Dent Today. 2010;29:104–5.
8. Bektas OO, Eren D, Akin EG, Akin H. Evaluation of a self-adhering flowable composite in terms of micro-shear bond strength and microleakage. Acta Odontol Scand. 2013;71:541–6.
9. Tay FR, Pashley DH. Dental adhesives of the future. J Adhes Dent. 2002;4:91–103.
10. Van Meerbeek B, Yoshihara K, Yoshida Y, Mine A, De Munck J, Van Landuyt KL. State of the art of self-etch adhesives. Dent Mater. 2011;27:17–28.
11. Van Meerbeek B, De Munck J, Yoshida Y, Inoue S, Vargas M, Vijay P, et al. Buonocore memorial lecture. Adhesion to enamel and dentin: current status and future challenges. Oper Dent. 2003;28:215–35.
12. Nakabayashi N, Kojima K, Masuhara E. The promotion of adhesion by the infiltration of monomers into tooth substrates. J Biomed Mater Res. 1982;16(3):265–73.
13. Yoshida Y, Nagakane K, Fukuda R, Nakayama Y, Okazaki M, Shintani H, et al. Comparative study on adhesive performance of functional monomers. J Dent Res. 2004;83:454–8.
14. Salz U, Mucke A, Zimmermann J, Tay FR, Pashley DH. pKa value and buffering capacity of acidic monomers commonly used in self-etching primers. J Adhes Dent. 2006;8:143–50.
15. Chan KM, Tay FR, King NM, Imazato S, Pashley DH. Bonding of mild self-etching primers/adhesives to dentin with thick smear layers. Am J Dent. 2003;16:340–6.
16. Peumans M, Kanumilli P, De Munck J, Van Landuyt K, Lambrechts P, Van Meerbeek B. Clinical effectiveness of contemporary adhesives: a systematic review of current clinical trials. Dent Mater. 2005;21:864–81.
17. Peumans M, De Munck J, Van Landuyt KL, Poitevin A, Lambrechts P, Van Meerbeek B. Eight-year clinical evaluation of a 2-step self-etch adhesive with and without selective enamel etching. Dent Mater. 2010;26:1176–84.
18. Peumans M, De Munck J, Van Landuyt K, Van Meerbeek B. Thirteen-year randomized controlled clinical trial of a two-step self-etch adhesive in non-carious cervical lesions. Dent Mater. 2015;31:308–14.
19. Boushell LW, Heymann HO, Ritter AV, Sturdevant JR, Swift EJ Jr, Wilder AD Jr, et al. Six-year clinical performance of etch-and-rinse and self-etch adhesives. Dent Mater. 2016;32:1065–72.
20. Yoshida Y, Inoue S. Chemical analyses in dental adhesive technology. Jpn Dent Sci Rev. 2012;48:141–52.
21. Perdigao J, Geraldeli S, Hodges JS. Total-etch versus self-etch adhesive: effect on postoperative sensitivity. J Am Dent Assoc. 2003;134:1621–9.
22. Unemori M, Matsuya Y, Akashi A, Goto Y, Akamine A. Self-etching adhesives and postoperative sensitivity. Am J Dent. 2004;17:191–5.

23. Tay FR, King NM, Chan KM, Pashley DH. How can nanoleakage occur in self-etching adhesive systems that demineralize and infiltrate simultaneously? J Adhes Dent. 2002;4:255–69.
24. Yoshida Y, Van Meerbeek B, Nakayama Y, Yoshioka M, Snauwaert J, Abe Y, et al. Adhesion to and decalcification of hydroxyapatite by carboxylic acids. J Dent Res. 2001;80:1565–9.
25. De Munck J, Vargas M, Van Landuyt K, Hikita K, Lambrechts P, Van Meerbeek B. Bonding of an auto-adhesive luting material to enamel and dentin. Dent Mater. 2004;20:963–71.
26. Van Landuyt KL, Yoshida Y, Hirata I, Snauwaert J, De Munck J, Okazaki M, et al. Influence of the chemical structure of functional monomers on their adhesive performance. J Dent Res. 2008;87:757–61.
27. Ferracane JL. Resin composite-state of the art. Dent Mater. 2011;27:29–38.
28. De Munck J, Vargas M, Iracki J, Van Landuyt K, Poitevin A, Lambrechts P, et al. One-day bonding effectiveness of new self-etch adhesives to bur-cut enamel and dentin. Oper Dent. 2005;30:39–49.
29. Yoshihara K, Yoshida Y, Nagaoka N, Fukegawa D, Hayakawa S, Mine A, et al. Nano-controlled molecular interaction at adhesive interfaces for hard tissue reconstruction. Acta Biomater. 2010;6:3573–82.
30. Yoshihara K, Yoshida Y, Hayakawa S, Nagaoka N, Torii Y, Osaka A, et al. Self-etch monomer-calcium salt deposition on dentin. J Dent Res. 2011;90:602–6.
31. Inoue S, Koshiro K, Yoshida Y, De Munck J, Nagakane K, Suzuki K, et al. Hydrolytic stability of self-etch adhesives bonded to dentin. J Dent Res. 2005;84:1160–4.
32. Yoshihara K, Yoshida Y, Hayakawa S, Nagaoka N, Irie M, Ogawa T, et al. Nanolayering of phosphoric acid ester monomer on enamel and dentin. Acta Biomater. 2011;7:3187–95.
33. Atai M, Nekoomanesh M, Hashemi SA, Amani S. Physical and mechanical properties of an experimental dental composite based on a new monomer. Dent Mater. 2004;20:663–8.
34. Matsui N, Takagaki T, Sadr A, Ikeda M, Ichinose S, Nikaido T, et al. The role of MDP in a bonding resin of a two-step self-etching adhesive system. Dent Mater J. 2015;34:227–33.
35. Erhardt MC, Pisani-Proenca J, Osorio E, Aguilera FS, Toledano M, Osorio R. Influence of laboratory degradation methods and bonding application parameters on microTBS of self-etch adhesives to dentin. Am J Dent. 2011;24:103–8.
36. Perdigao J, Kose C, Mena-Serrano AP, De Paula EA, Tay LY, Reis A, et al. A new universal simplified adhesive: 18-month clinical evaluation. Oper Dent. 2014;39:113–27.
37. Hanabusa M, Mine A, Kuboki T, Momoi Y, Van Ende A, Van Meerbeek B, et al. Bonding effectiveness of a new 'multi-mode' adhesive to enamel and dentine. J Dent. 2012;40:475–84.
38. Zhang ZY, Tian FC, Niu LN, Ochala K, Chen C, Fu BP, et al. Defying ageing: an expectation for dentine bonding with universal adhesives? J Dent. 2016;45:43–52.
39. Cardenas AM, Siqueira F, Rocha J, Szesz AL, Anwar M, El-Askary F, et al. Influence of conditioning time of universal adhesives on adhesive properties and enamel-etching pattern. Oper Dent. 2016;41(5):481–90.
40. El-Damanhoury HM, Gaintantzopoulou M. Effect of thermocycling, degree of conversion, and cavity configuration on the bonding effectiveness of all-in-one adhesives. Oper Dent. 2015;40:480–91.
41. Saikaew P, Chowdhury AF, Fukuyama M, Kakuda S, Carvalho RM, Sano H. The effect of dentine surface preparation and reduced application time of adhesive on bonding strength. J Dent. 2016;47:63–70.
42. Takamizawa T, Barkmeier WW, Tsujimoto A, Berry TP, Watanabe H, Erickson RL, et al. Influence of different etching modes on bond strength and fatigue strength to dentin using universal adhesive systems. Dent Mater. 2016;32:e9–e21.
43. Chen C, Niu LN, Xie H, Zhang ZY, Zhou LQ, Jiao K, et al. Bonding of universal adhesives to dentine—old wine in new bottles? J Dent. 2015;43:525–36.
44. Burgess JO. Materials you cannot work without - refining your tools for treatment. J Cosmet Dent. 2013;28:94–106.
45. Ferracane JL, Stansbury JW, Burke FJ. Self-adhesive resin cements - chemistry, properties and clinical considerations. J Oral Rehabil. 2011;38:295–314.
46. Martin R, Paul SJ, Luthy H, Scharer P. Dentin bond strength of Dyract Cem. Am J Dent. 1997;10:27–31.
47. Moodley D, Grobler SR, Rossouw RJ, Oberholzer TG, Patel N. In vitro evaluation of two adhesive systems used with compomer filling materials. Int Dent J. 2000;50:400–6.
48. Radovic I, Monticelli F, Goracci C, Vulicevic ZR, Ferrari M. Self-adhesive resin cements: a literature review. J Adhes Dent. 2008;10:251–8.
49. Grobler SR, Rossouw RJ, Van Wyk Kotze TJ. A comparison of fluoride release from various dental materials. J Dent. 1998;26:259–65.
50. Shaw AJ, Carrick T, McCabe JF. Fluoride release from glass-ionomer and compomer restorative materials: 6-month data. J Dent. 1998;26:355–9.
51. Chan DK. Making cementation simple and predictable with self-adhesive resin cements. Dental Economics. 2015. http://www.dentaleconomics.com/articles/print/volume-105/issue-11/science-tech/making-cementation-simple-and-predictable-with-self-adhesive-resin-cements.html. Accessed 9 Nov 2016.
52. Marcondes M, Souza N, Manfroi FB, Burnett LH Jr, Spohr AM. Clinical evaluation of indirect composite resin restorations cemented with different resin cements. J Adhes Dent. 2016;18:59–67.
53. Van Meerbeek B, Dhem A, Goret-Nicaise M, Braem M, Lambrechts P, VanHerle G. Comparative SEM and TEM examination of the ultrastructure of the resin-dentin interdiffusion zone. J Dent Res. 1993;72:495–501.

54. Charton C, Falk V, Marchal P, Pla F, Colon P. Influence of Tg, viscosity and chemical structure of monomers on shrinkage stress in light-cured dimethacrylate-based dental resins. Dent Mater. 2007;23:1447–59.
55. Ellakwa A, Cho N, Lee IB. The effect of resin matrix composition on the polymerization shrinkage and rheological properties of experimental dental composites. Dent Mater. 2007;23:1229–35.
56. Goncalves F, Pfeifer CS, Ferracane JL, Braga RR. Contraction stress determinants in dimethacrylate composites. J Dent Res. 2008;87:367–71.
57. Cramer NB, Stansbury JW, Bowman CN. Recent advances and developments in composite dental restorative materials. J Dent Res. 2011;90:402–16.
58. Pedreira AP, D'Alpino PH, Pereira PN, Chaves SB, Wang L, Hilgert L, et al. Effects of the application techniques of self-adhesive resin cements on the interfacial integrity and bond strength of fiber posts to dentin. J Appl Oral Sci. 2016;24:437–46.
59. Poitevin A, De Munck J, Van Ende A, Suyama Y, Mine A, Peumans M, et al. Bonding effectiveness of self-adhesive composites to dentin and enamel. Dent Mater. 2013;29:221–30.
60. Fukegawa D, Hayakawa S, Yoshida Y, Suzuki K, Osaka A, Van Meerbeek B. Chemical interaction of phosphoric acid ester with hydroxyapatite. J Dent Res. 2006;85:941–4.
61. Yoshioka M, Yoshida Y, Inoue S, Lambrechts P, Vanherle G, Nomura Y, et al. Adhesion/decalcification mechanisms of acid interactions with human hard tissues. J Biomed Mater Res. 2002;59:56–62.
62. Tay FR, Smales RJ, Ngo H, Wei SH, Pashley DH. Effect of different conditioning protocols on adhesion of a GIC to dentin. J Adhes Dent. 2001;3:153–67.
63. Mutluay MM, Zhang K, Ryou H, Yahyazadehfar M, Majd H, Xu HH, et al. On the fatigue behavior of resin-dentin bonds after degradation by biofilm. J Mech Behav Biomed Mater. 2013;18:219–31.
64. Toledano M, Osorio R, de Leonardi G, Rosales-Leal JI, Ceballos L, Cabrerizo-Vilchez MA. Influence of self-etching primer on the resin adhesion to enamel and dentin. Am J Dent. 2001;14:205–10.
65. Peumans M, De Munck J, Van Landuyt K, Lambrechts P, Van Meerbeek B. Five-year clinical effectiveness of a two-step self-etching adhesive. J Adhes Dent. 2007;9:7–10.
66. Ikeda T, De Munck J, Shirai K, Hikita K, Inoue S, Sano H, et al. Effect of fracture strength of primer-adhesive mixture on bonding effectiveness. Dent Mater. 2005;21:413–20.
67. Akinmade AO, Nicholson JW. Glass-ionomer cements as adhesives. Part I: Fundamental aspects and their clinical relevance. J Mater Sci Mater Med. 1993;4:95–101.
68. Lohbauer U. Dental glass ionomer cements as permanent filling materials?—properties limitations future trends. Materials. 2010;3:76–96.
69. Van Landuyt K, De Munck J, Coutinho E, Peumans M, Lambrechts P, Van Meerbeek B. Bonding to dentin: smear layer and the process of hybridization. In: Eliades G, Watts DC, Eliades T, editors. Dental hard tissues and bonding - interfacial phenomena and related properties. Berlin: Springer; 2005. p. 89–122.
70. Nicholson JW. Chemistry of glass-ionomer cements: a review. Biomaterials. 1998;19:485–94.
71. Trushkowsky RD. The role of glass ionomers in minimally invasive restorative dentistry. Dent Today. 2005;24:72–4. 6–7; quiz 7
72. Sidhu SK, Nicholson JW. A review of glass-ionomer cements for clinical dentistry. J Funct Biomater. 2016;7 doi:10.3390/jfb7030016.
73. Wilson AD, Prosser HJ, Powis DM. Mechanism of adhesion of polyelectrolyte cements to hydroxyapatite. J Dent Res. 1983;62:590–2.
74. Sahin G, Albayrak AZ, Bilgici ZS, Avci D. Synthesis and evaluation of new dental monomers with both phosphonic and carboxylic acid functional groups. J Polym Sci A Polym Chem. 2009;47:1953–65.
75. Adusei G, Deb S, Nicholson JW, Mou LY, Singh G. Polymerization behavior of an organophosphorus monomer for use in dental restorative materials. J Appl Polym Sci. 2003;88:565–9.
76. Vrochari AD, Eliades G, Hellwig E, Wrbas KT. Curing efficiency of four self-etching, self-adhesive resin cements. Dent Mater. 2009;25:1104–8.
77. Nakamura T, Wakabayashi K, Kinuta S, Nishida H, Miyamae M, Yatani H. Mechanical properties of new self-adhesive resin-based cement. J Prosthodont Res. 2010;54:59–64.
78. D'Alpino PH, Silva MS, Vismara MV, Di Hipolito V, Miranda Gonzalez AH, de Oliveira Graeff CF. The effect of polymerization mode on monomer conversion, free radical entrapment, and interaction with hydroxyapatite of commercial self-adhesive cements. J Mech Behav Biomed Mater. 2015;46:83–92.
79. Monticelli F, Osorio R, Mazzitelli C, Ferrari M, Toledano M. Limited decalcification/diffusion of self-adhesive cements into dentin. J Dent Res. 2008;87:974–9.
80. Di Hipólito V, Azevedo LD, Piveta FB, Vieira WS, Anauate-Netto C, Alonso RC, et al. Effect of dentinal surface preparation on the bonding of self-adhesive luting cements. J Adhes Sci Technol. 2014;28:1901–24.
81. Vaz RR, Hipolito VD, D'Alpino PH, Goes MF. Bond strength and interfacial micromorphology of etch-and-rinse and self-adhesive resin cements to dentin. J Prosthodont. 2012;21:101–11.
82. Gerth HU, Dammaschke T, Zuchner H, Schafer E. Chemical analysis and bonding reaction of RelyX Unicem and Bifix composites-a comparative study. Dent Mater. 2006;22:934–41.
83. Panigrahi A, Srilatha KT, Panigrahi RG, Mohanty S, Bhuyan SK, Bardhan D. Microtensile bond strength of embrace wetbond hydrophilic sealant in different moisture contamination: an in-vitro study. J Clin Diagn Res. 2015;9:ZC23–5.
84. Juloski J, Goracci C, Rengo C, Giovannetti A, Vichi A, Vulicevic ZR, et al. Enamel and dentin bond strength of new simplified adhesive materials with

and without preliminary phosphoric acid-etching. Am J Dent. 2012;25:239–43.
85. Fu J, Kakuda S, Pan F, Hoshika S, Ting S, Fukuoka A, et al. Bonding performance of a newly developed step-less all-in-one system on dentin. Dent Mater J. 2013;32:203–11.
86. Bayne SC, Thompson JY, Swift EJ Jr, Stamatiades P, Wilkerson M. A characterization of first-generation flowable composites. J Am Dent Assoc. 1998;129:567–77.
87. Eliades A, Birpou E, Eliades T, Eliades G. Self-adhesive restoratives as pit and fissure sealants: a comparative laboratory study. Dent Mater. 2013;29:752–62.
88. Sabbagh J, Ryelandt L, Bacherius L, Biebuyck JJ, Vreven J, Lambrechts P, et al. Characterization of the inorganic fraction of resin composites. J Oral Rehabil. 2004;31:1090–101.
89. Baroudi K, Rodrigues JC. Flowable resin composites: a systematic review and clinical considerations. J Clin Diagn Res. 2015;9:ZE18–24.
90. Alonso RC, Sinhoreti MA, Correr Sobrinho L, Consani S, Goes MF. Effect of resin liners on the microleakage of class V dental composite restorations. J Appl Oral Sci. 2004;12:56–61.
91. Chuang SF, Jin YT, Liu JK, Chang CH, Shieh DB. Influence of flowable composite lining thickness on Class II composite restorations. Oper Dent. 2004;29:301–8.
92. Salerno M, Derchi G, Thorat S, Ceseracciu L, Ruffilli R, Barone AC. Surface morphology and mechanical properties of new-generation flowable resin composites for dental restoration. Dent Mater. 2011;27:1221–8.
93. Labella R, Lambrechts P, Van Meerbeek B, Vanherle G. Polymerization shrinkage and elasticity of flowable composites and filled adhesives. Dent Mater. 1999;15:128–37.
94. Boaro LC, Goncalves F, Guimaraes TC, Ferracane JL, Versluis A, Braga RR. Polymerization stress, shrinkage and elastic modulus of current low-shrinkage restorative composites. Dent Mater. 2010;26:1144–50.
95. Ilie N, Hickel R. Investigations on a methacrylate-based flowable composite based on the SDR technology. Dent Mater. 2011;27:348–55.
96. Braun J. Top reasons why new liner/base materials should be considered for everyday use. 2013. http://www.dentalproductsreport.com/dental/article/top-reasons-why-new-linerbase-materials-should-be-considered-everyday-use. Accessed 2 Jan 2017.
97. Davidson CL, Feilzer AJ. Polymerization shrinkage and polymerization shrinkage stress in polymer-based restoratives. J Dent. 1997;25:435–40.
98. Millar BJ, Nicholson JW. Effect of curing with a plasma light on the properties of polymerizable dental restorative materials. J Oral Rehabil. 2001;28:549–52.
99. Darwell B. Resin restorative materials. In: Darwell B, editor. Materials science for dentistry. Cambridge, UK: Woodhead Publishing Ltd.; 2009. p. 115–45.
100. da Silva ACN, Melo PR, Oliveira SA, Gutknecht N. Evaluation of a self-adhesive composite in dentin surfaces. Laser. 2016;1:12–6.
101. Brueckner C, Schneider H, Haak R. Shear bond strength and tooth-composite interaction with self-adhering flowable composites. Oper Dent. 2017;42(1):90–100.
102. Celik EU, Kucukyilmaz E, Savas S. Effect of different surface pre-treatment methods on the microleakage of two different self-adhesive composites in Class V cavities. Eur J Paediatr Dent. 2015;16:33–8.
103. Celik EU, Aka B, Yilmaz F. Six-month clinical evaluation of a self-adhesive flowable composite in noncarious cervical lesions. J Adhes Dent. 2015;17:361–8.
104. Pacifici E, Chazine M, Vichi A, Grandini S, Goracci C, Ferrari M. Shear-bond strength of a new self-adhering flowable restorative material to dentin of primary molars. J Clin Pediatr Dent. 2013;38:149–54.
105. Frankenberger R, Lopes M, Perdigao J, Ambrose WW, Rosa BT. The use of flowable composites as filled adhesives. Dent Mater. 2002;18:227–38.
106. Carvalho RM, Pereira JC, Yoshiyama M, Pashley DH. A review of polymerization contraction: the influence of stress development versus stress relief. Oper Dent. 1996;21:17–24.
107. Andrzejewska E, editor. Kinetics of network formation during photopolymerization. Scientific insights into dental ceramics and photopolymer networks. Geneva, Switzerland: Academy of Dental Materials; 2004.
108. Malacarne J, Carvalho RM, de Goes MF, Svizero N, Pashley DH, Tay FR, et al. Water sorption/solubility of dental adhesive resins. Dent Mater. 2006;22:973–80.
109. Ferracane JL. Hygroscopic and hydrolytic effects in dental polymer networks. Dent Mater. 2006;22:211–22.
110. Pontes EC, Soares DG, Hebling J, Costa CA. Cytotoxicity of resin-based luting cements to pulp cells. Am J Dent. 2014;27:237–44.
111. King NM, Tay FR, Pashley DH, Hashimoto M, Ito S, Brackett WW, et al. Conversion of one-step to two-step self-etch adhesives for improved efficacy and extended application. Am J Dent. 2005;18:126–34.
112. Tay FR, Lai CN, Chersoni S, Pashley DH, Mak YF, Suppa P, et al. Osmotic blistering in enamel bonded with one-step self-etch adhesives. J Dent Res. 2004;83:290–5.
113. Tay FR, Pashley DH, Garcia-Godoy F, Yiu CK. Single-step, self-etch adhesives behave as permeable membranes after polymerization. Part II. Silver tracer penetration evidence. Am J Dent. 2004;17:315–22.
114. Sideridou I, Tserki V, Papanastasiou G. Study of water sorption, solubility and modulus of elasticity of light-cured dimethacrylate-based dental resins. Biomaterials. 2003;24:655–65.
115. Fiers W, Beyaert R, Declercq W, Vandenabeele P. More than one way to die: apoptosis, necrosis

and reactive oxygen damage. Oncogene. 1999;18: 7719–30.
116. D'Alpino PH, Araújo RP, Gonzalez AH, Di Hipolito V, Valduga CJ, Santos DY, et al. Inorganic characterizations and filler particles morphology of self-adhesive cements. Int J Adhes Adhes. 2016;68:62–9.
117. Black J. Does corrosion matter? J Bone Joint Surg. 1988;70:517–20.
118. da Fonseca Roberti Garcia L, Pontes EC, Basso FG, Hebling J, de Souza Costa CA, Soares DG. Transdentinal cytotoxicity of resin-based luting cements to pulp cells. Clin Oral Investig. 2016;20:1559–66.
119. Rueggeberg F. Contemporary issues in photocuring. Compend Contin Educ Dent. 1999;25:S4–S15.
120. Camilotti V, Grullon PG, Mendonca MJ, D'Alpino PH, Gomes JC. Influence of different light curing units on the bond strength of indirect resin composite restorations. Braz Oral Res. 2008;22:164–9.
121. Svizero Nda R, Silva MS, Alonso RC, Rodrigues FP, Hipolito VD, Carvalho RM, et al. Effects of curing protocols on fluid kinetics and hardness of resin cements. Dent Mater J. 2013;32:32–41.
122. D'Alpino PH, Caetano AF, Moura GEDD, Nascimento FD, Tersariol IL, editors. Cytotoxicity of self-adhesive resin cements as a function of the activation mode. Brazil: Brazilian Division of the I.A.D.R.; 2016.
123. Al-Hiyasat AS, Darmani H, Milhem MM. Cytotoxicity evaluation of dental resin composites and their flowable derivatives. Clin Oral Investig. 2005;9:21–5.
124. Baroudi K, Silikas N, Watts DC. In vitro pulp chamber temperature rise from irradiation and exotherm of flowable composites. Int J Paediatr Dent. 2009;19:48–54.
125. Xu HH, Weir MD, Sun L, Moreau JL, Takagi S, Chow LC, et al. Strong nanocomposites with Ca, PO(4), and F release for caries inhibition. J Dent Res. 2010;89:19–28.
126. Xu HH, Moreau JL, Sun L, Chow LC. Novel CaF(2) nanocomposite with high strength and fluoride ion release. J Dent Res. 2010;89:739–45.
127. Bansal R, Burgess J, Lawson NC. Wear of an enhanced resin-modified glass-ionomer restorative material. Am J Dent. 2016;29:171–4.
128. Pameijer CH, Garcia-Godoy F, Morrow BR, Jefferies SR. Flexural strength and flexural fatigue properties of resin-modified glass ionomers. J Clin Dent. 2015;26:23–7.
129. Bhat PK, Konde S, Raj SN, Kumar NC. Moisture-tolerant resin-based sealant: a boon. Contemp Clin Dent. 2013;4:343–8.
130. Hervas-Garcia A, Martinez-Lozano MA, Cabanes-Vila J, Barjau-Escribano A, Fos-Galve P. Composite resins. A review of the materials and clinical indications. Med Oral Patol Oral Cir Bucal. 2006;11:E215–20.
131. Taubock TT, Tarle Z, Marovic D, Attin T. Preheating of high-viscosity bulk-fill resin composites: effects on shrinkage force and monomer conversion. J Dent. 2015;43:1358–64.
132. Jackson RD. Class II composite resin restorations: faster, easier, predictable. Br Dent J. 2016;221:623–31.
133. Chirra HD, Desai TA. Emerging microtechnologies for the development of oral drug delivery devices. Adv Drug Deliv Rev. 2012;64:1569–78.

Part IV

Esthetics of Dental Composites

Esthetics of Dental Composites

11

Dayane Oliveira

11.1 Introduction

The word esthetics derives from the Greek "*aisthetikos,*" which means perceiving or noting. Esthetics is the branch of philosophy concerned with the nature and appreciation of beauty. In contemporary philosophy, there is a first concept that beauty can be objective and universal. However, there is also a second concept that involves the viewer's interpretation of beauty, which is subjective and can vary according to class, culture, and education.

Then, reproducing a biomimetic match between restorative materials and natural teeth involves not only knowledge and manual ability but also psychology and even philosophy. Many aspects are involved to perfectly reproduce a natural tooth, such as proper form, anatomy, contour, color, gloss, texture, translucency, fluorescence, and opalescence. This chapter provides general introduction to these aspects and how they can affect esthetics. Also, clinical tips are provided to achieve seamless transition between natural tooth and composite restorations.

> Perfect esthetic results are only reached when nobody can notice the difference from what is natural and what is not.

D. Oliveira
Department of Restorative Dentistry, Piracicaba Dental School—State University of Campinas, São Paulo, Brazil
e-mail: oliveira.day@icloud.com

11.2 Color and Its Dimensions

"Color is defined as the property of producing a visual perception as a result of the way an object reflects or emits light." Although it seems simple, color is best described as an abstract science in which it appears to be highly subjective.

In 2005, neuroscientists from the University of Rochester have found that the number of color-sensitive cells in the human retina differs among people by up to 40 times; yet people appear to perceive colors the same way. These findings indicated that visual perception of color is controlled much more by the human brain than the eyes [1].

A practical example of the influence of the human brain on visual perception is shown in Fig. 11.1. Observing the square, how many shades do you see? If you see two different shades of gray, cover the line blocking the darker and lighter shading across the middle and your

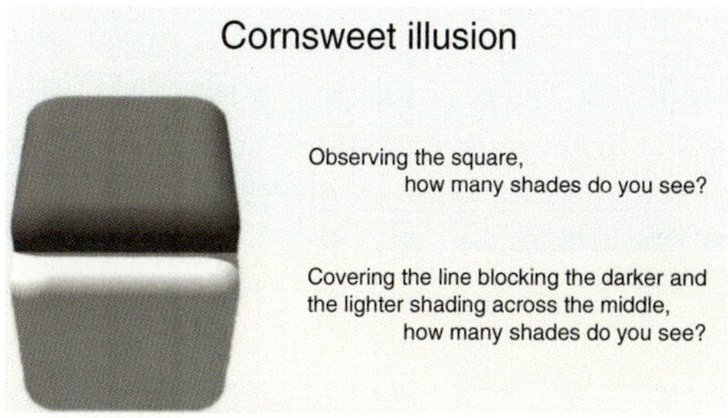

Fig. 11.1 Cornsweet illusion: color illusion designed by Tom Cornsweet

V. Miletic (ed.), *Dental Composite Materials for Direct Restorations*,
http://doi.org/10.1007/978-3-319-60961-4_11

brain will begin to realize that the cube actually has only one shade. This is a color illusion from Tom Cornsweet [2], who is best known for his work in visual perception. Color illusions are images where the surrounding colors trick the human brain into incorrect interpretation of color.

Indeed, the visual perception of different colors is a subjective process whereby the brain responds to the stimuli that are produced by color-sensitive cones localized in the human retina. But, it proves the importance of color education in dentistry [3].

Color can be specified based on three color appearance parameters, also known as the three color dimensions: hue, value (or lightness), and chroma (Fig. 11.2).

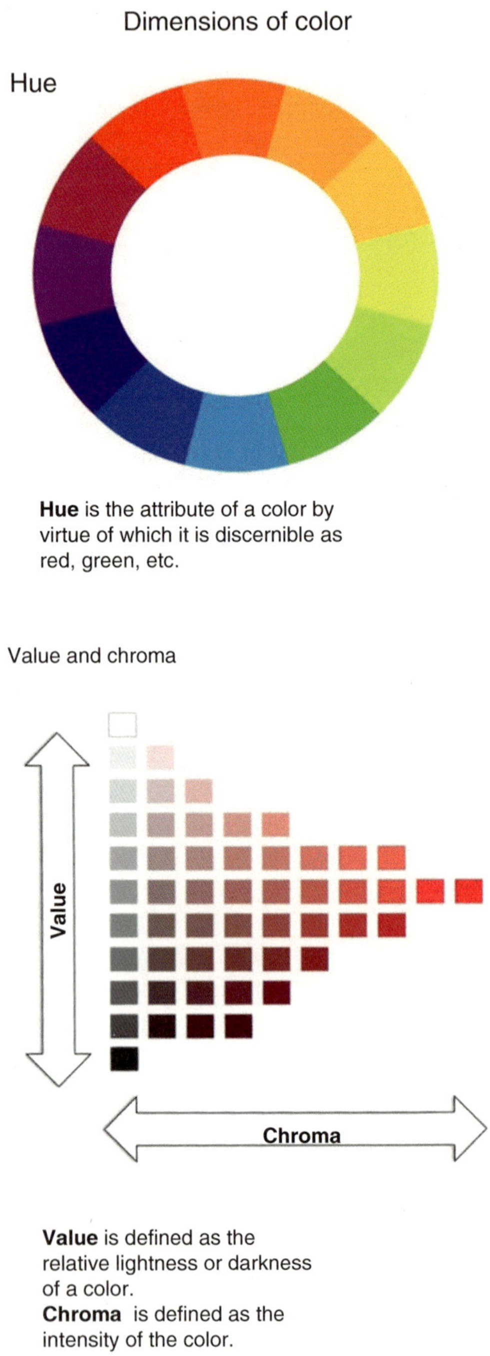

Fig. 11.2 Color dimensions: hue, value, and chroma

11.2.1 Hue

Hue is defined as the visual perception of the stimuli of a wavelength. As illustrated in Fig. 11.3, the main pure hues are red, blue, and yellow. The main pure hues are also called primary colors. However, the mixture of pure hues can generate different visual perception stimuli, also called secondary colors. For example, the mixture of blue (primary color) and yellow (primary color) generates the visual perception of green (secondary color). The mixture of a primary color and a secondary color can also generate a different visual perception stimulus, called a tertiary color.

11.2.2 Value

Value, also known as lightness or tone, is referred to the lightness or darkness of a color. In other words, it indicates the quantity of the light that is reflected.

11.2.3 Chroma

Chroma is defined as the purity, intensity, or saturation of a color. Thus, a lower chroma would indicate less intensity of the color, as in pastel colors, while a higher chroma is related to a more vivid color.

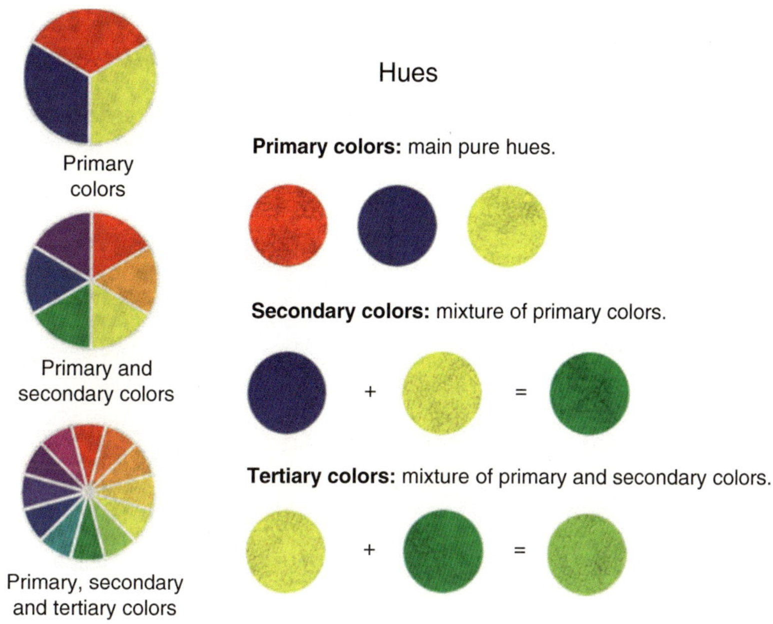

Fig. 11.3 Hues: primary, secondary, and tertiary colors

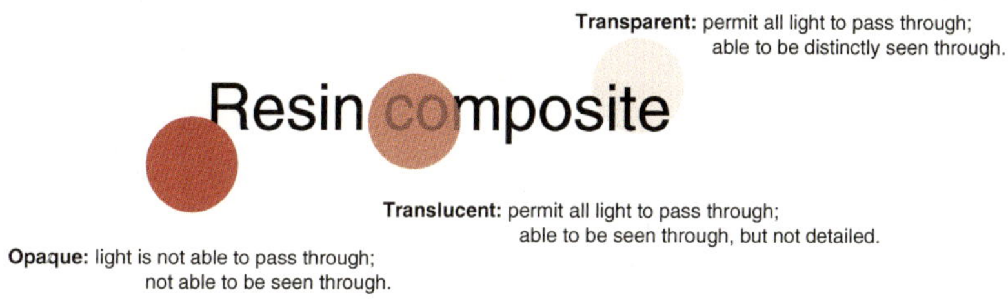

Fig. 11.4 Definition of transparency, translucency, and opacity

11.2.4 Translucency

Translucency is the physical property that allows light to pass through the material. The material can be considered transparent, translucent, or opaque according to the degree of light that is transmitted rather than absorbed or reflected (Fig. 11.4). When the material allows most light to pass through it, it is considered transparent. This means that it is possible to clearly see through it. On the other hand, when the material allows some light to pass through it, it is considered translucent. This means that it is still possible to see through it, but not as clearly. Last, when no light is able to pass through it, the material is considered opaque. This means that it is not possible to see through it.

Clearly, a mistake in translucency may compromise the natural appearance of a restoration in comparison to the natural teeth as the background changes [4]. This is the reason why some authors describe translucency as a fourth dimension of color.

11.3 Color Perception

Color is not a property of light, but the visual perception of light by an observer. In order for color to be perceived, three elements must be simultaneously present: illumination, an object and an observer.

11.3.1 Illumination

Although white light is colorless to the human eye, it contains all colors in the visible wavelength spectrum (Fig. 11.5). Thus, when the white light hits an object, the different wavelengths can be absorbed, transmitted, or reflected. The reflected wavelengths will be responsible for the color perception of the object (Fig. 11.6).

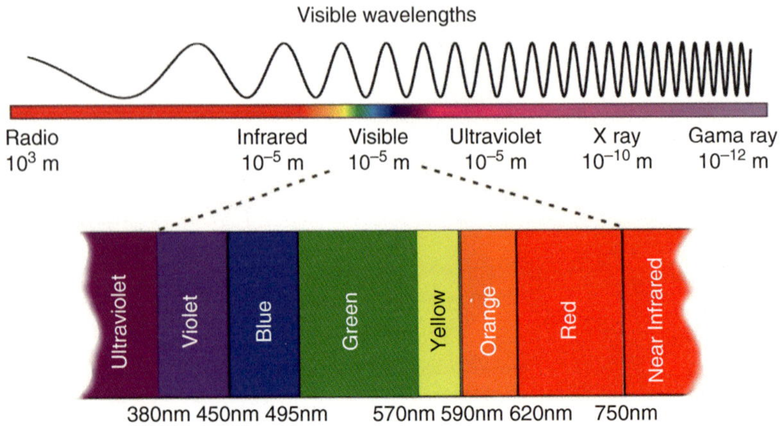

Fig. 11.5 Visible wavelength spectrums and color perception

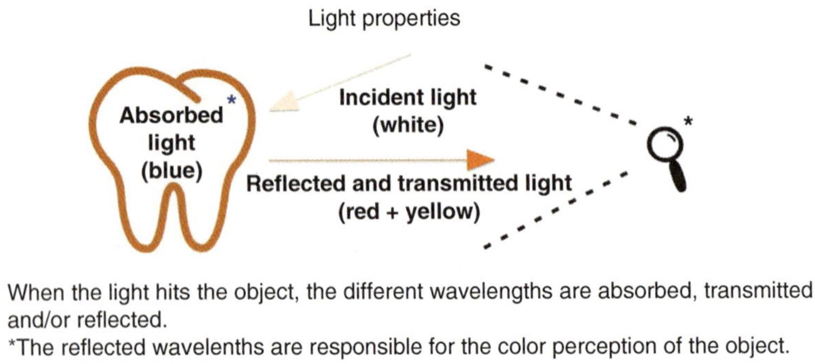

Fig. 11.6 Light reflection, absorption, and transmission and color perception

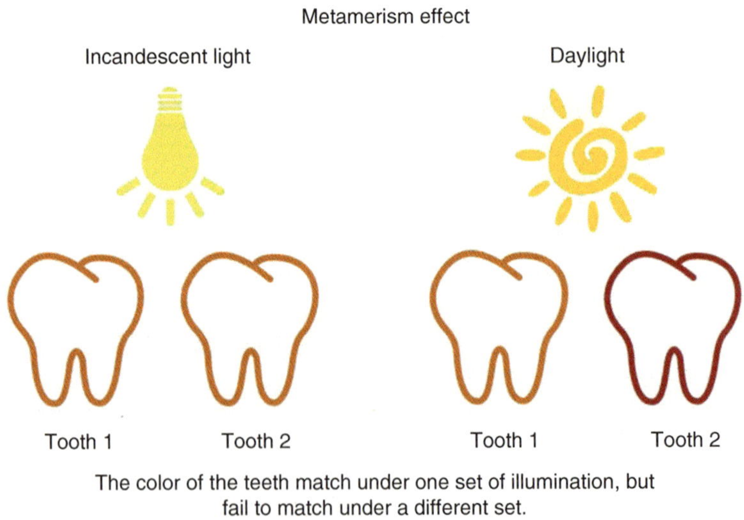

Fig. 11.7 Metamerism phenomenon

However, different light sources can emit different wavelengths. This means that not all visible wavelength spectra are being absorbed, transmitted, or reflected by the object under different light sources. Thus, the color of one object can look different under different illumination.

In some cases, the color of two different colored objects can match under one set of illumination, but fail to match under a different set (Fig. 11.7). This phenomenon is known as the metamerism effect [5, 6]. It shows the importance of illumination during color selection in dentistry [7].

People are usually exposed to different light sources during their routine: daylight, shady or cloudy sky, fluorescent light, incandescent light, etc. These different light sources have different color temperatures. The color temperature is related to the color appearance of the light emitted by the light source.

The color temperature is expressed in Kelvin (K). Color temperatures over 5000 K are called cool colors (blueish white), while lower color temperatures are called warm colors (yellowish white). Daylight, fluorescent light, and incandescent light, for example, are warm colors, while shady and cloudy sky are cooler colors (Fig. 11.8). Thus, the same object can have its color distorted when exposed to light sources with different color temperatures.

While low light intensity can affect hue perception, high light intensity can cause glare and result in fatigue to the eyes [8]. In dentistry, the recommended standard for color selection is a color temperature of 5500 K, which corresponds to an ideal natural daylight. However, natural light conditions vary from 3000 to 8000 K depending on the time (sunrise/sunshine) and the weather (sunny/cloudy). A practical way to have more success in color matching regardless of the natural conditions is to use a standardizing daylight lamp in the dental office. However, portable light-correcting devices are also available to assist chairside shade matching (Fig. 11.9). These devices also have a polarizing filter that eliminates reflection and enhances the visualization of internal details of the teeth (Fig. 11.10).

Hue perception can change as light intensity varies. This phenomenon is known as Bezold-Brucke shift [9, 10]. As the light intensity increases, the color perception shifts more toward blue or yellow depending on the original color of the object. Then, if the object is yellow, it tends to look more saturated than it really is (Fig. 11.11). It can influence the color selection to a more saturated color rather than the original color of the teeth. At lower intensities, however, the color perception shifts more toward the red/green axis.

Another phenomenon that can influence color perception is the absolute operatory field isolation [4]. As the rubber dam is usually brightly colored, it may alter the color perception of the tooth and lead to an incorrect color selection. The opponent color theory helps explain this phenomenon. The human eyes receive stimulus from different wavelengths by different sensory cells on the retina, the cones. There are specific selective cones for different wavelength ranges. However, when a specific selective cone is stimulated for prolonged viewing, it causes the fatigue of these cone cells. Then, the opponent

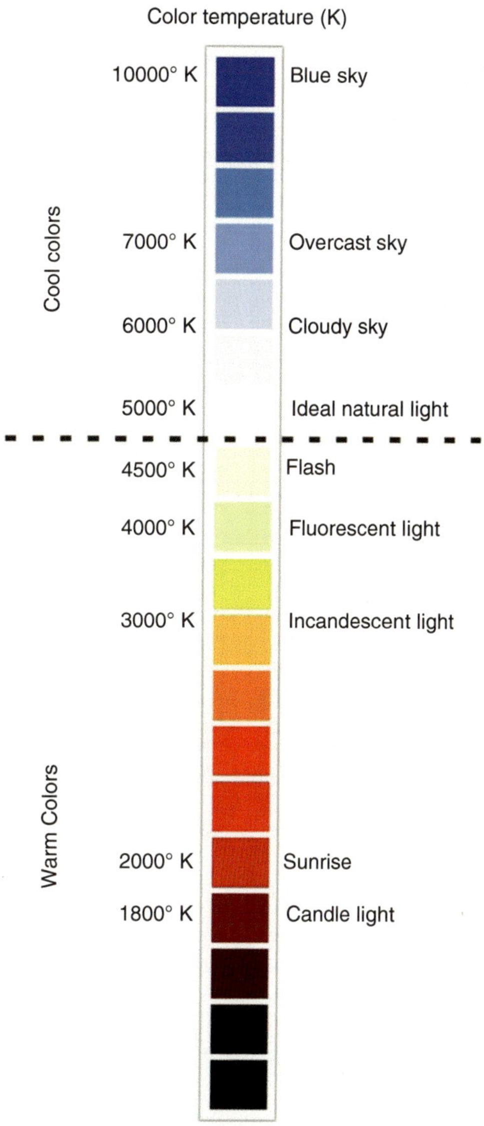

Fig. 11.8 Cool colors and warm colors: color temperature of different light sources

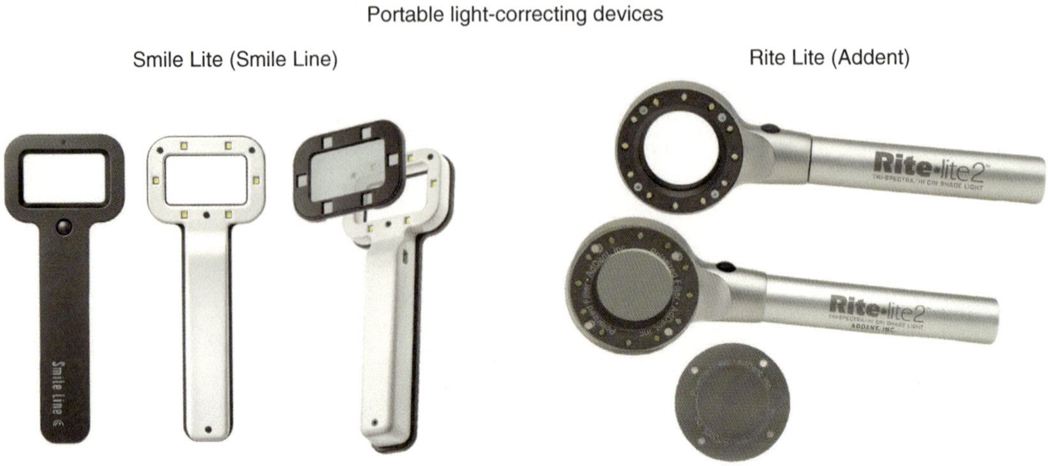

Fig. 11.9 Portable light-correcting devices: Smile Lite powered by Style Italiano and Rite-Lite (Addent)

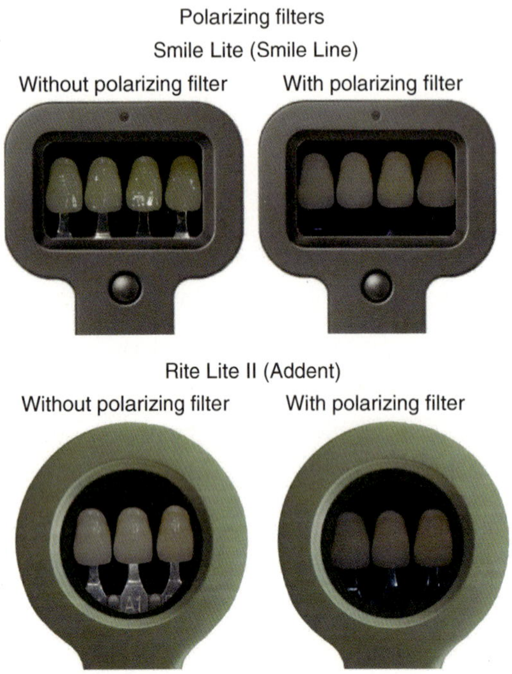

Fig. 11.10 Detail perception using light-correcting devices with and without polarizing filters

color receptor, which is not fatigued, receives the stimulus and the brain incorrectly perceives the opponent color. Thus, shade selection should be made before the dam is applied. Otherwise, prolonged exposure to the bright color of the dam can desensitize a specific selective cone and stimulate the opponent-specific selective cone when trying to select the color of the tooth under absolute operatory field isolation. The opponent colors are blue and yellow, red and green, and black and white (Fig. 11.12). Toward a better understanding of this theory, a practical example is given in Fig. 11.13.

The absolute operatory field isolation also causes the dehydration of the teeth. Natural teeth exhibit high gloss reflection when wet. Thus, color appearance looks vivid. However, in the absence of saliva, the roughness of the teeth surface scatters the light, and the color appearance looks more pastel [11].

11.3.2 Object (Light Reflection, Light Absorption, and Light Transmittance)

As previously explained, when the light hits an object, the different wavelengths can be absorbed, transmitted, or reflected, and the reflected wavelengths will be responsible for the color of the object (Fig. 11.6). It means that when the object is yellow, it absorbs and/or transmits all wavelengths, but yellow, which is reflected.

However, in highly translucent materials, the light that is scattered through the material can create a dichroism, in which the material appears blue from the front side (opalescence), but yellowish-red shines through back side

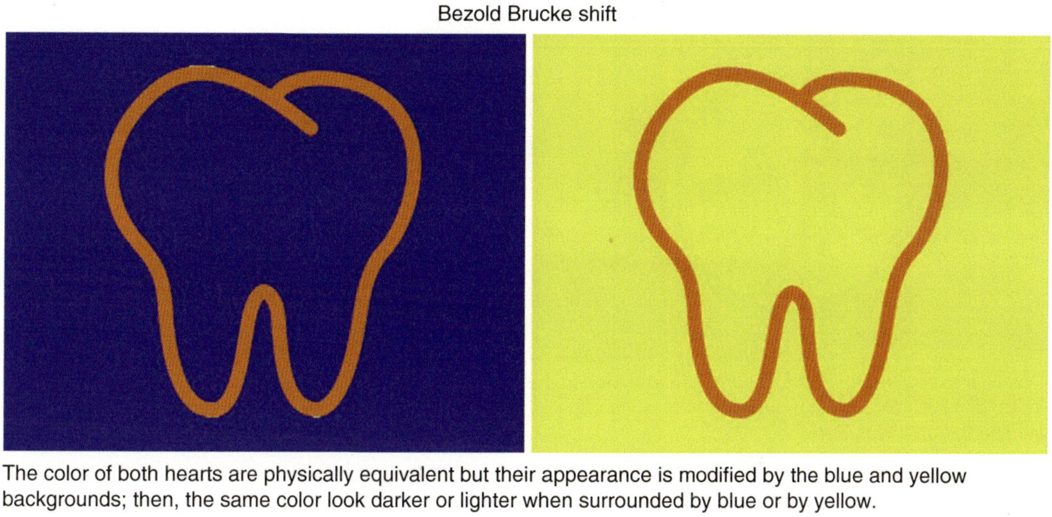

Fig. 11.11 Bezold-Brucke phenomenon

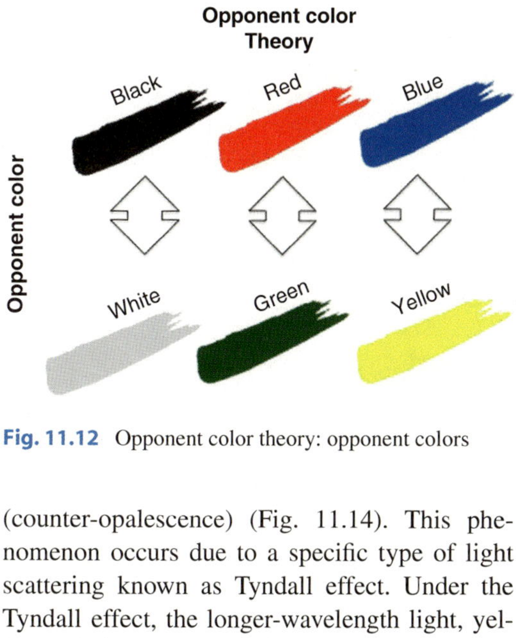

Fig. 11.12 Opponent color theory: opponent colors

(counter-opalescence) (Fig. 11.14). This phenomenon occurs due to a specific type of light scattering known as Tyndall effect. Under the Tyndall effect, the longer-wavelength light, yellow-red, is more transmitted while the shorter-wavelength light, blue, is more reflected.

Enamel is a highly translucent tissue responsible for the opalescence of the incisal halo [12]. This effect is not perceptible in the cervical and medium thirds of the teeth due to the presence of dentin in between, which is highly opaque. However, in the incisal third, it is possible to observe an opalescent halo that follows the incisal outline of the mamelon of dentin. Specific composites called "translucent" or "opalescent" can be used to reproduce this effect.

Also, the translucent multilayering characteristic of the teeth can make its color be perceived differently at different angles. This phenomenon is called as goniochromism [13].

Another natural effect that needs to be reproduced in the tooth is the fluorescence of the dentin. The fluorescence is the emission of a visible wavelength after absorption of radiation in the ultraviolet region of the spectrum, which is invisible to the human eye. Then, when exposed to ultraviolet light, the fluorescence of dentin gives a distinct color that glows. Thus, if the restorative material did not have this property, the difference from the natural teeth and the restorative material would be perceived, when exposed to ultraviolet light. However, nowadays, all dental composites have fluorescence properties due to the addition of rare earths to the composition.

11.3.3 Observer

The human eye is responsible for capturing stimulus from different wavelength spectra of light and discharging nerve impulses that are conducted to the brain. There are three types of cone cells in the human eye that are more sensitive to

Opponent-color theory test

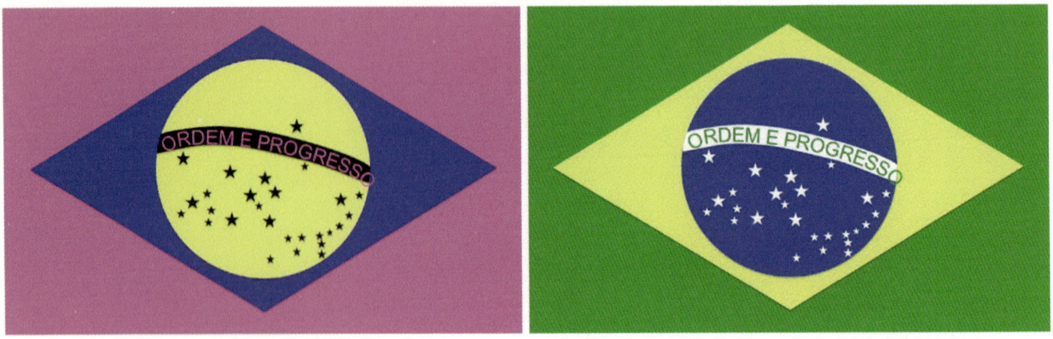

Practical example: Cover the second flag and look at the center of the first flag for approximately 30 seconds. Then, immediately look at a plain sheet of white paper and blink to see the Brazilian flag afterimage like the second flag that was covered.

Fig. 11.13 Opponent color theory test: practical example

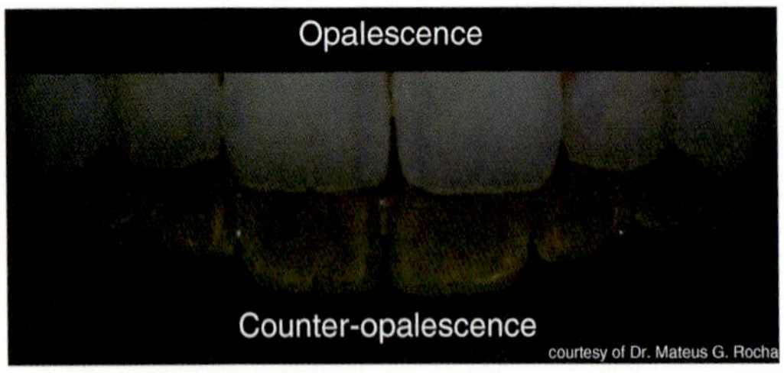

Fig. 11.14 Tyndall effect: opalescence and counter-opalescence

either short (blue), medium (green), or long (red) wavelengths (Fig. 11.15).

Despite being called "blue," "green," and "red" cone cells, each type of cell does not sense only one color, but a broad range of wavelengths in various degrees of sensitivity. Because of this, different specific selective cones can be stimulated by similar wavelength spectra, but in different levels. Thus, when the cone cells are exposed to a certain wavelength spectrum, the most sensitive cone cell for this specific wavelength spectrum is stimulated first.

However, as previously mentioned, when a specific selective cone is stimulated for prolonged viewing, it causes the fatigue of these cone cells. Then, the other color receptor, which is not fatigued, receives the stimulus and the brain incorrectly perceives the other color.

Human beings are capable of perceiving hundreds of shades equally; however, although findings are ambiguous, gender may have an influence on color perception [14, 15]. Thus, men and women may experience appearance of color differently. Generally, women are expected to experience more shades of color than men. What may be simple "purple" to a man could be "lavender" to a woman. Neuroscience says women are better at distinguishing among distinctions in color. On the other hand, linguistic researchers say that women possess a larger vocabulary of shades to describe color than men. But, women proved slightly better at detecting tiny differences between shades that look the same to men. The scientists believe the answer lies in the differences in men's and women's hormones that can alter development in the visual cortex. In contrast, children are more likely to sort the colors more randomly. However, the reason is probably due to the smaller exposure to color groups and general education of color.

The sensitivity of retinal cells declines with age, causing different shades of color to be less noticeable [16]. At the same time, certain neural pathways of the brain compensate it, so color perception remains constant over some time [17]. Because of this, color vision abnormalities are very uncommon in people younger than 70. However, as there is no treatment for this age-related loss of color perception, in mid-70s, dentists should be aware of this limitation.

Fig. 11.15 Different wavelength absorbance of sensory cells on human retina

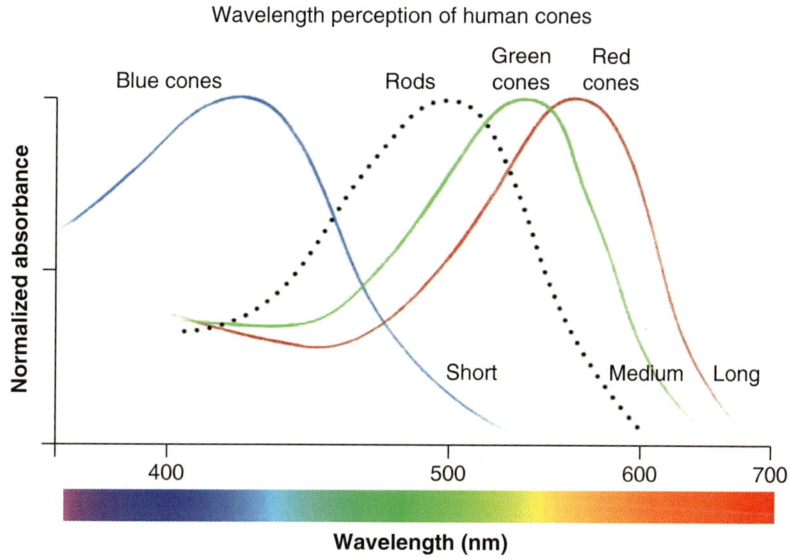

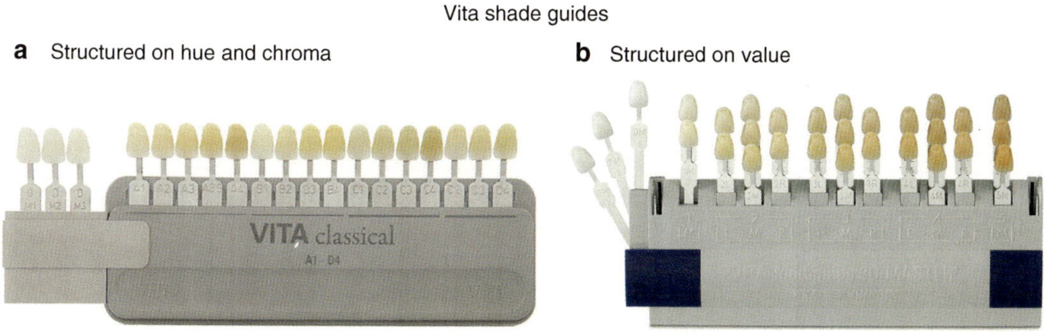

Fig. 11.16 Shade guides: (**a**) structured on hue and chroma (**b**) structured on value

11.4 Color Selection

Color selection is the first step before restoring a tooth. Different methods are described in literature to select color in dentistry [18]. The most traditionally used method is the visual analysis of color. This is a subjective simple method in which a standardized shade guide is compared with the natural tooth.

11.4.1 Shade Guides

Shade guides are the most common technique used to choose color in dentistry. In general, the shades of resin composites are described based on the VITA classical shade system. The arrangement of the shades in the VITA classical guide is a shade guide structured on hue and chroma (Fig. 11.16a). Hue can be identified according to the different letters, A (reddish-brownish), B (reddish-yellowish), C (greyish), and D (reddish-grey), and the chroma degree specified by numbers. The higher the number, the higher the chroma. Thus, observing VITA classical shade guide, it is possible to notice that A, B, and C represent different hues and also that letters (which indicate the hue) followed by number 1 are lighter than letters followed by numbers 2, 3, or 4.

When using VITA classical shade guide to choose color, it is recommended to choose the dentin/body shade according to the cervical

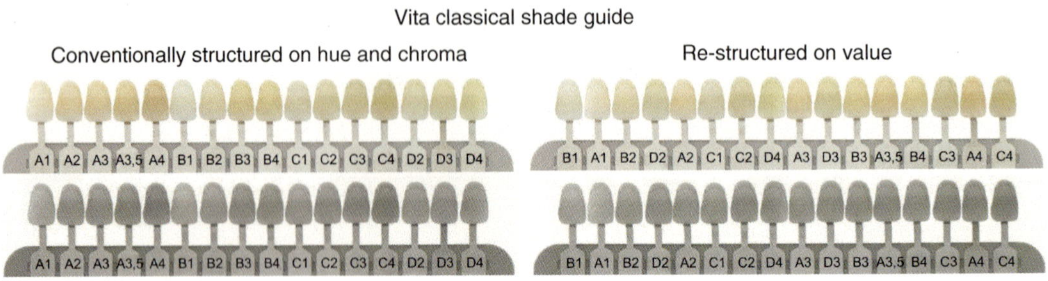

Fig. 11.17 Shade guide structured on hue and chroma repositioned in value order

portion of the tab, not the neck of the tab. To avoid confusion, grinding off the neck of the tab can be helpful. Likewise, it is recommended to choose the enamel shade according to the incisal portion of the tab from the shade guide.

The tabs of the VITA classical shade guide can also be repositioned in value order, B1, A1, B2, D2, A2, C1, C2, D4, A3, D3, B3, A3.5, B4, C3, A4, and C4, as shown in Fig. 11.17. In this way, the tabs will be reordered from the brighter to the darker shade. The VITA 3D-MASTER shade guide, however, already is shade guide structured on value (Fig. 11.16b). The VITA 3D-MASTER shade guide is based on the principle of choosing color in three quick steps:

First, selecting an appropriated value (from 1 to 5) according to the patient's tooth.

Then, selecting the corresponding chroma into that value. In this step, it is recommended to choose the middle hue group (M) to determine the chroma (from 1 up to 3).

Finally, choosing the final color, checking whether the patient's tooth is more reddish (R) or more yellowish (L) in comparison to the guide tab.

Although the shades of resin composites are described based on the VITA shade system, they are not part of the VITA shade guide [19–22]. Thus, it is not indicated to choose the resin composite shade using the VITA classical shade guide or the VITA 3D-MASTER shade guide. However, some manufactures provide information that allows choosing the right color according to the VITA shade system.

In general, the recommended way to choose color for direct restorations using resin composites is using the resin composite itself. Some manufactures provide their own shade guides. Even better, others provide plastic tabs that allow the dentist to place different resin composite types in different layers and simulate the restoration itself. It can be extremely useful to simulate polychromatic teeth with hypocalcification, stains, and/or translucent/opaque at the incisal edge.

However, it is important to notice that some manufacturers provide shade guides made of plastic. A discussion is held regarding plastic shade guides not being accurately similar to the resin composite, thus causing mismatch frequently.

11.4.2 Colorimeters and Spectrophotometers

Selecting color using shade guides, however, depends on the accuracy of human eyes [23]. Although the human eye is not always able to identify color accurately, it is a relatively simple task with a colorimeter or a spectrophotometer. While color is described verbally by subjective expressions, colorimeters and spectrophotometers express color numerically according to international standards.

Colorimeters and spectrophotometers process the light reflected from the tooth and calculate it into color parameters. In 1931, the Comission Internacionale de L'éclairage (CIE) quantitatively correlated the electromagnetic wavelengths in the visible spectrum and physiologically perceived color in human vision. As previously mentioned, the human eye has three types of cone cells with different spectral sensitivities: to blue, to green, or to red. The other colors are seen as a mixture of these primary colors. The L*a*b* color space, also known as CIELAB, is the most widely used space for measuring color. In this space, L* indicates lightness (value) and a* and b*, chromaticity. In the CIELAB diagram, the center is achromatic; but as a* and b* values increase, the saturation of the color increases. Positive and negative values for each color coordinates (a* and b*) indicate their chromaticity in different hues, +a* = red, −a* = green; +b* = yellow, −b* = blue, while for the L* coordinate, +L* = white, −L* = black.

Colorimeters therefore measure the light reflected from the object using three sensors filtered to the same sensitivity/color as the human eyes. Then, the values obtained are converted to a color space. In other words, a colorimeter identifies color the way the human eye does.

Spectrophotometers, on the other hand, not only obtain the numerical data of the color but also the full spectral reflectance graph for that color. It means that a spectrophotometer provides a full spectrum color analysis beyond that observable by the human eye.

A limitation of colorimeters in comparison to spectrophotometers is that colorimeters measure color against a standardized illuminant background to produce objective color data, while spectrophotometers can operate in multiple illuminant backgrounds, including ideal natural daylight. Thus, spectrophotometers are able to predict color more precisely for dental purposes. The use of spectrophotometers also avoids the probability of metamerism, once the illuminant used to choose color is similar to the natural daylight.

The L*a*b* color space data provided from colorimeters and spectrophotometers are scientifically employed to express color in numerical terms and to measure color differences between samples. Differences in lightness and darkness (*L** coordinate), red and green (*a** coordinate), and yellow and blue (*b** coordinate) are measured by reducing the final color coordinate value (*f*) from the initial baseline (*i*):

$$\Delta L = Lf - Li$$

$$\Delta a = af - ai$$

$$\Delta b = bf - bi$$

To measure the overall color difference between all three coordinates (ΔE), the CIELAB color difference formula from 1976 (ΔEab) [24] used to be the formula mostly applied in dental research:

$$\Delta Eab = \left[\Delta L^2 + \Delta a^2 + \Delta b^2\right]^{0.5}$$

However, since 2001, the Comission Internacionale de L'éclairage has been recommending the following color difference formula ($\Delta E00$), known as CIEDE2000 [25]:

$$\Delta E00 = \left[\left(\frac{\Delta L}{K_L} \times S_L\right)^2 + \left(\frac{\Delta C}{K_C} \times S_C\right)^2 + \left(\frac{\Delta H}{K_H} \times S_H\right)^2 + R_T \times \left(\frac{\Delta C}{K_C} \times S_C\right) \times \left(\frac{\Delta H}{K_H} \times S_H\right)\right]^{0.5}$$

where ΔL, ΔC, and ΔH are the differences in lightness, chroma, and hue and R_T is a function that accounts for the interaction between chroma and hue differences in the blue region. The weighting functions S_L, S_C, and S_H are used to adjust the total color difference for variations in the location of the color difference pair in *L**, *a**, and *b** coordinates. And, K_L, K_C, and K_H are correction terms for the experimental conditions [26]. Thus, a better correlation of perceptibility and acceptability thresholds can be obtained utilizing the concepts of hue, value, and chroma.

Spectrophotometers and colorimeters are mostly used in research on dental composites to evaluate color differences among resin composites, as well as their color stability in long term according to staining or degradation. Then, the data output conventionally used is expressed using the CIELAB color space in order to provide overall color difference in numbers as well as knowledge of each coordinate color change.

Although it seems complicated to use color space to reach the exact color of a tooth, dental colorimeters and spectrophotometers usually provide VITA shade system data as well. Thus, these devices are commonly used to select color for ceramics and compare shades during whitening processes [27].

Even though the shades of resin composites are not part of the VITA shade guide, the use of these devices can help to have a closer idea of the shade of the tooth when the manufacturer does not provide a specific shade guide for their product. Still, color checking after selecting the right shade will be necessary. If the manufacturer offers a shade guide, the color of the tooth can be checked and compared to the color of the color tab chosen from the shade guide.

11.4.3 Digital Cameras and Imaging Systems

Some software systems use high-resolution images to compare shades over the tooth with standard shade guides, such as VITA color systems. For this technique, high-resolution images are necessary [28–30]. In general, these images can be taken using digital cameras.

Digital cameras are cameras that present a digital imaging sensor as opposed to old photographic film. This difference permits the image to be saved as a bitmapped image (JPEG, PNG, GIF, TIFF, BMP, etc.) and transferred to a computer to be processed with a software system. Examples of digital cameras are point and shoot cameras and digital single-lens reflex cameras, also known as DSLR cameras.

Point and shoot cameras are highly recommended depending on the level of photography, the budget, and/or the purpose of the pictures. The advantages of point and shoot camera is that they are lightweight, compact, and work well for most simple clinical cases. DSLR cameras are cameras that have a removable lens with a reflex mirror, which allows live optical viewing through the lens that are taking the image. These cameras also permit the use of different lenses, such as a macro lens, which is suitable for taking close-up pictures with high resolution. And also, it includes port for flash or dual flash system that permits adjustment of lightening conditions to avoid under- or overexposure.

The use of DSLR can seem complicated for new users. However, the reduced cost of these cameras is worth the training. The two most popular brands of DSLR cameras in dentistry are Canon and Nikon (Fig. 11.18). However, all brands can take excellent extraoral and intraoral pictures.

The difference between a point and shoot camera and a DSLR camera is that point and shoot cameras have worse image quality. However, if the pictures will not be used for major enlargements or high level of esthetic cases, point and shoot cameras with 6 megapixels or higher are enough for the average user. Also, the imaging software that analyzes digital images compensates for different conditions and analyzes the data based on red, green, and blue (RGB) as well as black and white [31]. The software also analyzes all data to produce a shade map, which indicates all shade variations within the tooth.

There is also a smart digital camera designed exclusively for dentistry (Fig. 11.19). The dental digital camera is easy to handle and its program modes make most of the standard shots extremely simple. It is lightweight and scratch and scuff resistant, as well as water and chemical proof, which is essential for infection control in the dental office. However, despite the many advantages of this camera, it is much more expensive than a DSLR camera.

Smartphone cameras are also a welcome alternative for dental photography and photos can be taken at the tap of a finger. However, to overcome the bad reputation of smartphones in producing low-quality photos, some accessories are sometimes extremely helpful. For example, portable light-correcting devices are extremely helpful in giving adequate illumination. Also, other accessories have already been developed to facilitate the use of smartphones for dental photography. The Smile Line developed smartphone adapters to fix their portable light-correcting device in different types of smartphones. A calibration box is also available and permits setting the focusing distance of the smartphone camera to a fixed value for a very accurate color in every image (Fig. 11.20).

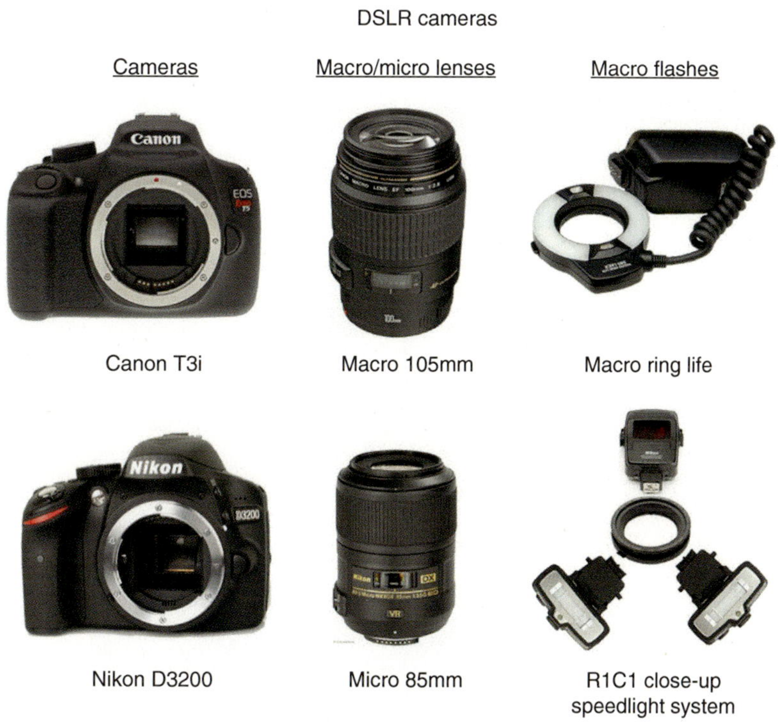

Fig. 11.18 DSLR cameras and accessories for dental photography

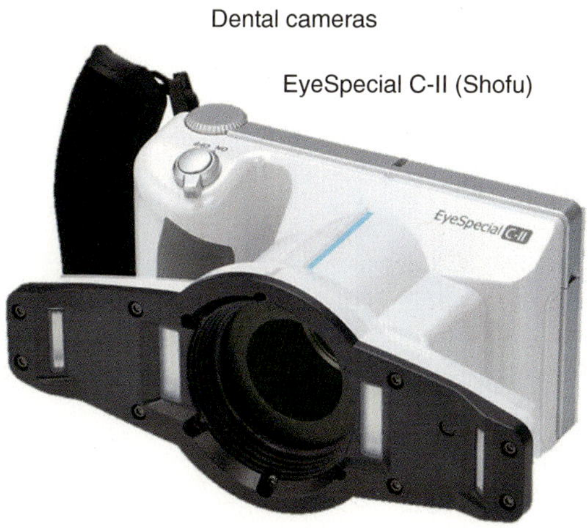

Fig. 11.19 Smart digital camera designed for dental photography

11.4.4 Clinical Techniques

About 28% of all visual shade measurements are not accurate. However, colorimeters, spectrophotometers, and imaging systems are expensive and time-consuming devices to have chairside in dental clinics that are not specialized in esthetics. Because of this, to achieve high esthetic levels, some clinical techniques are essential to avoid errors.

The majority of restorations can achieve an acceptable level of esthetic using only one shaded dentin and enamel type of a resin composite [32, 33]. However, it is extremely important to select the right shade to have success. An easy clinical technique to check whether the right shade was chosen or not is to place a small increment of the resin composite at the tooth and photoactivate it according to manufacturer's instructions. In this clinical technique, it is important to place each type of resin composite (dentin or enamel) at the right layer of the tooth (dentin or enamel) (Fig. 11.21). Also, this procedure should be performed before the isolation and preparation procedures. Otherwise, teeth will dry in absence of saliva and its shade will appear lighter than it really is [11]. Thus, disregarding selecting shade before isolation and preparation might affect the final color of the restoration. Also, depending on how the teeth dry during restoration procedures under isolation, the restoration might seem darker than the natural teeth. The rehydration shall be waited so the color of the restoration and the color of the teeth can match.

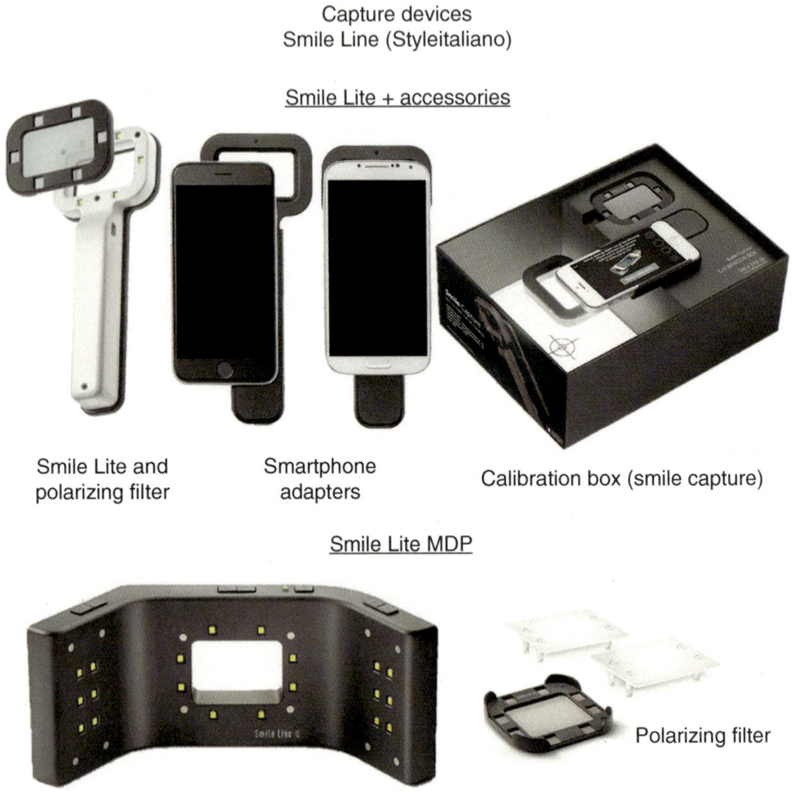

Fig. 11.20 Capture devices for smartphone cameras

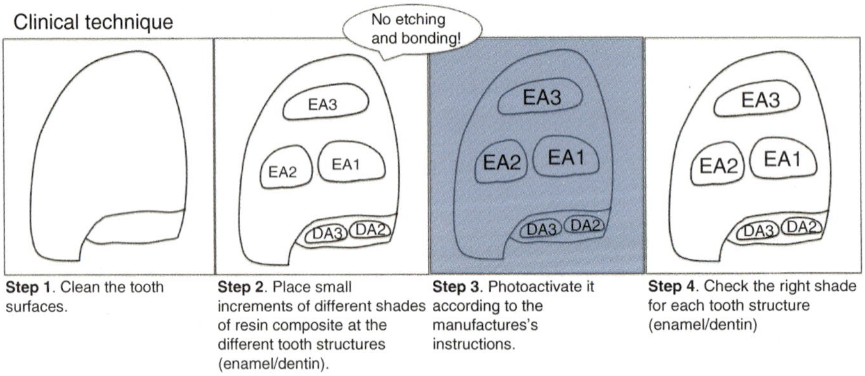

Fig. 11.21 Clinical technique using small increments of resin composites

Another point that should not be disregarded is to photoactivate the increment of resin composite. The resin composite that is not polymerized into the syringe is usually darker than the photopolymerized increment used during resin placement. These color differences are mainly caused by a decrease in lightness and chroma after photopolymerization.

In general, the decrease in lightness occurs because the monomers form polymers through the polymerization process. This reaction causes the reduction of their refractive indices, thus changing the way the light is transmitted, reflected, and refracted. The decrease in chroma, however, occurs due to the consumption of the photoinitiator during the photoactivation

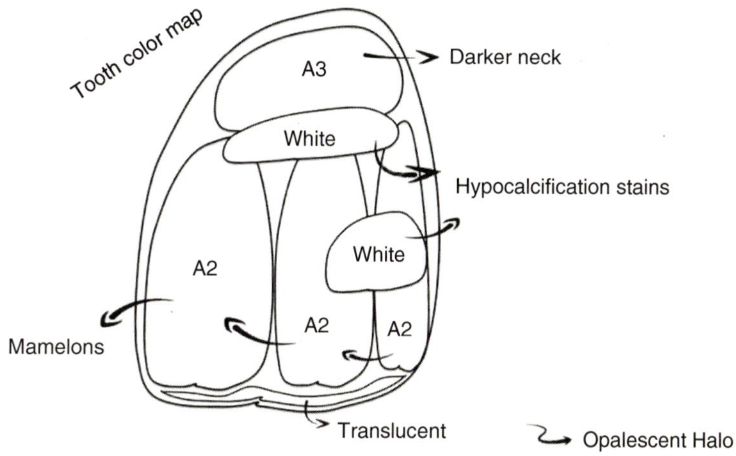

Fig. 11.22 Tooth color map draw

process. Camphorquinone is the most commonly used photoinitiator in dentistry. However, as a yellow colored molecule, after reacting, its consumption leads to a decrease in composite yellowness.

After checking the right shade of the tooth, sometimes we realize that just one shaded dentin and enamel type of resin composite is not enough to reproduce the polychromatic appearance of the natural tooth. However, a tooth color map enables to create an esthetically compatible reproduction. The tooth color map can be drawn in a paper with the different colors according to the different region of the tooth. Different characteristics or optical effects such as hypocalcifications, stains, and translucent and/or opaque halos shall also be drawn (Fig. 11.22). In these cases, different increments of resin composites are used in different regions of the tooth in order to identify the various shades within the tooth.

An intraoral direct resin composite mock-up can also be performed in an unetched tooth without using a bonding system. This technique allows checking whether the combination of the different shades that were chosen does really match with the polychromatic appearance of the natural tooth. This technique also helps to avoid goniochromism [13], once the different translucent layers are reproduced to confirm the final color of the restoration from different angles [34].

11.5 Resin Composite's Characteristics and Biomimetic of Natural Teeth

The smile is an important facial expression for a human being to transmit emotion and feelings. Restoring a tooth is extremely important not just to reestablish function but also to reestablish the social health of the individual.

Human teeth have different layers with different shades and translucencies [12, 35]. The presence of different layers also causes different optical effects that can have an influence on its color appearance. Thus, to restore a tooth, it is important to follow steps using different resin composite types.

11.5.1 Resin Composite Types × Esthetics

Resin composites are usually divided into four types: dentin; body, also called "universal"; enamel; and translucent. However, not all brands have all types of resin composites. The basic difference among the different types of resin composites is the translucency. In general, dentin and body types are more opaque than enamel and translucent types (Fig. 11.23). Thus, dentin and body types are used in deeper layers to substitute dentin, while enamel and translucent types are used in superficial layers to substitute enamel.

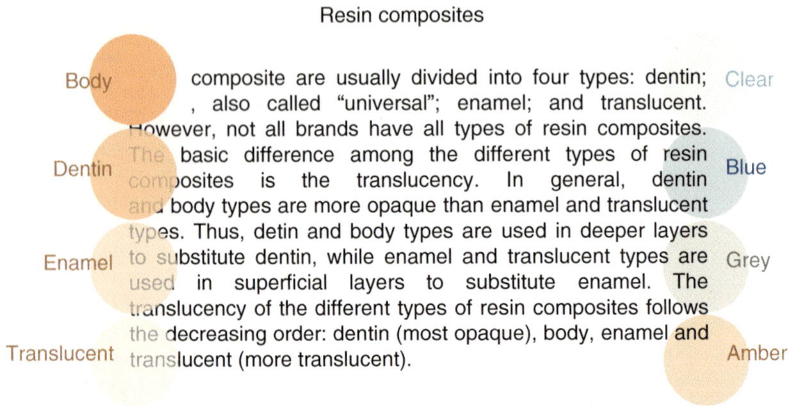

Fig. 11.23 Translucency of the different types of resin composites

The translucency of the different types of resin composites follows the decreasing order: dentin (most opaque), body, enamel, and translucent (more translucent).

The shades of dentin, body, and enamel types are available based on the VITA classical shade system. However, special shades for bleached teeth are also often available as white or extra white. The shades of the translucent type are usually clear, blue, gray, and amber, also called opalescent (Fig. 11.23). However, not all brands have all shades of the translucent types.

Beyond substituting dentin, more opaque types (dentin and body) can also be used to mimic hypocalcification stains or create an opaque halo sometimes present at the incisal edge of young individuals. The more translucent types, however, are indicated to mimic optical properties of the enamel in a high level of esthetic. Either clear, blue, or amber is frequently used to create the opalescent effect that often occurs at the incisal edge due to the high translucency of the natural enamel. But, it is important to notice that this opalescent effect can disappear over time due to enamel wear. Then, it is generally common to observe translucent and opaque halos at the incisal edge in young individuals, but almost rare in elders. Observing adjacent teeth or conferring teeth characteristics in old pictures is an important previous step to avoid the restoration looking artificial.

11.6 Surface Texture and Gloss

High gloss gives a natural esthetic appearance to a restoration. However, to achieve a natural esthetic gloss, polishing is extremely important to reduce roughness. Roughness is defined as the quantification of deviations in the normal vector of a real surface from its ideal form. Thus, if these deviations are large, the surface is considered rough. If these deviations are small, the surface is considered smooth. Gloss and roughness have an inverse linear relationship. As can be noticed in Fig. 11.24, the smoother the surface, the more light is reflected and thus the more glossy its appearance. First, the smoothness of the surface basically depends on the type of resin composite. As adjustments are always necessary for restorative procedures, finishing and polishing techniques can also influence the smoothness and gloss of direct restorations.

11.6.1 Resin Composite Type × Gloss

There are three basic types of resin composites: microfilled, nanofilled, and hybrid (Fig. 11.25). This classification is based on the type of filler that the resin composite contains. Differences in the filler content of resin composites can provide different levels of esthetics.

Microfilled resin composites contain silica fillers and prepolymerized resin fillers with size

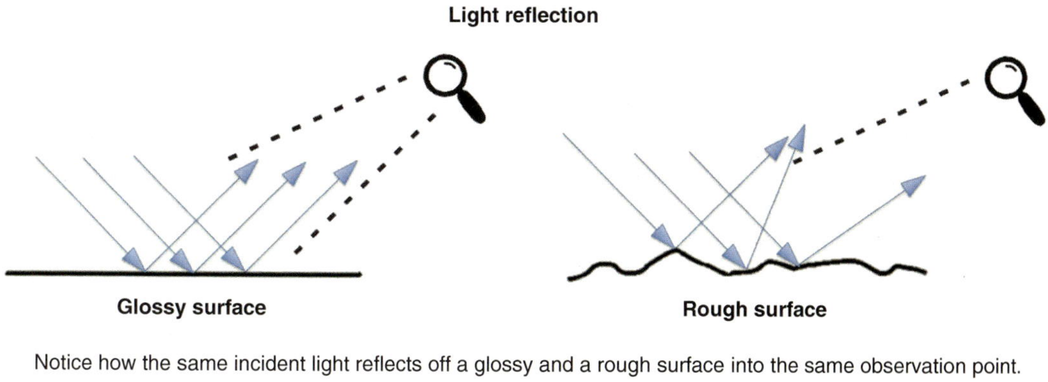

Fig. 11.24 Surface texture and gloss: light reflection of glossy and rough surfaces

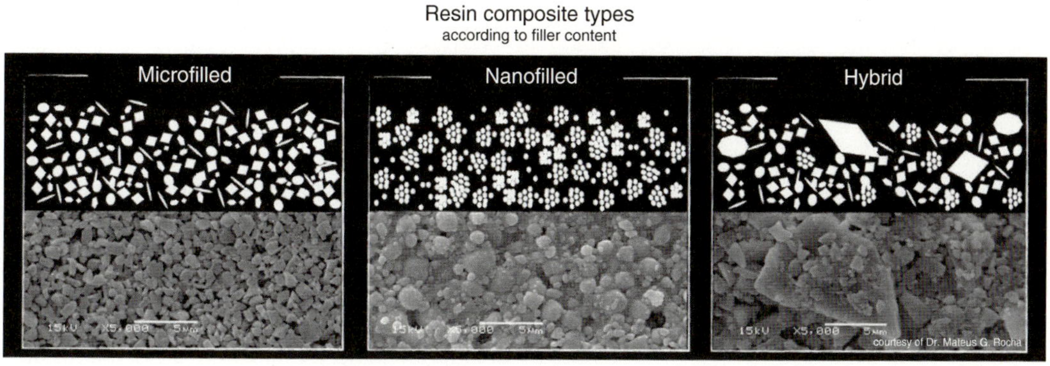

Fig. 11.25 Resin composite types according to filler content: microfilled, nanofilled, and hybrid

at the micron scale. These composites have excellent polishing due to the size of the particles but relatively weak mechanical properties due to the low concentration of fillers. For this reason, microfilled resin composites are indicated for esthetic areas, but not functional areas. On the other hand, hybrid resin composites contain particles with size at the micron and macro scales. These combinations of filler particles of different sizes allow high concentration of filler and enhanced mechanical properties in comparison to the microfilled resin composites. However, they do not allow the same polishing as microfilled resin composites. Thus, hybrid resin composites are conversely indicated for functional areas, but not esthetic areas.

The application of nanotechnology in dentistry, however, brought improvements to the resin composites. The development of nanofilled resin composites integrates a high concentration of nanoparticles with size into the nanometric scale. Thus, these resin composites not only have excellent polishing due to the size of the particles but also excellent mechanical properties due to the high concentration of fillers.

The difference in polishing of the different types of resin composites is due to the differences in size and shape of the fillers as well as the loading concentration. Resin composites with smaller filler particles are able to have a smoother finish. Then, nanofilled and microfilled resin composites are expected to have better polishing than hybrid resin composites. Moreover, during polishing, the particles can be worn away rather than plucked. The strongest is the matrix-filler integration; less will be the wear over time. Then, the defects will depend on the particle size and how strong is the filler-matrix integration. For these reasons, it is important to know the performance of different resin composites on the market over time beyond only its initial gloss appearance.

11.6.2 Finishing and Polishing × Gloss

Finishing systems are used for small adjustments after a direct restorative procedure. They are regularly used for reduction of excess material and contouring, correcting small defects of shape. Then, the polishing system is responsible for the smoothness of the final restoration by wearing down the micron defects of the surface.

In a metric scale, diamond- and carbide-finishing burs cause more roughness than polishers. Thus, this sequence should be respected in order to achieve a high smooth and glossy surface. A clinical tip is to place the resin composite into the correct anatomy but only slightly over contour. Then, polishing results will be easier achieved. However, if major adjustments are necessary, it is important to efficiently use finishing systems to gradually reduce the amount of roughness until starting to polish.

In turn, the polishing systems contain abrasives that are responsible for the wear. Commercially available polishing systems have a wide variety of abrasives, such as silicon oxide, aluminum oxide, and diamond dioxide, which are impregnated in rubber or discs. Polishing pastes are also available in order to be used with rubber, points, or felt or buff discs.

The polishing abrasives are expected to be harder than the resin composite in order to be efficient. On the contrary, the polisher would only remove the resin matrix and leave highly leveled fillers on the surface. In general, diamond dioxide and aluminum oxide are harder than silicon oxide, thus being expected to result in smoother surfaces than silicon oxide systems. However, diamond dioxide and aluminum oxide can provide different or similar polishing results. This is explained due to differences in the size of the abrasive particles of the different polishers on the market. Fine abrasive particles are expected to produce better polishing than larger abrasive particles. However, different brands can have different sizes of abrasive particles as well as different quality of polishers implying in different performances [36].

In the first part of this section, it was explained that resin composites with smaller filler particles are expected to have a smoother finish than resin composites with larger particles. However, despite the fact that nanofilled and microfilled resin composites have been showing better polishing results than hybrid resin composites, in general, nanofilled and microfilled resin composite seems to have similar initial smoothness after polishing. This fact, however, might be correlated to finishing/polishing systems available on the market. All polishing systems have abrasives into the micrometric scale. Thus, it is not unexpected that these abrasives do not have better polishing results in a nanofilled resin composite in comparison to a microfilled resin composite. However, it is expected that the finer the abrasive particle, the smoother the surface and the glossier the appearance of the restoration, regardless of the type of resin composite [37].

Liquid polishing systems are also commercially available. This system is a low-viscous light-cured resin that contains high molecular weight monomers diluted in a solvent. Thus, this low viscous liquid is capable of infiltrating in the surface porosities of the restoration. This way, after photoactivation, the restoration has a smoother and glossy surface. Although these liquid polishing systems have an easy and low-time-consuming technique as well as excellent initial smooth and gloss result, they have low wear resistance that leads to lower gloss retention in comparison to the other polishing systems.

Thus, for esthetics, the most important is not only to choose an adequate type of resin composite according to esthetical and functional needs but also to perform adequate finishing and polishing technique.

11.7 Color Change of Resin Composites

"Discoloration is defined as the process of changing to a different color." Discoloration of direct restorations with resin composite can be caused by intrinsic and extrinsic factors.

11.7.1 Intrinsic Factors

The intrinsic factors involve the discoloration of the material itself according to the degradation of its components over time [38–40]. The tertiary amines, however, are thought to be the major cause of intrinsic discoloration.

As previously explained, the tertiary amines are strong electron donors. In resin composites, the amines react with camphorquinone after photoactivation to generate free radicals that initiate the polymerization. However, when curing, only a portion of the amines actually reacts with a limited amount of camphorquinone. It occurs because the tertiary amine is usually added in excess in order to favor the reaction. Then, the unreacted amines that remain in the polymerized resin composite are still able to react with oxygen or other non-reacted compounds (such as non-reacted monomers). From these reactions, bigger conjugated systems are formed and responsible for the discoloration process over time.

The creation of a conjugated system increases the absorption of visible light in a specific region of the electromagnetic spectrum and, consequently, the reflection of the opponent region of the electromagnetic spectrum. In this case, the oxidation of the tertiary amine increases the absorption of visible light in the blue region of the electromagnetic spectrum and, thus, the reflection of visible light in the yellow region of the electromagnetic spectrum, causing the yellowing in the resin material over time.

The color stability of resin composites, however, can be improved depending on the type of tertiary amine present in its composition. In order to react with other compounds, first the tertiary amine needs to elevate its energy state by absorbing ultraviolet light. Then, these active molecules are capable of further reacting with other non-reacted molecules nearby. Different tertiary amines, however, have different absorbance in the ultraviolet region. Aliphatic tertiary amines, for example, have lower ultraviolet absorbance than aromatic tertiary amines. Consequently, aliphatic tertiary amines usually result in less discoloration over time in comparison to aromatic tertiary amines. Examples of tertiary amines present in dental resin composites are the 2-(dimethylamino)ethyl methacrylate (DMAEMA), which is aliphatic, and the ethyl 4(dimethylamino)benzoate (EDMAB), which is aromatic [39].

11.7.2 Extrinsic Factors

Extrinsic factors, on the other hand, involve staining by accumulation and absorption of staining colorants from exogenous sources, such as coffee, tea, wine, tobacco, and other foods and beverages [41–43]. The absorption of these staining colorants, however, is due to the staining susceptibility of resin composites. Resin composites are able to absorb water, as well as other fluids impregnated with colorants. Thus, the absorption of these fluids is a vehicle for stain penetration into the resin matrix.

The water sorption of resin composites depends on the composition of the resin matrix, as well as it concentration. The resin matrix is a polymer that is able to absorb water, while the filler particles are glasses that are unable to absorb water. Thus, the higher the concentration of the resin matrix in comparison to the filler content, the higher the probability of staining. However, different monomers from the resin matrix can also have different susceptibility to staining. The hydrophilic nature of the monomers directly influences on water sorption. Thus, the more hydrophilic the nature of the monomer, the more susceptible to water sorption and staining the resin matrix. In general, urethane dimethacrylate (UDMA), bisphenol A-glycidyl methacrylate (BisGMA), and triethylene glycol dimethacrylate (TEGDMA) follow an increase hydrophilic nature.

However, regardless the resin-based composite composition, different beverages are able to promote different levels of staining. In general, the higher the concentration of colorants in the beverage, the higher its staining potential. Thus, colorless beverages are expected not to produce visible color change in dental resin composites. Usually, the most staining beverages in regular diet are red wine, coffee, and tea. Red wines have high staining potential, while coffees and teas have medium to low staining potential depending on their type and "strength."

Soft drinks, however, do not directly implicate in discoloration of resin composite restorations. Despite the presence of colorant in its composition, its acidic pH causes the dissolution of the resin matrix present in the resin composite. Thus, during this dissolution process, it prevents the colorants to penetrate into the resin matrix. Another example of acidic drink that degrades the resin matrix rather than staining it is the sport drinks that are widely consumed by individuals highly involved in physical activities. High alcoholic drinks with high percentage of alcohol by volume (ABV), however, are also able to cause the dissolution of the resin matrix due to elution of alcohol that acts as a solvent.

However, it is important to notice that the consumption of these beverages can still affect the esthetical appearance of resin composite restorations. The dissolution of the resin matrix increases roughness, which directly affects the way light is scattered from the surface over time, progressively reducing its gloss. Also, as roughness is increased, staining susceptibility by other beverages over time is also increased, reducing the esthetic longevity of the restoration.

When roughness is increased, plaque and colorant retention is increased. Then, staining is not only caused by the absorption of the colorants during consumption but also by accumulation. The duration of the exposure to these colorants directly influences the susceptibility of staining. The higher the exposure to colorants, the higher the susceptibility of staining.

Staining colorants are also present or added to food. They are called food coloring or color additives. People unconsciously associate certain colors with certain flavors. Thus, in general, food coloring is added to food in order to make it more attractive and appetizing for the consumer.

The nicotine present in nicotine chewing gums and cigarettes is also capable of staining the teeth and resin composite restorations. Nicotine is the active principle of tobacco. Nicotine oxidizes in the presence of oxygen and becomes yellow. Thus, when tobacco is inhaled in the mouth, nicotine is oxidized and leached into microscopic porosities in the enamel or resin composite material, resulting in a yellow/brown discoloration of the tooth or the restoration surface. The nicotine stains, however, are harder to remove than most other surface stains.

11.7.3 Methods to Minimize Discoloration

A regular routine to minimize the effects of colorants on resin composite restorations is the use of toothbrush or mouth rinses after consumption of staining substances. To brush the teeth or to rinse the mouth eliminates most of the colorants that stay in the mouth. The toothbrush is also able to remove colorant substances that might stay retained in interproximal surfaces or rough surfaces of resin composite restorations.

Another regular routine that can prevent resin composite restoration from discoloration is the professional prophylaxis [44]. Professional prophylaxis is able to remove most of the colorants superficially absorbed by the resin matrix of the restorations. This procedure prevents from deeper staining that is more difficult or practically impossible to be removed.

Repolishing resin composite restoration each 6 months also prevents discoloration. Repolishing reduces roughness of the surface of the restoration [45, 46], reduces staining by accumulation and retakes the esthetic of a glossy surface, and then enhances the longevity and durability of the restoration as well as the comfort and satisfaction of the patient.

Regular dental routine appointments are extremely important for the maintenance of resin composite restorations.

Staining usually penetrates from 3 to 60 μm into resin composite restorations. The deeper the staining, the more difficult it is to be removed. Superficial staining can be easily removed during a repolishing procedure. Excessive interproximal staining can also be removed with polishing strip packed with polishing pastes. However, when staining reaches deep layers, it is more difficult to completely remove all the staining.

The bleaching procedure can be an alternative to minimize the appearance of discoloration [47, 48]. Bleaching or whitening is the process to make something appear whiter. In this process, bleaching agents based on peroxides (hydrogen or carbamide) are used. These agents are able to penetrate deep in the tooth or the resin composite and react with the stain, breaking it into small pieces, which make the color less concentrate.

Bleaching methods include in-office bleaching, during which the bleaching agent is applied by a dental professional, and at-home bleaching, which the individual carries out at home. In-office bleaching is more indicated for discoloration of resin composite restorations. In these cases, the bleaching agent is applied directly and exclusively to the stained surfaces. Usually three sessions reduce the staining to an acceptable color match between the tooth and the resin composite restoration.

However, it is important to point out that although effective, bleaching treatments are not able to reset the baseline color of the resin composite restoration. If color matching is not acceptable, repair or replacement should be considered according to the patient complaint [49].

References

1. Hofer H, Carroll J, Neitz J, Neitz M, Williams DR. Organization of the human trichromatic cone mosaic. J Neurosci. 2005;25(42):9669–79.
2. Cornsweet T. Visual perception. New York: Academic; 1970.
3. Ristic I, Stankovic S, Paravina RD. Influence of color education and training on shade matching skills. J Esthet Restor Dent. 2016;28(5):287–94.
4. Dudea D, Gasparik C, Botos A, Alb F, Irimie A, Paravina RD. Influence of background/surrounding area on accuracy of visual color matching. Clin Oral Investig. 2016;20(6):1167–73.
5. Feng X, Xu W, Han Q, Zhang S. LED light with enhanced color saturation and improved white light perception. Opt Express. 2016;24(1):573–85.
6. Kim SH, Lee YK, Lim BS, Rhee SH, Yang HC. Metameric effect between dental porcelain and porcelain repairing resin composite. Dent Mater. 2007;23(3):374–9.
7. Clary JA, Ontiveros JC, Cron SG, Paravina RD. Influence of light source, polarization, education and training on shade matching quality. J Prosthet Dent. 2016;116(1):91–7.
8. Penaorgias A, Kulikowski JJ, Parry NR, McKeefry DJ, Morray IJ. Phases of daylight and the stability of color perception in the near peripheral human retina. J Vis. 2012;12(3). doi: https://doi.org/10.1167/12.3.1.
9. Imhoff SM, Volbrecht VJ, Nerger JL. A new look at the Bezold-Brucke hue shift in the peripheral retina. Vis Res. 2004;44(16):1891–906.
10. Pridmore RW. Bezold–Brucke hue-shift as functions of luminance level, luminance ratio, interstimulus interval and adapting white for aperture and object colors. Vis Res. 1999;39(23):3873–91.
11. Burki Z, Watkins S, Wilson R, Fenlon M. A randomised controlled trial to investigate the effects of dehydration on tooth colour. J Dent. 2013;41(3):250–7.
12. Pop-Ciutrila IS, Ghinea R, Perez Gomez Mdel M, Colosi HA, Dudea D, Badea M. Dentin scattering, absorption, transmittance and light reflectivity in human incisors, canines and molars. J Dent. 2015;43(9):1116–24.
13. Chirdon WM, O'Brien WJ, Robertson RE. Mechanisms of goniochromism relevant to restorative dentistry. Dent Mater. 2009;25(6):802–9.
14. Abramov I, Gordon J, Feldman O, Chavarga A. Sex & vision I: spatio-temporal resolution. Biol Sex Differ. 2012;3(1):20.
15. Abramov I, Gordon J, Feldman O, Chavarga A. Sex & vision II: color appearance of monochromatic lights. Biol Sex Differ. 2012;3(1):21.
16. Haegerstrom-Portnoy G, Schneck ME, Lott LA, Hewlett SE, Brabyn JA. Longitudinal increase in anisometropia in older adults. Optom Vis Sci. 2014;91(1):60–7.
17. Wueger S. Colour constancy across the life span: evidence for compensatory mechanisms. PLoS One. 2013;8(5):e63921.
18. Chu SJ, Trushkowsky RD, Paravina RD. Dental color matching instruments and systems. Review of clinical and research aspects. J Dent. 2010;38(Suppl 2):e2–e16.
19. Barutcigil C, Harorli OT, Yildiz M, Ozcan E, Arslan H, Bayindir F. The color differences of direct esthetic restorative materials after setting and compared with a shade guide. J Am Dent Assoc. 2011;142(6):658–65.
20. Carney MN, Johnston WM. Appearance differences between lots and brands of similar shade designations of dental composite resins. J Esthet Restor Dent. 2017;29(2):E6–E14. https://doi.org/10.1111/jerd.12263.
21. Mikhail SS, Schricker SR, Azer SS, Brantley WA, Johnston WM. Optical characteristics of contemporary dental composite resin materials. J Dent. 2013;41(9):771–8.
22. Pecho OE, Pérez MM, Ghinea R, Della Bona A. Lightness, chroma and hue differences on visual shade matching. Dent Mater. 2016;32(11):1362–73.
23. Paravina RD, Ghinea R, Herrera LJ, Bona AD, Igiel C, Linninger M, Sakai M, Takahashi H, Tashkandi E, Perez Mdel M. Color difference thresholds in dentistry. J Esthet Restor Dent. 2015;27(Suppl 1):S1–9.
24. CIE (Comission Internationale de l'Eclairage). Colorimetry technical report. CIE Pub. No. 15. 2nd ed. Vienna, Austria: Bureau Central de La CIE; 1986.

25. CIE (Comission Internationale de I'Eclairage). Colorimetry technical report. CIE Pub. No. 15. 3rd ed. Vienna, Austria: Bureau Central da La CIE; 2004.
26. Sharma G, Wu WC, Daa EN. The CIEDE2000 color-difference formula: implementation notes, supplementary test data, and mathematical observations. Color Res Appl. 2005;30(1):21–30.
27. Ghinea R, Perez MM, Herrera LJ, Rivas MJ, Yebra A, Paravina RD. Color difference thresholds in dental ceramics. J Dent. 2010;38(Suppl 2):e57–64.
28. Tam WK, Lee HJ. Accurate shade image matching by using a smartphone camera. J Prosthodont Res. 2017;61(2):168–76.
29. Tam WK, Lee HJ. Dental shade matching using a digital camera. J Dent. 2012;40(Suppl 2):e3–e10.
30. Wee AG, Lindsey DT, Kuo S, Johnston WM. Color accuracy of commercial digital cameras for use in dentistry. Dent Mater. 2006;22(6):553–9.
31. Carney MN, Johnston WM. A novel regression model from RGB image data to spectroradiometric correlates optimized for tooth colored shades. J Dent. 2016;51:45–8.
32. Mikhail SS, Johnston WM. Confirmation of theoretical colour predictions for layering dental composite materials. J Dent. 2014;42(4):419–24.
33. Pecho OE, Ghinea R, do Amaral EA, Cardona JC, Della Bona A, Pérez MM. Relevant optical properties for direct restorative materials. Dent Mater. 2016;32(5):e105–12.
34. Miotti LL, Santos IS, Nicoloso GF, Pozzobon RT, Susin AH, Durand LB. The use of resin composite layering technique to mask discolored background: a CIELAB/CIEDE2000 analysis. Oper Dent. 2017;42(2):165–74.
35. Pop-Ciutrila IS, Ghinea R, Colosi HA, Dudea D. Dentin translucency and color evaluation in human incisors, canines, and molars. J Prosthet Dent. 2016;115(4):475–81.
36. Kemaloglu H, Karacolak G, Turkun LS. Can reduced-step polishers be as effective as multiple-step polishers in enhancing surface smoothness? J Esthet Restor Dent. 2017;29(1):31–40. https://doi.org/10.1111/jerd.12233.
37. Kaizer MR, de Oliveira-Ogliari A, Cenci MS, Opdam NJ, Moraes RR. Do nanofill or submicron composites show improved smoothness and gloss? A systematic review of in vitro studies. Dent Mater. 2014;30(4):e41–8.
38. De Oliveira DC, Ayres AP, Rocha MG, Giannini M, Puppin Rontani RM, Ferracane JL, Sinhoreti MA. Effect of different in vitro aging methods on color stability of a dental resin-based composite using CIELAB and CIEDE2000 color-difference formulas. J Esthet Restor Dent. 2015;27(5):322–30.
39. De Oliveira DC, Rocha MG, Gattia A, Correr AB, Ferracane JL, Sinhoreti MA. Effect of different photoinitiators and reducing agents on cure efficiency and color stability of resin-based composites using different LED wavelengths. J Dent. 2015;43(12): 1565–72.
40. De Oliveira DC, de Menzes LR, Gatti A, Correr Sobrinho L, Ferracane JL, Sinhoreti MA. Effect of nanofiller loading on cure efficiency and potential color change of model composites. J Esthet Restor Dent. 2016;28(3):171–7.
41. Alandia-Roman CC, Cruvinel DR, Sousa ABS, Pires-de-Souza FCP, Panzeri H. Effect of cigarette smoke on color stability and surface roughness of dental composites. J Dent. 2013;41(Suppl 3):73–9.
42. Antonov M, Lenhardt L, Manojlovic D, Milicevic B, Zekovic I, Dramicanin MD. Changes of color and fluorescence of resin composites immersed in beer. J Esthet Restor Dent. 2016;28(5):330–8.
43. Erdemir U, Yildiz E, Eren MM. Effects of sport drinks on color stability of nanofilled and microhybrid composites after long-term immersion. J Dent. 2016;40(Suppl 2):e55–63.
44. Samra APB, Ribeiro DG, Borges CPF, Kossatz S. Influence of professional prophylaxis on reducing discoloration of different aesthetic restorative materials. J Dent. 2012;40(Suppl 2):e71–6.
45. Anfe TE, Agra CM, Vieira GF. Evaluation of the possibility of removing staining by repolishing composite resins submitted to artificial aging. J Esthet Restor Dent. 2011;23(4):260–7.
46. De Oliveira AL, Botta AC, Campos JA, Garcia PP. Effects of immersion media and repolishing on color stability and superficial morphology of nanofilled composite resin. Microsc Microanal. 2014;20(4):1234–9.
47. Halacoglu DM, Yamanel K, Basaran S, Tuncer D, Celik C. Effects of staining and bleaching on a nanohybrid composite with or without surface sealant. Eur J Dent. 2016;10(3):361–5.
48. Lago M, Mozzaquatro LR, Rodrigues C, Kaizer MR, Mallmann A, Jacques LB. Influence of bleaching agents on color and translucency of aged resin composites. J Esthet Restor Dent. 2016. https://doi.org/10.1111/jerd.12261.
49. Demarco FF, Collares K, Coelho-de-Souza FH, Correa MB, Cenci MS, Moraes RR, Opdam NJ. Anterior composite restorations: a systematic review on long-term survival and reasons for failure. Dent Mater. 2015;31(10):1214–24.

Part V

Biological Considerations

12 Elution of Substances from Dental Composite Materials

Olga Polydorou

12.1 Introduction

Components of composite materials might be released under different circumstances in the oral cavity having consequences on the human health and on the materials themselves. The evaluation of the elution of substances from restorative materials presents an important parameter on the estimation of their biocompatibility. The mechanisms of cytotoxicity of composite materials concerning the released substances, as proposed by Goldberg [1], are determined firstly as their short-term release during the monomer-polymer conversion, taking place in the first hours after polymerization and secondly as the release of substances that can take place as a result of erosion and degradation over time.

Release of substances is a critical issue for dental materials. It can lead to important loss of material and probably also to failure of the restoration. Wear presents a progressive loss of the material or changes of the material surface after coming in contact with substances. Fatigue, abrasive, and/or chemical wear might result in changes in material structure and/or material surface. The eluted monomers might react with the bacteria in the oral cavity, which can have some biological implications after coming in contact with the pulp and/or gingival tissues, or exert systemic effects on human health [1]. Different routes of systemic intake of the released monomers are described including ingestion of the substances in the gastrointestinal tract, diffusion to the pulp through dentinal tubules, and uptake in the lungs [2]. Most research papers [3–11] are focused on the elution of monomers from composite materials; however the release of other components like filler particles should also be considered as they are not without negative consequences. Besides these, various additives, photoinitiators, and co-initiators have been shown to be eluted under different experimental conditions [3, 10].

12.2 Elution of Monomers from Composite Materials: What Is Eluted?

The content of the organic matrix of the composite materials plays an important role on the potential release of monomers. The composition and the amount of the eluates depend on the composition of the composite materials, their "chemistry," and the extraction medium used [12, 13]. Several additional factors influence the final amount of the eluted monomers. According to Ferracane [3], the elution of monomers from

O. Polydorou
Department of Operative Dentistry and Periodontology, Center for Dental Medicine, Medical Center—University of Freiburg, Faculty of Medicine, University of Freiburg, Hugstetter Straße 55, 79106 Freiburg, Germany
e-mail: olga.polydorou@uniklinik-freiburg.de

V. Miletic (ed.), *Dental Composite Materials for Direct Restorations*,
http://doi.org/10.1007/978-3-319-60961-4_12

composite materials relates to the following: the polymerization reaction, the kind of solvent used, and the size and kind of the eluted substances. Smaller molecules elute easier than the larger ones as the former show higher mobility.

More than 30 different compounds have been shown to be extracted from polymerized dental composites, and among those, major monomers, co-monomers, various additives, and reaction products have been detected [2, 3, 7, 10]. BisGMA (bisphenol-A glycol dimethacrylate Fig. 12.1), UDMA (urethane dimethacrylate, Fig. 12.2), and TEGDMA (triethylene glycol dimethacrylate, Fig. 12.3) are the most often investigated and detected monomers to be released from dental composites [2, 14–16]. In several studies it is reported that BisGMA was shown to be released in high rates [16–19], although it is a large molecule. It is suggested that this high elution rate of BisGMA is due to the fact that it is a rigid and highly viscous monomer with high transition temperature, resulting in its lower degree of conversion during polymerization [20]. Although HEMA does not present a component of modern composite materials nowadays, as it shows high cytotoxicity, it has been stated to be eluted from composite materials [2, 21]. The presence of HEMA has been explained by the

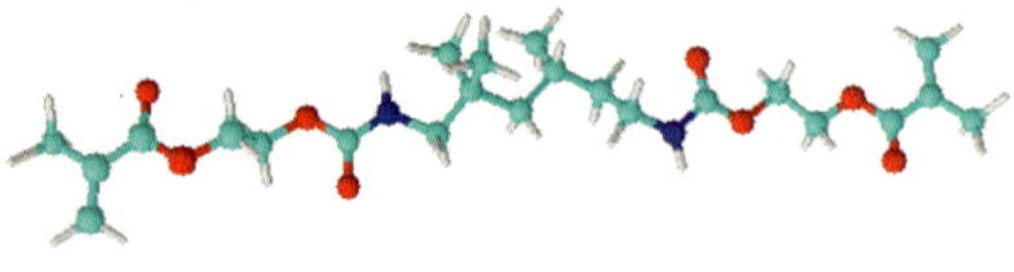

Fig. 12.1 BisGMA (bisphenol-A glycol dimethacrylate)

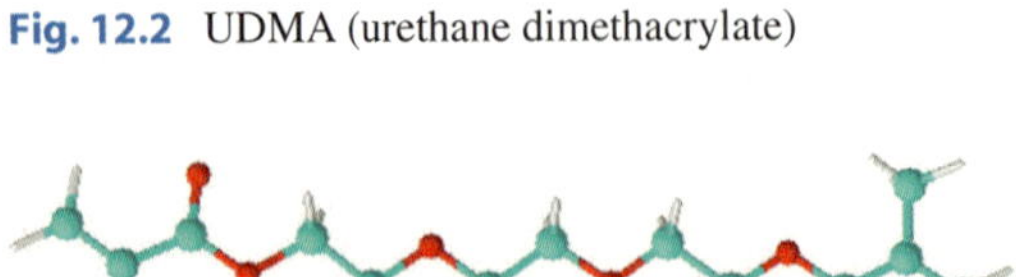

Fig. 12.2 UDMA (urethane dimethacrylate)

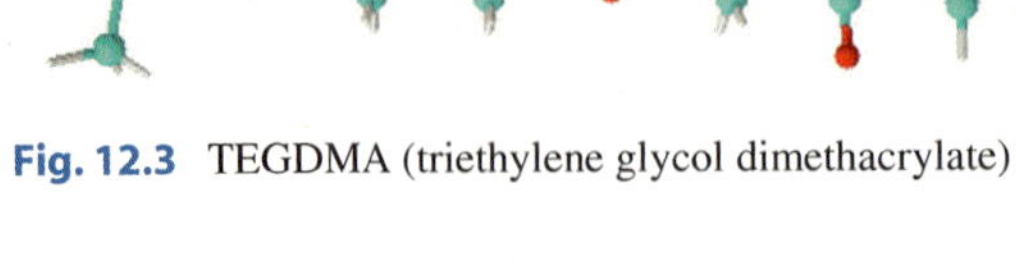

Fig. 12.3 TEGDMA (triethylene glycol dimethacrylate)

authors either as a part of the organic resin matrix of the composite materials or more probably as a by-product by the degradation of UDMA by the analytical process [22].

BisEMA and other derivatives of bisphenol A have been reported to release. Of high interest is the detection of small amounts of bisphenol A itself in the eluates of composite materials. This point will be discussed in detail in the following section. The release of degradation products of the monomers might also take place [7, 23, 24]. The eluted monomers might react with each other creating new by-products [25], which results in crucial problem in their analytical detection. Although it is mentioned that usually 5–10% of the unbound monomer is eluted [3], the eluted amount varies among the experimental studies, as the elution depends on the composition and structure of the composite material, on the curing process performed and additionally on the analytical method used.

12.2.1 Elution Rate of Monomers Over Time

In the past, it was thought that 50% of the eluted substances are extracted in water within 3 h, while in the same time 75% of the eluted monomers are extracted in 75% ethanol solution [14]. According to these, it was concluded that within 24 h almost all leachable substances are eluted and after that no further release of monomers takes place over time. It is definitely a fact that the elution of monomers is not linear over time. Some authors observed that the highest release takes place in the first week after polymerization [11, 26], while other authors have shown that the release of monomers continues over time, up to 30 days [16, 17, 19, 27] or even for 1 year after polymerization [15].

12.3 Parameters that Influence the Elution of Monomers

As it is mentioned above, reasons that can affect the release of monomers can be found in the material properties itself, the kind of storage media used, and the conditions in the environment of the oral cavity that might affect the composite filling surfaces.

In detail, the incomplete polymerization of the composite resins [28, 29], presenting usually a conversion rate, which varies between 35% and 77% [30–32], plays a role in the elution of monomers. This is due to the fact that a part of the monomers which remain unreacted after the polymerization reaction can be eluted from the polymerized structure. The degree of conversion is an important factor influencing the mechanical properties of the composite materials and additionally their biocompatibility [3, 33]. The composition of the composite materials in addition to the layer technique and the polymerization conditions used can influence the degree of conversion.

For a long time it was believed that the degree of conversion determines the elution of monomers from restorative materials. In some cases, a strong correlation was observed between the degree of conversion and the amount of eluted monomers for conventional materials, as the highest amount of eluted monomers (TEGDMA and BisGMA) was observed to be correlated to the lowest degree of conversion [34]. However, for some materials, the filler content was found to correlate to the elution of monomers so that materials with high filler content could show lower release of monomers, suggesting that the degree of conversion is not the only parameter that can influence the monomers' release [34]. Therefore the release of monomers cannot be predicted solely due to the degree of conversion. Pongprueksa et al. [26] observed no correlation between the degree of conversion and the elution of monomers from the composite materials tested. This is in accordance with other findings [17] in the literature. The authors [17] found that the composite and polymerization type (photo, chemical, or dual) are more important parameters for this elution. Materials with the same degree of conversion showed different elution rates, according to the kind of composite material. Dual-cured composite material revealed higher amounts of BisGMA and TEGDMA than the photo-cured material [17]. Interesting are the findings of studies where a correlation among the degree of conversion and monomers' release was found in the cases of suboptimal polymerization [35] or when changes on the composition of the materials took place [36]. Changes in the photoinitiator system were shown to affect the degree of conversion and the elution of monomers [37], verifying the strong inverse correlation among them. Replacing camphorquinone with Lucirin-TPO and using short curing times increased the degree of conversion and the elution of monomers remained stable or decreased.

According to literature data, it can be concluded that although the amount of the residual monomers might be influenced and correlated to the unreacted amount, the elutable residual monomer must be clearly differentiated from the amount of monomers that is not converted during the polymerization reaction, meaning that although the conversion rate might influence the eluted amount of monomers, it does not definitely determine it. Therefore, a direct correlation between the degree of conversion and elution of monomers is nowadays not justified, as the elution mechanism is also related to the molecular weight and the hydrophobicity of the substances as well as the filler content [34] and depends on the composite material used and the network characteristics of the resin matrix [26, 38].

12.3.1 Material Effect on the Elution of Monomers

Although there have been a great development concerning composite materials over the past decades and improvement of the conversion rate, as mentioned above, the elution of monomers is still a present problem. The composition of the composite materials has been shown to be more important for the polymerization success than the used polymerization unit or the kind the polymerization method used [39, 40]. A great effort has been performed by the industry to manufacture composite materials with a more complex network in order to prevent the direct elution of substances. It has been shown that the amount of monomers released from nanohybrid composite materials is higher than the one of ormocers [27]. The authors commented that a main part of the elution of substances takes place in the first 24 h. After this, the elution process becomes slower, while additional time is necessary where the swelling of the polymer chain takes place and then a further "extraction" of monomers happens. Storage media are shown to attack composite materials differently, depending on their chemistry. For materials with more complex chemistry, for example, ormocers, even if they do not show a better conversion rate compared to the hybrid composite materials, they do show less release of monomers due to the reduced initial contained amount and especially due to their complex three-dimensional network which does not allow the unbound monomers to elute easily [16, 17, 27]. Susila et al. [41] could show that ormocer and silorane materials elute less monomer and exert less cytotoxicity than conventional dimethacrylate-based composite materials.

In evaluating the data existing on the newest category of composite materials, the bulk-fill materials, the findings are controversial, as they state an inhomogeneous group of composite resins. In some cases [34], the amount of monomers (BisGMA and TEGDMA) released from the bulk-fill materials was lower than the one of the conventional materials, and in other cases [42], it was comparable with the conventional ones. High elution of monomers from bulk-fill materials was stated up to 30 days after polymerization and the elution was found to increase over time [43]. It is supposed that the use of the incremental application technique of composite materials may overwhelm some of their shortcomings, by achieving an adequate light penetration. For all conventional composite materials, the application of 2-mm layers is accepted as the best solution. In the case of using bulk-fill composite materials, a respective adequate depth cure is shown to be achieved by applying layers of 4 mm. By reducing the layer thickness of bulk-fill flowable materials, the released amount of substances can decrease [34]. However, the kind of composite material used was shown to be more important than the technique used. By increasing the filler/matrix ratio, it is demonstrated that the conversion decreases, as the presence of fillers states a problem for the polymeric chain propagation [44]. Flowable materials elute higher amount of their unreacted monomers [18] independently of the application method used (bulk-fill or layer technique) [26]. In addition to the filler amount in the composite materials, the light permeability of the fillers together with the monomer composition, the kind and amount of initiators, and the inhibitor/accelerator systems influence the degree of conversion of the composite resins [44]. The adhesion strength of the fillers in the organic matrix, due to the coupling agents, exerts an effect on the possible "washout" of the filler particles in the oral cavity.

Regarding the effect of material quality on monomer elution, the performance of low cost and not widely known brands of composites was compared to a standard widely used composite material [45]. Low-cost composite materials showed some shortcomings compared to the commonly used material, in terms of their mechanical and physical properties, as well as their monomers' release and potential cytotoxicity.

12.3.2 Effect of Curing Parameters on the Elution of Monomers

The curing mode, light curing time, and curing unit used are widely discussed in the literature concerning their effect on the elution of monomers from composite materials as they affect their polymerization degree. Polymerization of composite materials with different curing units and curing protocols results in different degrees of monomers' elution and softening in ethanol [46]. Additionally the energy density, power density, and mode of cure affect the softening and the elution of monomers from composite resins [47]. The higher the energy delivered to the material during the polymerization, the lower the degree of softening of the material and the eluted amount of monomers [48]. Different curing protocols can influence the solubility and water sorption of composite resins [48, 49]. Longer curing times were shown to result in lower solubility of the composite materials [50, 51]. Through the depth of the filling material, the light intensity is radically reduced. It must be taken into consideration that in addition to the altered properties of the materials caused by using shortened curing times, the increased solubility of the superficial layer is also a result of it. In the study of Kim et al. [50], composite materials with the same degree of conversion values showed different solubility values. The authors suggested that the difference in the functionality of the base monomers used among the tested composites, influencing the residual amount of monomers, is the reason of their findings.

The influence of curing time on the elution of monomers from composite materials has been widely studied in the literature [52–55]. A reduction of the curing times of the composite materials compared to the recommended curing times results in increased release of substances [53, 54]. The curing times recommended by the manufacturers were insufficient to minimize the release of substances [52, 53]. An increase of the curing time up to 200 s could not eliminate the eluted substances [53]. Although an increase of curing time is recommended by several studies [53, 55] in order to avoid the negative implication of the eluted substances, the rise of pulpal temperature due to increased curing time should be taken into consideration.

Not only the curing time but also the kind of curing unit and mode is of interest for achieving adequate polymerization. The compatibility of the material composition with the curing unit used seems to be important. The kind of the curing unit (halogen and LED) was not found to exert a determinative effect on the amount of eluted monomers [56], whereas the material itself was found to be more important than the curing unit used [57]. The effect of curing modes on composite materials has been shown to be material dependent, as the composition of the materials seems to be of higher importance concerning the effect on the polymerization reaction than the curing unit used [39, 40].

12.3.3 Effect of the Storage Medium on the Elution of Monomers

The release of monomers after polymerization is suggested to be influenced by the incomplete polymerization or additionally caused by the solvents in the oral cavity or the degradation of the materials after the initial polymerization. Regarding the chemical degradation of the composite materials in the oral cavity over time, this is thought to be caused by hydrolysis or enzymatic catalysis [58], through esterases from the human saliva.

The monomer elution is highly dependent on the hydrophobicity of the base monomers and the network characteristics of the resin matrix. Sorption and solubility of the dental composites are affected by factors like the hydrophilicity of the polymers and cross-linking density of the network [59]. Extraction media can be hydrophilic (e.g., physiological saline solution), hydrophobic (e.g., DMSO), or mixed (e.g., 75% ethanol and 25% water). Among the published studies, different media have been used in order to evaluate the elution of substances from composite materials: saliva or water in order to simulate the oral environment, culture media, and ethanol or acetone alone or in combination with saliva. Using ethanol, chloroform, or toluene as extraction medium can result in a high release of monomers [9]. The organic solutions can penetrate through the organic matrix easier than water, and therefore they can increase the elution of unreacted monomers [3]. It has been shown that the removal of leachable components from polymerized composites by the use of organic solvents drastically decreased cytotoxicity [9]. The effect of solvents on the composite materials in the oral cavity simulates some kind of erosion leading to weight loss of the polymer [60, 61]. It is mentioned that the solvent can penetrate the matrix, resulting in a change of the mass and the dimensions of the matrix. If the unreacted monomer is soluble in the solvent, it may be leached out of the polymer mass. Swelling and leaching both result from the process of diffusion. As the immersion solvent penetrates the matrix causing the opening between polymer chains, unreacted and leachable monomers may diffuse out [13]. Softening of the resin matrix allows the solvent to penetrate easier [60, 61] and might occur due to water sorption in wet oral environment, resulting in release of monomers. Water sorption can accelerate the degradation of dental composites [62, 63], influencing their physical and mechanical properties. First, the filler-resin matrix debonding is assumed [62], while after that the softening of dental resins through the plasticizing action of water occurs.

Food-simulated liquids have softening and hydrolyzing effects on dental composites which attribute to the degradation of the polymer matrix [39, 64, 65]. A lot of studies [13, 15, 16] have used ethanol 75% as extraction medium in order to simulate the clinical conditions in the oral cavity. Although ethanol 75% is thought to be a very aggressive medium, it is supposed by the Food and Drug Administration (FDA) of the USA to be a "food simulator and aging accelerator" [13]. An important factor that affects the release of monomers is the solubility parameters of the solvents. Weathering agents, such as ethanol, can accelerate the degradation of composite materials [66, 67]. Storage of composite samples in ethanol/water solution resulted in higher sorption values compared to artificial saliva and distilled water which both showed similar behavior [68]. Ethanol can penetrate easily into the resin matrix and therefore promote the release of substances. The highest solubility values of experimental composites were observed in ethanol 75%, while the solubility values in artificial saliva were a little higher than the ones found in distilled water [68]. Especially heavy monomers like UDMA and BisGMA are not able to be leached in aqueous media [69]. According to Ferracane [3], the oral environment is represented somewhere between the more aggressive organic solutions and water. Although a lot of media have been tested from time to time in order to evaluate the elution of monomers from composite materials, there is no systematic evaluation of them, which would make the comparison of the results of the different studies easier.

Besides ethanol 75%, by trying to evaluate clinically relevant media, artificial saliva, Dulbecco's Modified Medium (DMEM), and DMEM with 10% fetal bovine serum have been additionally investigated [70]. Although a higher release is usually observed in the case of ethanol 75%, TEGDMA as a small molecule can be eluted also in saliva and DMEM, suggesting that the solubility parameter of these solvents is very close to TEGDMA. Small molecules like TEGDMA have higher mobility and can elute faster than large molecules [11]. However, the elution of TEGDMA in DMEM 10% FCS solution is significantly lower than in saliva. TEGDMA seems to bind to albumin contained in serum resulting in different findings in the analytical process [69].

Authors have used methanol [10, 53] as extraction solvent in order to achieve a higher release of monomers. The extraction of photoinitiator (CQ), (co-)initiators, photostabilizers, and inhibitors took place in the case of methanol. Acetone was also used for evaluation of monomers' elution medium [45]. However, storing the samples for 7 days in acetone, which is a very aggressive medium, far away from the clinical conditions, resulted in a high elution of substances.

The oral cavity environment has an effect on the in vivo degradation of composite resins [71]. Human saliva presents the more clinically relevant medium in order to simulate the daily clinical conditions in oral cavity. Comparing human saliva to water and artificial saliva, the amount of monomers eluted is found to be lower when human saliva is used. Additionally the composition of human saliva might affect the elution rate [72]. Due to the presence of enzymes, human saliva seems to be more aggressive than the artificial one, being able to degrade the monomers of composite resins [18]. Components of human saliva (various salts and glycoproteins) have been suggested to bind comonomers of the composite materials [72]. Therefore it is assumed that using artificial saliva and water as extraction media, they do not represent the clinical situation in the oral cavity. The amount of small molecules like TEGDMA detected in human saliva was shown to be similar with the one released in ethanol 75% [16]. This correlation did not account for the larger molecules detected.

In order to evaluate the clinical relevance of the gained findings from studies using different storage media, the parameters used should be also taken into consideration, as they might influence the findings and generate correct or wrong assumptions for the dental composite restorations in the oral cavity. The preparation of the eluates presents an important parameter to affect the findings. Although there are instructions for the preparation of the eluates according to ISO 10993-12:2012 [73], most of the studies are performed under different conditions.

12.3.4 Methods for Analysis of the Eluted Monomers

Evaluating the available data in the literature, it is obvious that several different methods have been used from time to time in order to identify and quantify the eluted substances. Although all the available methods are thought to be able to determine the eluted substances, there is a big difference among them concerning their ability to identify unknown substances, to identify substances with high molecular weight (MW), to give the exact MW and amount of the identified substances, and, in the case of by-products or degradation products, to be able to differentiate the substance from which the identified substances came from.

The qualitative and quantitative methods for the analysis of the monomers and degradation products include gas chromatography (GC), high-performance liquid chromatography (HPLC) [7, 20, 74–77], gas chromatography/mass spectrometry [5, 10, 78], and electrospray ionization/mass spectrometry [6, 20].

HPLC analysis is usually preferred to gas chromatography, because it gives a greater level of control over the separation process in this case since the monomers are soluble in the mobile phase. Gas chromatography (GC) is usually used for detection of small molecules. Bulky matrix monomers can be identified by GC only in the case of combining it with mass spectrometry (MS) as GC/MS detects substances by their decomposition products and fragmentation pattern [10, 79], and therefore it is not suitable for analyzing molecules with high molecular weight [80]. Large base monomers, like UDMA, decompose in GC. The proposed analytical methods used in HPLC techniques may vary between the different studies, due to the conditions established for determination of residual monomers. Although most of the studies have used HPLC as a tool to investigate the elution of monomers from the composite resin materials, it has been pointed out [79] that this method alone is not appropriate.

Several parameters involved in the analytical procedure influence the findings of each study, starting from the selection of the substances that are used as external references in order to be able to qualify and quantify the eluted monomers [81]. In the case of HPLC, these pure components are necessary for the identification and quantification of the eluted components. However, as has been reported [79] when HPLC was used alone as analytical method, it has some disadvantages as it is not suitable to give an exact identification of the substances eluted and the references used. In detail, during the analysis of the eluted substances with HPLC alone, the reference standards of the monomers that are expected to be eluted are needed for two purposes: The first is in order to be able to determine the amount of the detected substances through the use of the calibration standard curves of peak areas versus monomer concentration of each substance. A linear curve for each monomer is necessary at known concentrations. Secondly, the chromatogram of each reference substance is of importance in order to determine the mass(es) and the peaks (and their retention time) that are characteristic for each monomer. This step is very important as different peaks for different masses might be present for one monomer by its chromatogram. Usually in most of the published data, it is mentioned that the MW of each expected substance is used for the qualification process. The mass that should be used for the detection of the expected molecule is not necessary the one represented with the higher peak, and in order to be able to give adequate results, it might be necessary to use different peaks for qualification and quantification

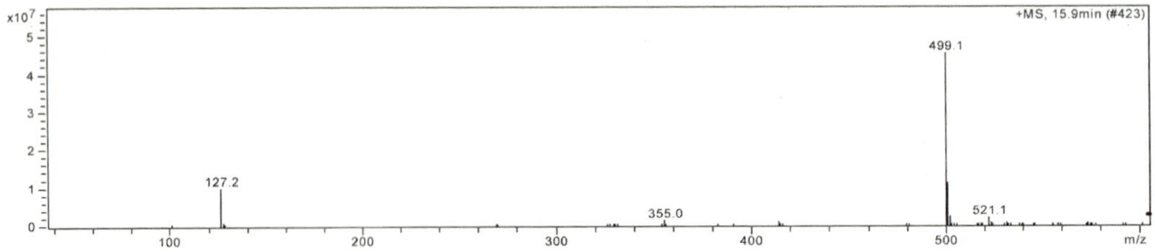

Fig. 12.4 Identification of substances with HPLC-MS/MS. Here is a given example of the spectrum of one form of UDMA using HPLC-MS/MS (*Polydorou O, König A, Hellwig E, Kümmerer K. Urethane dimethacrylate: a molecule that may cause confusion in dental research. J Biomed Mater Res B Appl Biomater. 2009 Oct;91(1):1–4. doi:10.1002/jbm.b.31383*)

processes. Additionally, due to the analysis of the reference standards, it is possible to evaluate the stability of respective substances and therefore explain some findings wherein some eluted substances might be unstable after their elution or they might also react with other eluted substances resulting in by-products. In all these cases, the use of HPLC alone to the analytical progress is not adequate to identify all eluted substances. With this method and a very good and appropriate use of the reference standards, it is possible to evaluate only the elution of expected substances. A combination of HPLC with mass spectrometry (LC-MS or LC-MS/MS) (Fig. 12.4) can be used in these cases for a highly specific and accurate identification of the compounds eluted [26, 79, 82]. This method is a very sensitive method being able to identify additional substances to the ones used as references. A mass scanning of the reference standards and the samples prepared for the analysis can give important information about by-products, degradation products, or the possible reaction of eluted substances. In a recent study of Schulz et al. [25], the authors could show that eluted substances can react with each other when they are in the same solution. After mixing three basic monomers, an additional high peak of a molecule with higher mass and lower polarity than the basic monomers was detected (Figs. 12.5 and 12.6) suggesting that some kind of interaction has taken place among the eluted monomers of the composite materials causing difficulties during the analysis process. This can be avoided by selecting the appropriate analytical method and careful performance of the analysis. An additional challenge for the analytical methods is the decomposing of molecules like UDMA. It can decompose to HEMA, affecting the analytic findings if the appropriate method is not used [22].

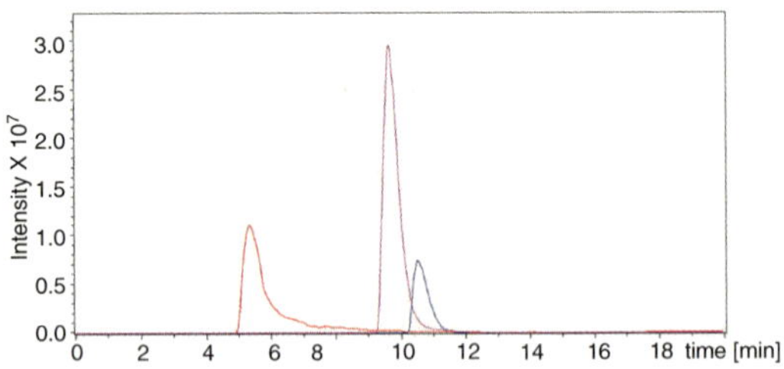

Fig. 12.5 Retention time of three standards: [BisGMA (*1*), TEGDMA (*2*), and UDMA (*3*)] (Simon Daniel Schulz, Tobias Laquai, Klaus Kümmerer, Richard Bolek, Volker Mersch-Sundermann, and Olga Polydorou, "Elution of Monomers from Provisional Composite Materials," International Journal of Polymer Science, vol. 2015, ArticleID617407,7pages,2015.doi:10.1155/2015/617407)

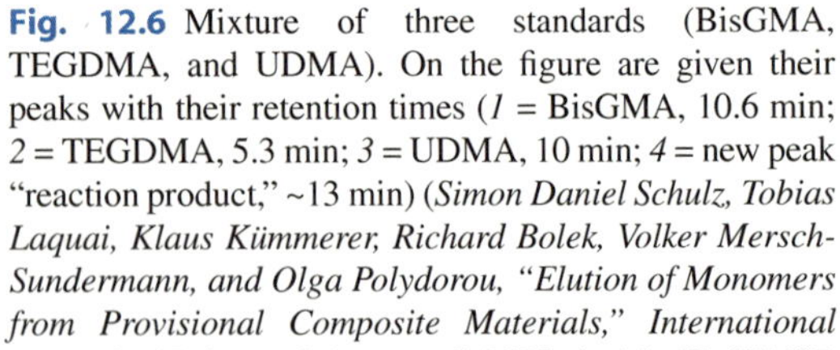

Fig. 12.6 Mixture of three standards (BisGMA, TEGDMA, and UDMA). On the figure are given their peaks with their retention times (*1* = BisGMA, 10.6 min; *2* = TEGDMA, 5.3 min; *3* = UDMA, 10 min; *4* = new peak "reaction product," ~13 min) (*Simon Daniel Schulz, Tobias Laquai, Klaus Kümmerer, Richard Bolek, Volker Mersch-Sundermann, and Olga Polydorou, "Elution of Monomers from Provisional Composite Materials," International Journal of Polymer Science, vol. 2015, Article ID 617407, 7 pages, 2015. doi:10.1155/2015/617407*)

In addition, the selection of the substances needed as references in a study is an important parameter that can influence the findings, as this might result in misleading findings. The selection of the pure chemicals as reference standards gained by the chemical industry is commonly done when planning a study as these are supposed to be used for the manufacturing of the composite materials. However, not all companies use the pure monomers for manufacturing dental composites, but some modifications might take place before their use, resulting in substances with differences in MW and altered chemical structure compared to the original ones. The use of the original monomers taken from the chemical industry as reference standards in analytical studies results in failed detection of eluted substances when modified monomers are contained in the materials that are under examination. Additional confusion is caused by the fact that usually these modified substances continue to be labeled like the original monomer. Appropriate evaluation of the composition of the examined composite materials is necessary in order to be able to give adequate and correct findings. The ideal situation is the use of monomers given by the company manufacturing the composite materials that are under evaluation.

Additional attempts have been made to improve the analytical methods for better detection. High-temperature GC (HT-GC) in combination with MS has also been suggested [35] to detect BisEMA homologues in the eluates of composite materials. The use of the high-temperature columns, which can be heated up to 400 °C, was suggested to be able to vaporize the low volatile BisEMA homologues. However, the difficulties of using the appropriate reference standards remained as limitation. The use of ultra UHPLC in combination with tandem MS detector as suggested in new studies appears to be an adequate sensitive method to analyze the eluted substances [83, 84] in different extraction solvents like ethanol, water, and artificial saliva.

Summarizing the data in the literature, the combination of HPLC-MS/MS presents at the moment the most accurate method of performing precise analysis of the eluted substances, under the condition that appropriate reference materials have been used and a clinical relevant preparation of the samples has taken place. Actual data are promising for a more standardized qualification in the near future.

12.4 Elution of Bisphenol A from Dental Composite Materials

Bisphenol A (BPA) is the common name for 2,2-bis(4-hydroxyphenyl)propane. It is an organic compound, produced by the reaction of two phenols with one acetone catalyzed by a cation exchange resin. BPA is a xeno-estrogen, a known endocrine disruptor showing similar estrogenic activity like the normal estrogens after binding to human estrogenic receptors. BPA and its release from dental composite materials are widely discussed in literature. The discussion and concern about BPA have been induced due to one of the first reports [85] evidencing the release of BPA from dental materials under different circumstances and commenting the possible estrogenicity of dental composite and sealants. This report has been discussed and commented widely up to date concerning the method and the conditions used in the study, like the hydrolysis in alkaline ($pH = 13$) and acid media ($pH = 1$) after heating to 100 °C for 30 min.

Several studies have been performed concerning the possible implications of BPA on human health [86–89]. BPA has been shown to have estrogenic activity even at concentration lower than 1 μg/m^3 [90]. Recently the European Food Safety Authority (EFSA) has lowered the tolerable daily intake (TDI) from 50 μg/kg/bw/day (microgram/kilogram/(body weight/day) to 4 μg/kg/bw/day [91].

BPA is used in the manufacturing process for polycarbonate plastic products, food packaging, as inner coating of many food cans, and is also used for synthetization of monomers like BisGMA and BisEMA used in composite materials. The main exposure of the population is definitely through the plastics and food packaging.

Among the published data in the literature, the findings concerning the release of BPA from dental

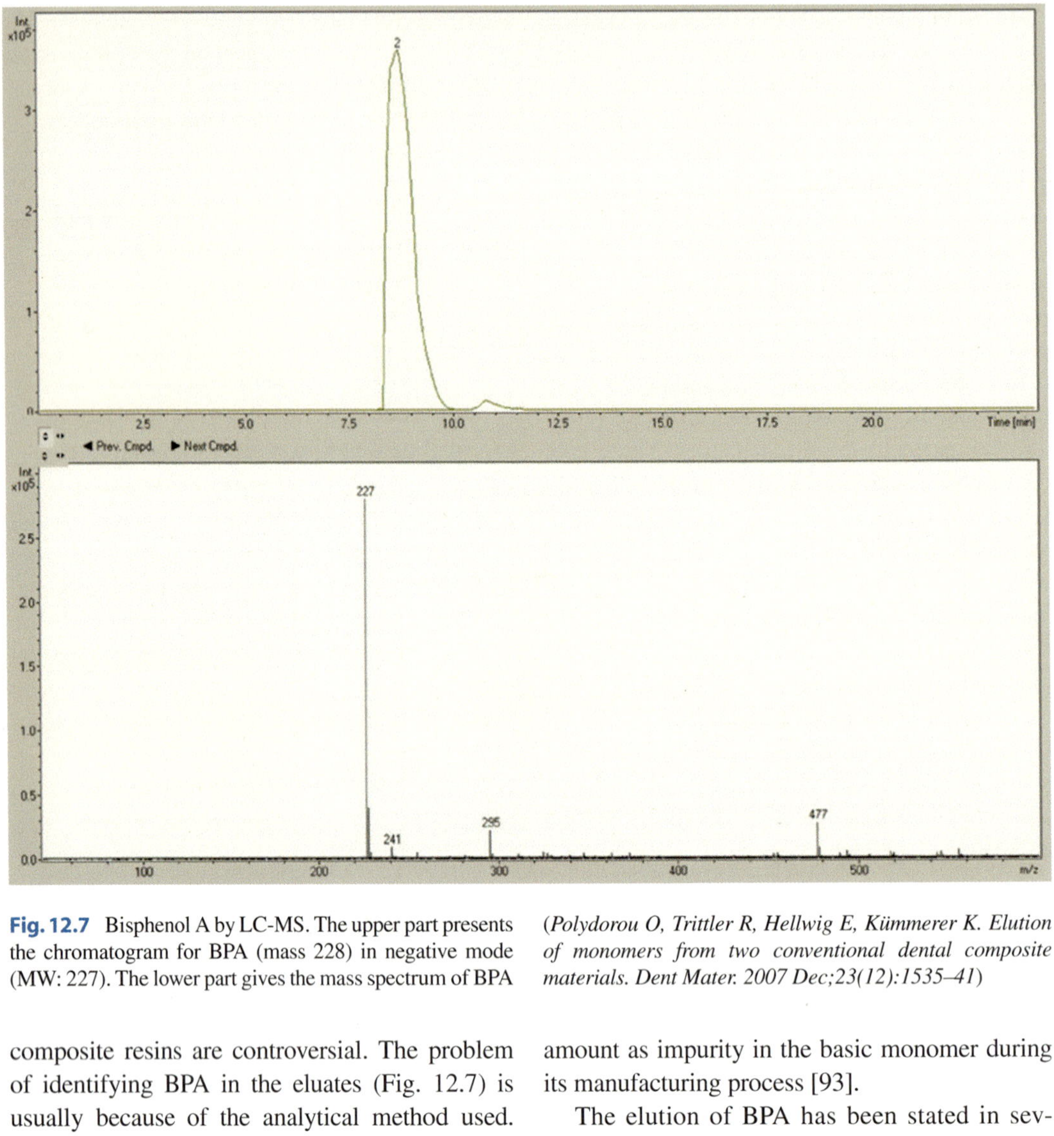

Fig. 12.7 Bisphenol A by LC-MS. The upper part presents the chromatogram for BPA (mass 228) in negative mode (MW: 227). The lower part gives the mass spectrum of BPA (*Polydorou O, Trittler R, Hellwig E, Kümmerer K. Elution of monomers from two conventional dental composite materials. Dent Mater. 2007 Dec;23(12):1535–41*)

composite resins are controversial. The problem of identifying BPA in the eluates (Fig. 12.7) is usually because of the analytical method used. A very sensitive precise method with very low qualification/quantification limit is necessary as in the case that BPA is eluted, it will happen in very small amounts. Due to the different methods used, it happens very often that different findings are mentioned for the same composite materials causing confusion on this serious subject of BPA. The release of BPA from composite materials was thought to be due to these monomers, and a possible degradation of them was assumed. However, this is not totally accepted as the degradation of these monomers is not really documented [92]. Another suggestion was that the eluted BPA from composite materials comes through residual amount as impurity in the basic monomer during its manufacturing process [93].

The elution of BPA has been stated in several studies [16, 26, 70, 94, 95]. Mainly this release was shown in ethanol 75%. The released amount of BPA was material dependent, and in most cases, the maximum amount was after 7 days of storage [26, 94], while a longer release up to 28 days after polymerization has been also mentioned [95]. As far as the importance of the eluted amount is concerned, it is suggested [2] that the released amount of BPA in a period of 24 h is probably important in the case of several large fillings in the oral cavity. However, the present studies [2, 26] mention that the detected amount of BPA in composite materials' eluates is lower than the tolerable daily intake determined by EFSA assuming that these are safe for the human health.

Interesting is the finding of Yin et al. [96], who evaluated the associations of blood mercury, inorganic mercury, methyl mercury, and BPA with dental restoration in US population. Significant decreases were found in urinary BPA for both evaluated periods 2003–2004 and 2011–2012, especially for individuals under the age of 12 years. This signalizes the efforts to reduce the BPA exposure over the last years. No significant association was found between urinary BPA and dental surface restorations. Based on their findings, the authors suggested that the use of composite materials for dental restorations does not have any effect on the long-term urinary amount of BPA. Other daily used products should be reconsidered as the sources for the BPA exposure. However, no information exist up to date concerning the short-term effect of BPA on human health directly after the application of the filling material as other published data reveal a significant increase in the urinary or salivary BPA in short time after the filling application [97, 98]. Further research is necessary in order to be able to evaluate the estrogenic potential of the composite materials' eluates, under the consideration that BPA is a substance that has been shown to exert effects by low-dose exposure. Development of materials free of substances with estrogenic potential should be considered.

12.5 Elution of Particles from Composite Materials

Besides the elution of monomers, the solubility of filler particles containing zinc, barium, strontium, silicon, boron, and sodium in aqueous solutions was also reported [99, 100]. In 1990 [101], it was reported that leaching of silica and barium did not decrease in the evaluation time period of 6 months. It was suggested that among other filler compositions, the filler content and the filler treatment might influence the amount of eluted substances [101].

During the development of composite materials, in the area of filler particles, much effort has been made in order to produce new composite materials with better properties. Although the use of nanoparticles in composite materials is not new, their use was extended over the past years, using also ceramic nanofiller resins in order to improve their physical/mechanical properties developing materials with better esthetics, better surface properties, and increased strength and durability.

Although the use and incorporation of nanoparticles/fillers in the composite materials seems to improve their properties having better clinical performance, the nanoscale size has the potential to alter physicochemical properties from the bulk form of any substance [102]. The size of the filler particles contained varies among the different categories of composite materials however; a lot of modern composite materials contain nanosized particles. Modern composites might contain high amounts of nanoparticles (<100 nm). Although modern composite materials nowadays contain radio-opaque glass fillers (with elements like barium, zirconium, strontium, or ytterbium) which are larger than 0.4–1 μm, they additionally contain smaller particles (<100 nm) in order to improve the properties of the materials. Only few data exist in the literature concerning the release of particles, especially nanoparticles, from dental composite materials, as it might take place during the abrasive procedures like cutting, shaping, finishing, or also removing of composite restorations.

In the past years, the possible health risks by using nanoparticles have been widely discussed. Usually particles under 100 nm are thought to present a risk for human health [103–105]; however, it must be taken into consideration that particles up to 300 nm exhibit nanospecific properties and should be treated as nanoparticles. Additionally, nanoparticles might build agglomerates and/or aggregates (>100 nm) which have reactive single particles on their surface [106]. Nanoparticles with a diameter of 50 nm, for example, are able to penetrate the cell membrane [107] increasing the considerations for their possible negative health impacts. Although inhalation of silica might take place by dental personnel, the size of the considered particles is thought to be larger than the dangerous size [108]. A recent perspective about the toxicity of nanomaterials claims that there is actually up to date no evidence that nanomaterials exhibit novel toxic mechanisms [109, 110], and similar conventional particles should be evaluated as far as their toxicology is concerned [109, 110].

Van Landuyt et al. [111] evaluated the release of "dust" from composite materials. Under standardized in vitro conditions to simulate the worst case clinical situations, the authors could detect micro-particles (<1 μm) and nanoparticles (<100 nm), suggesting that without water cooling, dust inhalation might be hazardous for the human health. The detected amount of the submicron particles differed among the composite materials. The same authors in another study [112] with more clinically relevant conditions were able to identify high concentrations of nanoparticles (<100 nm) to be set free in the air after grinding composite materials with dental burs. Although the present literature data are very scarce, they indicate that the dental procedures might result in increased release of nanoparticles which can be inhaled. The use of water cooling during composite grinding, finishing, and polishing might release this potential. However, no data exist up to date about the toxicological potential of such particles.

12.5.1 Methods to Evaluate the Release of Particles from Composite Materials

By evaluating the release of particles from dental composite materials, the determination of their size is of great importance, but besides this, their identification plays an important role in order to be able to certify their possible impact on human health.

In literature, the most suggested methods for the analysis of nanoparticles are the nanoparticle tracking analysis (NTA), dynamic light scattering (DLS), scanning electron microscopy (SEM), size exclusion chromatography (SEC), gel electrophoresis, asymmetrical flow field-flow fractionation (AF4), and analytical ultracentrifugation (AUC) [113–116]. DLS is a powerful and accessible tool and has become the preferred technique to routinely determine the size of nanoparticles. It has the advantage to detect small amounts of large particles. NTA is an innovative technique for sizing particles from about 30 to 1000 nm, with the lower detection limit being dependent on the refractive index of the nanoparticles, being able to identify and track individual nanoparticles moving under Brownian motion and relate the movement to a particle size [113]. Besides this, a scanning mobility particle sizer (SMPS) was suggested for measuring submicron particle distributions in combination with an electrostatic precipitator (ESP) for electron microscopic characterization [112]. The chemical analysis of the released particles can be performed by SEM and electron dispersive X-ray (EDX).

12.6 Conclusions and Future Perspectives

Taken into consideration the data in the literature, it is to assume that composite materials release respective amounts of monomers over time, stating this way a potential risk for human health, in the case that the detected amounts of eluted substances would represent the real clinical situation. Even if the in vitro studies are performed in respect of the clinical circumstances, they are not able to imitate the in vivo situation representing usually the worst case scenarios. Great differences exist in the sample preparation among studies. Using thin layers of composite materials like 1 mm definitely influences their polymerization degree and the elution of substances. Not only the thickness but also the diameter of the composite samples can affect clearly these properties. Diameter of samples larger than the tip of the polymerization unit will definitely negatively affect the elution of monomers. Although the information gained from these studies is worth full presenting an important screening of the potential release of monomers from the available composite materials, it is not clearly proven up to date that the eluted amounts can generally cause detrimental effects on human health. A direct correlation of the detected amounts of substances with the biological reactions caused is of great importance. The present data give some evidence of possible effects on human respective cell cultures however; the interpretation of these data in the in vivo situation needs further investigation. Of importance is the presence of BPA in the eluates of composite materials, as this substance exerts biological effects after low-dose exposure. Further research in this area is necessary concerning the uptake of BPA of composite materials and the factors that can influence it in addition to the evaluation of the estrogenic potential of the composite eluates in order to be able to develop appropriate materials.

Summarizing the data cornering the parameters that can influence the monomers' release, the composition and the chemistry of the composite are the most important parameters. Factors like the degree of conversion; curing times, curing modes, and curing units; and also handling modes of the restorative materials seem to be important, being able to improve in some cases the performance of the applied materials; however, they seem not the ones that can regulate the elution of monomers. In addition to these, it has to be mentioned that it is not possible to generalize the findings of the composite materials evaluated in the literature for all composite materials existing nowadays, as due to the rapid development in material science, modern restorative materials with improved properties and chemistry are available nowadays which have been shown to be beneficial concerning the monomers' release. Systematic and standardized screening of modern materials is always necessary in order to be able to estimate their real potential risk.

Besides monomer elution, scarce literature data reveal a release of nanoscale particles from composite materials through grinding and cutting procedures, independently of their composition. Although particles in this size are thought to exert biological effects, parameter size solely is not the one determining the potential effects, as the characterization of the particles is of great importance. Clinical relevant risk assessment of the released particles should be addressed before the composite materials are accused of having detrimental effects on patients and dental practitioners.

The release of monomers and nanoparticles is not only of great importance in respect of the oral cavity and their effects directly on human individuals, but additionally the environmental aspects should be taken strongly into consideration.

The potential environmental pollution through restorative materials is beyond amalgam. The release of BPA and nanoparticles in the wastewater through dental daily clinical procedures will probably become a topic in the future, and it would be in interest of all to act earlier preventing additional environmental pollution.

References

1. Goldberg M. In vitro and in vivo studies on the toxicity of dental resin components: a review. Clin Oral Investig. 2008;12:1–8. Review.
2. Van Landuyt KL, Nawrot T, Geebelen B, De Munck J, Snauwaert J, Yoshihara K, Scheers H, Godderis L, Hoet P, Van Meerbeek B. How much do resin-based dental materials release? A meta-analytical approach. Dent Mater. 2011;27:723–47.
3. Ferracane JL. Elution of leachable components from composites. J Oral Rehabil. 1994;21:441–52.
4. Komurcuoglu E, Olmez S, Vural N. Evaluation of residual monomer elimination methods in three different fissure sealants in vitro. J Oral Rehabil. 2005;32:116–21.
5. Lee SY, Greener EH, Menis DL. Detection of leached moieties from dental composites in fluids stimulating food and saliva. Dent Mater. 1995;11:348–53.
6. Mazzaoui SA, Burrow MF, Tyas MJ, Rooney FR, Capon RJ. Long-term quantification of the release of monomers from dental resin composites and a resin-modified glass ionomer cement. J Biomed Mater Res. 2002;63:299–305.
7. Pelka M, Distler W, Petschelt A. Elution parameters and HPLC-detection of single components from resin composite. Clin Oral Investig. 1999;3:194–200.
8. Pulgar R, Olea-Serrano MF, Novillo-Fertrell A, Rivas A, Pazos P, Pedraza V, Navajas JM, Olea N. Determination of Bisphenol A and related aromatic released from Bis-GMA-based composites and sealants by high performance liquid chromatography. Environ Health Perspect. 2000;108:21–7.
9. Rathbun MA, Craig RG, Hanks CT, Filisko FE. Cytotoxicity of a BIS-GMA dental composite before and after leaching in organic solvents. J Biomed Mater Res. 1991;25:443–57.
10. Spahl W, Budzikiewicz H, Geurtsen W. Determination of leachable components from four commercial dental composites by gas and liquid chromatography/mass spectrometry. J Dent. 1998;26:137–45.

11. Tanaka K, Taira M, Shintani H, Wakasa K, Yamaki M. Residual monomers (TEGDMA and Bis-GMA) of a set visible-light-cured dental composite resin when immersed in water. J Oral Rehabil. 1991;18:353–62.
12. Al-Hiyasat AS, Darmani H, Elbetieha AM. Leached components from dental composites and their effects on fertility of female mice. Eur J Oral Sci. 2004;112:267–72.
13. Sideridou ID, Achilias DS. Elution study of unreacted Bis-GMA, TEGDMA, UDMA, and Bis-EMA from light-cured dental resins and resin composites using HPLC. J Biomed Mater Res B Appl Biomater. 2005;74:617–26.
14. Ferracane JL, Condon JR. Rate of elution of leachable components from composite. Dent Mater. 1990;6:282–7.
15. Polydorou O, König A, Hellwig E, Kümmerer K. Long-term release of monomers from modern dental-composite materials. Eur J Oral Sci. 2009;117:68–75.
16. Polydorou O, Huberty C, Wolkewitz M, Bolek R, Hellwig E, Kümmerer K. The effect of storage medium on the elution of monomers from composite materials. J Biomed Mater Res B Appl Biomater. 2012;100:68–74.
17. Polydorou O, Hammad M, König A, Hellwig E, Kümmerer K. Release of monomers from different core build-up materials. Dent Mater. 2009;25:1090–5.
18. Tabatabaee MH, Mahdavi H, Zandi S, Kharrazi MJ. HPLC analysis of eluted monomers from two composite resins cured with LED and halogen curing lights. J Biomed Mater Res B Appl Biomater. 2009;88:191–6.
19. Tabatabaei MH, Sadrai S, Bassir SH, Veisy N, Dehghan S. Effect of food stimulated liquids and thermocycling on the monomer elution from a nanofilled composite. Open Dent J. 2013;7:62–7.
20. Sideridou I, Tserki V, Papanastasiou G. Effect of chemical structure on degree of conversion in light-cured dimethacrylate-based dental resins. Biomaterials. 2002;23:1819–29.
21. Rothmund L, Reichl FX, Hickel R, Styllou P, Styllou M, Kehe K, Yang Y, Högg C. Effect of layer thickness on the elution of bulk-fill composite components. Dent Mater. 2017;33:54–62.
22. Michelsen VB, Moe G, Skålevik R, Jensen E, Lygre H. Quantification of organic eluates from polymerized resin-based dental restorative materials by use of GC/MS. J Chromatogr B Analyt Technol Biomed Life Sci. 2007;850:83–91.
23. Ortengren U, Langer S, Göransson A, Lundgren T. Influence of pH and time on organic substance release from a model dental composite: a fluorescence spectrophotometry and gas chromatography/mass spectrometry analysis. Eur J Oral Sci. 2004;112:530–7.
24. Yap AU, Lee HK, Sabapathy R. Release of methacrylic acid from dental composites. Dent Mater. 2000;16:172–9.
25. Schulz SD, Laquai T, Kümmerer K, Bolek R, Mersch-Sundermann V, Polydorou O. Elution of monomers from provisional composite materials. Int J Polym Sci. 2015;2015:617407.
26. Pongprueksa P, De Munck J, Duca RC, Poels K, Covaci A, Hoet P, Godderis L, Van Meerbeek B, Van Landuyt KL. Monomer elution in relation to degree of conversion for different types of composite. J Dent. 2015;43:1448–55.
27. Manojlovic D, Radisic M, Vasiljevic T, Zivkovic S, Lausevic M, Miletic V. Monomer elution from nanohybrid and ormocer-based composites cured with different light sources. Dent Mater. 2011;27:371–8.
28. Ruyter IE, Svendsen SA. Remaining methacrylate groups in composite restorative materials. Acta Odontol Scand. 1978;36:75–82.
29. Ruyter E. Composite dental filling materials. Tandlakartidningen. 1984;76:1207–10.
30. Ruyter IE, Oysaed H. Composites for use in posterior teeth: composition and conversion. J Biomed Mater Res. 1987;21:11–23.
31. Chung K, Greener EH. Degree of conversion of seven visible light-cured posterior composites. J Oral Rehabil. 1988;15:555–60.
32. Eliades GC, Vougiouklakis GJ, Caputo AA. Degree of double bond conversion in light-cured composites. Dent Mater. 1987;3:19–25.
33. Ferracane JL, Greener EH. The effect of resin formulation on the degree of conversion and mechanical properties of dental restorative resins. J Biomed Mater Res. 1986;20:121–31.
34. Lempel E, Czibulya Z, Kovács B, Szalma J, Tóth Á, Kunsági-Máté S, Varga Z, Böddi K Degree of conversion and BisGMA, TEGDMA, UDMA elution from Flowable bulk fill composites. Int J Mol Sci. 2016;17:pii:E732.
35. Durner J, Obermaier J, Draenert M, Ilie N. Correlation of the degree of conversion with the amount of elutable substances in nano-hybrid dental composites. Dent Mater. 2012;28:1146–53.
36. Pongprueksa P, Miletic V, Janssens H, Van Landuyt KL, De Munck J, Godderis L, Van Meerbeek B. Degree of conversion and monomer elution of CQ/amine and TPO adhesives. Dent Mater. 2014;30:695–701.
37. Randolph LD, Palin WM, Bebelman S, Devaux J, Gallez B, Leloup G, Leprince JG. Ultra-fast light-curing resin composite with increased conversion and reduced monomer elution. Dent Mater. 2014;30:594–604.
38. Al-Ahdal K, Ilie N, Silikas N, Watts DC. Polymerization kinetics and impact of post polymerization on the degree of conversion of bulk-fill resin-composite at clinically relevant depth. Dent Mater. 2015;31:1207–13.
39. Yap AU, Wong NY, Siow KS. Composite cure and shrinkage associated with high intensity curing light. Oper Dent. 2003;28:357–64.
40. Christensen RP, Palmer TM, Ploeger BJ, Yost MP. Resin polymerization problems–are they caused by resin cur-

ing lights, resin formulations, or both? Compend Contin Educ Dent Suppl. 1999; (25):S42–54; quiz S74.
41. Susila AV, Balasubramanian V. Correlation of elution and sensitivity of cell lines to dental composites. Dent Mater. 2016;32:e63–72.
42. Alshali RZ, Salim NA, Sung R, Satterthwaite JD, Silikas N. Analysis of long-term monomer elution from bulk-fill and conventional resin-composites using high performance liquid chromatography. Dent Mater. 2015;31:1587–98.
43. Cebe MA, Cebe F, Cengiz MF, Cetin AR, Arpag OF, Ozturk B. Elution of monomer from different bulk fill dental composite resins. Dent Mater. 2015;31: e141–9.
44. Nomoto R, Hirasawa T. Residual monomer and pendant methacryloyl group in light-cured composite resins. Dent Mater J. 1992;11:177–88.
45. Johnsen GF, Thieu MK, Hussain B, Pamuła E, Reseland JE, Lyngstadaas SP, Haugen H. Own brand label restorative materials-a false bargain? J Dent. 2017;56:84–98.
46. Moon HJ, Lee YK, Lim BS, Kim CW. Effects of various light curing methods on the leachability of uncured substances and hardness of a composite resin. J Oral Rehabil. 2004;31:258–64.
47. Benetti AR, Asmussen E, Munksgaard EC, Dewaele M, Peutzfeldt A, Leloup G, Devaux J. Softening and elution of monomers in ethanol. Dent Mater. 2009;25:1007–13.
48. Hofmann N, Markert T, Hugo B, Klaiber B. Effect of high intensity vs. soft-start halogen irradiation on light-cured resin-based composites. Part II: hardness and solubility. Am J Dent. 2004;17:38–42.
49. Hofmann N, Renner J, Hugo B, Klaiber B. Elution of leachable components from resin composites after plasma arc vs standard or soft-start halogen light irradiation. J Dent. 2002;30:223–32.
50. Kim JG, Chung CM. Elution from light-cured dental composites: comparison of trimethacrylate and dimethacrylate as base monomers. J Biomed Mater Res B Appl Biomater. 2005;72:328–33.
51. Pearson GJ, Longman CM. Water sorption and solubility of resin-based materials following inadequate polymerization by a visible-light curing system. J Oral Rehabil. 1989;16:57–61.
52. Polydorou O, Trittler R, Hellwig E, Kümmerer K. Elution of monomers from two conventional dental composite materials. Dent Mater. 2007;23:1535–41.
53. Högg C, Maier M, Dettinger-Maier K, He X, Rothmund L, Kehe K, Hickel R, Reichl FX. Effect of various light curing times on the elution of composite components. Clin Oral Investig. 2016;20:2113–21.
54. Durner J, Schrickel K, Watts DC, Ilie N. Determination of homologous distributions of bisEMA dimethacrylates in bulk-fill resin-composites by GC-MS. Dent Mater. 2015;31:473–80.
55. Sajnani AR, Hegde MN. Leaching of monomers from bulk-fill composites: an in vitro study. J Conserv Dent. 2016;19:482–6.
56. Nalçaci A, Ulusoy N, Atakol O. Time-based elution of TEGDMA and BisGMA from resin composite cured with LED, QTH and high-intensity QTH lights. Oper Dent. 2006;31:197–203.
57. Polydorou O, König A, Altenburger MJ, Wolkewitz M, Hellwig E, Kümmerer K. Release of monomers from four different composite materials after halogen and LED curing. Am J Dent. 2011;24:315–21.
58. Göpferich A. Mechanisms of polymer degradation and erosion. Biomaterials. 1996;17:103–14. Review.
59. Lee SY, Huang HM, Lin CY, Shih YH. Leached components from dental composites in oral simulating fluids and the resultant composite strengths. J Oral Rehabil. 1998;25:575–88.
60. Finer Y, Santerre JP. Salivary esterase activity and its association with the biodegradation of dental composites. J Dent Res. 2004;83:22–6.
61. Finer Y, Jaffer F, Santerre JP. Mutual influence of cholesterol esterase and pseudocholinesterase on the biodegradation of dental composites. Biomaterials. 2004;25:1787–93.
62. Toledano M, Osorio R, Osorio E, Fuentes V, Prati C, Garcia-Godoy F. Sorption and solubility of resin-based restorative dental materials. J Dent. 2003 Jan;31(1):43–50.
63. Ortengren U, Wellendorf H, Karlsson S, Ruyter IE. Water sorption and solubility of dental composites and identification of monomers released in an aqueous environment. J Oral Rehabil. 2001;28: 1106–15.
64. Asmussen E. Softening of BISGMA-based polymers by ethanol and by organic acids of plaque. Scand J Dent Res. 1984;92:257–61.
65. Lee SY, Greener EH, Mueller HJ, Chiu CH. Effect of food and oral simulating fluids on dentine bond and composite strength. J Dent. 1994;22:352–9.
66. McKinney JE, Wu W. Chemical softening and wear of dental composites. J Dent Res. 1985;64:1326–31.
67. Wu W, McKinney JE. Influence of chemicals on wear of dental composites. J Dent Res. 1982;61:1180–3.
68. Zhang Y, Xu J. Effect of immersion in various media on the sorption, solubility, elution of unreacted monomers, and flexural properties of two model dental composite compositions. J Mater Sci Mater Med. 2008;19:2477–83.
69. Moharamzadeh K, Van Noort R, Brook IM, Scutt AM. HPLC analysis of components released from dental composites with different resin compositions using different extraction media. J Mater Sci Mater Med. 2007;18:133–7.
70. Tsitrou E, Kelogrigoris S, Koulaouzidou E, Antoniades-Halvatjoglou M, Koliniotou-Koumpia E, van Noort R. Effect of extraction media and storage time on the elution of monomers from four contemporary resin composite materials. Toxicol Int. 2014;21:89–95.
71. Akova T, Ozkomur A, Aytutuldu N, Toroglu MS. The effect of food simulants on porcelain-composite bonding. Dent Mater. 2007;23:1369–72.

72. Rothmund L, Shehata M, Van Landuyt KL, Schweikl H, Carell T, Geurtsen W, Hellwig E, Hickel R, Reichl FX, Högg C. Release and protein binding of components from resin based composites in native saliva and other extraction media. Dent Mater. 2015;31:496–504.
73. ISO 10993-12:2012. Biological evaluation of medical devices – Part 12: Sample preparation and reference materials.
74. Bagis YH, Rueggeberg FA. The effect of post-cure heating on residual, unreacted monomer in a commercial resin composite. Dent Mater. 2000;16:244–7.
75. Munksgaard EC, Peutzfeldt A, Asmussen E. Elution of TEGDMA and BisGMA from a resin and a resin composite cured with halogen or plasma light. Eur J Oral Sci. 2000;108:341–5.
76. Noda M, Komatsu H, Sano H. HPLC analysis of dental resin composites components. J Biomed Mater Res. 1999;47:374–8.
77. Viljanen EK, Langer S, Skrifvars M, Vallittu PK. Analysis of residual monomers in dendritic methacrylate copolymers and composites by HPLC and headspace-GC/MS. Dent Mater. 2006;22:845–51.
78. Michelsen VB, Lygre H, Skålevik R, Tveit AB, Solheim E. Identification of organic eluates from four polymer-based dental filling materials. Eur J Oral Sci. 2003;111:263–71.
79. Geurtsen W. Substances released from dental resin composites and glass ionomer cements. Eur J Oral Sci. 1998;106:687–95. Review.
80. Michelsen VB, Kopperud HB, Lygre GB, Björkman L, Jensen E, Kleven IS, Svahn J, Lygre H. Detection and quantification of monomers in unstimulated whole saliva after treatment with resin-based composite fillings in vivo. Eur J Oral Sci. 2012;120:89–95.
81. Polydorou O, König A, Hellwig E, Kümmerer K. Urethane dimethacrylate: a molecule that may cause confusion in dental research. J Biomed Mater Res B Appl Biomater. 2009;91:1–4.
82. Jaffer F, Finer Y, Santerre JP. Interactions between resin monomers and commercial composite resins with human saliva derived esterases. Biomaterials. 2002;23:1707–19.
83. Cokic SM, Duca RC, Godderis L, Hoet PH, Seo JW, Van Meerbeek B, Van Landuyt KL. Release of monomers from composite dust. J Dent. 2017;60:56–62.
84. Putzeys E, Cokic SM, Chong H, Smet M, Vanoirbeek J, Godderis L, Van Meerbeek B, Van Landuyt KL, Duca RC. Simultaneous analysis of bisphenol A based compounds and other monomers leaching from resin-based dental materials by UHPLC-MS/MS. J Sep Sci. 2017;40:1063–75.
85. Olea N, Pulgar R, Pérez P, Olea-Serrano F, Rivas A, Novillo-Fertrell A, Pedraza V, Soto AM, Sonnenschein C. Estrogenicity of resin-based composites and sealants used in dentistry. Environ Health Perspect. 1996;104:298–305.
86. Kawai K, Murakami S, Senba E, Yamanaka T, Fujiwara Y, Arimura C, Nozaki T, Takii M, Kubo C. Changes in estrogen receptors alpha and beta expression in the brain of mice exposed prenatally to bisphenol A. Regul Toxicol Pharmacol. 2007;47:166–70.
87. Susiarjo M, Hassold TJ, Freeman E, Hunt PA. Bisphenol A exposure in utero disrupts early oogenesis in the mouse. PLoS Genet. 2007;3:e5.
88. Barrett ES, Sobolewski M. Polycystic ovary syndrome: do endocrine-disrupting chemicals play a role? Semin Reprod Med. 2014;32:166–76.
89. Frye CA, Bo E, Calamandrei G, Calzà L, Dessì-Fulgheri F, Fernández M, Fusani L, Kah O, Kajta M, Le Page Y, Patisaul HB, Venerosi A, Wojtowicz AK, Panzica GC. Endocrine disrupters: a review of some sources, effects, and mechanisms of actions on behaviour and neuroendocrine systems. J Neuroendocrinol. 2012;24:144–59. Review.
90. Careghini A, Mastorgio AF, Saponaro S, Sezenna E. Bisphenol A, nonylphenols, benzophenones, and benzotriazoles in soils, groundwater, surface water, sediments, and food: a review. Environ Sci Pollut Res Int. 2015;22:5711–41.
91. EFSA. Scientific opinion on the risks to public health related to the presence of bisphenol A (bpa) in foodstuffs. EFSA J. 2015;13:3978.
92. Schmalz G, Preiss A, Arenholt-Bindslev D. Bisphenol-A content of resin monomers and related degradation products. Clin Oral Investig. 1999;3:114–9.
93. Söderholm KJ, Mariotti A. BIS-GMA – based resins in dentistry: are they safe? J Am Dent Assoc. 1999;130:201–109. Review.
94. Malkiewicz K, Owoc A, Kluska M, Grzech-Leśniak K, Turło J. HPLC analysis of potentially harmful substances released from dental filing materials available on the EU market. Ann Agric Environ Med. 2014;21:86–90.
95. Polydorou O, Beiter J, König A, Hellwig E, Kümmerer K. Effect of bleaching on the elution of monomers from modern dental composite materials. Dent Mater. 2009;25:254–60.
96. Yin L, Yu K, Lin S, Song X, Yu X. Associations of blood mercury, inorganic mercury, methyl mercury and bisphenol A with dental surface restorations in the U.S. population, NHANES 2003-2004 and 2010-2012. Ecotoxicol Environ Saf. 2016;134P1:213–25.
97. Fung EY, Ewoldsen NO, St Germain HA Jr, Marx DB, Miaw CL, Siew C, Chou HN, Gruninger SE, Meyer DM. Pharmacokinetics of bisphenol A released from a dental sealant. J Am Dent Assoc. 2000;131:51–8.
98. Joskow R, Barr DB, Barr JR, Calafat AM, Needham LL, Rubin C. Exposure to bisphenol A from bis-glycidyl dimethacrylate-based dental sealants. J Am Dent Assoc. 2006;137:353–62.
99. Oysaed H, Ruyter IE. Water sorption and filler characteristics of composites for use in posterior teeth. J Dent Res. 1986;65:1315–8.
100. Söderholm KJ, Zigan M, Ragan M, Fischlschweiger W, Bergman M. Hydrolytic degradation of dental composites. J Dent Res. 1984;63:1248–54.

101. Söderholm KJ. Filler leachability during water storage of six composite materials. Scand J Dent Res. 1990;98:82–8.
102. Subramani K, Ahmed W, Hartsfield LK, editors. Nanobiomaterials in clinical dentistry. Waltham (USA); Oxford (UK): Elsevier; 2013.
103. Kunzmann A, Andersson B, Thurnherr T, Krug H, Scheynius A, Fadeel B. Toxicology of engineered nanomaterials: focus on biocompatibility, biodistribution and biodegradation. Biochim Biophys Acta. 2011;1810:361–73.
104. Oberdörster G, Maynard A, Donaldson K, Castranova V, Fitzpatrick J, Ausman K, Carter J, Karn B, Kreyling W, Lai D, Olin S, Monteiro-Riviere N, Warheit D, Yang H, ILSI Research Foundation/Risk Science Institute Nanomaterial Toxicity Screening Working Group. Principles for characterizing the potential human health effects from exposure to nanomaterials: elements of a screening strategy. Part Fibre Toxicol. 2005;2:8.
105. Napierska D, Thomassen LC, Lison D, Martens JA, Hoet PH. The nanosilica hazard: another variable entity. Part Fibre Toxicol. 2010;7:39. Review.
106. Borm PJ, Robbins D, Haubold S, Kuhlbusch T, Fissan H, Donaldson K, Schins R, Stone V, Kreyling W, Lademann J, Krutmann J, Warheit D, Oberdorster E. The potential risks of nanomaterials: a review carried out for ECETOC. Part Fibre Toxicol. 2006;3:11.
107. Shang L, Nienhaus K, Nienhaus GU. Engineered nanoparticles interacting with cells: size matters. J Nanobiotechnology. 2014;12:5.
108. Sivakumar I, Arunachalam KS, Solomon E. Occupational health hazards in a prosthodontic practice: review of risk factors and management strategies. J Adv Prosthodont. 2012;4:259–65.
109. Boverhof DR, Bramante CM, Butala JH, Clancy SF, Lafranconi M, West J, Gordon SC. Comparative assessment of nanomaterial definitions and safety evaluation considerations. Regul Toxicol Pharmacol. 2015;73:137–50.
110. Donaldson K, Poland CA. Nanotoxicity: challenging the myth of nano-specific toxicity. Curr Opin Biotechnol. 2013;24:724–34.
111. Van Landuyt KL, Yoshihara K, Geebelen B, Peumans M, Godderis L, Hoet P, Van Meerbeek B. Should we be concerned about composite (nano-) dust? Dent Mater. 2012;28:1162–70.
112. Van Landuyt KL, Hellack B, Van Meerbeek B, Peumans M, Hoet P, Wiemann M, Kuhlbusch TA, Asbach C. Nanoparticle release from dental composites. Acta Biomater. 2014;10:365–74.
113. Filipe V, Hawe A, Jiskoot W. Critical evaluation of nanoparticle tracking analysis (NTA) by NanoSight for the measurement of nanoparticles and protein aggregates. Pharm Res. 2010;27:796–810.
114. Bootz A, Vogel V, Schubert D, Kreuter J. Comparison of scanning electron microscopy, dynamic light scattering and analytical ultracentrifugation for the sizing of poly(butyl cyanoacrylate) nanoparticles. Eur J Pharm Biopharm. 2004;57:369–75.
115. Brown PH, Schuck P. Macromolecular size-and-shape distributions by sedimentation velocity analytical ultracentrifugation. Biophys J. 2006;90:4651–61.
116. Fraunhofer W, Winter G, Coester C. Asymmetrical flow field-flow fractionation and multiangle light scattering for analysis of gelatin nanoparticle drug carrier systems. Anal Chem. 2004;76:1909–20.

Part VI

Clinical Considerations

13 Bonding to Tooth Tissues

Vesna Miletic and Salvatore Sauro

13.1 Current Adhesive Approaches

Apart from self-adhesive (self-adhering) composites, all contemporary composites bond to tooth tissues via adhesive systems. Current classification of adhesive systems is based on their interaction with the smear layer, adhesive composition and clinical application steps: (1) 3-step etch-and-rinse (3ER), (2) 2-step etch-and-rinse (2ER), (3) 2-step self-etch (2SE) and (4) 1-step self-etch (1SE) [1]. A new 'class' of dental adhesives has recently attracted interest of both researchers and practitioners—'universal' adhesives. These are recommended not only for bonding to tooth tissues and composites but also materials for indirect restorations (e.g. metal alloys, zirconia and glass-ceramics) without the use of separate priming step.

Two main application approaches determined by the adhesive systems, *etch-and-rinse* and *self-etch*, differ primarily in the use of phosphoric acid etchants. Clinically, 32–37% phosphoric acid is used to remove the smear layer and demineralize the surface of enamel and dentin, by which the micro-retentive surface is created for adhesive infiltration. In the ER approach, adhesive primer and bond are applied to the acid-etched enamel and dentin, either as separate (3ER) or as one clinical step (2ER). In the SE approach, acidic functional monomers in SE adhesive systems 'replace' phosphoric acid by partially demineralizing dental tissues followed by separate or simultaneous infiltration of bonding agent (2SE and 1SE, respectively). In general, acidic monomers are less effective on enamel than phosphoric acid due to their pH and shallower demineralization; this results in lower bond strength [2, 3]. Therefore, the third clinical approach—*selective-etch*—is now an accepted concept for enamel bonding of SE and 'universal' adhesives. In the selective-etch approach, enamel is etched using phosphoric acid followed by the application of SE or 'universal' adhesives to the entire cavity. Figure 13.1 summarizes the adhesive systems for bonding direct composites to tooth tissues.

V. Miletic
DentalNet Research Group, School of Dental Medicine, University of Belgrade, Belgrade, Serbia

S. Sauro (✉)
Departamento de Odontología, Facultad de Ciencias de la Salud, Universidad CEU-Cardenal Herrera, Valencia, Spain

Biomaterials, Biophotonics and Tissue Engineering, King's College London Dental Institute, London, UK
e-mail: salvatore.sauro@uchceu.es

V. Miletic (ed.), *Dental Composite Materials for Direct Restorations*,
http://doi.org/10.1007/978-3-319-60961-4_13

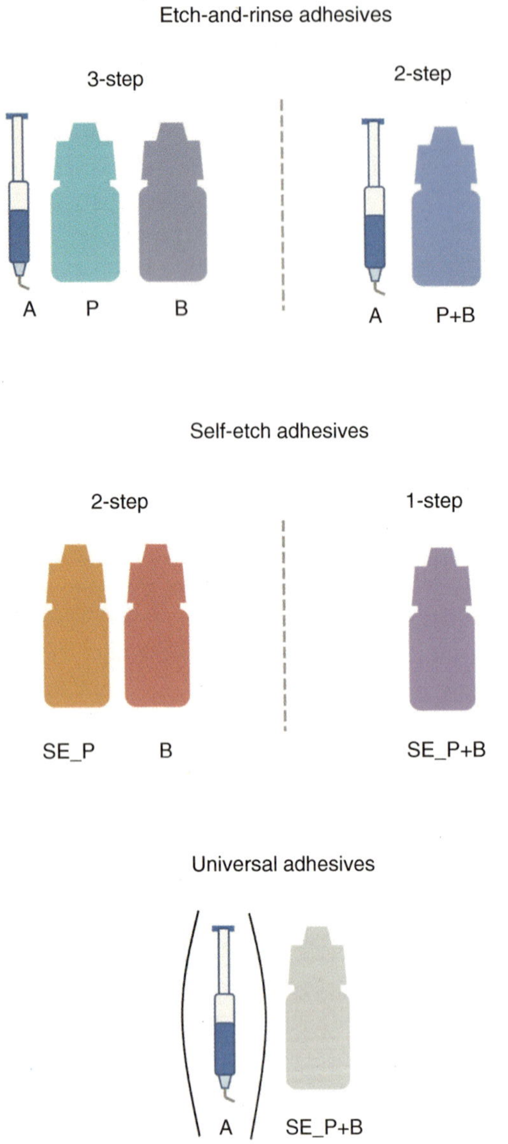

Fig. 13.1 Current adhesive systems. Brackets depict that universal adhesives may be used with or without phosphoric acid, making them essentially 2-step etch-and-rinse or 1-step self-etch adhesives. *A* acid, *P* primer, *B* bond, *SE* 'self-etch'

13.2 Characteristics of the Tooth-Adhesive Bond

13.2.1 Mechanisms of Adhesion

The primary mechanism of adhesion to enamel and dentin is attributed to micromechanical interlocking between the adhesive resin and apatite crystallites in enamel or the exposed collagen fibril network in dentin. The micromechanical interlocking was classified as 'hybridization' to highlight the formation of a distinctive layer ('hybrid layer') comprising of adhesive resin and natural tissue with unique properties [4]. The hybrid layer in dentin may be considered a form of tissue engineering according to Pashley et al. [5]. However, the interfibrillar porosities within the collagen network of 10–30 nm serving as a sort of scaffold for adhesive resin infiltration are far smaller than 5–20 μm porosities in most bioengineering scaffolds [5].

Additional interlocking at dentin is achieved as resin monomers penetrate into dentinal tubules and form resin tags upon polymerization. The resin tags are considered a contributing factor to the overall retention and resin-dentin seal [6]. The micromorphology of resin tags generally differs in ER and SE systems in that the ER adhesives form cone-shaped, thicker tags with evident later branching, whereas the SE adhesives form thinner, cylindrical tags with scarce lateral branching [7] (Fig. 13.2).

Secondary mechanisms of adhesion comprise chemical and physical interaction between adhesive monomers and tooth tissues. Chemical bonding was confirmed between certain functional monomers (10-MDP, 4-MET and phenyl-P) and Ca^{2+} in hydroxyapatite [8]. It was also shown that hydrolytic stability of the formed ionic salts determines the stability of the chemical bond

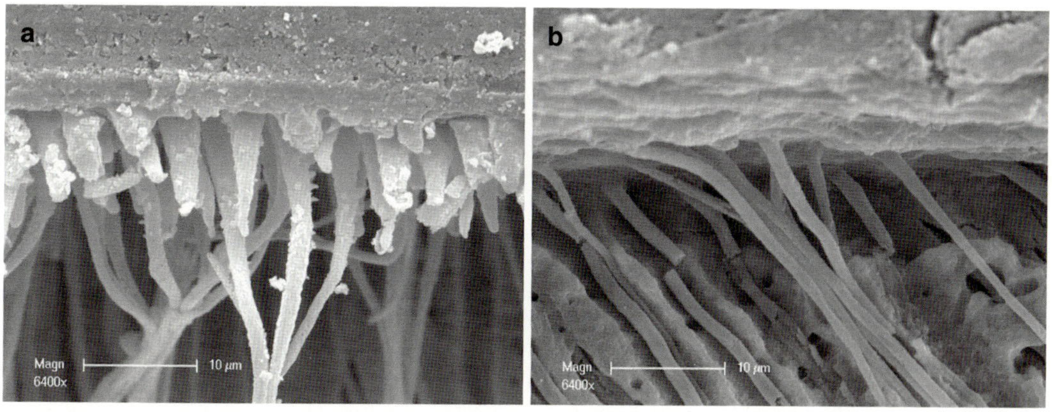

Fig. 13.2 Representative SEM images of the adhesive-dentin interface of (**a**) an ER and (**b**) an SE adhesive

according to the 'adhesion-decalcification (AD) concept' suggested by Yoshida et al. [9]. A stable chemical bond was confirmed between 10-MDP monomer and hydroxyapatite, further creating a unique regular pattern of 10-MDP-Ca salts, the phenomenon called 'nano-layering' [10]. It is suggested that nano-layering may contribute to the hydrolytic resistance of the resin-dentin bond and overall bond durability [11].

Cohesive forces may occur in the form of intermolecular hydrogen bonds between amide or carboxylic groups of functional resin monomers and amino acids of collagen peptides [12, 13]. Furthermore, adhesion through van der Waals and electrostatic interactions of functional monomers and collagen fibrils was proposed to contribute to bond strength and marginal sealing [14].

13.2.2 Characteristics of the Hybrid Layer

Microscopy studies, SEM as well as TEM, allow detailed insight into the micromorphology of the hybrid layer. The thickness of the hybrid layer is mostly between 5 and 8 µm in ER [5] and less than 3–4 µm in SE adhesives, with ultra-mild adhesives creating less than 1-µm-thick hybrid layer [11]. The hybrid layer formed by ER adhesives generally consists of collagen fibrils within demineralized dentin infiltrated and encapsulated by resin monomers [5]. Conversely, the hybrid layer of the SE adhesives is more complex due to partial demineralization of dentin hydroxyapatite. In addition to closely packed collagen fibrils, partially demineralized hydroxyapatite crystals encapsulated by adhesive resin appear in deeper parts of the hybrid layer [15, 16]. Water-rich and resin-poor zones were identified within the hybrid layer using water-soluble tracers, such as ammoniacal silver nitrate; this phenomenon is known as 'nanoleakage' [17, 18].

Micro-Raman spectroscopy is a non-destructive tool for chemical characterization of the hybrid layer complementing the well-established and widely used SEM and TEM techniques. Micro-Raman spectroscopic studies have shown evidence of phase separation between hydrophilic and hydrophobic monomers, primarily HEMA and BisGMA, within the hybrid layer indicating differences in the ability of these monomers to effectively infiltrate dentin [19]. Furthermore, differences between the extent of dentin demineralization and subsequent adhesive penetration were reported by Santini and Miletic [20]. This discrepancy is likely pronounced with ER adhesives due to the more aggressive etching effect of the phosphoric acid compared to milder acidic functional monomers in SE adhesives (Fig. 13.3) [20]. An example is given in Fig. 13.3.

The depth of dentine demineralization and adhesive penetration in μm

	Dentine demineralization		Adhesive penetration	
Group	Mean	SD	Mean	SD
Excite	12.5	0.8	8.0	3.0
AdheSE	6.0	1.7	5.9	1.9
AdheSE One	3.0	0.8	2.8	1.7

SD, standard deviation.

Fig. 13.3 The depth of dentin demineralization and adhesive penetration determined in situ using micro-Raman spectroscopy. Excite is a 2-step ER adhesive, AdheSE is a 2-step SE adhesive and AdheSe One is a 1-step SE adhesive (*Reprinted with permission from Santini A, Miletic V. Eur J Oral Sci 2008;116:177–183*)

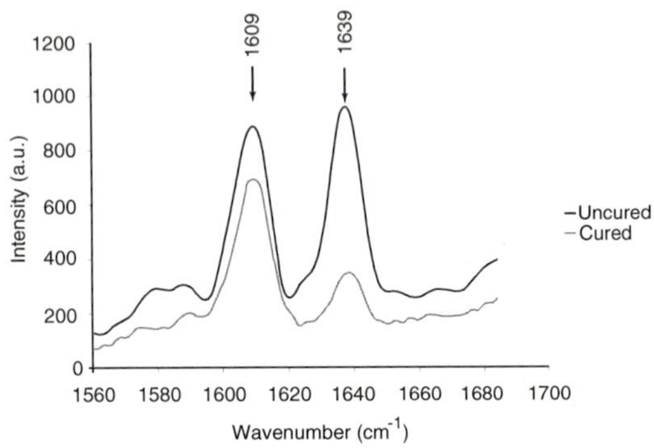

Fig. 13.4 Micro-Raman spectra of uncured and cured adhesive. The peak at 1639 cm^{-1} corresponds to the vinyl (aliphatic) C=C bonds that convert to C-C single bonds during polymerization. The peak at 1609 cm^{-1} corresponds to the aromatic C=C bonds which do not change during polymerization (internal standard). The DC is calculated as the ratio of 1639/1609 cm^{-1} peak intensities in cured and uncured materials: $DC = \left(1 - \frac{R_{cured}}{R_{uncured}}\right) \times 100$

13.2.3 Polymerization of Adhesive Resin

As the quality of polymerization is a major determinant of the properties of composite materials, the same is true for the adhesive itself and the adhesive-enamel/adhesive-dentin bond. It is widely accepted that the greater the polymerization, the better the material properties. Adequate polymerization of adhesive resin contributes to adhesive bond stability and resistance to polymer degradation processes. Hybridization of tooth tissues by adhesive resin indicates that tooth substrate (enamel and dentin) influences monomer-to-polymer conversion, in addition to material- and light-source-related factors determining conversion of composites. It is well known that water (moisture) impairs polymerization of resin monomers. Residual water within interfibrillar spaces of the hybrid layer that is not replaced by resin monomers during adhesive infiltration may play a critical role in suboptimal monomer-to-polymer conversion of dental adhesives.

Polymerization kinetics of adhesive systems may be quantified using differential scanning calorimetry [21, 22] or real-time spectroscopy methods [23]. The degree of conversion (DC) may be determined in situ using micro-Raman spectroscopy [20, 24–27] or in bulk material using micro-Raman but also FTIR spectroscopy [28–33]. Figure 13.4 illustrates the changes in the intensity of 1639 cm^{-1} peak associated with C = C double bonds before and after polymerization.

The reported DC values of adhesive systems vary considerably from less than 50% [23, 28, 34] to 60–95% [26, 30, 34]. Post-polymerization or 'dark cure' occurs in adhesives during the first 24 h, similarly to composites; however, the extent is variable as the previously mentioned range of DC is also quite variable in adhesives [30, 34]. Large compositional differences between ER, SE and 'universal' adhesives do not allow any conclusive statements about cause and effect regarding differences in the DC values. However, several factors influencing the DC have been clearly identified.

The DC of commercial adhesives is positively related to curing time [35, 36] and light irradiance [23, 28]. Overall, the type of commonly used light sources does not seem to influence conversion as inconsistent differences or the lack of differences was reported for LED and halogen light-curing units [23, 28, 36, 37]. A negative effect of increased curing distance was reported for conventional-intensity (~500 mW/cm^2) light-curing units [38], whereas no differences occurred up to 7–8 mm distance for high-intensity (>1000 mW/cm^2) light-curing units [39]. Excess amount of solvent in adhesive composition also negatively affects the DC [29, 40].

The effect of initiators and coinitiators in adhesives on monomer conversion is largely influenced by compatibility of the photoinitiator system with the acidic adhesive monomers and the presence of water. Water-compatible photoinitiators, such as TPO or CQ/EDMAB system, have shown favourable effects on monomer conversion in aqueous and acidic adhesive formulations [41]. A common CQ/DMAEMA system with quite low conversion in the presence of water has shown a significant improvement with the addition of an iodonium salt (DPIHP), most likely due to the increase of active phenyl radicals [42].

The relationship between the DC and adhesive bond strength to dentin has not been clearly established. Whilst positive correlation was found for a number of SE and ER adhesives and shear bond strength [30, 38], no correlation could be found for ER and SE adhesives and microtensile bond strength to dentin [34]. 'Universal' adhesives have shown improved monomer conversion and microshear bond strength to enamel following the ER compared to the SE approach [27]. In dentin, monomer conversion of 'universal' adhesives could not be associated with either the ER or the SE approach, but it was shown to be material-dependent with no direct association with bond strength to dentin [26].

13.2.4 Clinical Factors Affecting the Adhesive-Dentin Bond

Application protocols and curing parameters clearly influence the quality of polymerization of adhesive resin in clinical conditions. Clinicians should be aware of the negative effects that alterations to the recommended clinical protocol may have on the quality of the adhesive polymer network and the durability of the adhesive-dentin bond: (1) excess moisture on the substrate and/or within the dentin hybrid layer due to insufficient air-drying, (2) excess solvent in the adhesive following application and inadequate solvent evaporation by air-drying and (3) insufficient light energy delivered by the light source due to its low irradiance, inadequate position of the light-curing tip in terms of distance and angle and/or interference between the light tip and the applied adhesive, as well as insufficient curing time.

Another important factor in the quality of the adhesive-dentin bond is the microarchitecture of the collagen network following acid etching and prior to the adhesive application in the ER approach. Clinical rinsing-and-drying phase completely lacks standardization. The amount of residual water in the interfibrillar spaces of the exposed collagen network supporting collagen fibrils remains unknown in the drying phase. It is generally accepted that there is a relatively small window of opportunity for optimal substrate conditions as insufficient drying leads to excess residual water whilst overdrying results in the collapse of the collagen fibrils followed by insufficient adhesive infiltration. Therefore, 'wet bonding' proposed by Kanca [43] remains the most desirable clinical approach. It is recommended to apply the adhesive primer (and bond, if in one solution) to the visibly moist dentin in order to prevent the collagen network collapse. Furthermore, the HEMA-/water-based primers may be able to partially re-expand the collapsed collagen [44] allowing adhesive infiltration and the formation of hybrid layers.

The technique of application of SE and 'universal' adhesives may influence the depth of partial demineralization, the adhesive infiltration and the thickness of the hybrid layer. Active adhesive application improves bonding performance at dentin and enamel of SE and 'universal' adhesives [27, 45] due to the enhanced effect of acidic primers. As self-etch priming requires time, manufacturers recommend applying SE and 'universal' adhesives to the cavity for about 10–20 s to achieve partial demineralization. Clinicians should be aware that shorter application times of SE and 'universal' adhesives followed by rapid polymerization may result in shallow and insufficient hybridization and poor adhesive performance.

13.3 Characteristics of the Composite-Adhesive Bond

Similar monomer content of adhesives and composites based on dimethacrylate cross-linking monomers allows chemical bonding of the two

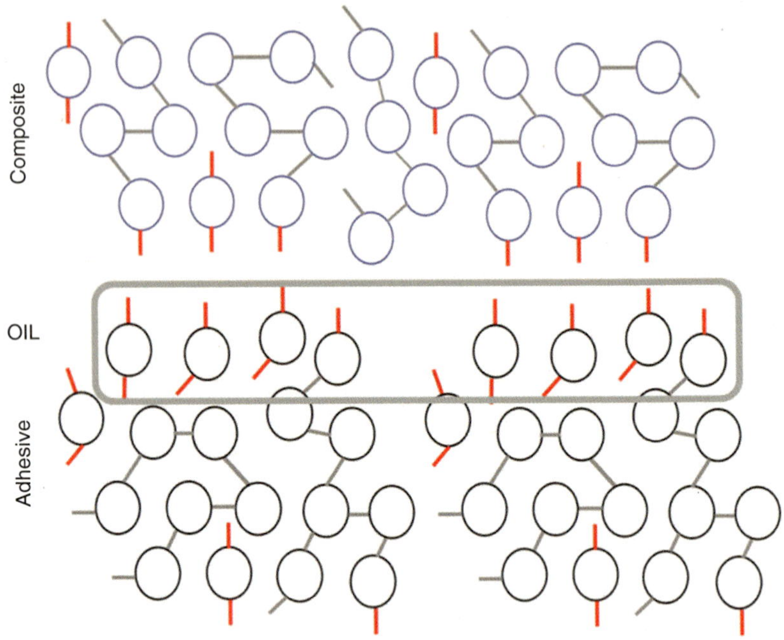

Fig. 13.5 The oxygen-inhibition layer (OIL) at the top of the adhesive layer contains multiple C=C double bonds available for chemical bonding with the same groups in the overlying composite. These C=C double bonds appear in the form of uncured monomer and pendant groups within the polymer

materials. It is widely known that a so-called oxygen-inhibition layer forms on the surface of resin-based materials due to the adverse effect of atmospheric oxygen on polymerization. The formation of the oxygen-inhibition layer on the surface of adhesives applied to tooth tissues was confirmed by Endo et al. [46]; the thickness of the oxygen-inhibition layer in four SE adhesives was below 25 μm. The C=C double bonds in the form of uncured monomer and pendant groups within the polymer enable the formation of covalent bonds between the adhesive layer and the overlying composite material (Fig. 13.5).

Effects of the oxygen-inhibition layer on composite-adhesive bond have been scarcely addressed in the literature. Its limited effect on shear bond strength to enamel and dentin was reported for SE adhesives [46]. A stronger positive relationship was found between the presence of the oxygen-inhibition layer and microtensile [35] or shear bond strength to dentin [47]. No effect of the oxygen-inhibition layer on bonding to enamel and dentin was found for a chemically cured composite and an SE adhesive in another study [48].

Koga et al. [47] showed that the oxygen-inhibition layer on the surface of the cured SE adhesive reduces surface-free energy and changes the acid-base interactions towards Lewis base component. The Lewis base component acts as an electron donor capable of accelerating the subsequent polymerization reaction at the adhesive-composite interface [47]. This might be the reason for improved bonding at the adhesive-composite interface and overall higher-bond strength in the composite-adhesive-tooth assembly observed in the presence of the oxygen-inhibition layer.

13.4 Mechanisms of Hybrid Layer Degradation

Degradation of the hybrid layer remains an important issue in clinical dentistry as it drastically reduces the lifetime of tooth-colored resin composite restorations. There is a persuasive necessity to understand the underlying mechanisms behind the degradation of the resin-dentin interface in order to extend its durability. Nowadays, it is well known that the main mechanisms responsible for the degradation of resin-dentin interfaces are (1) enzyme-mediated dentin collagen degradation [e.g. matrix metalloproteinases (MMPs) and cysteine cathepsins

(CTPs) (intrinsic or proteolytic degradation of the organic matrix)] and (2) extrinsic hydrolysis of the polymeric matrix. This latter also includes hydrolysis of the silane-coupling molecule (Si-O-Si), which may cause debonding of the fillers from the polymer matrix. These degradation processes may occur simultaneously and reduce the durability of resin-dentin bonds as well as the prognosis of the tooth [49, 50].

13.4.1 Hydrolytic Degradation of the Resin Matrix

Adhesive systems are not able to infiltrate completely the demineralized collagen matrix (i.e. acid-etched dentin) due to the inability of resin monomers to displace water. This leads to micro (e.g. micropermeability) and/or nano-phase separation (e.g. nanoleakage) within the hybrid layer (Figs. 6a, b); these represent the critical sites where the hydrolytic degradation can occur causing decrease of the durability of the resin-dentin bond [51, 52].

This represents a clear problem that challenges the clinical success of resin-based dental restorations. Indeed, most adhesive systems produce very good immediate bond strengths, but the long-term strengths are a cause for concern [52].

However, hydrolysis of resin matrices occurs both in self-etch (SE) and etch-and-rinse (ER) adhesives, and it is related to their degree of hydrophilicity [53] and, thus, to the amount of water sorption within the hybrid layer [54]. Subsequent to water sorption, these materials are subject to both hygroscopic and hydrolytic effects, which may influence their mechanical properties, dimensional stability and biocompatibility [54].

Polymer chains within light-cured adhesives absorb water and undergo volumetric changes such as swelling and physical changes such as plasticization/softening and chemical degradation through two main mechanisms: (1) passive hydrolysis and (2) enzymatic reaction.

Indeed, dental polymer networks may undergo hydroperoxidation reactions that cause scission of the polymer chain (breakdown of double covalent bonds). Furthermore, saliva contains several esterases (e.g. cholesterol esterase and pseudocholinesterase) that may cause esterification of methacrylates; extent of the enzymatic degradation is related to the degree of cure of resin monomers at the resin-dentin interface. Loosely cross-linked resin networks (i.e. 'poor' polimerized hybrid layers) are characterized by the presence of ester groups that may be more susceptible to degradation [55].

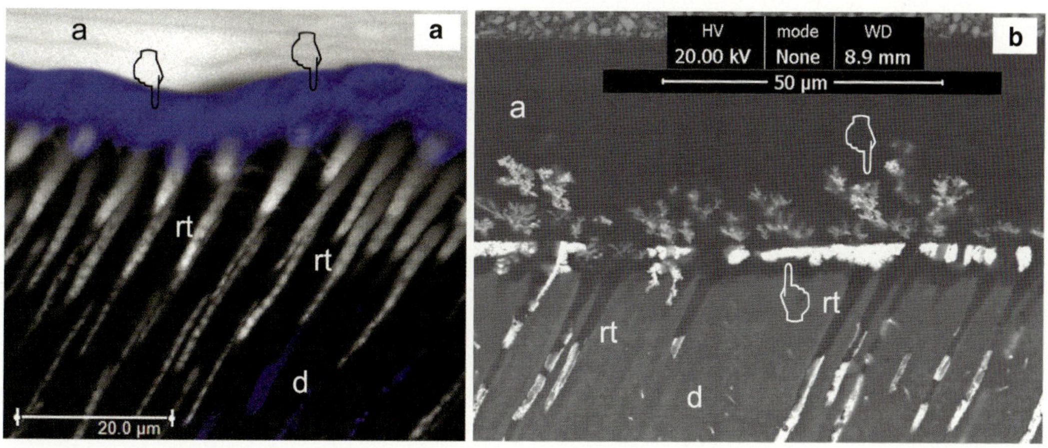

Fig. 13.6 (**a**) Representative dye-assisted confocal image of the adhesive-dentin interface showing micropermeability at the hybrid layer (*pointer*) and resin tags penetrating several microns into dentinal tubules (rt). (**b**) Representative SEM image showing nanoleakage at the adhesive-dentin interface (*pointer*) and resin tags penetrating into dentinal tubules (rt)

The degradation of the polymer matrix is also related, along with the degree of polymerization achieved in a clinically relevant time (20–60 s), to the chemical composition of the different adhesives (the balance between hydrophilic and hydrophobic components plays an impotant rule in such a situation). The higher the amount of hydrophilic monomers, the lower the degree of conversion. The higher the amount of hydrophilic monomers, the greater the water sorption/hydrolysis [56, 57].

Unfortunately, the increased demand for more 'user-friendly' adhesive protocols has led to the production of adhesive systems with fewer application steps, such as all-in-one SE, 2-step ER and, more recently, universal adhesives. Such systems usually exhibit lower bond strength over time and less predictable clinical results compared to the more complex adhesive protocols [58]. Such simplified adhesives are too hydrophilic and allow water sorption, which leads to more drastic hydrolytic degradation of the resin matrix [51, 53, 58].

Conversely, it is widely accepted that 3-step ER and 2-step SE adhesive systems can be considered as the 'gold standard' in dental adhesion. The reason being that is the placement of a hydrophobic adhesive over a primered dentin that reduces water sorption within the resin-dentin interface [52, 53]. Moreover, 2-step SE adhesives have been shown to be less technique-sensitive and therefore may be more recommendable than 3-step ER adhesives [58, 59].

13.4.2 Enzyme-Mediated Collagen Degradation

The bulk of the tooth is made of dentin, which is constituted by a mineral component of up to 70 vol% calcium-deficient/carbonate-rich hydroxyapatite [HAP: $Ca_{10}(PO_4)_6(OH)_2$] and 4–5 vol% of carbonates. Dentin also contains up to 20 vol% of 'free' (e.g. intratubular fluid) and bound water. However, the most important constituent of the dentin is represented by the of organic components (up to 30 vol%), that is made of 90% collagen fibrils (mainly type I and very minimal amounts of type III and V) and 10% water-rich non-collagenous proteins (NCPs) such as proteoglycans, glycosaminoglycans, phospholipids and enzymes [60]. These latter are essentially endogenous MMPs and cysteine cathepsins (e.g. cathepsin K) proteases bonded to the collagen matrix as inactive enzymes pro-forms and fossilized within the mineralized dentin [61, 62].

When matrix endopeptidases (e.g. MMP-2, MMP-9) are exposed and activated during restorative procedures using acid etchants (ER bonding approaches) or SE adhesives [63, 64], these become able to cleave the helical and telopeptide segments of the demineralized collagen matrix within the hybrid [65]. Moreover, it has been demonstrated that acidic resin monomers contained in mild SE adhesives can inhibit TIMPs and thus allow MMPs to become active [66].

Mazzoni et al. [67] showed significant gelatinolytic activity when using 2-step ER systems and suggested a 2-step activation process of dentin proteases: (1) enzyme activation due to initial demineralization and exposure of collagen fibres and (2) enzyme activation due to the acidity of the bonding agents employed. These authors also provided evidence that proteolytic and gelatinolytic activity may destroy collagen fibrils at the bottom of the hybrid layer, if not completely infiltrated by resin monomers. Moreover, increased dentinal fluid flow towards the resin-dentin interface would exacerbate the degradation process, in particular within the upper regions of the hybrid layer.

Cathepsin K has also been postulated to cause hybrid layer degradation [68]. Tezvergil-Mutluay et al. [69] showed in vitro that the release of ICTP telopeptides fragments following MMP-mediated degradation is higher than CTX fragments released by the proteolytic activity of cathepsin K. This could be explained by the fact that the pH of the incubation media was neutral and the optimum pH for MMPs to function at near maximum rates is between 7.2 and 7.5, while the optimum pH for cathepsin K is around 5.0 [70].

Nevertheless, there is no information about the synergic role of these two enzymes in a clinical scenario; hence, further studies are required to clarify which of the two families of enzymes play the most significant role in reducing the longevity of composite restorations in vivo. One more aspect to elucidate is if the salivary proteases and those potentially created by a biofilm may contribute to the degradation of hybrid layers.

However, there is a consensus within authorities in adhesive dentistry that collagen degradation is more evident with ER approaches, as the use of phosphoric acid-etchant demineralizes more the dentin, leaving collagen matrices exposed and making them more susceptible to proteolytic degradation by endogenous enzymes [71].

SE adhesives etch and infiltrate the dental substrate simultaneously preventing complete exposure of collagen fibres and removal of smear plugs from dentinal tubules. Therefore, the main reason why mild SE adhesives degrade less ER adhesives is that collagen fibrils remain protected by HAP crystallites and because there is less water sorption from the pulpal chamber (i.e. micropermeability) [53, 72].

Nevertheless, mild SE systems are still vulnerable to degradation, as their hydrophilicity will allow water sorption and cause enzymatic hydrolysis of ester bonds over time. Moreover, it is possible that during their application, such systems will not completely remove the water within the demineralized dentin collagen and replace it with resin; this is a possible reason why degradation may still arise in simplified (all in one/universal) as well as in mild 2-step self-etch systems [59, 72].

13.5 Strategies for Improved Durability of Resin-Dentin Bond

13.5.1 Inhibition of Enzyme-Mediated Collagen Degradation

One of the most encouraging methods to inhibit enzyme-mediated collagen degradation for a relatively long-term period is based on the incorporation of specific MMP (e.g. BB94 and GM6001) and/or cathepsin K inhibitors within the formulation of adhesive systems [73]. The most common method advocated to preserve the durability of resin-dentin bonds is by using chlorhexidine (CHX), a strong bisbiguanide antimicrobial agent. For instance, in vitro studies showed that CHX inhibited MMP-2, MMP-8, MMP-9 [74] as well as dentinal cysteine cathepsins [75]. Moreover, in vivo studies confirmed that CHX could increase the long-term dentin bond strength of simplified 2-step ER adhesives [76, 77].

In particular, Carrilho et al. [76] showed in vivo that when using a 2-step ER adhesive applied onto acid-etched dentin that was pretreated with 2% CHX (60 s), it was possible to preserve the resin-dentin bond strength as well as a sound structure of the hybrid layer. Conversely, the use of CHX in combination with SE adhesives has not been extensively tested, although few in vitro studies showed dentin pretreatment using CHX 1% or 2% could preserve the bond strength of SE adhesive systems [78, 79].

Even though the myriad of CHX protocols proposed to preserve the integrity of hybrid layers, it is mostly accepted that the pretreatment of acid-etched dentin with CHX 2% for 1 min might provide excellent immediate [79] and long-lasting bond strength results [80]. CHX may also be incorporated into dental adhesives in order to achieve a potential inhibition of collagenolytic activity. In particular, Zhou et al. [81] incorporated varying concentrations of CHX (0.5%, 1% and 2%) into a 2-step SE adhesive system and found that CHX 1% and 2% produced more favourable bonding longevity.

The use of CHX may offer noteworthy benefits in slowing down the proteolytic degradation at the bottom of the hybrid layer, although it may move the chief site of failure up towards the adhesive and composite resin areas [76, 82]. Moreover, it seems that the main problem associated with the incorporation of CHX within the compositions of adhesive systems is that it may leak out of the hybrid layer after 18–24 months; thus, it may not be an enduring solution to protect the hybrid layer [82]. Additional studies should be performed to clarify this problem, as well as obtain further information about the effect of

CHX application with SE adhesives. An effort should be also made to simplify the protocols to decrease the risk of operator error.

Quaternary ammonium compounds (QACs), like CHX, are positively charged molecules, and they represent a further class of antimicrobial agents that may reduce the enzyme-mediated collagen degradation within the hybrid layer. However, since QACs are smaller than CHX molecules (lower molecular weight), it has been hypothesized that they penetrate better within the demineralized dentin and lead to more stability of the molecule within the hybrid layer [83].

Light-curable quaternary ammonium methacrylates (QAMs) have also shown encouraging results in decreasing the degradation of resin-dentin bonds. For instance, methacryloyloxydodecylpyridinium bromide (MDPB) was able to inhibit bacterial growth on its surface and thus able to nullify invading bacteria in gaps so reducing the risk of secondary caries [84]. Nevertheless, it has been reported that its antibacterial activity may last only for 14 days [85]. Further studies demonstrated that when using a 2-step SE adhesive continuing such a 'therapeutic' monomer, it was possible to accomplish long-lasting bond strength to both enamel and dentin [84, 85]. However, some concerns have been raised over the clinical safety of MDPB molecules because they may be 'cytotoxic to human pulp cells' [85].

Benzalkonium chloride (BAC) is another antibacterial quaternary ammonium compound (QAC) that has been incorporated into phosphoric acid etchants. However, although the anti-proteolytic efficacy of BAC in an etchant is questionable as it may be rinsed away before adhesive placement, the individual use of either a BAC-containing etchant or a BAC-containing adhesive showed positive effects on bond strength in an in vitro study [84]. More studies are required to prove the efficacy of BAC and to present any potential advantages over MDPB-based adhesives. QACs have been used for a long time in dentistry and have only been tested to prevent proteolytic degradation of the hybrid layer for the past 10 years. While the concept and multiple in vitro studies are very promising, more in vivo studies should be carried out to gain more knowledge about clinical results.

It has been advocated that fluoride might also inhibit MMP-2 and MMP-9 from human saliva [86]. Brackett et al. [87] showed that 150 ppm of NaF could inhibit both soluble and matrix-bound MMPs. Moreover, fluoride ions could chelate calcium and zinc on MMPs and alter their three-dimensional configuration; this structural alteration leads to the inhibition of their enzymatic activity [88].

Fluoride has been demonstrated to be effective in impeding the proteolytic activity of human cathepsin K and B [89]. Altinci et al. [90] demonstrated that it is possible to inhibit matrix-bound cathepsin-mediated dentin matrix degradation using a minimum concentration of NaF (≥120 mM). However, the mechanism of inhibition offered by fluoride on cathepsin K is still unclear; thus, this issue should be further investigated in future studies.

13.5.2 Cross-Linking Agents for Collagen Strengthening

Collagen cross-linking agents have been advocated as a potential alternative to achieve a long-term protection of hybrid layers. However, various collagen cross-linking agents require more than 1 h to take effect; thus, many studies are focusing on acceptable clinical application times, combined with an improvement in bond strength durability and resin-dentin interface stability [91].

The rationale behind the use of collagen cross-linking agents is to enhance the inter- and intramolecular collagen cross-linking and improve the structural stability of collagen matrices to resistant to degradation over time [92]. This stability would potentially inactivate endogenous proteases (e.g. MMPs and cathepsins) bound to the collagen matrix in an enduring way [93]. For instance, the application of glutaraldehyde onto demineralized dentin to encourage collagen cross-linking succeeded in vitro. However, this substance may have cytotoxic effects on the pulp, perhaps the main reason why it never achieved so much popularity in clinical dentistry [94]. Conversely, several in vitro studies showed that grape seed extract (e.g. proanthocyanidin) could be biocompatible and increase the modulus of elasticity of demineralized dentin matrices much more than glutaraldehyde [94, 95].

Furthermore, it was shown using SEM that the application of proanthocyanidin (120 s) could create a homogenous and regular collagen network in demineralized dentin [96]. Although such a natural collagen cross-linker presents very promising results, there is a lack of long-term in vitro and in vivo studies on its stability; it may also stain the dentin brown [91, 96].

Another strategy that has been suggested to improve the durability of resin-dentin bonds through collagen cross-linking is the application of 1-ethyl-3-carbodiimide (EDC). Indeed, Mazzoni et al. [93] demonstrated improved bond stability after 1 year with the use of a 0.3 M EDC post-etchant conditioner for 1 min. The same study also showed through zymography that 0.3 M EDC could completely inhibit the dentinal gelatinases (MMP-2 and MMP-9).

Riboflavin (0.1%), combined with UVA irradiation (2 min), has also been tested to improve collagen cross-linking. The theory behind the use of riboflavin is that the UVA disrupts the weak intrinsic cross-links within collagen matrix and the riboflavin can encourage the formation of new and more stable cross-links. Unfortunately, the use of UVA in the clinic is a concern, as its safety is questionable. Moreover, additional light-curing steps may result unsuitable for some clinicians in their daily practice [92]. A further study tested the use of a tungsten-halogen dental light to activate riboflavin, and although UVA produced better results, the blue light could obtain better bonding performance compared to specimens that were pretreated with no cross-linker [97].

Collagen cross-linking agents are providing very promising results in increasing the durability of resin-dentin bonds. Nevertheless, future studies are required to assess long-term results and to promote the use of these agents in clinical practice.

13.5.3 Hydrophobic Hybrid Layers and Improved Polymerization

As previously mentioned, a critical issue in contemporary dentin adhesion is represented by the inability of both ER and SE adhesives to replace free and loosely bound water from the demineralized collagen matrix [98]. Mineral-depleted collagen fibrils within demineralized dentin are characterized by a hydrogel of highly hydrated proteoglycans that impede the penetration of large hydrophobic monomers (e.g.

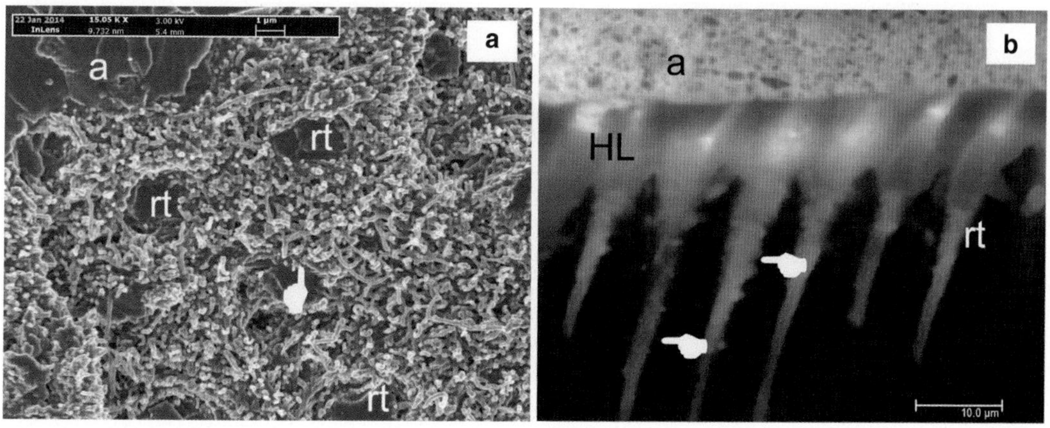

Fig. 13.7 (**a**) Representative SEM image showing acid-etched dentin collagen fibrils not properly infiltrated by the adhesive system (*pointer*) and fractured adhesive (a) and resin tags (rt) inside dentinal tubules after microtensile bond strength (rt). (**b**) Representative dye-assisted confocal image of the adhesive-dentin interface created with the ethanol wet-bonding technique showing no micropermeability at the hybrid layer (HL) but only between resin tags (rt) and the intra-tubular dentin (*pointer*)

BisGMA, UDMA) [99] (Fig. 13.7a). Conversely, only smaller water-soluble monomer such as HEMA can penetrate such demineralized dentin to form a very hydrophilic HEMA-rich hybrid layer. This type of hybrid layer may absorb a great deal of fluids both from the pulpal chamber and enamel marginal gaps, which can induce fast degradation of the resin-dentin interface [53].

A possible solution to allow better penetration of hydrophobic monomers into acid-etched dentin and create hybrid layers less porous (Fig. 13.7b) and less prone to uptake water, and thus less susceptible to hydrolytic degradation, is represented by the ethanol wet-bonding technique in combination with hydrophobic adhesives [100].

In this way, it will be possible to create more hydrophobic and durable hybrid layers with decreases water sorption/solubility, resin plasticization and enzyme-mediated degradation of collagen. [101, 102] Moreover, it is possible to solvate hydrophobic resins (BisGMA/UDMA/TEGDMA) in 50–70 vol% absolute ethanol to render the parameters of solubility of such resins closer to those of ethanol-saturated dentin; the probability that hydrophobic monomers can coax into a demineralized collagen matrix will be greater [103]. However, rather than using the classic time-consuming ethanol wet-bonding technique (5 min application), it is possible to use a simplified technique where absolute ethanol is applied to water-saturated acid-etched dentin in a more clinically relevant time (1 min) [104, 105].

Ethanol wet-bonding technique is extremely technique-sensitive and does not completely reduce dentin permeability nor replace the water contamination caused by outward fluid flow (Fig. 13.8a) [105]. Conversely, pretreatment of acid-etched dentin with oxalic acid prior to the application of the ethanol wet-bonding technique can reduce the risk for such contamination (Fig. 13.8b) of the hybrid layer caused by pulpal fluid pressure during bonding procedures in vital teeth [106].

Since the application of hydrophobic resins onto acid-etched dentin may result substantially challenging, an alternative version of the ethanol wet-bonding technique, based on the application of conventional hydrophilic adhesives (simplified and multistep systems), can be employed. Hybrid layers created with such technique showed, compared to water-wet bonding, less nanoleakage and more durable bond strength after ageing [107].

Although the presence of ethanol may increase the degree of conversion of the hydrophilic adhesives, its incomplete removal from the hydrophilic adhesives may interfere with their polimerization and make them more susceptible

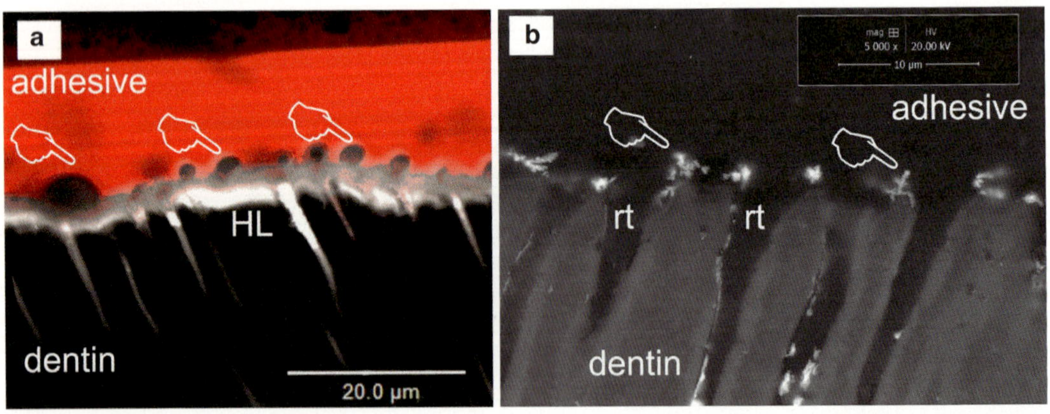

Fig. 13.8 (**a**) Representative dye-assisted confocal image of the adhesive-dentin interface created with the ethanol wet-bonding technique in dentin under simulated pulpal pressure. Note the severe micropermeability at the hybrid layer (HL) and the phase separation induced by the tubular fluid. (**b**) Representative SEM image of a specimen created with the ethanol wet-bonding technique in dentin pretreated with oxalic acid and submitted to simulated pulpal pressure. Very little nanoleakage can be appreciated within the resin-dentin interface as well as between dentin and resin tags (rt)

to water sorption [108]. Hence, such possible solutions have been recommended: (1) use less hydrophilic resins in dental adhesives to create more reliable and durable resin-dentin interface and (2) employ adhesives containing new-generation hydrophilic photoinitiators.

As already mentioned, resin degradation is directly related to the extent of water absorbed by the adhesive system employed during bonding procedures. Camphorquinone is a hydrophobic photoinitiator that in the presence of residual water and/or acidity environment does not induce ideal polymerization of modern hydrophilic adhesives [109]. Conversely, the incorporation of hydrophilic photoinitiators such as QTX [2-hydroxy-3-(3,4-dimethyl-9-oxo-9H-thioxanthen-2-yloxy)-N,N,N-trimethyl-1-propanaminium chloride] or TPO [diphenyl(2,4,6-trimethylbenzoyl)-phosphine oxide may improve the polymerization reaction in more hydrophilic conditions [109, 110]. The presence of sodium acylphosphine oxide as coinitiator may also improve the polymerization of hydrophilic adhesives in the presence of water and in a more acidic environment [111].

Intensification of the polymerization in mono/dimethacrylate monomers may reduce the number of unreacted pendant functional groups and increase their resistance to hydrolytic degradation. Moreover, it is also possible to enhance the mechanical properties of the resin-dentin interface [110].

It is important to consider that this strategy based on alternative photoinitiators cannot advantage the ability of adhesive monomers to infiltrate a mineral-depleted dentin substrate, especially in the presence of water-saturated collagen fibrils. On the other hand, the ethanol wet-bonding technique discussed above may not be properly suitable in all clinical situations; indeed, it remains a bonding philosophy rather than a bonding approach. Thus, it is still necessary to find a bonding strategy based on the use of 'smart' materials that able to induce replacement of the lost mineral phase within the demineralized dentin and collagen protection by entombing MMPs and cysteine cathepsins. This might represent a possible critical approach to create 'self-healing' restorations that can preserve the integrity and the longevity of the resin-dentin interface over time.

13.5.4 Therapeutic Remineralization of Resin-Dentin Interfaces

Therapeutic remineralization of the resin-dentin interface can be achieved through biomimetic/bioactive processes that may restore the biomechanical properties of mineral-depleted dentin within hybrid layers and/or caries-affected dentin [112, 113].

To re-establish the mechanical properties of demineralized dentin matrices, specific ions such as calcium and phosphates must infiltrate the nanometric-sized areas within demineralized dentin collagen fibrils [114]; calcium-phosphate (Ca/P) precipitants bigger than 40 nm may not 'fit' into such demineralized collagen matrices. This is exactly how current remineralising techniques employed nowadays (i.e. glass ionomer cements and calcium-silicate cements) "remineralize" the mineral-depleted bonding interface. Indeed, self-adhesive glass ionomer (GIC) and resin-modified glass ionomer cements (RMGIC) bonded to dentin can induce partial remineralization of the resin-bonded interface [115]; however, the therapeutic remineralization activity of such materials can be enhanced if applied after air-abrasion performed with bioactive glasses [116, 117]. Conversely, calcium-silicate MTA-like cements may cause a caustic degradation of dentin collagen fibrils at the interface due to their pronounced alkalising activity (pH > 10); collagen is then supplanted by calcium carbonates or by apatite-like crystals if immersed in phosphate-rich solutions (i.e. saliva, blood) [118, 119].

Moreover, esthetic resin-based materials (e.g. resin composites) as well as conventional adhesive systems have no remineralizing ability on poorly resin-infiltrated hybrid layers and/or caries-affected dentin underneath the hybrid layers; such interfaces are characterized by poor durability [120, 121]. One of the main reasons why this degradation occurs so quickly at the resin-dentin interface is because multilayer composite-dentin restorations are characterized by very different gradation of stiffness; application of stress creates high stress concentrations where the difference in stiffness are greatest (e.g. resin-dentin interface) [112].

However, a recent investigation has demonstrated that amorphous calcium and phosphates can move into collagen fibrils in the presence of biomimetic phosphoproteins' analogs (e.g. polyvinyl-phosphonic acid and trimetaphosphate) and calcium-sequestering agents such as polyaspartic and polyacrylic acid that control the size of polyanion-stabilized calcium and phosphate ions (i.e. amorphous calcium phosphate) [112, 113].

Such minerals will slowly replace water within the mineral-depleted resin-dentin interface, and the stiffness of the resin-infiltrated dentin (i.e. hybrid layer) will increase to 10–15 GPa. As the therapeutic resin-based material releases calcium and phosphates, apatite crystals would ultimately occupy the resin-dentin interface so that the stiffness of the remineralized dentin can reach a stiffness of 18–20 GPa [121] and the endogenous proteases re-fossilized/inactivated on collagen to which they are bound (Fig. 13.9a, b) [91].

This 'reparative' process is known as 'bottom-up' remineralization, and it is opposite to the 'top-down' remineralization that is typically obtained when one tries to deposit minerals on the moist dentin surface using only ion-releasing materials such as GIC and RMGIC. Moreover, such resin-dentin interfaces remineralized by experimental ion-releasing resin used in combination with primers containing biomimetic analogs (TMP and PASA) show no significant reduction of the bond strength after 3–6 months of storage in artificial saliva and collagen nanocrystals deposition both at interfibrillar and intra-fibrillar level [122].

From a clinical point of view, there is actually no restorative material able to remineralise hybrid layers and completely restore the mechanical properties of mineral-depleted dental structures within resin-bonded interfaces. In such circumstances, collagen will quickly degrade if not protected through the application of cross-liking [123] anti-MMPs [124] agents such as those commercially available based on glutaraldehyde/2-hydroxyethylmethacrylate (Figure 13.9c, d).

Nowadays clinicians may perform restorations that can remineralise resin-dentin interfaces, prevent the reoccurrence of secondary carious lesions and maintain a prolonged bonding performance [125]. For instance, clinicians may use bioactive glass powders (e.g. Bioglass 45S5) in air-abrasion units to perform a selective caries removal or a final polishing of the cavity dentin. This alternative procedure will create a 'bioactive' smear layer on the dentin surface that can protect the bonded interface and preserve the adhesion performance of RMGIC [116] and self-etching adhesives [117].

In case one is dealing with the restoration of deep cavity lesions, close to the pulp chamber, it would also be appropriate to apply quick-setting calcium-silicate cements in combination with a selective caries removal and with a modified stepwise restorative technique. With such technique, it will be necessary at a partial removal of the cement (~1–2 mm) at the final step, followed by the application of an adhesive system and aesthetic composite [126].

The rationale behind the use of such bioactive cements is that it can cause a caustic degradation of the caries-affected/caries-infected dentin left inside the cavity, along with a strong antibacterial effect. This caries-affected/caries-infected dentin will be strengthened with calcium carbonates and/or apatite-like crystallisation at the interface [118], and the cement will also bio-stimulate pulpal cells to produce reparative dentin along the walls of the pulpal chamber (reparative dentin bridge) [127]. This is an alternative way to perform a minimal intervention treatment, which might save the vitality of the tooth and avoid root-canal treatments.

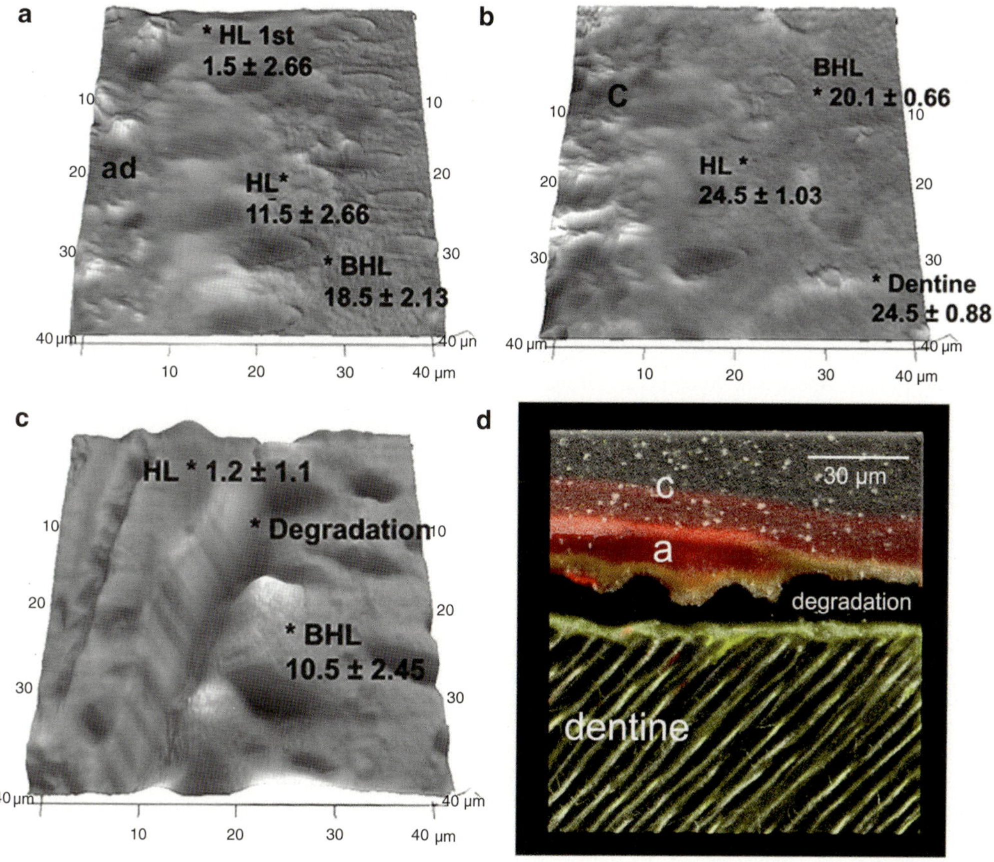

Fig. 13.9 (**a**) AFM image showing the resin-dentin interface after 24 h of AS storage created with an experimental ion-releasing adhesive applied onto acid-etched dentin. The initial values of elasticity of a sound hybrid layer (HL), bottom of hybrid layer (BHL) and sound dentin are shown digitally. (**b**) AFM image showing the resin-dentin interface after 90 days of AS storage created with the experimental ion-releasing adhesive applied to acid-etched dentin. Note that neither the hybrid layer (HL) nor the adhesive layer shows any sign of degradation but re-establishment of the modulus of elasticity of middle and bottom of hybrid layer (BHL) compared to the same specimen after 24 h AS storage (**a**). (**c**) AFM image showing the resin-dentin interface after 90 days of AS storage created with a simplified etch-and-rinse adhesive. Note the resin-dentin interface characterised by a gap as a sign of hybrid layer degradation. (**d**) CLSM 3D projection captured after 90 days of AS immersion in reflection/fluorescence showing the resin-dentin interface created with a simplified etch-and-rinse adhesive. The resin-dentin interface presents a clear gap as a sign of degradation between the adhesive (**a**) and the dentin. *Modified with permission from: [112]. Sauro S, Pashley DH. Strategies to stabilise dentin-bonded interfaces through remineralising operative approaches–State of The Art. Int J Adhes Adhes 2016;69, 39–57*

References

1. Van Meerbeek B, De Munck J, Yoshida Y, Inoue S, Vargas M, Vijay P, et al. Buonocore memorial lecture. Adhesion to enamel and dentin: current status and future challenges. Oper Dent. 2003;28:215–35.
2. Gregoire G, Ahmed Y. Evaluation of the enamel etching capacity of six contemporary self-etching adhesives. J Dent. 2007;35:388–97.
3. Hanabusa M, Mine A, Kuboki T, Momoi Y, Van Ende A, Van Meerbeek B, et al. Bonding effectiveness of a new 'multi-mode' adhesive to enamel and dentin. J Dent. 2012;40:475–84.
4. Nakabayashi N, Pashley DH. Hybridization of dental hard tissues. Tokyo: Quintessence Publishing Co, Ltd; 1998.
5. Pashley DH, Tay FR, Breschi L, Tjaderhane L, Carvalho RM, Carrilho M, et al. State of the art etch-and-rinse adhesives. Dent Mater. 2011;27:1–16.

6. Carrilho MR, Tay FR, Sword J, Donnelly AM, Agee KA, Nishitani Y, et al. Dentin sealing provided by smear layer/smear plugs vs. adhesive resins/resin tags. Eur J Oral Sci. 2007;115:321–9.
7. Miletic V. Micro-Raman spectroscopic studies on the adhesive-dentin interface and the degree of conversion of dental adhesives [Ph.D. thesis]. Edinburgh: The University of Edinburgh; 2010. https://www.era.lib.ed.ac.uk/handle/1842/4415.
8. Yoshida Y, Nagakane K, Fukuda R, Nakayama Y, Okazaki M, Shintani H, et al. Comparative study on adhesive performance of functional monomers. J Dent Res. 2004;83:454–8.
9. Yoshida Y, Van Meerbeek B, Nakayama Y, Yoshioka M, Snauwaert J, Abe Y, et al. Adhesion to and decalcification of hydroxyapatite by carboxylic acids. J Dent Res. 2001;80:1565–9.
10. Yoshida Y, Yoshihara K, Nagaoka N, Hayakawa S, Torii Y, Ogawa T, et al. Self-assembled Nano-layering at the adhesive interface. J Dent Res. 2012;91: 376–81.
11. Van Meerbeek B, Yoshihara K, Yoshida Y, Mine A, De Munck J, Van Landuyt KL. State of the art of self-etch adhesives. Dent Mater. 2011;27:17–28.
12. Nishiyama N, Asakura T, Suzuki K, Sato T, Nemoto K. Adhesion mechanisms of resin to etched dentin primed with N-methacryloyl glycine studied by 13C-NMR. J Biomed Mater Res. 1998;40:458–63.
13. Nishiyama N, Suzuki K, Asakura T, Komatsu K, Nemoto K. Adhesion of N-methacryloyl-omega-amino acid primers to collagen analyzed by 13C NMR. J Dent Res. 2001;80:855–9.
14. Vaidyanathan TK, Vaidyanathan J. Recent advances in the theory and mechanism of adhesive resin bonding to dentin: a critical review. J Biomed Mater Res B Appl Biomater. 2009;88:558–78.
15. Milia E, Santini A. Ultrastructural transmission electron microscopy (TEM) study of hybrid layers formed beneath a one-bottle adhesive system using the total-etch technique and a self-etching system. Quintessence Int. 2003;34:447–52.
16. Van Meerbeek B, Dhem A, Goret-Nicaise M, Braem M, Lambrechts P, VanHerle G. Comparative SEM and TEM examination of the ultrastructure of the resin-dentin interdiffusion zone. J Dent Res. 1993;72:495–501.
17. Sano H, Takatsu T, Ciucchi B, Horner JA, Matthews WG, Pashley DH. Nanoleakage: leakage within the hybrid layer. Oper Dent. 1995;20:18–25.
18. Tay FR, Pashley DH, Yoshiyama M. Two modes of nanoleakage expression in single-step adhesives. J Dent Res. 2002;81:472–6.
19. Wang Y, Spencer P, Yao X. Micro-Raman imaging analysis of monomer/mineral distribution in intertubular region of adhesive/dentin interfaces. J Biomed Opt. 2006;11:024005.
20. Santini A, Miletic V. Quantitative micro-Raman assessment of dentin demineralization, adhesive penetration, and degree of conversion of three dentin bonding systems. Eur J Oral Sci. 2008;116:177–83.
21. Breschi L, Cadenaro M, Antoniolli F, Sauro S, Biasotto M, Prati C, et al. Polymerization kinetics of dental adhesives cured with LED: correlation between extent of conversion and permeability. Dent Mater. 2007;23:1066–72.
22. Cadenaro M, Antoniolli F, Sauro S, Tay FR, Di Lenarda R, Prati C, et al. Degree of conversion and permeability of dental adhesives. Eur J Oral Sci. 2005;113:525–30.
23. Ye Q, Wang Y, Williams K, Spencer P. Characterization of photopolymerization of dentin adhesives as a function of light source and irradiance. J Biomed Mater Res B Appl Biomater. 2007;80:440–6.
24. Miletic V, Santini A, Trkulja I. Quantification of monomer elution and carbon-carbon double bonds in dental adhesive systems using HPLC and micro-Raman spectroscopy. J Dent. 2009;37:177–84.
25. Navarra CO, Cadenaro M, Armstrong SR, Jessop J, Antoniolli F, Sergo V, et al. Degree of conversion of Filtek Silorane adhesive system and Clearfil SE bond within the hybrid and adhesive layer: an in situ Raman analysis. Dent Mater. 2009;25:1178–85.
26. Munoz MA, Luque I, Hass V, Reis A, Loguercio AD, Bombarda NH. Immediate bonding properties of universal adhesives to dentin. J Dent. 2013;41:404–11.
27. Loguercio AD, Munoz MA, Luque-Martinez I, Hass V, Reis A, Perdigao J. Does active application of universal adhesives to enamel in self-etch mode improve their performance? J Dent. 2015;43:1060–70.
28. Arrais CA, Pontes FM, Santos LP, Leite ER, Giannini M. Degree of conversion of adhesive systems light-cured by LED and halogen light. Braz Dent J. 2007;18:54–9.
29. Giannini M, Arrais CA, Vermelho PM, Reis RS, dos Santos LP, Leite ER. Effects of the solvent evaporation technique on the degree of conversion of one-bottle adhesive systems. Oper Dent. 2008;33:149–54.
30. Kanehira M, Finger WJ, Hoffmann M, Endo T, Komatsu M. Relationship between degree of polymerization and enamel bonding strength with self-etching adhesives. J Adhes Dent. 2006;8:211–6.
31. Shin DH, Rawls HR. Degree of conversion and color stability of the light curing resin with new photoinitiator systems. Dent Mater. 2009;25:1030–8.
32. Miletic V, Pongprueksa P, De Munck J, Brooks NR, Van Meerbeek B. Monomer-to-polymer conversion and micro-tensile bond strength to dentin of experimental and commercial adhesives containing diphenyl(2,4,6-trimethylbenzoyl)phosphine oxide or a camphorquinone/amine photo-initiator system. J Dent. 2013;41(10):918–26. doi:10.1016/j.jdent.2013.07.007.
33. Pongprueksa P, Miletic V, De Munck J, Brooks NR, Meersman F, Nies E, et al. Effect of evaporation on the shelf life of a universal adhesive. Oper Dent. 2014;39:500–7.
34. Sadek FT, Calheiros FC, Cardoso PE, Kawano Y, Tay F, Ferrari M. Early and 24-hour bond strength and degree of conversion of etch-and-rinse and self-etch adhesives. Am J Dent. 2008;21:30–4.

35. Kim JS, Choi YH, Cho BH, Son HH, Lee IB, Um CM, et al. Effect of light-cure time of adhesive resin on the thickness of the oxygen-inhibited layer and the microtensile bond strength to dentin. J Biomed Mater Res B Appl Biomater. 2006;78:115–23.
36. Miletic V, Santini A. Micro-raman assessment of the ratio of carbon-carbon double bonds of two adhesive systems cured with LED or halogen light-curing units. J Adhes Dent. 2010;12:461–7.
37. D'Alpino PH, Svizero NR, Pereira JC, Rueggeberg FA, Carvalho RM, Pashley DH. Influence of light-curing sources on polymerization reaction kinetics of a restorative system. Am J Dent. 2007;20:46–52.
38. Xu X, Sandras DA, Burgess JO. Shear bond strength with increasing light-guide distance from dentin. J Esthet Restor Dent. 2006;18:19–27. discussion 8
39. Wegehaupt FJ, Lunghi N, Belibasakis GN, Attin T. Influence of light-curing distance on degree of conversion and cytotoxicity of etch-and-rinse and self-etch adhesives. BMC Oral Health. 2016;17:12.
40. Cadenaro M, Breschi L, Antoniolli F, Navarra CO, Mazzoni A, Tay FR, et al. Degree of conversion of resin blends in relation to ethanol content and hydrophilicity. Dent Mater. 2008;24:1194–200.
41. Cadenaro M, Antoniolli F, Codan B, Agee K, Tay FR, Dorigo Ede S, et al. Influence of different initiators on the degree of conversion of experimental adhesive blends in relation to their hydrophilicity and solvent content. Dent Mater. 2010;26:288–94.
42. Guo X, Peng Z, Spencer P, Wang Y. Effect of initiator on photopolymerization of acidic, aqueous dental model adhesives. J Biomed Mater Res A. 2009;90(4):1120–7.
43. Kanca J III. Improving bond strength through acid etching of dentin and bonding to wet dentin surfaces. J Am Dent Assoc. 1992;123:35–43.
44. Nakaoki Y, Nikaido T, Pereira PN, Inokoshi S, Tagami J. Dimensional changes of demineralized dentin treated with HEMA primers. Dent Mater. 2000;16:441–6.
45. do Amaral RC, Stanislawczuk R, Zander-Grande C, Michel MD, Reis A, Loguercio AD. Active application improves the bonding performance of self-etch adhesives to dentin. J Dent. 2009;37:82–90.
46. Endo T, Osada T, Finger WJ, Hoffmann M, Kanehira M, Komatsu M. Effect of oxygen inhibition of self-etching adhesives on enamel-dentin polymer bond. J Adhes Dent. 2007;9:33–8.
47. Koga K, Tsujimoto A, Ishii R, Iino M, Kotaku M, Takamizawa T, et al. Influence of oxygen inhibition on the surface free-energy and dentin bond strength of self-etch adhesives. Eur J Oral Sci. 2011;119:395–400.
48. Endo T, Finger WJ, Hoffmann M, Kanehira M, Komatsu M. The role of oxygen inhibition of a self-etch adhesive on self-cure resin composite bonding. Am J Dent. 2007;20:157–60.
49. Wood JD, Sobolewski P, Thakur V, Arola D, Nazari A, Tay FR, Pashley DH. Measurement of micro-strain across resin-dentin interfaces using microscopic moiré interferometry. Dent Mater. 2008;24:859–66.
50. Hickel R, Manhart J. Longevity of restorations in posterior teeth and reasons for failure. J Adhes Dent. 2001;3:45–64.
51. Perdigão J, Reis A, Loguercio AD. Dentin adhesion and MMPs: a comprehensive review. J Esthet Restor Dent. 2013;25:219–41.
52. Sauro S, Pashley DH, Mannocci F, Tay FR, Pilecki P, Sherriff M, Watson TF. Micropermeability of current self-etching and etch-and-rinse adhesives bonded to deep dentin: a comparison study using a double-staining/confocal microscopy technique. Eur J Oral Sci. 2008;116:184–93.
53. Sauro S, Pashley DH, Montanari M, Chersoni S, Carvalho RM, Toledano M, Osorio R, Tay FR, Prati C. Effect of simulated pulpal pressure on dentin permeability and adhesion of self-etch adhesives. Dent Mater. 2007;23:705–13.
54. Anchieta RB, Machado LS, Martini AP, Dos Santos PH, Giannini M, Janal M, et al. Effect of long-term storage on nanomechanical and morphological properties of dentin-adhesive interfaces. Dent Mater. 2015;31:141–53.
55. Lee SY, Greener EH, Mueller HJ. Effect of food and oral simulating fluids on structure of adhesive composite systems. J Dent. 1995;23:27–35.
56. Ferracane JL. Hygroscopic and hydrolytic effects in dental polymer networks. Dent Mater. 2006;22:211–22.
57. Schneider LF, Pfeifer CS, Consani S, Prahl SA, Ferracane JL. Influence of photoinitiator type on the rate of polymerization, degree of conversion, hardness and yellowing of dental resin composites. Dent Mater. 2008;24:1169–77.
58. Breschi L, Mazzoni A, Ruggeri A, Cadenaro M, Di Lenarda R, De Stefano Dorigo E. Dental adhesion review: aging and stability of the bonded interface. Dent Mater. 2008;24:90–101.
59. De Munck J, Van Landuyt K, Peumans M, Poitevin A, Lambrechts P, Braem M, Van Meerbeek B. A critical review of the durability of adhesion to tooth tissue: methods and results. J Dent Res. 2005;84:118–32.
60. Agee KA, Prakki A, Abu-Haimed T, Naguib GH, Nawareg MA, Tezvergil-Mutluay A, Scheffel DL, Chen C, Jang SS, Hwang H, Brackett M, Grégoire G, Tay FR, Breschi L, Pashley DH. Water distribution in dentin matrices: bound vs. unbound water. Dent Mater. 2015;31:205–16.
61. Palosaari H, Pennington CJ, Larmas M, Edwards DR, Tjäderhane L, Salo T. Expression profile of matrix metalloproteinases (MMPs) and tissue inhibitors of MMPs in mature human odontoblasts and pulp tissue. Eur J Oral Sci. 2003;111:117–27.
62. Pashley DH, Tay FR, Yiu C, Hashimoto M, Breschi L, Carvalho RM, et al. Collagen degradation by host-derived enzymes during aging. J Dent Res. 2004;83:216–21.
63. Lehmann N, Debret R, Roméas A, Magloire H, Degrange M, Bleicher F, et al. Self-etching increases matrix metalloproteinase expression in the dentin-pulp complex. J Dent Res. 2009;88:77–82.

64. Nishitani Y, Yoshiyama M, Wadgaonkar B, Breschi L, Mannello F, Mazzoni A, et al. Activation of gelatinolytic/collagenolytic activity in dentin by self-etching adhesives. Eur J Oral Sci. 2006;114:160–6.
65. Fedarko NS, Jain A, Karadag A, Fisher LW. Three small integrin binding ligands N-linked glycoproteins (SIBLINGS) bind and activate specific matrix metalloproteinases. FASEB J. 2004;18:734–6.
66. Sulkala M, Wahlgren J, Larmas M, Sorsa T, Teronen O, Salo T, et al. The effects of MMP inhibitors on human salivary MMP activity and caries progression in rats. J Dent Res. 2001;80(6):1545–9.
67. Mazzoni A, Nascimento FD, Carrilho M, Tersariol I, Papa V, Tjäderhane L, et al. MMP activity in the hybrid layer detected with *in situ* Zymography. J Dent Res. 2012;91:467–72.
68. Nascimento FD, Minciotti CL, Geraldeli S, Carrilho MR, Pashley DH, Tay FR, et al. Cysteine cathepsins in human carious dentin. J Dent Res. 2011;90:506–11.
69. Tezvergil-Mutluay A, Seseogullari-Dirihan R, Feitosa VP, Tay FR, Watson TF, Pashley DH, Sauro S. Zoledronate and ion-releasing resins impair dentin collagen degradation. J Dent Res. 2014;93:999–1004.
70. Holman CM, Kan CC, Gehring MR, Van Wart HE. Role of His-224 in the anomalous pH dependence of human Stromelysin-1. Biochemistry. 1999;28:677–81.
71. Hashimoto M. A review – micromorphological evidence of degradation in resin-dentin bonds and potential preventional solutions. J Biomed Mater Res B Appl Biomater. 2010;92:268–80.
72. Nakabayashi N, Kojima K, Masuhara E. The promotion of adhesion by the infiltration of monomers into tooth substrates. J Biomed Mater Res. 1982;16:265–73.
73. Almahdy A, Koller G, Sauro S, Bartsch JW, Sherriff M, Watson TF, Banerjee A. Effects of MMP inhibitors incorporated within dental adhesives. J Dent Res. 2012;91:605–11.
74. Gendron R, Grenier D, Sorsa T, Mayrand D. Inhibition of the activities of matrix metalloproteinases 2, 8, and 9 by Chlorhexidine. Clin Diagn Lab Immunol. 1999;6:437–9.
75. Scaffa PM, Vidal CM, Barros N, Gesteira TF, Carmona AK, Breschi L, et al. Chlorhexidine inhibits the activity of dental cysteine cathepsins. J Dent Res. 2012;91:420–5.
76. Breschi L, Cammelli F, Visintini E, Mazzoni A, Vita F, Carrilho M, et al. Influence of chlorhexidine concentration on the durability of etch- and-rinse dentin bonds: a 12-month in vitro study. J Adhes Dent. 2009;11:191–8.
77. Carrilho MR, Geraldeli S, Tay F, de Goes MF, Carvalho RM, Tjäderhane L, et al. In vivo preservation of the hybrid layer by chlorhexidine. J Dent Res. 2007;86:529.
78. Campos EA, Correr GM, Leonardi DP, Barato-Filho F, Gonzaga CC, Zielak JC. Chlorhexidine diminishes the loss of bond strength over time under simulated pulpal pressure and thermo-mechanical stressing. J Dent. 2009;37:108–14.
79. Yiu CK, Hiraishi N, Tay FR, King NM. Effect of chlorhexidine into dental adhesive resin on durability of resin-dentin bond. J Adhes Dent. 2012;14:355–62.
80. Montagner AF, Sarkis-Onofre R, Pereira-Cenci T, Cenci MS. MMP inhibitors on dentin stability: a systematic review and meta- analysis. J Dent Res. 2014;93:733.
81. Zhou J, Tan J, Yang X, Xu X, Li D, Chen L. MMP-inhibitory effect of chlorhexidine applied in a self-etching adhesive. J Adhes Dent. 2011;13:111–5.
82. Ricci HA, Sanabe ME, de Souza Costa CA, Pashley DH, Hebling J. Chlorhexidine increases the longevity of in vivo resin-dentin bonds. Eur J Oral Sci. 2010 Oct;118:535.
83. Pupo YM, Farago PV, Nadal JM, Simão LC, Esmerino LA, Gomes OMM, et al. Effect of a novel quaternary ammonium methacrylate polymer (QAMP) on adhesion and antibacterial properties of dental adhesives. Int J Mol Sci. 2014;15:8998–9015.
84. Imazato S, Kuramoto A, Takahashi Y, Ebisu S, Peters MC. In vitro antibacterial effects of dentin primer of Clearfil Protect Bond. Dent Mater. 2006;22: 527–32.
85. Sabatini C, Patel SK. Matrix metalloproteinase inhibitory properties of benzalkonium chloride stabilizes adhesive interfaces. Eur J Oral Sci. 2013;121: 610–6.
86. Feuerstein O, Matalon S, Slutzky H, Weiss EI. Antibacterial properties of self-etching dental adhesive systems. J Am Dent Assoc. 2007;138:349–54.
87. Brackett MG, Agee KA, Brackett WW, Key WO, Sabatini C, Kato MT, Buzalaf MA, Tjäderhane L, Pashley DH. Effect of sodium fluoride on the endogenous MMP activity of dentin matrices. J Nat Sci. 2015;1:e118.
88. Kato MT, Bolanho A, Zarella BL, Salo T, Tjäderhane L, Buzalaf MAR. Sodium Fluoride Inhibits MMP-2 and MMP-9. J Dent Res 2013;93(1):74–77.
89. Altinci P, Mutluay M, Seseogullari-Dirihan R, Pashley D, Tjäderhane L, Tezvergil-Mutluay A. NaF inhibits matrix-bound Cathepsin-mediated dentin matrix degradation. Caries Res. 2016;50: 124–32.
90. Mei ML, Ito L, Cao Y, Li QL, Chu CH, Lo EC. The inhibitory effects of silver diamine fluorides on cysteine cathepsins. J Dent. 2014;42:329–35.
91. Tjäderhane L, Nascimento FD, Breschi L, Mazzoni A, Tersariol ILS, Geraldeli S, et al. Strategies to prevent hydrolytic degradation of the hybrid layer – a review. Dent Mater. 2013;29:999–1011.
92. Chiang YS, Chen YL, Chuang SF, Wu CM, Wei PJ, Han CF, et al. Riboflavin-ultraviolet-A-induced collagen cross-linking treatments in improving dentin bonding. Dent Mater. 2013;29:682–92.
93. Mazzoni A, Angeloni V, Apolonio FM, Scotti N, Tjäderhane L, Tezvergil-Mutluay A, et al. Effect of carbodiimide (EDC) on the bond stability of etch-and-rinse adhesive systems. Dent Mater. 2013;29: 1040–7.

94. Bedran-Russo AK, Pashley DH, Agee K, Drummond JL, Miescke KJ. Changes in stiffness of demineralized dentin following application of collagen crosslinkers. J Biomed Mater Res B Appl Biomater. 2008;86:330–4.
95. Fang M, Liu R, Xiao Y, Li F, Wang D, Hou R, et al. Biomodification to dentin by a natural crosslinker improved the resin-dentin bonds. J Dent. 2012;40:458–66.
96. Scheffel DL, Hebling J, Scheffel RH, Agee K, Turco G, de Souza Costa CA, et al. Inactivation of matrix-bound matrix metalloproteinases by crosslinking agents in acid-etched dentin. Oper Dent. 2014;39:152–8.
97. Fawzy AS, Nitisusanta LI, Iqbal K, Daood U, Neo J. Riboflavin as a dentin crosslinking agent: ultraviolet A versus blue light. Dent Mater. 2012;28:1284–91.
98. Kim J, Gu L, Breschi L, Tjäderhane L, Choi KK, Pashley DH, et al. Implication of ethanol wet-bonding in hybrid layer remineralization. J Dent Res. 2010;89:575–80.
99. Pashley DH, Agee KA, Wataha JC, Rueggeberg F, Ceballos L, Itou K, et al. Viscoelastic properties of demineralized dentin matrix. Dent Mater. 2003;19:700–6.
100. Pashley DH, Tay FR, Carvalho RM, Rueggeberg FA, Agee KA, Carrilho M, et al. From dry bonding to water-wet bonding to ethanol-wet bonding. A review of the interactions between dentin matrix and solvated resins using a macromodel of the hybrid layer. Am J Dent. 2007;20:7–20.
101. Hosaka K, Nishitani Y, Tagami J, Yoshiyama M, Brackett WW, Agee KA, et al. Durability of resin-dentin bonds to water- vs. ethanol saturated dentin. J Dent Res. 2009;88:146–51.
102. Sadek FT, Mazzoni A, Breschi L, Tay FR, Braga RR. Six-month evaluation of adhesives interface created by a hydrophobic adhesive to acid-etched ethanol-wet bonded dentin with simplified dehydration protocols. J Dent. 2010;38:276–83.
103. Tay FR, Pashley DH, Kapur RR, Carrilho MR, Hur YB, Garrett LV, et al. Bonding BisGMA to dentin—a proof of concept for hydrophobic dentin bonding. J Dent Res. 2007;86:1034–9.
104. Nishitani Y, Yoshiyama M, Donnelly AM, Agee KA, Sword J, Tay FR, et al. Effects of resin hydrophilicity on dentin bond strength. J Dent Res. 2006;85:1016–21.
105. Sauro S, Toledano M, Aguilera FS, Mannocci F, Pashley DH, Tay FR, et al. Resin-dentin bonds to EDTA-treated vs. acid-etched dentin using ethanol wet-bonding. Dent Mater. 2010;36:368–79.
106. Sadek FT, Pashley DH, Ferrari M, Tay FR. Tubular occlusion optimizes bonding of hydrophobic resins to dentin. J Dent Res. 2007;86:524–8.
107. Sauro S, Watson TF, Mannocci F, Miyake K, Huffman BP, Tay FR, et al. Two-photon laser confocal microscopy of micropermeability of resin-dentin bonds made with water or ethanol wet bonding. J Biomed Mater Res B Appl Biomater. 2009;90:327–37.
108. Malacarne-Zanon J, Pashley DH, Agee KA, Foulger S, Alves MC, Breschi L, et al. Effects of ethanol addition on the water sorption solubility and percent conversion of comonomers in model dental adhesives. Dent Mater. 2009;25:1275–84.
109. Ye Q, Park J, Topp E, Spencer P. Effect of photoinitiators on the in vitro performance of a dentin adhesive exposed to simulated oral environment. Dent Mater. 2009;25:452–8.
110. Park J, Ye Q, Topp EM, Misra A, Kieweg SL, Spencer P. Effect of photoinitiator system and water content on dynamic mechanical properties of a light-cured bisGMA/HEMA dental resin. J Biomed Mater Res A. 2010;93:1245–51.
111. Ikemura K, Ichizawa K, Fuchigami K, Ito S, Endo T. Design of a new dental adhesive—effect of a water-soluble sodium acylphosphine oxide with crown ether on adhesion to dental hard tissues. Dent Mater J. 2009;28:267–76.
112. Sauro S, Pashley DH. Strategies to stabilise dentin-bonded interfaces through remineralising operative approaches–state of the art. Int J Adhes Adhes. 2016;69:39–57.
113. Tay FR, Pashley DH. Biomimetic remineralization of resin-bonded acid-etched dentin. J Dent Res. 2009;88:719–24.
114. Kinney JH, Habelitz S, Marshall SJ, Marshall GW. The importance of intrafibrillar mineralization of collagen on the mechanical properties of dentin. J Dent Res. 2003;82:957–61.
115. Kim YK, Yiu CK, Kim JR, Gu L, Kim SK, Weller RN, Pashley DH, Tay FR. Failure of a glass ionomer to remineralise apatite-depleted dentin. J Dent Res. 2010;89:230–5.
116. Sauro S, Watson TF, Thompson I, Toledano M, Nucci C, Banerjee A. Influence of air-abrasion executed with polyacrylic acid-bioglass 45S5 on the bonding performance of a resin-modified glass ionomer cement. Eur J Oral Sci. 2012;120: 168–77.
117. Sauro S, Watson TF, Thompson I, Banerjee A. One-bottle self-etching adhesives applied to dentin air-abraded using bioactive glasses containing polyacrylic acid: an in vitro microtensile bond strength and confocal microscopy study. J Dent. 2012;40:896–905.
118. Atmeh AR, Chong EZ, Richard G, Festy F, Watson TF. Dentin-cement interfacial interaction: calcium silicates and polyalkenoates. J Dent Res. 2012;91:454–9.
119. Watson TF, Atmeh AR, Sajini S, Cook RJ, Festy F. Present and future of glass-ionomers and calcium-silicate cements as bioactive materials in dentistry: biophotonics-based interfacial analyses in health and disease. Dent Mater. 2014;30:50–61.
120. Nakajima M, Kunawarote S, Prasansuttiporn T, Tagami J. Bonding to caries-affected dentin. Jpn Dent Sci Rev. 2011;47:102–14.
121. Sauro S, Osorio R, Watson TF, Toledano M. Influence of phosphoproteins' biomimetic

analogs on remineralization of mineral-depleted resin-dentin interfaces created with ion-releasing resin-based systems. Dent Mater. 2015;31:759–77.
122. Abuna G, Feitosa VP, Correr AB, Cama G, Giannini M, Sinhoreti MA, Pashley DH, Sauro S. Bonding performance of experimental bioactive/biomimetic self-etch adhesives doped with calcium-phosphate fillers and biomimetic analogs of phosphoproteins. J Dent. 2016;52:79–86.
123. Al-Ammar A, Drummond JL, Bedran-Russo AK. The use of collagen cross-linking agents to enhance dentin bond strength. J Biomed Mater Res B Appl Biomater. 2009;91:419–24.
124. Sabatini C, Scheffel DL, Scheffel RH, Agee KA, Rouch K, Takahashi M, Breschi L, Mazzoni A, Tjäderhane L, Tay FR, Pashley DH. Dent Mater. 2014;30:752–8.
125. Peters MC, Mclean ME. Minimally invasive operative care. II. Contemporary techniques and materials: an overview. J Adhes Dent. 2001;3:17–31.
126. Bjørndal L, Reit C, Bruun G, Markvart M, Kjaeldgaard M, Näsman P, Thordrup M, Dige I, Nyvad B, Fransson H, Lager A, Ericson D, Petersson K, Olsson J, Santimano EM, Wennström A, Winkel P, Gluud C. Treatment of deep caries lesions in adults: randomized clinical trials comparing stepwise vs direct complete excavation, and direct pulp capping vs. partial pulpotomy. Eur J Oral Sci. 2010;118:290–7.
127. Bortoluzzi EA, Niu LN, Palani CD, El-Awady AR, Hammond BD, Pei DD, Tian FC, Cutler CW, Pashley DH, Tay FR. Cytotoxicity and osteogenic potential of silicate calcium cements as potential protective materials for pulpal revascularization. Dent Mater. 2015;31:1510–22.

Polymerization Shrinkage Stress

14

Luis Felipe Schneider and Rafael R. Moraes

14.1 Introduction

Resin composite has been widely used and is the first choice as restorative material in dentistry due to the possibility to perform minimally invasive, or noninvasive, treatments associated with favorable properties and reliable clinical performance.

Despite many advantages, some drawbacks have been described in the scientific literature, and "shrinkage stress" has been widely cited as one of the most problematic ones [1, 2]. Basically, the shrinkage-derived stress is a resultant phenomenon from the polymerization process, which involves mass densification resultant from the molecular approximation of monomers when carbon double bonds are converted into single ones. Due to the clinical situations and restriction for material's flow by vitrification—such as the boundary conditions imposed by the surrounding cavity walls that were previously treated with an adhesive layer—the deformation of the growing polymer is restricted, and consequently, stress arises in the whole system [3, 4]. Therefore, a list of clinical consequences has been cited through the years in publications derived from numerous in vitro and few in vivo data. A recent study called into question how deleterious this phenomenon might be for long-term success of restorative procedures in a realistic clinical setting [5]. This doubt comes from the fact that it has not been possible to confirm a direct relationship between in vivo and in vitro data. Furthermore, recent publications have demonstrated that other factors related to personal and clinical conditions might overcome the importance of the polymerization shrinkage stress [6–11]. Nevertheless it is necessary to consider the importance of polymerization shrinkage stress and clarify its real effects on the resin composite restoration during function and, more importantly, to intensify knowledge transfer in education at all levels.

Over the last 10–15 years, extensive research in this field has been summarized in several literature reviews containing valuable data considering origins, ways of evaluation, and management of stress and is a mandatory source for those who seek a deeper insight [1–4, 12]. Polymerization stress is not a myth nor is its clinical significance even though state-of-the-art resin composites may exert fewer problems and consequences than did previous composite materials. The aim of this chapter is to provide a critical overview and, somehow, raise in readers' minds the

L.F. Schneider (✉)
Veiga de Almeida University, Rio de Janeiro, Brazil

School of Dentistry, Federal Fluminense University, Niterói, Brazil
e-mail: felipefop@gmail.com

R.R. Moraes
Graduate Program in Dentistry, Federal University of Pelotas, Pelotas, Brazil

V. Miletic (ed.), *Dental Composite Materials for Direct Restorations*,
http://doi.org/10.1007/978-3-319-60961-4_14

question "what are we looking for when considering stress?"

14.2 Origins of Stress

The shrinkage stress phenomenon may be associated with two main origins: the polymerization process and clinical situations. Resin composites are typically formulated with ceramic-derived filler particles, treated with a coupling agent, dispersed into a resinous matrix usually formulated with methacrylate monomers. These monomers typically appear in the fluid state and need to be rapidly converted into rigid polymers through a polymerization process during the material's clinical application [13]. By using an initiator—photoinitiators are regularly used to facilitate materials handling and clinical applications—reactive radicals react with monomer molecules. Active centers are then created and propagate the polymerization process. The propagation reaction involves polymer chain growth by rapid sequential addition of monomer to the active centers via covalent bonds until the maximum degree of conversion of C=C double bond into C–C bond is achieved. During the polymerization process, van der Waals forces are substituted by covalent bonds, and the distances is reduced from 4 to approximately 1.5 Å, and, consequently, volumetric shrinkage occurs [14].

Besides shrinkage, the polymerization process also involves elastic modulus development, meaning that materials' flowability becomes restricted due to polymer chains' growth and vitrification and, thus, stress release becomes also reduced [3, 4]. It has also been considered that thermal variations may play an important role in material deformation during the polymerization reaction. It is of fundamental importance to consider that the polymerization process is dynamic and that the effect of speed of reaction, the rate of polymerization, has also been evaluated but with conflicting results [15–18].

In clinical situations, resin composites usually have to be placed inside cavities and are bonded to the surrounding walls. Therefore, the material deformation is restricted in these constrained conditions, thereby developing stresses. In 1987, Feilzer, de Gee, and Davidson [19] developed the well-known theory of the "configuration factor," or "C-factor", an approach considering that the ratio between bonded and unbonded surfaces might predict the relationship between confinement and stress development. Afterward, authors have demonstrated that the C-factor should not be solely considered, since the materials' used volume (the "V-factor"), or mass, and the condition—the compliance—of the surrounded areas of the remaining tooth need to be considered [20–23]. Han et al. [23] suggest the C-factor is a valid parameter in comparisons of restorations of identical shapes and volumes.

Some other issues regarding origins of stress must be addressed when considering the multiple situations that clinicians have to deal in the daily practice. It was demonstrated that increasing the local temperature and humidity might increase post-gel shrinkage and cusp deformation with higher shrinkage stresses at the tooth structure and tooth/restoration interface [24]. Also important are those factors that might occur just after the materials' final placement or as the patients leave the dental office. For example, Bicalho et al. [25] demonstrated that the contact on the tooth/composite restoration margin increases the stresses around the margins of the restoration. Another research has shown that relaxation of the shrinkage-derived stress might occur due to material expansion caused by liquid uptake (water, saliva, etc.) that might compensate the negative effects of stress [26].

14.3 Consequences

It has been suggested that polymerization-derived stresses might cause deleterious effects on the bonding area (with consequent formation of gaps, lack of adaptation, infiltration, "leakage," "secondary/recurrent caries"), cusp deflection (with tooth fracture as an extreme possible consequence), postoperative sensitivity, and reduction of clinical lifespan of composite restorations. However, questions have arisen over the true clinical significance of such possible shortcomings. Numerous papers have reported on in vitro evaluations, but very rarely have the data been derived from clinically-based systematic observations.

14.3.1 Consequences Related to the Bonding Area

It is believed that polymerization shrinkage leads to a competition between the internal composite stresses and the bonded interface, potentially leading to gap formation and consequent "microleakage" and "secondary," or "recurrent," caries lesions and/or marginal staining.

With the current data available in the literature, it is not possible to clearly state that the presence of "micro-gaps" would result in the formation of new caries lesions [27–31]. Besides, educators and researchers who deal with dental materials should keep in mind that caries is a behavioral disease and, undoubtedly, a question of patient's behavior and way of life, and then efforts must be driven to habit modifications. If not, we will continuously observe dental companies and researchers aiming to develop better materials to compensate the lack of proper education at all levels in dentistry. And, to date, no material is able to replace enamel and dentin as nature created these tissues. In addition, the clinical effectiveness of antibacterial adhesives and composites has not been confirmed.

Unlike "secondary caries," the resultant gap formation is clearly associated with higher marginal staining incidence [32]. Unfortunately, marginal staining is frequently associated with secondary/recurrent caries by many clinicians and subsequent repair or—much worse—premature substitution of the restoration [33]. Therefore, clinicians should be aware of stress management when dealing with composites, and it is of paramount importance that educators include teaching appropriate methods to determine the need for restorations' substitutions based on systematic criteria, considering not only the restoration per se but also patients' and clinicians' behavior and preferences. Another important aspect of marginal staining relies on the proper bonding procedures, as the adhesive layer is, unfortunately, semipermeable to oral fluids and, consequently, to infiltration of pigments during the years of service.

14.3.2 Cusp Deflection, Tooth Cracking, and Postoperative Sensitivity

Cusp deflection, tooth cracking, and postoperative sensitivity have been cited as the main consequences of volumetric shrinkage when the bond strength is superior to the developed stress [34]. Cusp deflection and tooth fracture are directly associated with the quality of the remaining surrounding area; thus, clinicians should be aware about the quality of the remaining tissues and cavity designs. It is obvious that within the perspective of minimally invasive dentistry, all efforts should be aimed at healthy tooth tissue preservation. However, both clinicians and patients must consider that premature failure might occur due to the unfavorable cavity design.

A recent publication demonstrates that the third most common reason for failure of posterior composite restorations during the 2006–2016 decade was tooth fracture, which changed from 3.45% in 1995–2005 to 23.76% in 2006–2016 [35]. The authors also state that fracture of restoration and of the tooth, together, represents 62.83% of failures in the 2006–2016 period compared with 32.29% in the 1995–2005 period. It could be hypothesized that such differences could be due to the use of more powerful light sources, but an increase in materials' fracture ratio has also been reported. The authors attribute this change to the increased and wider use of composite materials in complex and multi-surface cavities, which are known to be more prone to tooth and restoration fracture [35].

Postoperative sensitivity has been traditionally described in publications as a potential problem associated with stress. However, this aspect has to be critically analyzed, and nowadays postoperative sensitivity seems more related to difficulties in obtaining a proper hybrid layer in dentin [5, 27]. Postoperative sensitivity is not described as a common cause of premature failure in recent systematic reviews [10, 36]. Considering the approach by Alvanforoush et al. [35] who compared the clinical success of direct composite restorations in vital posterior teeth in two different time periods, it is possible to verify that the incidence of postoperative sensitivity decreased from 11.60% in studies published between 1995 and 2005 to 0.96% in studies published between 2006 and 2016. It is necessary to consider the fact that when resin composites were introduced for posterior restorations, general knowledge about bonding procedures, especially wet bonding associated with the total etch technique, and stress management was not sufficient and consequent pain was probably more frequent. Additionally, Alvanforoush's study [35] shows that different materials were used in the two decades, so we can speculate that the reduction in postoperative sensitivity over the last decade might also be associated with materials' improvements in terms of lower volumetric shrinkage.

14.3.3 What Is the Effect of Stress over the Restoration Longevity?

With the current data available in the literature, it is not possible to clearly state the real effect of stress on the final restoration longevity. However, recent findings on the long-term success of composite restorations show that some factors commonly associated with material properties might not be crucial for real clinical lifespan or could be suppressed by other factors that are out of clinician's control, such as patients' general behavior and socioeconomic status [7, 8].

Publications considering more than 20 or even 30 years of follow-up demonstrate that when the patients' conditions are favorable—i.e., low caries risk and no parafunctional habits—the annual failure rate is low, usually between 1% and 4% [7, 9, 36–38]. On the other hand, the annual failure rate varied between 2.3 and 7.9% in a recent study about longevity of direct restorations performed by Dutch dental practitioners [39]. Instead of claiming that material associated properties affect clinical lifespan, or that the amount of stress development may directly affect the clinical lifespan of a composite restoration, one should consider that education in dentistry has to be improved instead of solely relying on materials' development. There is also the possibility that such differences among clinicians might be related to differences in stress management.

14.4 Methods for Shrinkage and Stress Evaluation

Since polymerization stress is considered one of the main drawbacks of resin composites, a series of methods have been used throughout the years to determine strain and stress, and numerous publications with detailed explanations may be found in the literature.

A general list of methodologies used to determine shrinkage/strain must include the mercury dilatometer [40] (Fig. 14.1), the bonded-disc method developed by Watts and Cash [41] (Fig. 14.2), the strain gauges [42, 43], and the linometer [44]. More recently, some complex methods have been based on video and digital images [45–47]: laser speckle contrast analysis [48], the mathematical and computational models [49, 50], the X-ray microtomography [51–53], and optics [54, 55].

Stress development is not a material property but a consequence of multiple factors, and specific research methods have been used including the ring-slitting method [56, 57], photoelastic analysis [58, 59], finite element analysis [60, 61], mathematical models [45], force transducers [4, 19, 62–66], and, more recently, crack propagation in ceramics [67–69].

Force transducers have been widely used as the main method of stress development analyses. Although the basic principle is the same for all force transducers, there are different measurement approaches for each system, the instrument compliance being the most significant one [2].

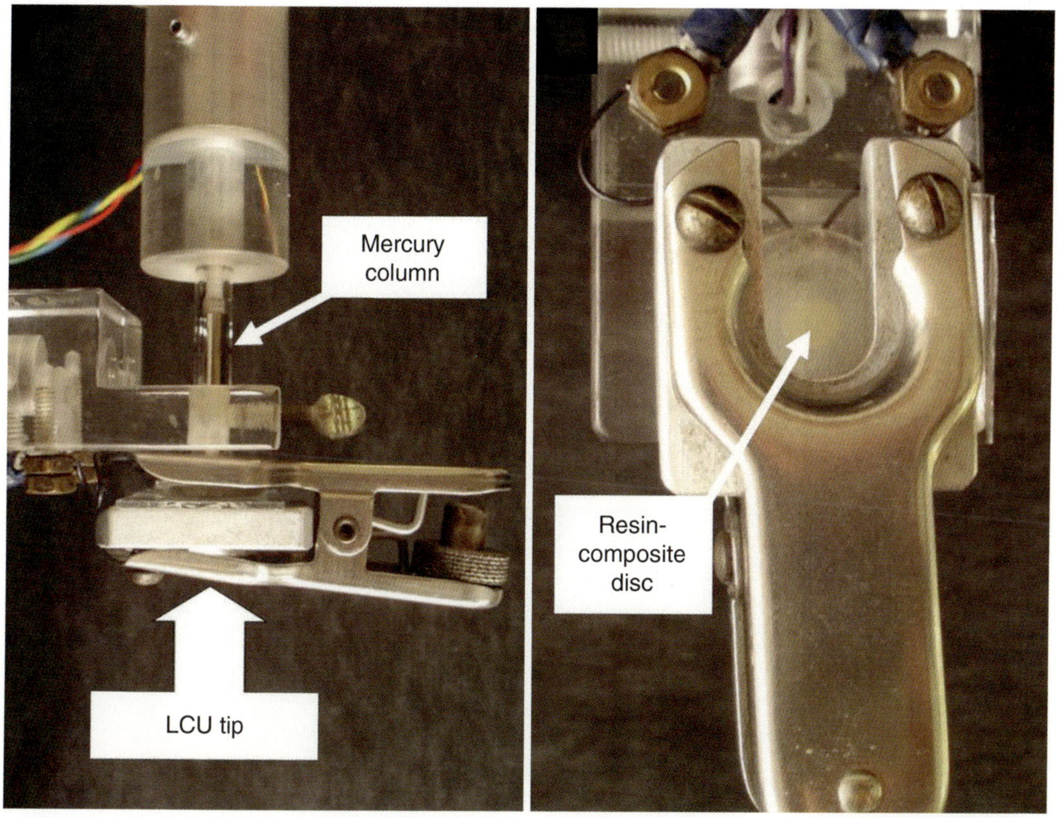

Fig. 14.1 (**a**) Mercury dilatometer. The figure shows a mercury column and the clasp that holds the resin composite sample and (**b**) the place where the LCU is positioned. These pictures were kindly donated by Dr. Carmen Silvia C. Pfeifer. Equipment is from the Division of Biomaterials and Biomechanics, School of Dentistry, Oregon Health & Sciences University (Portland, USA). The original picture was published in "Shrinkage Stresses Generated during Resin-Composite Applications: A Review. Schneider LF, Cavalcante LM, Silikas N. 2010; doi:10.4061/2010/131630"

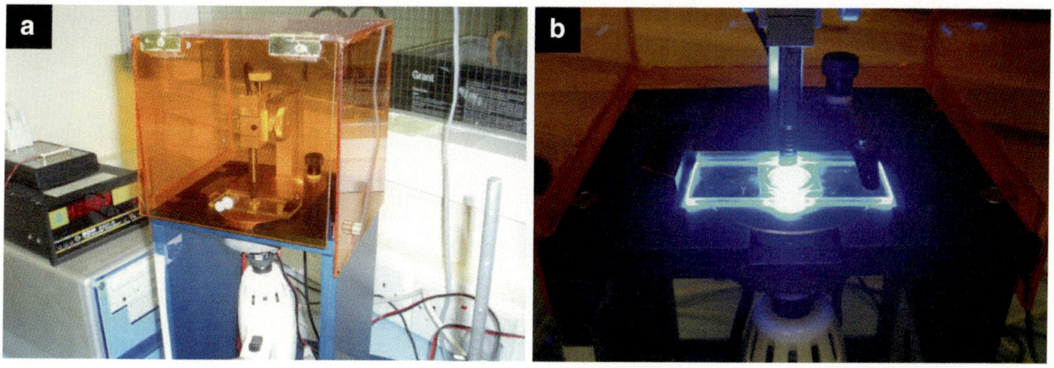

Fig. 14.2 The "Bonded-disc" apparatus. (**b**) A close view of the LVDT probe in contact with the glass slide during the resin composite photoactivation. Equipment is from the Biomaterials Research Group, School of Dentistry, University of Manchester (Manchester, UK). The original picture was published in "Shrinkage Stresses Generated during Resin-Composite Applications: A Review. Schneider LF, Cavalcante LM, Silikas N. 2010; doi:10.4061/2010/131630"

Universal testing machines modified with extensometers connected to a computer unit are very precise and can identify movement of extension caused by the polymerization shrinkage and by feedback response compensate deformations, while the sample's length remains constant (Fig. 14.3). This system does not allow material deformation, and consequently, the registered values of stress tend to be higher than by more compliant methods [70]. Some variations exist within this method, and a significant one is the kind of substrate to which the resin composite sample is attached [71].

There are also force transducers adapted to systems with unknown or calculated compliance [18, 21, 22, 49, 64, 72, 73] (Figs. 14.4 and 14.5). Unfortunately, besides variations in the final stress values, the comparisons among different materials can also be affected [2], and different interpretations about a given aspect may also vary when all these methods are used. Therefore, it must be clear that care should be taken when analyzing stress data, since the system compliance should also be considered. As the final objective of the in vitro research is to provide valid data that simulate the clinical

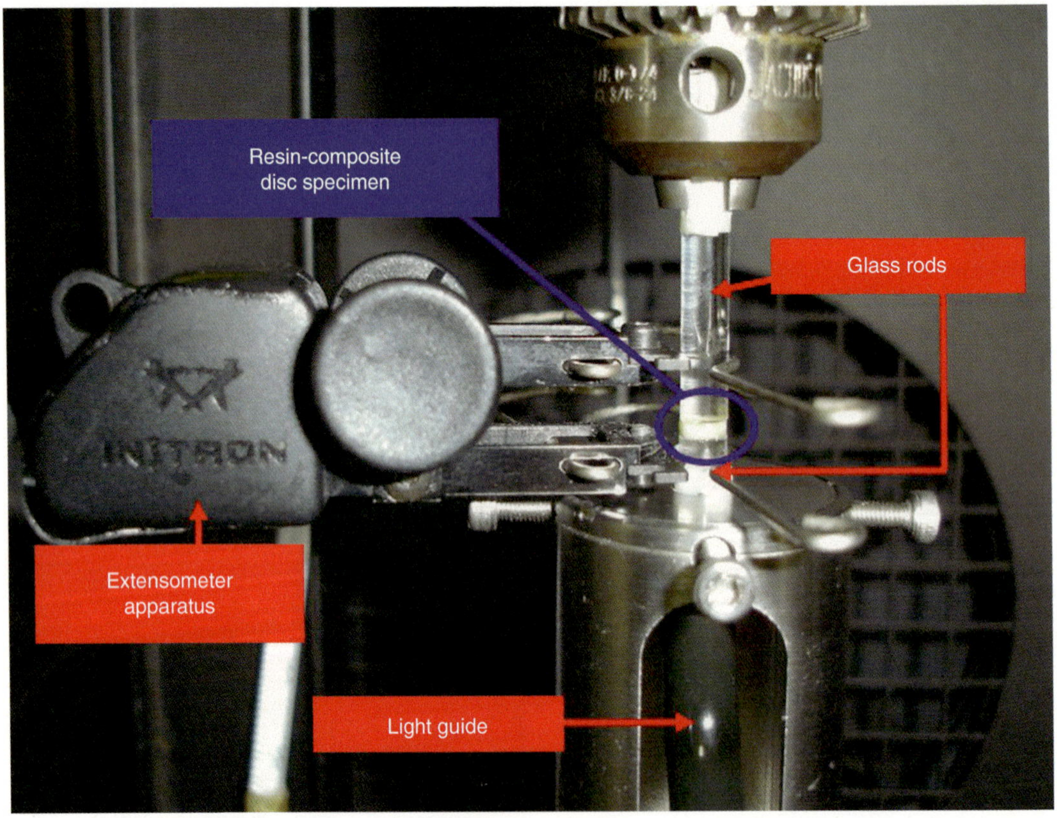

Fig. 14.3 Extensometer apparatus connected to a universal testing machine. As a feedback response, the system compensates deformations, and the sample remains constant. Consequently, this kind of method is known as a "low-compliant method." Pictures kindly donated by Dr. Carmen Silvia C. Pfeifer. Equipment is from the School of Dentistry, University of São Paulo (São Paulo, Brazil). The original picture was published in "Shrinkage Stresses Generated during Resin-Composite Applications: A Review. Schneider LF, Cavalcante LM, Silikas N. 2010; doi:10.4061/2010/131630"

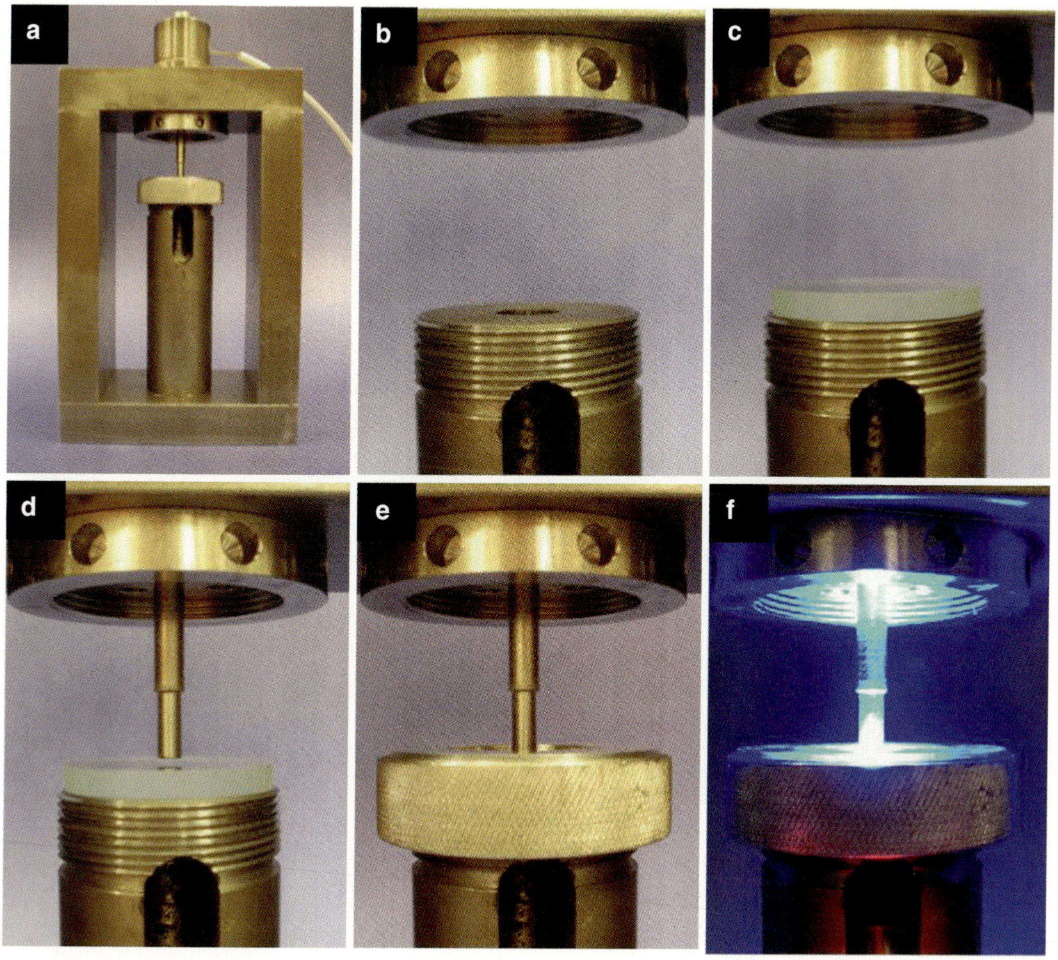

Fig. 14.4 Controlled compliance apparatus for contraction stress test. (**a**) The entire apparatus with a view of the steel frame and the upper load cell holder; (**b**) slot for light guide; (**c**) glass plate positioned; (**d**) steel piston in position and the space where the resin composite specimen is positioned; (**e**) equipment ready for use and (**f**) light-curing procedure during an experiment. These pictures were kindly donated by Dr. Carmen Silvia C. Pfeifer. Equipment is from Division of Biomaterials and Biomechanics, the School of Dentistry, Oregon Health & Sciences University (Portland, USA). The original picture was published in "Shrinkage Stresses Generated during Resin-Composite Applications: A Review. Schneider LF, Cavalcante LM, Silikas N. 2010; doi:10.4061/2010/131630"

situations, instrument compliance should be similar to that of the prepared tooth [20]. Wang and Chiang recently demonstrated that the correlation between polymerization shrinkage stress and the C-factor [21] and also the effect of composite filler content on stress development depend on the compliance of the testing instrument [22]. Unfortunately, to date, there are no studies on the validation of polymerization stress analysis based on clinical conditions.

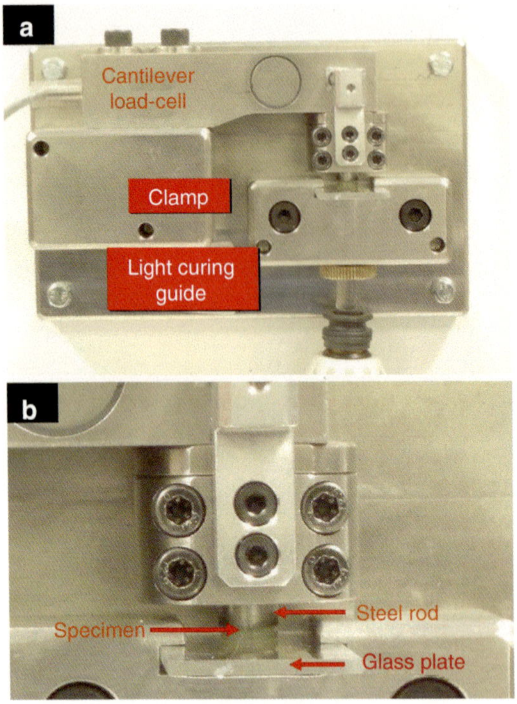

Fig. 14.5 (**a**) The Bioman stress measurement device. (**b**) A close view of the resin composite specimen. Equipment is from the Biomaterials Research Group, School of Dentistry, University of Manchester (Manchester, UK). The original picture was published in "Shrinkage Stresses Generated during Resin-Composite Applications: A Review. Schneider LF, Cavalcante LM, Silikas N. 2010; doi:10.4061/2010/131630"

14.5 Stress Control by Clinical Management

Several attempts have been suggested to control or reduce stress development during placement of resin composites. The placement, or filling, technique—incremental vs. bulk—and the photoactivation protocols are under clinicians' control and have been widely advocated. The use of stress-absorbing layers and thermally modified composites theoretically could reduce stress development, but these two approaches have not become the standard of care. Model and experimental materials have been extensively used to understand the stress phenomenon and to find ways of reduction. Nevertheless only a few new formulations have become commercially available but without guarantees of stress reduction, such as "ormocers," dimer acid, and "silorane"-based materials [74, 75].

14.5.1 Placement Techniques

The incremental layering techniques have been advocated due to the inherent confinement of cavities. The rationale is that shrinkage may be less detrimental when there are fewer bonded cavity walls involved at each stage of the restoration procedures. Furthermore, such techniques also enhance the degree of conversion as thin sections undergo higher degree of cure due to lower light attenuation, yielding better mechanical properties [76].

For a long time, the filling technique has been a matter of discussion [34, 60, 77] and came to focus again with the launch of bulk-fill resin composites, which will be addressed further below. The literature is not conclusive concerning the advantages promoted by the incremental layering technique over the effects of resin composite polymerization shrinkage. Versluis et al. [60] assessed the developing stress fields for different incremental filling techniques by finite element analysis (FEA) and concluded that the incremental filling technique increased the deformation of the restored tooth and could actually produce higher polymerization stresses at the restoration interface compared with bulk filling, particularly when many small increments and consecutive light activations are used [78, 79]. Additionally, multiple increments showed to induce greater cuspal movement than a bulk increment in cuspal deflection measurements of premolars [80]. Loguercio et al. [81] reported that some evaluated effects of polymerization shrinkage such as gap width, adhesive bond strength, and the cohesive strength of the resin composite were not reduced by the filling technique under the different C-factor cavities. Lee et al. [82] observed that cusp deflection increased with increasing cavity dimension and C-factor; thus, the use of an incremental filling technique or an indirect composite inlay restoration could reduce the cuspal strain. Conversely, Park et al. [76] found that the bulk-filling technique yielded significantly more cuspal deflection than the incremental filling techniques, concluding that cuspal deflection resulting from polymerization shrinkage can be reduced by incremental filling techniques to obtain optimal outcomes in clinical situations.

Despite the controversy over the advantages of incremental buildup of resin composites, this technique has been broadly recommended for direct resin composite restorations to assure sufficient polymerization in deep cavities with the traditional materials [83].

14.5.2 Photoactivation Protocols

Photoactivation protocols that were theoretically able to control or reduce stress were strongly suggested in the past. The explanation is that stress release is possible by viscous flow before the vitrification stage, popularly called as the pre-gel state, without compromising the final polymer properties and became very popular with clinicians [84–86]. It has been accepted that initial light exposure at lower irradiance values would lead to the formation of a reduced number of polymer growth centers, slowing down the reaction and decreasing the rate and the final stress development due to increased time for polymer relaxation. Some outcomes suggest that a possible stress reduction is derived from lower degree of conversion [87].

Despite large breadth of in vitro studies about curing protocols such as soft-start and pulse-delay, scientific literature lacks data from clinical trials. A few studies have suggested that those alternative protocols do not have a measurable effect on the longevity of composite restorations [88–91]. In another publication, the significance of the C-factor has been questioned in a scenario with low failure after 12 years in cavities with a high C-factor [6]. However, Ferracane and Hilton [5] suggest that the excellent outcomes found by van Dijken [6] also "resulted from the efforts to reduce or minimize stress by the curing methods used."

By careful analyses of articles derived from clinical trials, it is possible to relate scientific evidence of certain material properties with clinical outcomes. In a 30-year follow-up of three dental composites, it was found that the chemically-cured resin composites showed better performance than the light-cured composite [38] contrary to expectations. However, the rate of polymerization for chemically-cured materials is known to be lower than that of photoactivated, and, therefore, stress release would be possible. It is also necessary to consider the chance of poor conversion of the photoactivated material, especially considering the light sources available 30 years ago and the lack of familiarity in clinical use of light-curable composites for posterior restorations by clinicians at that time.

14.5.3 Stress-Absorbing Layers

The suggested use of flowable composites as "stress-absorbing layers" is based on the "elastic cavity wall concept." Although controversial, this concept suggests that the shrinkage stress generated by a subsequent layer of higher modulus resin composite can be absorbed by an elastic intermediary layer, thereby reducing the stress at the tooth-restoration interface manifested clinically as a reduction in cuspal deflection [92–95]. However, van Dijken and Pallesen [96] found that flowable resin composite as an intermediate layer did not result in improved effectiveness in Class II restorations during a 7-year evaluation period.

A different approach is the use of glass ionomer cements to replace part of the tooth and reduce the amount of the shrinkable composite. However, the systematic review by Opdam et al. [10] clearly demonstrated no benefits of using this technique. In fact, a possibility of higher prevalence of fractures was suggested due to differences of elastic moduli and consequent fatigue over time.

14.5.4 Pre-warming Composites

The idea behind pre-warming composites is that increased temperature decreases system viscosity and enhances radical mobility, resulting in additional polymerization and higher conversion [97, 98]. At raised temperatures, in theory, it would be possible to obtain higher degree of conversion before the vitrification point, decreasing the magnitude of stress [99]. In a recent study by Tauböck et al. [98], the authors demonstrated that composite pre-warming reduced the shrinkage stress formation of high-viscosity bulk-fill and conventional resin composites while maintaining or increasing degree of conversion. Apart from in vitro data, there are no published clinical data. It should be pointed out that such pre-warming composites could increase technique sensitivity/variability or only be useful for marketing new gadgets.

14.6 Stress Development Understanding and Control Related to Material Composition

Undoubtedly serious academic research in the field of dental materials science has provided theories and knowledge that have become widely accepted in both the academic and clinical community, improving education of dentists and clinical practice as well as development of new materials. At this point, a few questions should be pointed out: how many "experimental materials" do indeed find their way to the market? And do those marketed materials indeed affect the final clinical outcome? Is this a cost-effective model?

Since Bowen's pioneering work resulting in BisGMA-based formulations, the basic principles of dental composites have changed very little. But it was from the industry that we saw the evolution from paste-to-paste mixed formulations to nowadays materials that facilitate clinicians' work and improved restoration general qualities. Nevertheless, stress development reduction is still a matter of concern, and dental industry has launched the so-called low-shrinkage materials over the years. However, there is no evidence that such "improvements" do have a positive effect on the performance of composite restorations. In a fierce competition on the dental market, the manufacturers are sometimes urged by marketing rather than scientific needs to launch new materials. Yet it is the duty of the scientific community to critically ascertain new materials and their effects on clinical practice.

14.6.1 Model and Experimental Composites

Model composites are valuable means to systematically understand the effect of materials' components on their final properties and behavior [100–104]. One very interesting study, for example, was published by Gonçalves et al. [103]. By using different concentrations of BisGMA and TEGDMA and/or BisEMA as comonomers, the authors analyzed the contraction stress determinants in dimethacrylate composites and demonstrated that the association between polymerization stress and conversion ($R^2 = 0.905$) was higher than stress and shrinkage ($R^2 = 0.825$) and stress and elastic modulus ($R^2 = 0.623$).

Recent studies have shown that ester-free thiol-ene derivatives exhibit lower shrinkage stress and moisture absorption than conventional BisGMA/TEGDMA resin and that low viscosity allows high filler content [105, 106]. Thio-urethane oligomers improved conversion and mechanical properties with reduced shrinkage and stress of model resin cements in a study by Bacchi et al. [107]. As stated by the authors, the success was accomplished by the use of photoinitiators commonly applied in commercial materials, which facilitates the benchtop to chairside implementation of such additives without changing common operatory procedures. Improved conversion and mechanical properties allied with lower stress values were also found for restorative composite by the same group [108]. Although promising, there is a long way until such innovations become potentially useful for the market.

14.6.2 Commercially Available Materials

Methacrylate-based materials represent the vast majority of commercially available materials and have been used to systematically understand shrinkage stress phenomenon through in vitro tests

[74, 75]. Considering clinical data within systematic reviews, methacrylate-based hybrid composites have demonstrated the best performance over the years [7, 33, 109]. At this point, a question may be asked: if such materials are still the gold standard and several developments were claimed over the last years, why do we not see major clinical success? A possible explanation may be the fact that clinical trials are often performed in very well-controlled conditions, such as experienced operators with proper time for careful execution of all procedures, highly motivated patients with low caries risk, etc. The question is whether or not the new materials would impact the clinical performance in not so well-controlled conditions. Anyway, it may be assumed that clinical success is possible with materials available on the market in the last 10 years.

Silorane-based materials and bulk-fill composites represent two interesting groups of commercially available materials that caught attention of the scientific community. Silorane-based materials were launched promising less than 1% volumetric shrinkage and quickly became largely investigated materials [75, 110, 111]. It is possible to find more than 300 articles published over the past 10 years on PubMed by simple typing "silorane AND dental." Unfortunately, silorane-based materials failed to produce significant improvements in both in vitro and in vivo studies and are off the market today. In addition, a recent systematic review of clinical studies showed no gain in clinical performance of silorane compared with methacrylate-based resin composites [112].

Currently "bulk-fill" composites are in focus of a number of studies [113–117]. Although dental companies might claim certain innovative components—like specific photoinitiators and polymerization modulators—these materials are, in fact, derived from a combination of well-known possibilities. The use of UDMA-based molecules, the better matching of refractive indexes from monomers and filler particles, and the affordable high-intensity light sources are some of them. It should be highlighted that the use of bulk-fill composites is encouraged on the notion that stress development would not be a detrimental adverse effect. Only few studies have been conducted with such materials and have provided good results in the studies with no more than 5-6 years [118, 119]. More clinical data is necessary to answer those questions arising from in vitro studies [113–116].

14.7 Final Thoughts: What Do We Need to Look For?

Longevity of direct restorations is related to many factors including patient's general and health conditions and the clinical condition of the tooth to be restored—such as the volume of remaining walls, previous endodontic treatment, and others—but also the clinician who executes the procedure. The understanding of materials handling characteristics is crucial for the success of any clinical procedure pointing to the need for better teaching strategies.

The present discussion has not the intention to underestimate the importance of polymerization shrinkage stress in direct restorations since this phenomenon was part of a series of industrial developments and academic research over the last years leading to the current state of dental composites. However, the lack of clear clinical evidence about the effect of shrinkage stress on the restoration longevity suggests that shrinkage stress alone may not be of such a great interest. Clinical trials comparing a wide range of materials have hardly shown differences that might be related to shrinkage stress. A slow decline in the volume of published data on the phenomenon, even in vitro studies, also suggests that this topic may not be the main problem of resin composites as it was believed in recent past. It is, however, important to keep an open mind with regard to those aspects that clearly influence the treatment immediate success and restoration longevity. Although this entire chapter aimed to address direct restorations, researchers and clinicians should be aware of potential negative effects of polymerization stress when resin composites are applied as luting materials (as resin cements, flowable composites or thermally-modified resin composites) for indirect restorations - specially those fabricated with ceramics - due to the very high constriction and low compliant situation.

References

1. Ferracane JL. Developing a more complete understanding of stresses produced in dental composites during polymerization. Dent Mater. 2005;21(1):36–42.
2. Ferracane JL. Buonocore Lecture. Placing dental composites – a stressful experience. Oper Dent. 2008;33(3):247–57.
3. Braga RR, Ferracane JL. Alternatives in polymerization contraction stress management. Crit Rev Oral Biol Med. 2004;15(3):176–84.
4. Braga RR, Ballester RY, Ferracane JL. Factors involved in the development of polymerization shrinkage stress in resin-composites: a systematic review. Dent Mater. 2005;21(10):962–70.
5. Ferracane JL, Hilton TJ. Polymerization stress – is it clinically meaningful? Dent Mater. 2016;32(1):1–10.
6. van Dijken JW. Durability of resin composite restorations in high C-factor cavities: a 12-year follow-up. J Dent. 2010;38(6):469–74.
7. Demarco FF, Corrêa MB, Cenci MS, Moraes RR, Opdam NJ. Longevity of posterior composite restorations: not only a matter of materials. Dent Mater. 2012;28(1):87–101.
8. Correa MB, Peres MA, Peres KG, Horta BL, Barros AJ, Demarco FF. Do socioeconomic determinants affect the quality of posterior dental restorations? A multilevel approach. J Dent. 2013;41(11):960–7.
9. van de Sande FH, Opdam NJ, Rodolpho PA, Correa MB, Demarco FF, Cenci MS. Patient risk factors' influence on survival of posterior composites. J Dent Res. 2013;92(7 Supplement):78S–83S.
10. Opdam NJM, van de Sande FH, Bronkhorst E, Cenci MS, Bottenberg P, Pallesen U, Gaengler P, Lindberg A, Huysmans MCDNJM, van Dijken JWV. Longevity of posterior composite restorations: a systematic review and meta-analysis. J Dent Res. 2014;93(10):943–9.
11. van Dijken JW, Lindberg A. A 15-year randomized controlled study of a reduced shrinkage stress resin composite. Dent Mater. 2015;31(9):1150–8.
12. Cramer NB, Stansbury JW, Bowman CN. Recent advances and developments in composite dental restorative materials. J Dent Res. 2011;90(4):402–16.
13. Schneider LF, Cavalcante LM, Silikas N. Shrinkage stresses generated during resin-composite applications: a review. J Dent Biomech. 2010:1–14. doi:10.4061/2010/131630.
14. Loshaek S, Fox TG. Cross-linked polymers. I. Factors influencing the efficiency of cross-linking in copolymers of methyl methacrylate and glycol dimethacrylate. J Am Chem Soc. 1953;75(14):3544–50.
15. Cunha LG, Alonso RC, Pfeifer CS, Correr-Sobrinho L, Ferracane JL, Sinhoreti MA. Modulated photoactivation methods: influence on contraction stress, degree of conversion and push-out bond strength of composite restoratives. J Dent. 2007;35(4):318–24.
16. Pfeifer CS, Ferracane JL, Sakaguchi RL, Braga RR. Factors affecting photopolymerization stress in dental composites. J Dent Res. 2008;87(11):1043–7.
17. Palin WM, Hadis MA, Leprince JG, Leloup G, Boland L, Fleming GJ, Krastl G, Watts DC. Reduced polymerization stress of MAPO-containing resin composites with increased curing speed, degree of conversion and mechanical properties. Dent Mater. 2014;30(5):507–16.
18. Wang Z, Landis FA, Giuseppetti AA, Lin-Gibson S, Chiang MY. Simultaneous measurement of polymerization stress and curing kinetics for photopolymerized composites with high filler contents. Dent Mater. 2014;30(12):1316–24.
19. Feilzer AJ, De Gee AJ, Davidson CL. Setting stress in composite resin in relation to configuration of the restoration. J Dent Res. 1987;66(11):1636–9.
20. Watts DC, Satterthwaite JD. Axial shrinkage-stress depends upon both C-factor and composite mass. Dent Mater. 2008;24(1):1–8.
21. Wang Z, Chiang MY. Correlation between polymerization shrinkage stress and C-factor depends upon cavity compliance. Dent Mater. 2016;32(3):343–52.
22. Wang Z, Chiang MY. System compliance dictates the effect of composite filler content on polymerization shrinkage stress. Dent Mater. 2016;32(4):551–60.
23. Han SH, Sadr A, Tagami J, Park SH. Internal adaptation of resin composites at two configurations: influence of polymerization shrinkage and stress. Dent Mater. 2016;32(9):1085–94.
24. Bicalho AA, de Souza SJ, de Rosatto CM, Tantbirojn D, Versluis A, Soares CJ. Effect of temperature and humidity on post-gel shrinkage, cusp deformation, bond strength and shrinkage stress – construction of a chamber to simulate the oral environment. Dent Mater. 2015;31(12):1523–32.
25. Bicalho AA, Tantbirojn D, Versluis A, Soares CJ. Effect of occlusal loading and mechanical properties of resin composite on stress generated in posterior restorations. Am J Dent. 2014;27(3):129–33.
26. Suiter EA, Watson LE, Tantbirojn D, Lou JS, Versluis A. Effective expansion: balance between shrinkage and hygroscopic expansion. J Dent Res. 2016;95(5):543–9.
27. Sarrett DC. Clinical challenges and the relevance of materials testing for posterior composite restorations. Dent Mater. 2005;21(1):9–20.
28. Cenci MS, Tenuta LM, Pereira-Cenci T, Del Bel Cury AA, ten Cate JM, Cury JA. Effect of microleakage and fluoride on enamel-dentine demineralization around restorations. Caries Res. 2008;42(5):369–79.
29. Cenci MS, Pereira-Cenci T, Cury JA, Ten Cate JM. Relationship between gap size and dentine secondary caries formation assessed in a microcosm biofilm model. Caries Res. 2009;43(2):97–102.
30. Nedeljkovic I, Teughels W, De Munck J, Van Meerbeek B, Van Landuyt KL. Is secondary caries with composites a material-based problem? Dent Mater. 2015;31:e247–77.
31. Jokstad A. Secondary caries and microleakage. Dent Mater. 2016;32:11–25.

32. Ferracane JL, Mitchem JC. Relationship between composite contraction stress and leakage in Class V cavities. Am J Dent. 2003;16(4):239–43.
33. Heintze SD, Rousson V, Hickel R. Clinical effectiveness of direct anterior restorations – a meta-analysis. Dent Mater. 2015;31(5):481–95.
34. Rosatto CM, Bicalho AA, Veríssimo C, Bragança GF, Rodrigues MP, Tantbirojn D, Versluis A, Soares CJ. Mechanical properties, shrinkage stress, cuspal strain and fracture resistance of molars restored with bulk-fill composites and incremental filling technique. J Dent. 2015;43(12):1519–28.
35. Alvanforoush N, Palamara J, Wong R, Burrow MF. A Comparison between published clinical success of direct resin composite restorations in vital posterior teeth in 1995–2005 and 2006–2016 periods. Aust Dent J. 2017;62(2):132–45. doi:10.1111/adj.12487.
36. Demarco FF, Collares K, Coelho-de-Souza FH, Correa MB, Cenci MS, Moraes RR, Opdam NJ. Anterior composite restorations: a systematic review on long-term survival and reasons for failure. Dent Mater. 2015;31(10):1214–24.
37. Da Rosa Rodolpho PA, Donassollo TA, Cenci MS, Loguércio AD, Moraes RR, Bronkhorst EM, Opdam NJ, Demarco FF. 22-year clinical evaluation of the performance of two posterior composites with different filler characteristics. Dent Mater. 2011;27(10):955–63.
38. Pallesen U, van Dijken JW. A randomized controlled 30 years follow up of three conventional resin composites in Class II restorations. Dent Mater. 2015;31(10):1232–44.
39. Laske M, Opdam NJ, Bronkhorst EM, Braspenning JC, Huysmans MC. Longevity of direct restorations in Dutch dental practices. Descriptive study out of a practice based research network. J Dent. 2016;46:12–7.
40. de Gee AJ, Davidson CL, Smith A. A modified dilatometer for continuous recording of volumetric polymerization shrinkage of composite restorative materials. J Dent. 1981;9(1):36–42.
41. Watts DC, Cash AJ. Determination of polymerization shrinkage kinetics in visible-light-cured materials: methods development. Dent Mater. 1991;7(4):281–7.
42. Sakaguchi RL, Sasik CT, Bunczak MA, Douglas WH. Strain gauge method for measuring polymerization contraction of composite restoratives. J Dent. 1991;19(5):312–6.
43. Sakaguchi RL, Peters MC, Nelson SR, Douglas WH, Poort HW. Effects of polymerization contraction in composite restorations. J Dent. 1992;20(3):178–82.
44. de Gee AF, Feilzer AJ, Davidson CL. True linear polymerization shrinkage of unfilled resins and composites determined with a linometer. Dent Mater. 1993;9(1):11–4.
45. Li J, Li H, Fok SL. A mathematical analysis of shrinkage stress development in dental composite restorations during resin polymerization. Dent Mater. 2008;24(7):923–31.
46. Miletic V, Manojlovic D, Milosevic M, Mitrovic N, Stankovic TS, Maneski T. Analysis of local shrinkage patterns of self-adhering and flowable composites using 3D digital image correlation. Quintessence Int. 2011;42(9):797–804.
47. Fok AS. Shrinkage stress development in dental composites – an analytical treatment. Dent Mater. 2013;29(11):1108–15.
48. Sato T, Miyazaki M, Rikuta A. Real-time dimensional change in light-cured composites at various depths using laser speckle contrast analysis. Eur J Oral Sci. 2004;112(6):538–44.
49. Sakaguchi RL, Wiltbank BD, Murchison CF. Prediction of composite elastic modulus and polymerization shrinkage by computational micromechanics. Dent Mater. 2004;20(4):397–401.
50. Atai M, Watts DC. A new kinetic model for the photopolymerization shrinkage-strain of dental composites and resin-monomers. Dent Mater. 2006;22(8):785–91.
51. Kakaboura A, Rahiotis C, Watts DC, Silikas N, Eliades G. 3D-marginal adaptation versus setting shrinkage in light-cured microhybrid resin composites. Dent Mater. 2007;23(3):272–8.
52. Sun J, Eidelman N, Lin-Gibson S. 3D mapping of polymerization shrinkage using X-ray micro-computed tomography to predict microleakage. Dent Mater. 2009;25(3):314–20.
53. Van Ende A, Van de Casteele E, Depypere M, De Munck J, Li X, Maes F, Wevers M, Van Meerbeek B. 3D volumetric displacement and strain analysis of composite polymerization. Dent Mater. 2015;31(4):453–61.
54. Kweon HJ, Ferracane J, Kang K, Dhont J, Lee IB. Spatio-temporal analysis of shrinkage vectors during photo-polymerization of composite. Dent Mater. 2013;29(12):1236–43.
55. Tantbirojn D, Pfeifer CS, Amini AN, Versluis A. Simple optical method for measuring free shrinkage. Dent Mater. 2015;31(11):1271–8.
56. Park JW, Ferracane JL. Measuring the residual stress in dental composites using a ring slitting method. Dent Mater. 2005;21(9):882–9.
57. Park JW, Ferracane JL. Residual stress in composites with the thin-ring-slitting approach. J Dent Res. 2006;85(10):945–9.
58. Ernst CP, Meyer GR, Klöcker K, Willershausen B. Determination of polymerization shrinkage stress by means of a photoelastic investigation. Dent Mater. 2004;20(4):313–21.
59. Kinomoto Y, Torii M. Photoelastic analysis of polymerization contraction stresses in resin composite restorations. J Dent. 1998;26(2):165–71.
60. Versluis A, Douglas WH, Cross M, Sakaguchi RL. Does an incremental filling technique reduce polymerization shrinkage stresses? J Dent Res. 1996;75(3):871–8.
61. Versluis A, Tantbirojn D, Douglas WH. Do dental composites always shrink toward the light? J Dent Res. 1998;77(6):1435–45.
62. Davidson CL, de Gee AJ. Relaxation of polymerization contraction stresses by flow in dental composites. J Dent Res. 1984;63(2):146–8.

63. Condon JR, Ferracane JL. Assessing the effect of composite formulation on polymerization stress. J Am Dent Assoc. 2000;131(4):497–503.
64. Watts DC, Marouf AS, Al-Hindi AM. Photo-polymerization shrinkage-stress kinetics in resin-composites: methods development. Dent Mater. 2003;19(1):1–11.
65. Braga RR, Ferracane JL. Contraction stress related to degree of conversion and reaction kinetics. J Dent Res. 2002;81(2):114–8.
66. Braga RR, Boaro LC, Kuroe T, Azevedo CL, Singer JM. Influence of cavity dimensions and their derivatives (volume and 'C' factor) on shrinkage stress development and microleakage of composite restorations. Dent Mater. 2006;22(9):818–23.
67. Yamamoto T, Ferracane JL, Sakaguchi RL, Swain MV. Calculation of contraction stresses in dental composites by analysis of crack propagation in the matrix surrounding a cavity. Dent Mater. 2009;25(4):543–50.
68. Yamamoto T, Kubota Y, Momoi Y, Ferracane JL. Polymerization stresses in low-shrinkage dental resin composites measured by crack analysis. Dent Mater. 2012;28(9):e143–9.
69. Yamamoto T, Hanabusa M, Momoi Y, Sakaguchi RL. Polymerization stress of dental resin composite continues to develop 12 hours after irradiation. J Esthet Restor Dent. 2015;27(1):44–54.
70. Witzel MF, Ballester RY, Meira JB, Lima RG, Braga RR. Composite shrinkage stress as a function of specimen dimensions and compliance of the testing system. Dent Mater. 2007;23(2):204–10.
71. Gonçalves F, Pfeifer CS, Ferracane JL, Braga RR. Contraction stress determinants in dimethacrylate composites. J Dent Res. 2008;87(4):367–71.
72. Miguel A, de la Macorra JC. A predictive formula of the contraction stress in restorative and luting materials attending to free and adhered surfaces, volume and deformation. Dent Mater. 2001;17(3):241–6.
73. Lu H, Stansbury JW, Bowman CN. Towards the elucidation of shrinkage stress development and relaxation in dental composites. Dent Mater. 2004;20(10):979–86.
74. Boaro LC, Gonçalves F, Guimarães TC, Ferracane JL, Versluis A, Braga RR. Polymerization stress, shrinkage and elastic modulus of current low-shrinkage restorative composites. Dent Mater. 2010;26(12):1144–50.
75. Bacchi A, Feitosa VP, da Silva Fonseca AS, Cavalcante LM, Silikas N, Schneider LF. Shrinkage, stress, and modulus of dimethacrylate, ormocer, and silorane composites. J Conserv Dent. 2015;18(5):384–8.
76. Park J, Chang J, Ferracane J, Lee IB. How should composite be layered to reduce shrinkage stress: incremental or bulk filling? Dent Mater. 2008;24(11):1501–5.
77. Kim YJ, Kim R, Ferracane JL, Lee IB. Influence of the compliance and layering method on the wall deflection of simulated cavities in bulk-fill composite restoration. Oper Dent. 2016;41(6):e183–94.
78. Bicalho AA, Pereira RD, Zanatta RF, Franco SD, Tantbirojn D, Versluis A, Soares CJ. Incremental filling technique and composite material – part I: cuspal deformation, bond strength, and physical properties. Oper Dent. 2014;39(2):E71–82.
79. Bicalho AA, Valdívia AD, Barreto BC, Tantbirojn D, Versluis A, Soares CJ. Incremental filling technique and composite material – part II: shrinkage and shrinkage stresses. Oper Dent. 2014;39(2):E83–92.
80. Abbas G, Fleming GJ, Harrington E, Shortall AC, Burke FJ. Cuspal movement and microleakage in premolar teeth restored with a packable composite cured in bulk or in increments. J Dent. 2003;31(6):437–44.
81. Loguercio AD, Reis A, Ballester RY. Polymerization shrinkage: effects of constraint and filling technique in composite restorations. Dent Mater. 2004;20(3):236–43.
82. Lee MR, Cho BH, Son HH, Um CH, Lee IB. Influence of cavity dimension and restoration methods on the cusp deflection of premolars in composite restoration. Dent Mater. 2007;23(3):288–95.
83. Frauscher KE, Ilie N. Depth of cure and mechanical properties of nano-hybrid resin-based composites with novel and conventional matrix formulation. Clin Oral Investig. 2012;16(5):1425–34.
84. Sakaguchi RL, Berge HX. Reduced light energy density decreases post-gel contraction while maintaining degree of conversion in composites. J Dent. 1998;26(8):695–700.
85. Sakaguchi RL, Wiltbank BD, Murchison CF. Contraction force rate of polymer composites is linearly correlated with irradiance. Dent Mater. 2004;20(4):402–7.
86. Pfeifer CS, Braga RR, Ferracane JL. Pulse-delay curing: influence of initial irradiance and delay time on shrinkage stress and microhardness of restorative composites. Oper Dent. 2006;31(5):610–5.
87. Lu H, Stansbury JW, Bowman CN. Impact of curing protocol on conversion and shrinkage stress. J Dent Res. 2005;84(9):822–6.
88. Oberländer H, Friedl KH, Schmalz G, Hiller KA, Kopp A. Clinical performance of polyacid-modified resin restorations using "softstart-polymerization". Clin Oral Investig. 1999;3(2):55–61.
89. Brackett WW, Covey DA, St Germain HA Jr. One-year clinical performance of a self-etching adhesive in class V resin composites cured by two methods. Oper Dent. 2002;27(3):218–22.
90. Chan DC, Browning WD, Frazier KB, Brackett MG. Clinical evaluation of the soft-start (pulse-delay) polymerization technique in Class I and II composite restorations. Oper Dent. 2008;33(3):265–71.
91. van Dijken JW, Pallesen U. A 7-year randomized prospective study of a one-step self-etching adhesive in non-carious cervical lesions. The effect of curing modes and restorative material. J Dent. 2012;40(12):1060–7.
92. Oliveira LC, Duarte S Jr, Araujo CA, Abrahão A. Effect of low-elastic modulus liner and base as stress-absorbing layer in composite resin restorations. Dent Mater. 2010;26(3):e159–69.
93. Choi KK, Condon JR, Ferracane JL. The effects of adhesive thickness on polymerization contraction stress of composite. J Dent Res. 2000;79(3):812–7.

94. Braga RR, Hilton TJ, Ferracane JL. Contraction stress of flowable composite materials and their efficacy as stress-relieving layers. J Am Dent Assoc. 2003;134(6):721–8.
95. Cara RR, Fleming GJ, Palin WM, Walmsley AD, Burke FJ. Cuspal deflection and microleakage in premolar teeth restored with resin-based composites with and without an intermediary flowable layer. J Dent. 2007;35(6):482–9.
96. van Dijken JW, Pallesen U. Clinical performance of a hybrid resin composite with and without an intermediate layer of flowable resin composite: a 7-year evaluation. Dent Mater. 2011;27(2):150–6.
97. Daronch M, Rueggeberg FA, De Goes MF. Monomer conversion of pre-heated composite. J Dent Res. 2005;84(7):663–7.
98. Tauböck TT, Tarle Z, Marovic D, Attin T. Preheating of high-viscosity bulk-fill resin composites: effects on shrinkage force and monomer conversion. J Dent. 2015;43(11):1358–64.
99. Jongsma LA, Kleverlaan CJ. Influence of temperature on volumetric shrinkage and contraction stress of dental composites. Dent Mater. 2015;31(6):721–5.
100. Schneider LF, Consani S, Sakaguchi RL, Ferracane JL. Alternative photoinitiator system reduces the rate of stress development without compromising the final properties of the dental composite. Dent Mater. 2009;25(5):566–72.
101. Gonçalves F, Pfeifer CC, Stansbury JW, Newman SM, Braga RR. Influence of matrix composition on polymerization stress development of experimental composites. Dent Mater. 2010;26(7):697–703.
102. Gonçalves F, Kawano Y, Braga RR. Contraction stress related to composite inorganic content. Dent Mater. 2010;26(7):704–9.
103. Gonçalves F, Azevedo CL, Ferracane JL, Braga RR. BisGMA/TEGDMA ratio and filler content effects on shrinkage stress. Dent Mater. 2011;27(6):520–6.
104. Satterthwaite JD, Maisuria A, Vogel K, Watts DC. Effect of resin-composite filler particle size and shape on shrinkage-stress. Dent Mater. 2012;28(6):609–14.
105. Podgórski M, Becka E, Claudino M, Flores A, Shah PK, Stansbury JW, Bowman CN. Ester-free thiol-ene dental restoratives – Part A: Resin development. Dental Materials. 2015;31:1255–62.
106. Podgórski M, Becka E, Claudino M, Flores A, Shah PK, Stansbury JW, Bowman CN. Ester-free thiol-ene dental restoratives – Part B: composite development. Dent Mater. 2015;31(11):1263–70.
107. Bacchi A, Consani RL, Martim GC, Pfeifer CS. Thio-urethane oligomers improve the properties of light-cured resin cements. Dent Mater. 2015;31(5):565–74.
108. Bacchi A, Nelson M, Pfeifer CS. Characterization of methacrylate-based composites containing thio-urethane oligomers. Dent Mater. 2016;32(2):233–9.
109. Heintze SD, Rousson V. Clinical effectiveness of direct class II restorations - a meta-analysis. J Adhes Dent. 2012;14(5):407–31.
110. Almeida e Silva JS, Rolla JN, Baratieri LN, Monteiro S Jr. The influence of different placement techniques on the microtensile bond strength of low-shrink silorane composite bonded to Class I cavities. Gen Dent. 2011;59(6):e233–7.
111. Arrais CA, Oliveira MT, Mettenburg D, Rueggeberg FA, Giannini M. Silorane- and high filled-based "low-shrinkage" resin composites: shrinkage, flexural strength and modulus. Braz Oral Res. 2013;27(2):97–102.
112. Magno MB, Nascimento GC, Rocha YS, Ribeiro BD, Loretto SC, Maia LC. Silorane-based composite resin restorations are not better than conventional composites – a meta-analysis of clinical studies. J Adhes Dent. 2016;18(5):375–86.
113. Yamasaki LC, De Vito Moraes AG, Barros M, Lewis S, Francci C, Stansbury JW, Pfeifer CS. Polymerization development of "low-shrink" resin composites: reaction kinetics, polymerization stress and quality of network. Dent Mater. 2013;29(9):e169–79.
114. Kim RJ, Kim YJ, Choi NS, Lee IB. Polymerization shrinkage, modulus, and shrinkage stress related to tooth-restoration interfacial debonding in bulk-fill composites. J Dent. 2015;43(4):430–9.
115. Guo Y, Landis FA, Wang Z, Bai D, Jiang L, Chiang MY. Polymerization stress evolution of a bulk-fill flowable composite under different compliances. Dent Mater. 2016;32(4):578–86.
116. Al Sunbul H, Silikas N, Watts DC. Polymerization shrinkage kinetics and shrinkage-stress in dental resin-composites. Dent Mater. 2016;32(8):998–1006.
117. Kalliecharan D, Germscheid W, Price RB, Stansbury J, Labrie D. Shrinkage stress kinetics of bulk fill resin-based composites at tooth temperature and long time. Dent Mater. 2016;32(11):1322–31.
118. van Dijken JW, Pallesen U. Posterior bulk-filled resin composite restorations: a 5-year randomized controlled clinical study. J Dent. 2016;51:29–35.
119. van Dijken JW, Pallesen U. Bulk-filled posterior resin restorations based on stress-decreasing resin technology: a randomized, controlled 6-year evaluation. Eur J Oral Sci. 2017;125 (4):303–309

Secondary Caries 15

Ivana Nedeljkovic and Kirsten L. Van Landuyt

Secondary or recurrent caries is defined as a new caries lesion developing at the margin of an existing restoration [1] (Fig. 15.1). As opposed to the residual caries, which is left behind after cavity preparation, secondary caries develops de novo next to a restoration. Nevertheless, in clinical practice it is most often not possible to distinguish between these two entities.

Secondary caries (SC) has been receiving an increasing attention over the last 10 years and has become a matter of concern in restorative dentistry, since it has been recognized as the most common reason for premature failure of composite restorations [2]. In a recent Delphi survey on the directions and trends in restorative dentistry and dental materials over the next 20 years, prevention of SC was identified as one of the top priorities [3].

The prevalence and the incidence of SC are, however, not completely clear from the literature, and there are several reasons for that. First, as many researchers pointed out, it seems that there is a lack of standardized diagnostic criteria for SC [4]. In addition, there are broad differences in decision-making among dentists, which may lead to many false-positive diagnoses of SC and unnecessary restoration replacements [5]. This may not only explain the high variability of SC incidences reported in the literature, but to a certain extent also the higher SC incidence in practice-based studies with a high number of non-calibrated operators than in academic studies [6, 7]. On the other hand, prevalence and incidence of SC in controlled clinical trials (CCTs) may not be representative for daily dental practice. The investigators in such academic studies are usually well trained and calibrated to assess clinical performance of the restorations, including the presence of SC, and in CCTs typically only low-caries risk and highly compliant patients are included. Therefore, the median SC incidence with posterior direct composite restorations measured in long-term (follow-up period of 5 years and longer) university-based clinical trials is predictably much lower (0.7%) compared to that in practice-based studies (7.1%) (Fig. 15.2) [6].

Apart from the study setup (university/practice-based), certain clinical parameters, such as restoration location (anterior/posterior/cervical) and type (class I/class II), also seem to affect the incidence of SC, as SC occurs more frequently with posterior compared to anterior and cervical composite restorations, and with class II compared to class I restorations (Fig. 15.3) [6].

I. Nedeljkovic (✉)
Department of Dental Material Sciences, Academic Center for Dentistry Amsterdam (ACTA), University of Amsterdam and Vrije Universitetit Amsterdam, Amsterdam, The Netherlands
e-mail: ivkagm86@gmail.com

K.L. Van Landuyt
Department of Oral Health Sciences, BIOMAT, KU Leuven (University of Leuven), Leuven, Belgium

Dentistry, University Hospitals Leuven (UZ Leuven), Leuven, Belgium

V. Miletic (ed.), *Dental Composite Materials for Direct Restorations*,
http://doi.org/10.1007/978-3-319-60961-4_15

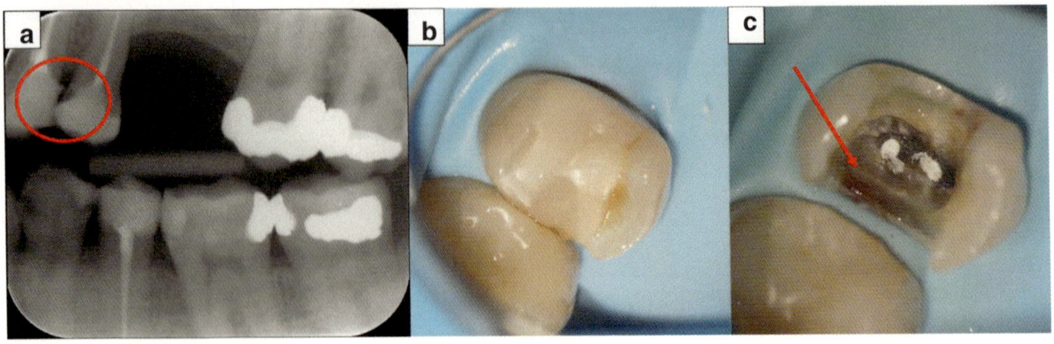

Fig. 15.1 In the bitewing radiograph (**a**), a secondary caries lesion on the distal gingival margin of a composite restoration could be observed. After removal of the composite restoration (**b**), an active caries lesion is disclosed (**c**)

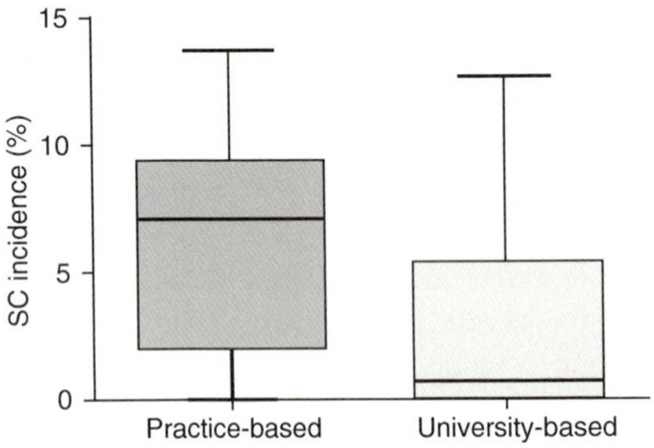

Fig. 15.2 Incidence of SC in long-term studies (at least 5 years of follow-up) with posterior composite restorations. Median SC incidence calculated in practice-based studies (7.1%) is about ten times higher compared to university-based studies (0.7%) (Based on data from Nedeljkovic et al., 2015 [6])

Nevertheless, a growing body of evidence shows that composites are twice more affected by SC than dental amalgams [8, 9], which are in some countries still used as a standard restorative material. In addition, composites seem to be much more vulnerable to SC compared to glass-ionomer cements, particularly in high-caries-risk patients [10].

The reasons for the higher vulnerability of composites to SC are still not entirely clear, and there has been an ongoing discussion whether SC is a material-based problem after all [6]. Secondary caries is in essence the same disease as primary caries, which is a localized dissolution and demineralization of hard tooth tissues by acids produced by the metabolic activity of the

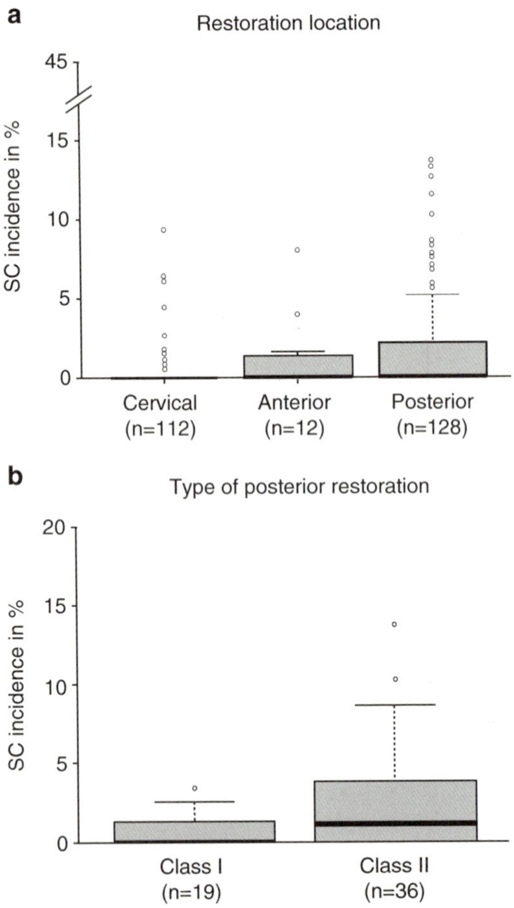

Fig. 15.3 Median SC incidence is higher with posterior than with anterior and cervical restorations (**a**). When only posterior composites are considered, class II restorations seem to be more prone to SC than class I restorations (**b**). (Adapted from Nedeljkovic et al., 2015 [6]). Reprinted with permission from Elsevier

plaque covering the affected site. Therefore, all the **factors playing a role in the development of caries lesions** in general, are also the primary determinants of the development of an SC lesions. However, it could easily be perceived that in case of SC, **a restoration** should be considered as an additional factor, since it considerably changes the local environment compared to an intact tooth. As it was mentioned above, certain ***clinical characteristics of the restoration,*** such as restoration type, size, and the location, seem to affect the SC occurrence. In addition, certain ***properties of a restorative material*** can potentially interfere with the carious process and either facilitate it, which makes a material more vulnerable to SC, or exhibit a cariostatic effect. We can, therefore, say that secondary caries is a multifactorial problem, and all the mentioned factors that might affect its development are summarized in Fig. 15.4.

General factors influencing carious process are certainly beyond the scope of this book; nevertheless, the restoration-related factors, including material properties that can contribute to the development of SC next to composite restorations, will be discussed in more detail in the following paragraphs.

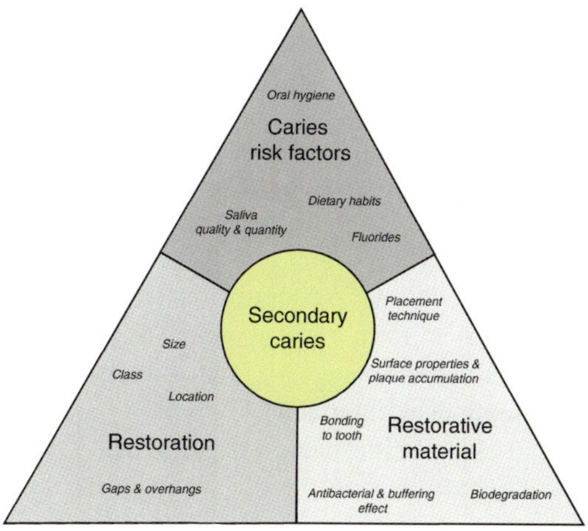

Fig. 15.4 Factors influencing secondary caries (SC) development next to a restoration. The factors determining the caries process in general are decisive and thus are placed at the top of the pyramid. Nevertheless, factors related to the presence of the restoration and to the properties of the restorative material can significantly influence this process

15.1 Interfacial Gaps and Microleakage

For a long time, the presence of a gap at the tooth-restoration interface and subsequent leakage of bacteria and their metabolites have been considered to be the main reason and the prerequisite for SC, irrespective of the restorative material [11]. Almost 40 years ago, Hals et al. described SC lesions as consisting of an outer and a cavity wall lesion. While the outer lesion is the result of a cariogenic attack taking place at the outer tooth surface, a cavity wall lesion results from a cariogenic attack and demineralization taking place at the interface, as a direct consequence of microleakage [12, 13]. However, the microleakage theory has recently been challenged by many cariologists, who argue that SC is nothing but a "primary caries at the filling margin" driven by the activity of the biofilm on the tooth surface, while the presence of gap and microleakage is irrelevant [14, 15]. In addition, it was suggested that the wall lesion does not exist as a separate entity but is formed after the outer lesion is extended in the direction of the enamel prisms [1, 16]. Nevertheless, recent research on the role of interfacial gaps in SC by Kuper et al. provides strong evidence that the presence of a gap indeed predisposes composite restorations to SC, especially in case of high caries risk patients. It was shown that an interfacial space of only 70 μm can lead to the demineralization of the tooth-restoration interface and the formation of the wall lesion [17, 18]. This gap size threshold is much lower than previously reported (around 225 μm) [19]. Furthermore, it has been demonstrated that failed bonded interfaces and nonbonded interfaces without an adhesive layer at the dentin surface allow the development of a wall lesion under cariogenic challenge [20]. It is therefore clear from these results that the integrity of tooth-restoration interface may be of great importance for the development of SC around composite restorations.

An important issue to be discussed here is under which circumstances gaps large enough to predispose the restoration to SC might occur in vivo. In the first instance, they may occur already **during the composite placement procedure**, due to its relatively high technique sensitivity. There are several critical issues that deserve special attention during the composite placement procedure in order to reliably seal the tooth cavity and avoid initial gap formation and microleakage, thereby decreasing the risk of SC.

15.1.1 Technique Sensitivity of the Adhesive Procedure

Application of an adhesive prior to the composite placement is generally considered to be a very technique-sensitive procedure. Insufficient or over-extended etching, inadequate wetting or penetration, and curing of the bonding agent may compromise good adhesion, by which micro- and nanoleakage due to inadequate bonding may occur [21–23]. In this regard, simplified adhesives may allegedly have an advantage, because they require fewer steps in their application, which means lower risk of making application errors [24]. On the other hand, each step of a multi-step adhesive system has its particular function. Additionally, a manipulation error in one of the steps may even be compensated by the next steps [25]. Finally, it is of utmost importance for good adhesion to avoid contamination of the cavity by saliva or blood, which is not always easy in clinical circumstances.

15.1.2 Composite Adaptation into the Cavity

Not only is the adhesion procedure critical for the acquisition of a good seal but also the adaptation of the material into the cavity. Opdam et al. showed that it is challenging to restore the tooth with composite without the formation of porosities and voids inside of material, some of which very often exceed 1 mm in size [26]. It could easily be perceived that this kind of voids at the outer margin may compromise the cavity sealing and make the restoration more prone to SC. Therefore, more attention should be given to the composite insertion and adaptation techniques in order to prevent the formation of voids and gaps at the cavity margins.

15.1.3 Polymerization Shrinkage

As discussed in Chap. 14, one of the inherent shortcomings of composites that can significantly affect their sealing ability is the volumetric shrinkage upon polymerization, which was reported to be in the range of 1.5–5% [27]. As the adhesion to the cavity walls poses a confinement to the shrinkage, shrinkage stresses in composite material are generated, which can lead to the formation of so-called stress-relieving gaps at the tooth-restoration interface and subsequent microleakage [28, 29]. It is still not clear, however, whether these gaps could exceed the clinically relevant gap width of around 70 μm and predispose the restoration margin to demineralization and SC [30, 31]. In order to control the development of shrinkage stresses, several specific placement and curing procedures have been proposed, including the well-known incremental technique, which is able to considerably reduce shrinkage stresses [32, 33].

Nevertheless, if used properly by a skilled clinician, composites can form an excellent bond to the tooth tissues and reliably seal the tooth cavity. However, **during restoration's service** in the mouth, tooth-composite adhesive interface undergoes **degradation and deterioration** [34]. This is, on the other hand, not the case with other restorative materials, such as dental amalgams, which are, in spite of their "macro-mechanical" retention in the cavity and the lack of real bonding to tooth tissues, considered to have a "self-sealing" ability, thanks to the deposition of corrosion products at the tooth-amalgam interface over time [35]. Also, glass-ionomer cements are considered to be "self-adhesive" restorative materials, due to their ability to form a real chemical (ionic) bond with tooth hard tissues [36]. Two main modes of tooth-composite interfacial degradation are biodegradation and mechanical degradation.

15.1.4 Biodegradation

Biodegradation of composite-tooth adhesive interface includes hydrolytic and enzymatic degradation. Salivary enzymes from the class of esterases, such as cholesterol esterase (CE) and pseudocholinesterase

(PCE), can degrade BisGMA-based dental adhesives extensively enough to allow bacterial leakage into the interface [37]. In addition, it was demonstrated in vitro that cariogenic species *Streptococcus mutans* has a similar esterase activity as saliva and may as well partake in the degradation of the tooth-composite interface [38].

15.1.5 Mechanical Degradation

Occlusal stresses generated during mastication and especially during parafunctional activities, such as bruxism, were shown to have a deleterious effect on the marginal adaptation of composites, in particular at the gingival margin [39, 40]. These mechanical stresses repeated over time lead to fatigue or weakening of the interface, and once the concentrated stresses exceed the interfacial fracture toughness, a crack could form, which may further lead to gap formation and micro-leakage [24]. In addition to occlusal stresses, thermal stresses generated by intra-oral temperature changes exert a similar effect on the composite-tooth interface because composites and adhesives have a higher thermal contraction/expansion coefficient than hard tooth tissues [41].

Not only through the formation of a gap at the interface may the occlusal load and thermal contraction or expansion contribute to the development of SC next to composites but also through the percolation phenomenon. Both occlusal loading and thermal cycling subject the restoration's margins to opening and closing forces, which could cause flow of the oral fluids in and out of the gap [41]. In this way, demineralization products may actively be removed from the gap, allowing SC lesions to develop faster [42].

15.2 Physicochemical Properties of Composites and Interactions with Dental Plaque

Apart from the quality of the tooth-restoration interface, physicochemical properties of the restorative material and its biological effects are also important when it comes to the restoration's vulnerability to SC. A restored tooth surface represents a new substrate to which dental biofilm or plaque attaches. As the presence and metabolic activity of dental plaque are the main etiological factors in caries, the interactions between the restorative material and bacteria from dental plaque might affect the development of SC around the restoration. Some of the properties of dental composites that might contribute to their higher vulnerability to SC through the interactions with bacteria from dental plaque are discussed in the following paragraphs.

15.2.1 Surface Properties of Composites and Plaque Accumulation

It has been suggested that dental composites accumulate more plaque on their surface compared to other restorative materials and the tooth enamel [43, 44] and that this could be a reason for their higher vulnerability to SC. Bacterial attachment and accumulation are complex processes and depend on various surface properties of the material, such as surface roughness, hydrophobicity/hydrophilicity, charge and chemical composition, as well as on different environmental factors, such as shear forces, pH, temperature, etc. [45]. The relationship between **surface roughness** and bacterial adhesion has been well established, and smoother surfaces are known to accumulate less plaque. Contemporary composites have considerably high polishability, and with current polishing techniques and composite materials, it is possible to achieve a highly smooth and shiny restored surface for a long period of time [46]. However, it has been determined that there is a surface roughness threshold below which no further decrease in bacterial accumulation can be achieved, which corresponds to the average roughness (Ra) value of about 0.2 μm [47]. Below the mentioned threshold, other surface physicochemical characteristics play a dominant role in bacterial adhesion and accumulation. It is considered that increased **surface free energy** facilitates biofilm formation on the material's surface [48]. In other words, materials with hydrophobic properties should accumulate less plaque. In this regard, special attention was paid to silorane-based composites, which were shown to have the lowest susceptibility to oral streptococci adhesion after in vitro evaluation [49]. This was assigned to their high hydrophobicity imparted by the siloxane backbone. However, a recent in situ study showed that even though silorane-based composites are indeed more hydrophobic than methacrylate-based composites, they are equally susceptible to biofilm accumulation [50]. However, it seems that the relationship between the material's hydrophobicity/hydrophilicity and bacterial adhesion is not so straightforward and that this also depends on the properties of the bacterial cell wall and is specific for a bacterial strain [51, 52]. The presence of certain chemical groups at the material surface, or material **surface chemistry**, as well has an impact on the bacterial adhesion. It has been shown that certain bacterial species have the affinity to adhere to filler particles, rather than to the resinous matrix [53]. In addition, different composite resin formulations can influence bacterial attachment to the composite surface, although the underlying mechanisms are not entirely clear [54, 55].

15.2.2 The Release of Composite Compounds Due to Incomplete Polymerization

It has been reported that unreacted monomers released from incompletely polymerized composite restorations could stimulate the growth of certain cariogenic bacterial species, such as *Streptococcus sobrinus* and *Lactobacillus acidophilus*, which could lead to higher cariogenicity of plaque covering composite restorations [56]. However, these findings are controversial, since there are several studies disputing this [57, 58]. In addition, it is not known whether relatively high concentrations of methacrylate monomers used in the in vitro studies are representative of those in the plaque in vivo. Nevertheless, proper polymerization of composites is of great importance not only because of the putative stimulatory effect of the released monomers on the growth of cariogenic bacteria, but also because it has been shown that composites which were not fully polymerized accumulate more biofilm on their surface, even after the unreacted monomers have leached out [59].

15.2.3 Lack of Antibacterial Effect of the Material

Another property of composites that contributes to their vulnerability to SC is the fact that conventional composites do not possess any antibacterial properties. This characteristic distinguishes them from other commonly used restoratives, such as amalgams, which contain metal ions with antibacterial effect such as Ag, Hg, and Cu, and glass-ionomers with their well-documented antibacterial effect due to fluorides release [60]. As a result, unlike glass-ionomer-based materials and amalgams, composites do not have the ability to prevent or to reduce the formation of the biofilm and to retard the progression of the SC [61]. In recent years, much effort has been invested to produce dental composites and adhesives with antibacterial properties, which would help prevent the development of SC around a restoration [62–64]. Several products with antibacterial effect appeared on the market, such as 12-methacryloyloxydodecylpyridinium bromide (MDPB)—containing adhesives, which exhibit contact inhibition of the attached bacterial cells, and so-called giomers, which contain surface pre-reacted glass-ionomer (S-PRG) particles capable of accumulating and releasing fluorides. Their effect against cariogenic bacteria has been confirmed in a number of in vitro as well as in situ studies; however, there are still no clinical data supporting their protective effect against SC [65, 66]. Clinical studies on the performance of these materials are necessary to determine whether this strategy can result in an improved resistance to SC and greater longevity of composites.

15.2.4 Lack of Buffering Properties

Aside from the antibacterial effect, another property of a restorative material that could affect the composition and cariogenicity of the overlying plaque is its buffering ability, or the ability to increase the local pH in plaque toward more neutral values. The pH of the overlying plaque is important in two aspects. First, its value is critical for the demineralization and remineralization processes taking place at the tooth surface, and second, it directly affects the bacterial composition of the plaque, since a lower pH promotes the growth of more aciduric and acidogenic bacteria, which have the highest cariogenic potential [67]. It has been shown that plaque formed on composites contains more cariogenic species, such as mutans streptococci and lactobacilli, than plaque covering intact enamel [68]. Furthermore it was demonstrated that this selection of cariogenic species might stem from the lack of buffering abilities of composite restorations, which allows the local pH of the plaque to stay low for a longer period of time. In contrast, dental amalgams and glass-ionomer cements, apart from their antibacterial effect, have the ability to counteract the local acidity, which is another cariostatic property of these materials [61].

Conclusions

Secondary caries is the most common reason for the failure of composite restorations and as such is the main culprit for their shorter longevity compared to amalgams. The factors contributing to the higher vulnerability of composites to SC are multiple and not entirely clear. However, one should be aware of all the clinical and material-related factors that could have an impact on caries development around a restoration, especially of those that could easily be controlled in practice. Careful application of the adhesive system and adaptation of the composite into the tooth cavity, along with good control of salivary or blood contamination, proper light curing, and finishing and polishing of the restoration will allow achieving stronger and more durable bonding of the restoration to the tooth tissues and minimize the plaque retention on the restored tooth. As for improvement of the restorative material composition, such as the incorporation of various antibacterial compounds in composites and adhesives, results of laboratory studies suggest that it is a promising strategy to increase the resistance of composites against cariogenic challenges. However, there are to date no clinical data available about the anticariogenic effect of these materials in vivo.

References

1. Mjor IA, Toffenetti F. Secondary caries: a literature review with case reports. Quintessence Int. 2000;31(3):165–79.
2. Opdam NJ, et al. Longevity of posterior composite restorations: a systematic review and meta-analysis. J Dent Res. 2014;93(10):943–9.
3. Seemann R, et al. Restorative dentistry and restorative materials over the next 20 years: a Delphi survey. Dent Mater. 2014;30(4):442–8.
4. Mjor IA. Clinical diagnosis of recurrent caries. J Am Dent Assoc. 2005;136(10):1426–33.
5. Bader JD, Shugars DA. Understanding dentists' restorative treatment decisions. J Public Health Dent. 1992;52(2):102–10.
6. Nedeljkovic I, et al. Is secondary caries with composites a material-based problem? Dent Mater. 2015;31(11):e247–77.
7. Mjor IA. The location of clinically diagnosed secondary caries. Quintessence Int. 1998;29(5):313–7.
8. Rasines Alcaraz MG, et al. Direct composite resin fillings versus amalgam fillings for permanent or adult posterior teeth. Cochrane Database Syst Rev. 2014;3:CD005620.
9. Moraschini V, et al. Amalgam and resin composite longevity of posterior restorations: a systematic review and meta-analysis. J Dent. 2015;43(9):1043–50.
10. McComb D, et al. A clinical comparison of glass ionomer, resin-modified glass ionomer and resin composite restorations in the treatment of cervical caries in xerostomic head and neck radiation patients. Oper Dent. 2002;27(5):430–7.
11. Kidd EA. Microleakage in relation to amalgam and composite restorations. A laboratory study. Br Dent J. 1976;141(10):305–10.
12. Hals E, Nernaes A. Histopathology of in vitro caries developing around silver amalgam fillings. Caries Res. 1971;5(1):58–77.
13. Hals E, Andreassen BH, Bie T. Histopathology of natural caries around silver amalgam fillings. Caries Res. 1974;8(4):343–58.

14. Barata JS, et al. Influence of gaps in adhesive restorations in the development of secondary caries lesions: an in situ evaluation. Am J Dent. 2012;25(4):244–8.
15. Fejerskov O, Kidd EAM. Dental caries: the disease and its clinical management. 2nd ed. Oxford; Ames, Iowa: Blackwell Munksgaard; 2008. 616 p.
16. Gilmour AS, Edmunds DH. The polarized light microscopic appearance of caries-like lesions adjacent to restored cavities in the crowns and roots of extracted human teeth. J Oral Rehabil. 1998;25(12):929–39.
17. Diercke K, et al. Isolated development of inner (wall) caries like lesions in a bacterial-based in vitro model. Clin Oral Investig. 2009;13(4):439–44.
18. Kuper NK, et al. Gap size and wall lesion development next to composite. J Dent Res. 2014;93(7 suppl):108S–13S.
19. Thomas RZ, et al. Approximal secondary caries lesion progression, a 20-week in situ study. Caries Res. 2007;41(5):399–405.
20. Montagner AF, et al. Behavior of failed bonded interfaces under in vitro cariogenic challenge. Dent Mater. 2016;32(5):668–75.
21. Tay FR, et al. Variability in microleakage observed in a total-etch wet-bonding technique under different handling conditions. J Dent Res. 1995;74(5):1168–78.
22. Hilton TJ. Can modern restorative procedures and materials reliably seal cavities? In vitro investigations. Part 1. Am J Dent. 2002;15(3):198–210.
23. Pioch T, et al. Nanoleakage at the composite-dentin interface: a review. Am J Dent. 2001;14(4):252–8.
24. De Munck J, et al. A critical review of the durability of adhesion to tooth tissue: methods and results. J Dent Res. 2005;84(2):118–32.
25. Van Landuyt KL, et al. Are one-step adhesives easier to use and better performing? Multifactorial assessment of contemporary one-step self-etching adhesives. J Adhes Dent. 2009;11(3):175–90.
26. Opdam NJ, et al. Porosities and voids in class I restorations placed by six operators using a packable or syringable composite. Dent Mater. 2002;18(1):58–63.
27. Ferracane JL. Developing a more complete understanding of stresses produced in dental composites during polymerization. Dent Mater. 2005;21(1):36–42.
28. Braga RR, Ballester RY, Ferracane JL. Factors involved in the development of polymerization shrinkage stress in resin-composites: a systematic review. Dent Mater. 2005;21(10):962–70.
29. Ferracane JL, Mitchem JC. Relationship between composite contraction stress and leakage in class V cavities. Am J Dent. 2003;16(4):239–43.
30. Moreira da Silva E, et al. The influence of C-factor, flexural modulus and viscous flow on gap formation in resin composite restorations. Oper Dent. 2007;32(4):356–62.
31. Bakhsh TA, et al. Concurrent evaluation of composite internal adaptation and bond strength in a class-I cavity. J Dent. 2013;41(1):60–70.
32. Park J, et al. How should composite be layered to reduce shrinkage stress: incremental or bulk filling? Dent Mater. 2008;24(11):1501–5.
33. Lu H, Stansbury JW, Bowman CN. Impact of curing protocol on conversion and shrinkage stress. J Dent Res. 2005;84(9):822–6.
34. Hashimoto M, et al. In vivo degradation of resin-dentin bonds in humans over 1 to 3 years. J Dent Res. 2000;79(6):1385–91.
35. Ben-Amar A, Cardash HS, Judes H. The sealing of the tooth/amalgam interface by corrosion products. J Oral Rehabil. 1995;22(2):101–4.
36. Van Meerbeek B, et al. Buonocore memorial lecture. Adhesion to enamel and dentin: current status and future challenges. Oper Dent. 2003;28(3):215–35.
37. Kermanshahi S, et al. Biodegradation of resin-dentin interfaces increases bacterial microleakage. J Dent Res. 2010;89(9):996–1001.
38. Bourbia M, et al. Cariogenic bacteria degrade dental resin composites and adhesives. J Dent Res. 2013;92(11):989–94.
39. Qvist V. The effect of mastication on marginal adaptation of composite restorations in vivo. J Dent Res. 1983;62(8):904–6.
40. Francisconi LF, et al. The effects of occlusal loading on the margins of cervical restorations. J Am Dent Assoc. 2009;140(10):1275–82.
41. Gale MS, Darvell BW. Thermal cycling procedures for laboratory testing of dental restorations. J Dent. 1999;27(2):89–99.
42. Kuper NK, et al. Hydrodynamic flow through loading and in vitro secondary caries development. J Dent Res. 2013;92(4):383–7.
43. Konishi N, et al. Confocal laser scanning microscopic analysis of early plaque formed on resin composite and human enamel. J Oral Rehabil. 2003;30(8):790–5.
44. de Fucio SB, et al. Analyses of biofilms accumulated on dental restorative materials. Am J Dent. 2009;22(3):131–6.
45. Song F, Koo H, Ren D. Effects of material properties on bacterial adhesion and biofilm formation. J Dent Res. 2015;94(8):1027–34.
46. Kaizer MR, et al. Do nanofill or submicron composites show improved smoothness and gloss? A systematic review of in vitro studies. Dent Mater. 2014;30(4):e41–78.
47. Bollen CM, Lambrechts P, Quirynen M. Comparison of surface roughness of oral hard materials to the threshold surface roughness for bacterial plaque retention: a review of the literature. Dent Mater. 1997;13(4):258–69.
48. Teughels W, et al. Effect of material characteristics and/or surface topography on biofilm development. Clin Oral Implants Res. 2006;17(Suppl 2):68–81.
49. Buergers R, et al. Streptococcal adhesion to novel low-shrink silorane-based restorative. Dent Mater. 2009;25(2):269–75.
50. Claro-Pereira D, et al. In situ evaluation of a new silorane-based composite resin's bioadhesion properties. Dent Mater. 2011;27(12):1238–45.

51. van Loosdrecht MC, et al. The role of bacterial cell wall hydrophobicity in adhesion. Appl Environ Microbiol. 1987;53(8):1893–7.
52. Hahnel S, et al. Surface properties and in vitro Streptococcus Mutans adhesion to dental resin polymers. J Mater Sci Mater Med. 2008;19(7):2619–27.
53. Yamamoto K, et al. Adherence of oral streptococci to composite resin of varying surface roughness. Dent Mater J. 1996;15(2):201–4.
54. Ruttermann S, et al. Bacterial viability on surface-modified resin-based dental restorative materials. Arch Oral Biol. 2012;57(11):1512–21.
55. Ikeda M, et al. Effect of surface characteristics on adherence of *S. mutans* biofilms to indirect resin composites. Dent Mater J. 2007;26(6):915–23.
56. Hansel C, et al. Effects of various resin composite (co)monomers and extracts on two caries-associated micro-organisms in vitro. J Dent Res. 1998;77(1):60–7.
57. Takahashi Y, et al. Influence of resin monomers on growth of oral streptococci. J Dent Res. 2004;83(4):302–6.
58. Nedeljkovic I, et al. No evidence for the growth-stimulating effect of monomers on cariogenic streptococci. Clin Oral Investig. 2017;21(5):1861–9.
59. Brambilla E, et al. The influence of light-curing time on the bacterial colonization of resin composite surfaces. Dent Mater. 2009;25(9):1067–72.
60. Beyth N, Domb AJ, Weiss EI. An in vitro quantitative antibacterial analysis of amalgam and composite resins. J Dent. 2007;35(3):201–6.
61. Nedeljkovic I, et al. Lack of buffering by composites promotes shift to more cariogenic bacteria. J Dent Res. 2016;95(8):875–81.
62. Imazato S. Antibacterial properties of resin composites and dentin bonding systems. Dent Mater. 2003;19(6):449–57.
63. Chen L, Shen H, Suh BI. Antibacterial dental restorative materials: a state-of-the-art review. Am J Dent. 2012;25(6):337–46.
64. Wang Z, Shen Y, Haapasalo M. Dental materials with antibiofilm properties. Dent Mater. 2014;30(2):e1–e16.
65. Saku S, et al. Antibacterial activity of composite resin with glass-ionomer filler particles. Dent Mater J. 2010;29(2):193–8.
66. van de Sande FH, et al. The influence of different restorative materials on secondary caries development in situ. J Dent. 2014;42(9):1171–7.
67. Marsh PD. Microbial ecology of dental plaque and its significance in health and disease. Adv Dent Res. 1994;8(2):263–71.
68. Thomas RZ, et al. Bacterial composition and red fluorescence of plaque in relation to primary and secondary caries next to composite: an in situ study. Oral Microbiol Immunol. 2008;23(1):7–13.

Repair of Direct Resin Composite Restorations

16

Neslihan Arhun and Duygu Tuncer

A chain is no stronger than its weakest link.

16.1 Introduction

No one can deny that esthetics is a major demand in the modern world. Along with this epidemic esthetic expectation and environmental concern about mercury and amalgam toxicity arguments, different types of esthetic restorative materials have been evolved. Resin composites have been introduced to the restorative dentistry to minimize the disadvantages of amalgam and earlier esthetic materials like silicate cements and acrylic resins in the 1940s [1–3]. In recent years, the use of resin composites increased its acceptance which may be based on continuing developments in material's esthetic and physical properties, handling properties, adhesive techniques, minimal intervention dentistry strategies, and curing refinements to fulfill this expectation.

Although the ultimate aim of restorative dentistry is to perform superior lifelong restorations without sacrificing healthy tooth tissue more than required [4–6], the real situation is not in this way. When placing a direct resin composite restoration, every clinician should be aware of the fact that every restoration in the mouth is prone to degradation [7]. Although the Academy of Operative Dentistry European Section (AODES) considers resin composites of appropriate composition and properties to be the "material of choice" for using in direct minimal intervention approaches to the restoration of posterior teeth, the AODES acknowledges that resin composites are still lacking and suffer certain limitations. In fact, the AODES highlights the importance of performing refurbishment and repair techniques to extend longevity of restorations [8].

It is a universal reality that operative dentistry remains the mainstay of dental practice [9]. Tyas et al. and Mjör et al. updated this ratio and estimated that half of the general practitioners' time is spent on "replacement" dentistry [10, 11].

16.2 Terminology

The management of defective restorations was subcategorized into four approaches by the World Dental Federation (FDI) [12, 13]:

- *No treatment* (*monitoring*): Minor defects around margins (minor discoloration or ditching) that are clinically acceptable and may not result in impaired function may be left untreated and monitored [14].
- *Refurbishment:* The defects may be corrected without damage to the tooth (removal of overhangs, recontouring the surface, removal of discoloration) and without adding new restorative material [15, 16].
- *Repair:* Repair is a minimally invasive approach and includes the placement of a new

N. Arhun (✉) • D. Tuncer
Department of Restorative Dentistry, School of Dentistry, Baskent University, Ankara, Turkey
e-mail: neslihan@baskent.edu.tr

V. Miletic (ed.), *Dental Composite Materials for Direct Restorations*,
http://doi.org/10.1007/978-3-319-60961-4_16

partial restoration, with or without a preparation in the defective part of a restoration and/or adjacent tooth tissues while leaving the intact part in place [12, 17].

- *Replacement*: Replacement is the removal of an entire restoration with generalized or severe problems including any bases, liners and secondary caries, and tooth tissue followed by the placement of a new restoration when repair is not feasible or reasonable [9].

Contemporary dental treatment strategies advise repair of questionable restorations when evaluating different treatment options [7, 13]. Besides, as "Minimal Intervention Dentistry" concept spreads, repair of restorations has gained popularity over the last two decades [10, 18]. Restorative materials based on different kinds of resin monomers can be adhesively adhered to enamel, dentin, cast metal alloys, ceramic materials, and composite resins, depending on the surface preparation techniques. This material-specific possibility offers new options for repair restoration in diverse fields.

Advantages of repair:

- A less invasive procedure with decreased tooth loss avoiding weakening and overtreatment of tooth.
- Avoid "restoration repetitive cycle" [19, 20].
- Reduction in patient and third-party payers' cost and time, since the intact part of the restoration can be maintained [21, 22].
- Prevention of further stimulation of pulp [6, 23] and iatrogenic damage to the neighboring teeth.
- The need for local anesthesia may be reduced [7, 13].
- Less traumatic or stressful than replacement for patients with good acceptance [24, 25].
- Increased the longevity of the existing restoration.

16.3 Indications and Contraindications of Repair

Notwithstanding the advantages of repair, the decision to repair rather than replace is complex and multifactorial. These variables yield the 3 ft of a tripod which completely rely on optimization of pros and cons based on future risk assessments.

Indications of repair:

- Patients who attend to the dental clinics regularly with high motivation are favorable candidates for this minimal intervention. However, it should be kept in mind that it is essential to obtain an informed consent for this repair procedure. The clinician should explain the consequences and possible prognosis of both options [7].
- Patients who necessitate limited chair time with limited cooperation are the other nominees for the repair procedure. These may be geriatric patients or patients with complex medical histories. Thus, the nature of treatment options should be restricted to be short and simple without any complex options [7].
- The presence of secondary caries does not necessarily mean that the restoration is clinically unacceptable and inevitably requires urgent replacement (Fig. 16.1). When diagnosed, the subsequent decision relies on caries risk assessment of the patient. A low caries-risk patient may be the most appropriate candidate with the best prognosis [7].

Diagnosis of secondary caries may be challenging for many dentists and "false-negative" diagnosis sometimes hamper the treatment outcome [26], resulting in the decision that is often not based on objective criteria [27]. When the dentist hesitates about the presence of secondary caries, he adopts a "defensive dentistry" approach by choosing replacement [7].

The presence of excess filling materials, a deficient restoration around the margin, and the formation of gaps may cause marginal defects in anterior restoration [28]. However, it is important to realize that the presence of marginal defects does not always indicate the presence of secondary caries [7] (Fig. 16.2). Besides, poor etching ability of self-etching adhesives at the enamel margins may also trigger marginal defects [29–32]. These margins are prone to pick up exogenous stain, which jeopardizes esthetic appearance. The treatment approach may include

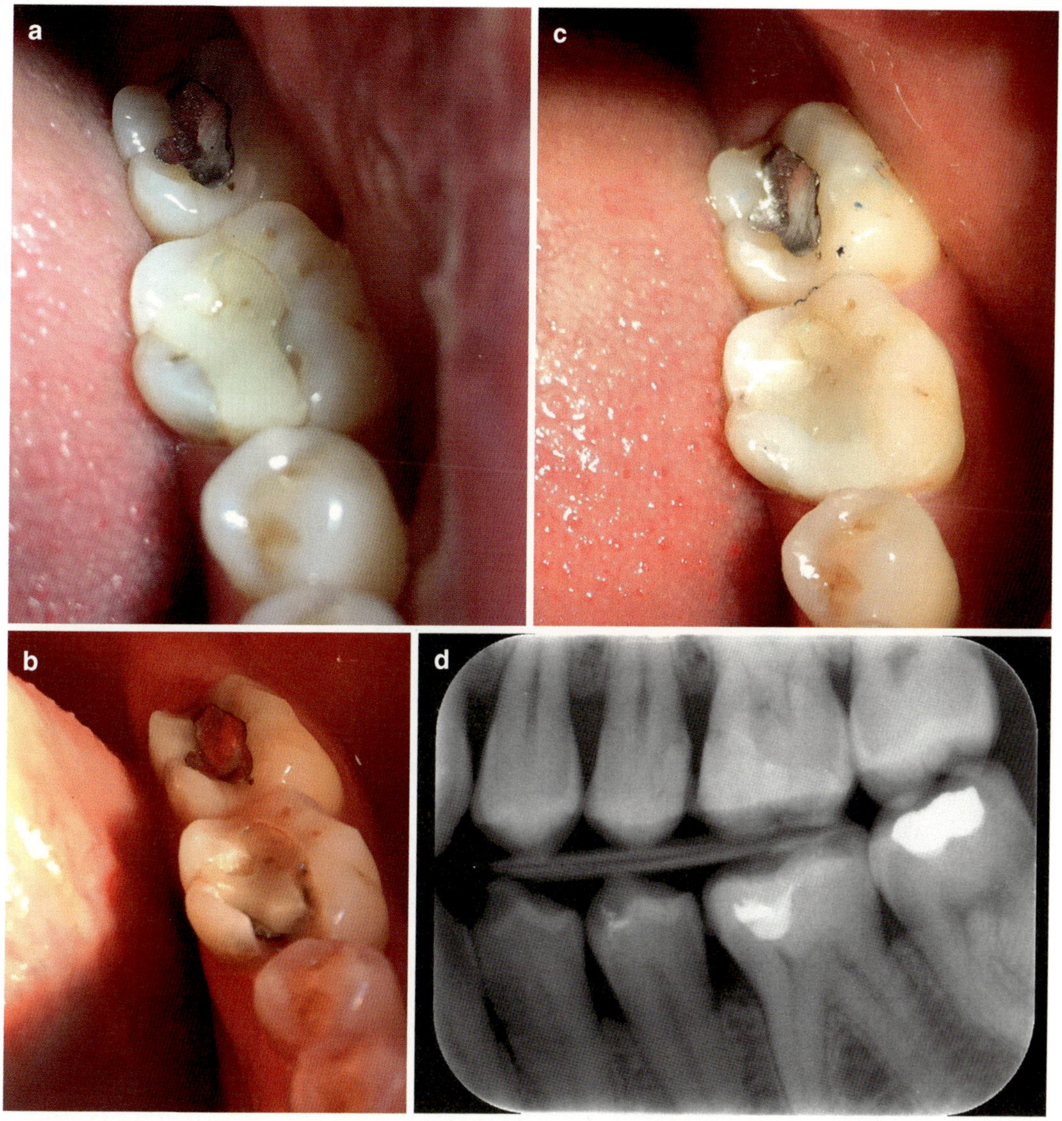

Fig. 16.1 Repair of a defective restoration with secondary caries. (**a**) Secondary caries and marginal defects adjacent to the restoration in tooth number 36. (**b**) Secondary caries and defected parts were cleaned. (**c**) The restoration was repaired with the aid of adhesive system and resin composite. (**d**) Postoperative radiograph

refinishing with refurbishment of the restoration for a longer survival period. However, if the defect is found to be heavy penetrating, restoration replacement may be inevitable [7].

Most defects in restorations, except acute trauma, progress in extended periods of time [33] allowing dentists to eliminate the cause and perform minimal intervention treatments to prolong survival expectancy (Fig. 16.3).

- Bruxism-related occlusal wear of a resin composite restoration may also be repaired by adding new material to the occlusal surface of the existing restoration if there is adequate space [7].
- The presence of premature fractures of recent restorations, color mismatch between restoration and the tooth, deficient contact point, or inadequate anatomy necessitates the addi-

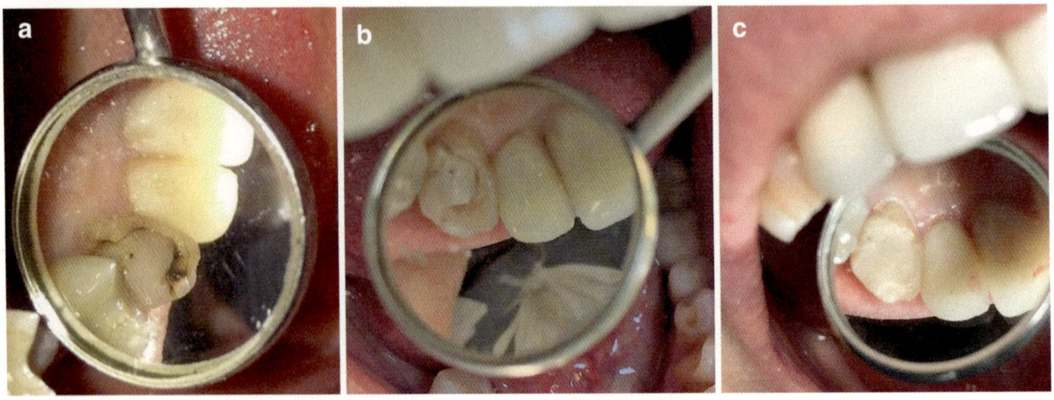

Fig. 16.2 Extensive marginal defects of an existing composite restoration but with no secondary caries that was repaired. (**a**) Marginal defects and gap formation on tooth no. 13. (**b**) The defective parts of the restoration were removed and/or prepared. (**c**) The margins were acid etched, and an appropriate adhesive system and microhybrid composite were used to repair the defective parts

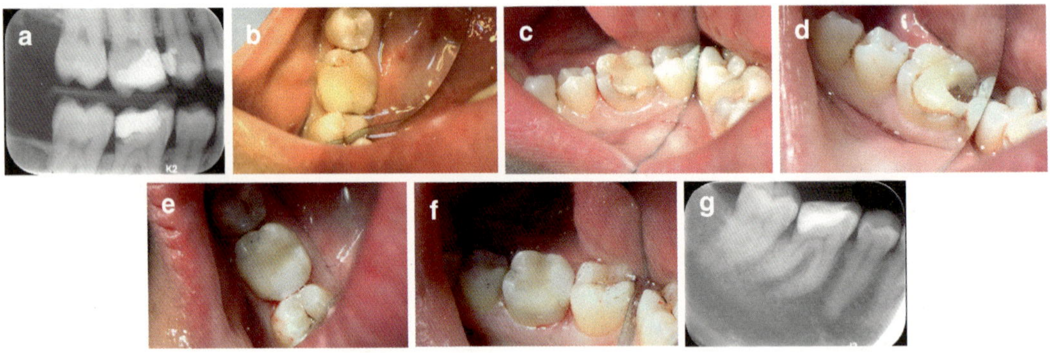

Fig. 16.3 Repair of a composite restoration on tooth no. 46. (**a**) A defective resin composite restoration on tooth no. 46 with secondary caries in the gingival region. (**b**) Clinical examination revealed marginal defects and a faulty contact. (**c**) Buccal view of the defective restoration. (**d**) Secondary caries and the defective margins were cleaned. (**e**) The repaired restoration. (**f**) Buccal view of the repaired restoration. (**g**) Postoperative radiographic view

tion of more resin composite to the initial restoration [34].

- Dentists may sometimes experience bulk fracture of a recent restoration or an old restoration. This may be the result of stress fatigue within the restorative material. Existing reports suggest that repair approach is indicated if the bulk fracture comprises of less than half of the restoration and only if the remaining portion of the restoration is intact [35–37].
- Polymerization shrinkage stresses during polymerization or acute/chronic trauma may cause fractures of the tooth tissues adjacent to the restoration. The restoration may be repaired without impairing the integrity of the restoration [7].

Contraindications of repair:

- Patient unwilling to accept a repair instead of replacement.
- Low-motivated patients who do not regularly visit dentists.
- Patients with high caries risk.
- Presence of caries undermining a large portion of the existing restoration.
- Presence of unsuccessful previous repair.

In a recent publication, Schwendicke et al. emphasized "retreatment of restorations should aim to repair by resealing, refurbishing, or repolishing where possible, and replacement should be last resort (strong recommendation)" in "Consensus Recommendations on Carious Tissue Removal" [38].

16.4 Repair Mechanisms

Some clinical situations may involve immediate repair of a composite restoration. If a clinician determined that an inadequate restoration was placed (open margin, inadequate proximal contact) and enough time remained in the appointment, then the clinician may decide to perform an immediate repair.

Immediate repair of freshly cured resin composites does not pose any challenge to the clinician as free radicals that are readily present on the surface of the cured composite contribute to the bonding between the layers of available composite and repair composite. The presence of oxygen inhibition layer thus facilitates bonding between two methacrylate-based composite layers [39]. Rinastiti et al. [40] reported that the application of an adhesive system when performing immediate repair may not be necessary as the survival rate of free radicals in polymerized resin composite is 14 days. Therefore, a sufficient amount of unreacted carbon–carbon double bonds remains available for bonding with the repair composite in an immediate repair.

Repairs of composite restorations are usually performed months or years after the initial placement. These restorations are exposed to dynamic oral environment conditions including saliva, bacteria, enzymes, and dietary and temperature fluctuations. When considering repair of aged resin composite restoration, the clinician should bear in mind that these aging conditions pose several changes to the vast majority of resin-based composites, such as water sorption, chemical degradation, and leaching of some constituents [41, 42], which diminish the reactivity of the remaining material [39]. This hydrolytic degradation also leads to swelling and crack propagation within the matrix and breakdown of the coupling agent, resulting in loss of filler particles [43]. The amount of unreacted methacrylate groups and presence of the oxygen-inhibited layer of unpolymerized resin available for bonding on the surface of a composite decrease significantly after 24 h [44, 45]. Furthermore, volatile sulfur compounds that are responsible for oral malodor may diffuse into composite restorations with oral fluids contributing to a compromised bond between aged and repair composites [46]. As a result, prognosis of bonding to aged or contaminated composite is unpredictable [41, 47].

The interface between the aged and repair composite material can be considered as "the weakest link." Therefore, it is of utmost importance to increase the bond strength between the old and new resin composite and to obtain complete adaptation between them to prevent microleakage [48]. The presence of this interface forms a fragile point to withstand intraoral forces [49].

It is difficult to state a threshold bond strength value required for proper composite repair. A repair bond strength equal to the bond strength of resin composite to etched enamel is assumed to be clinically sufficient [50]. The minimum repair bond strength should not be less than 15–30 MPa which is the bond strength of composite to the etched enamel [51]. Theoretically, the adhesion to the aged composite should reach up to the cohesive strength of the composite to reestablish its original properties and guarantee its survival [52, 53]. Although the importance of a proper bond between the aged and repair composite has been emphasized numerous times, repair bond strengths have been found to be variable and unpredictable. Literature offers a wide range of repair bond strength values ranging from 20% to 82% of the cohesive strength of bulk materials [49, 54, 55]. Several authors found that different repair techniques achieved similar bond strengths to the cohesive one [55, 56].

An adequate surface treatment of the old resin, selection of the adhesive system, and restorative material are fundamentals of a successful repair. A deficient repair is inevitable when the dentist fails at one of these stages. Despite available repair strategies, there is still no agreement on the most efficient protocol [4, 57–59]. All the available surface treatment strategies aim to prepare a clean surface with high surface energy to provide better wettability with adequate surface roughness and surface area by removing the superficial layer of the aged composite [60].

Brosh et al. [61] reported that the repair of the old and new composite resin is achieved by three mechanisms: chemical bonding with the organic matrix, chemical bonding with the exposed filler particles, and macro/micromechanical retention [61].

The most important factor for improving the repair bond strength is surface roughening of the old composite by creating micro- and macro-mechanical retention and broadening the surface area available for adhesion [51, 62, 63]. Moreover, trimming a layer of resin may expose a rough and fresh surface that might improve the bond strength [62]. Macro-mechanical retention can be achieved by creating retention holes and undercuts or by just roughening the surface with a coarse diamond bur and lasers; micromechanical retention is created by etching (e.g., phosphoric acid or hydrofluoric acid or acidulated phosphate fluoride) or air abrasion with alumina or alumina particles coated with silica particles. Interlocking roughness is a critical constituent of micromechanical retention apart from macro-mechanical retention [64]. Micro-retentive interlocking has been reported to be the most important factor for providing an adequate repair bond strength and is likely more important than chemical bonding to the resin matrix or to the exposed filler particles [65].

16.4.1 Surface Roughening by Acid Etching

Etching of substrates is typically achieved by phosphoric or hydrofluoric acid. However, the literature contains contradictory data about the effectiveness of acid etching on the bond strength of repaired surfaces. Phosphoric acid is a weak acid and insufficient to create surface roughness on the composite resin surface [49]. Likewise, surface imaging performed by Fawzy et al. demonstrated no significant change in the composite's surface morphology after acid etching [47]. Literature consists of various in vitro reports demonstrating the insufficient effect of acid etching on the repair bond strength [53, 55, 66]. However, repairing a composite resin restoration involves not only removing a portion of the restoration but also adjacent enamel and dentin [53]. Phosphoric acid is effective on enamel and dentin but has no direct effect on surface characteristics of composites, ceramics, and metals. It may only be a superficial cleanser [48, 63]. In fact, the main purpose of acid etching is to cleanse the material surface from debris/smear layer after preparation, expose the surface irregularities left by wear, increase surface energy for better wetting, remove surface contamination by saliva or other agents, and help to increase contact between the fresh resin [67–69].

Gupta et al. compared 10% hydrofluoric acid, 30% citric acid, 7% maleic acid, and 37% phosphoric acid in the repair mechanism, and hydrofluoric acid yielded the best repair bond strength [59]. Unlike phosphoric acid, hydrofluoric acid attacks the exposed glass particles and dissolves them, thereby reducing the irregularities available for silane coupling, leaving the resin matrix unaffected. Therefore, it is important to realize that the effect of hydrofluoric acid is largely dependent on the composition of the filler particles in the material. Composite resins containing zirconium clusters or quartz fillers, for instance, will react less upon hydrofluoric acid etching than composite resins consisting of barium-glass fillers [57]. Also, it was observed that hydrofluoric acid (9.6%) dissolves a silica phase and dislodges the zirconia filler part from the resin matrix nanofilled composite [57]. Thus, etching with hydrofluoric acid is reasonable for the composite repair. The adequate concentration is found to be between 4% and 10% to achieve proper repair bond strength values [59].

The limitation of the use of hydrofluoric acid is the hazards associated with the intraoral use of hydrofluoric acid [70]. It not only jeopardizes the bond strengths of resin composites to dentin but forms a calcium fluoride (CaF_2) precipitate on dentin and enamel [71]. The precipitate of CaF_2

could then prevent the infiltration of adhesive resin in the opened dentin tubuli, resulting in poor adhesion of composite to the contaminated enamel or dentin [71, 72]. Contamination of the skin or mucosa with hydrofluoric acid is painless but may result in tissue necrosis in the deeper layers of the tissue [73].

16.4.2 Surface Roughening by Air Abrasion

Airborne-particle abrasion is typically applied using chairside air abrasion devices for intraoral repairs operating under a pressure between 2 and 3 bars. The substrate material to be conditioned, metal, ceramic, composite, or amalgam, is abraded for approximately 10 s from approximately 10 mm distance to achieve a clean and rough surface. Prolonged duration of air abrasion may be needed for zirconia [74]. The abrasion particles consist of 30–50 μm or aluminum oxide particles coated with a silicon dioxide layer, where the latter is referred to as "silicoating" or "tribochemical surface conditioning" [75]. Alumina or silica particles coat the surface, which then make covalent bonds through the siloxane layer with the silane coupling agent. Given that one disadvantage of air abrasion is the aerosol with abrasive particles, a good suction device is mandatory to prevent aspiration of these particles. The CoJet particles are designed to penetrate and be embedded in the surface of the substrate and leave it partially coated with silica [76]. It is possible that the embedded particles act as microretention sites for the new composite, explaining the improved bond strength. Besides, Da Silva et al. speculate that an effective surface treatment, such as sandblasting or aluminum oxide silica coating, may prevent negative effects of biofilm acids on composite repair [77]. However, the silica coating has been suggested to reduce the bond strength between enamel and dentin and the repair composite within the repair zone [78].

In literature, there are numerous in vitro reports evaluating the effect of sandblasting/air abrasion with other surface treatment methods and reported different results. It was reported that the repair of several composite brands only achieved bond strengths closer to the cohesive one after sandblasting with 50 μm alumina particles [57]. Various reports confirm satisfactory bond strength values for 50 μm aluminum oxide sandblasting repair [50, 79–83]. Another study reported the superiority of 50 μm aluminum oxide sandblasting over chemical treatments as it provides increased surface roughness and wetting potential of the repair composite and improved bond strength for composite repair [22, 84]. Several research groups have found that bond strength values obtained by air abrasion were not significantly different from the results obtained with diamond bur grinding [85, 86].

The bond strength following air abrasion using 50 μm aluminum oxide was found to be similar to tribochemical silica coating (30 μm alumina particles coated with silica) [22, 79, 84, 87]. It was postulated that similar surface roughness pattern resulted in similar mechanical retention. Likewise, Passos et al. reported that treatment with 50 μm aluminum oxide air abrasion followed by 37% phosphoric acid etching and the application of one-step total-etch adhesive resulted in the highest μTBS values in the repair zone [88]. However, a good suction device is necessary to avoid aspiration of these particles.

In addition to favorable repair bond strength, Celik et al. reported that air abrasion produced the lowest microleakage values regardless of the adhesive systems and the existing resin composite type [89].

16.4.3 Surface Roughening by Bur Cutting

Diamond burs are commercially available with different diamond grit sizes. Abrasive granulometry influences the cutting efficiency of the burs, potentially affecting the composite surface micromorphology and interlocking with the repair material [90]. As the resin phase and the inorganic particles differ in hardness, their abrasion rate is not uniform, leaving a retentive pattern on the surface. The cutting efficiency and the ability to remove material from the composite surface are different, depending on the diamond bur grit size, affecting the profile left on the composite for mechanical interlocking [90]. Previous studies have indicated that diamond grit sizes may interfere with the thickness and morphology of the smear layer and bonding to dentin [91, 92]. Treatment of aged composites using diamond burs before restoration repair could also be influenced by the diamond grit size.

The use of diamond burs as a surface preparation approach at the repair zone revealed contradictory results [63, 93, 94]. Bonstein et al. indicated that surface treatment by diamond bur led to higher bond strength compared to other techniques [63]. However, similar bond strength values or wetting characteristics of roughening with diamond burs alone or with sandblasting wetting were reported as well [52, 60, 84, 95, 96]. This approach with the application of an adhesive provides an efficient, clinically applicable, and cost-effective procedure for repair of aged composite restorations [90]. Surface roughening using burs is an easy and cost-effective procedure that does not necessitate the use of additional equipment or chemical substances. Nevertheless, from a clinical perspective, hydrofluoric acid application and sandblasting are not as safe and convenient as surface roughening with diamond burs [94]. Covalcanti et al. reported that surface treatment of direct composite with air abrasion led to higher repair bond strength values compared with diamond burs [55].

Valente et al. observed similar surface roughness for the no-treatment and extra-fine grit groups, despite the higher bond strength for the extra-fine grit group [90]. Therefore, other physicochemical properties of the treated surface (aside from surface roughness) should be considered in any explanation of the results. Wettability of the adhesive on the surface is one aspect that could play a role in improving the repair bond strength to bur-roughened restoratives. It was expected that rougher surfaces would show a lower contact angle, because coarser topography could affect the critical value of surface tension and coefficient of friction. As a result, attraction between water molecules and rougher surfaces would be increased, improving wettability. However, no significant differences in contact angle were observed between surface treatments. In contrast, the contact angle formed on the aged composite was lower than on the fresh composite, which might be linked to the absorption of water and hydrolytic effects occurring during aging, making the surface more polar [90].

16.4.4 Surface Roughening by Laser

The purpose of using lasers in resin repairs is similar to other mechanical surface treatment modalities aiming to increase surface roughness and energy to deliver adequate surface topography for bonding [79, 97–100].

Laser is also accepted to be more conservative than other mechanical treatment alternatives [99]. Among different lasers used in dentistry, erbium lasers are considered as the best option for caries removal and cavity preparation. This family of lasers has two wavelengths including Er:YAG laser (erbium-doped: yttrium-aluminum-garnet) (2940 nm) and erbium, chromium-doped yttrium scandium gallium garnet (Er,Cr:YSGG) laser (2780 nm) [101, 102]. Enhancements in laser technology enabled Er:YAG laser usage as a surface treatment approach [103]. The Waterlase laser cuts the tooth tissues with highly energized water particles [104, 105]. Lately, Er:YAG laser has been indicated in the repair process as a surface treatment modality [106]. Energized water molecules abrade the composite surface without increasing the surface temperature avoiding the formation of subsurface microcracks which might act as stress concentration zones [104, 105]. The ablation process with energized water molecules provides clean surface without any composite debris [104, 105].

As laser technology marks a new era in operative dentistry, there are numerous studies in dental literature about the effect of lasers on the repair process demonstrating variable results. The topography of the ablated resin composite surface depends not only on the power setting of the Er:YAG laser but also the composition of the resin composite [107]. Consequently, it is obvious that these parameters affect bonding mechanisms between the resin composites [108]. Murray et al. and Cho et al. reported that reduced output power was associated with better bonding conditions [79, 109]. Etemadi et al. reported that with the increasing output power of Er:YAG laser, the composite surface became unsuitable due to excessive material deterioration, but powers below 5 W produced retentive surface that can interact with composite resin [110]. Lizarelli et al. concluded that microfilled and hybrid resin composite were more prone to ablation than condensable counterparts [107].

The ablation process on the surface of the resin composite produces an ablated diameter depending on the energy per pulse [111]. As the ablation diameter, depth, and volume increases, the adhesion of the repair resin composite decreases. Similarly, Duran et al. found out that 75 mJ Er:YAG resulted in the highest repair bond strength, whereas 200 and 300 mJ test groups had lower bond strengths [108]. However, Tugut et al. reported that 300 mJ presented high bond strength values than 100, 200 (short and long pulses), and 400 mJ Er:YAG laser irradiation. They explained the increased bond strength with the increased surface area produced by the ablation caused instant vaporization of water [112]. Likewise, Gokce et al. demonstrated that 300 mJ produced higher shear bond strength values than 600–900 mJ power settings. Decreased bond strength values were thought to be related with heat-damaged layer [111].

Oskoee et al. evaluated the efficacy of different lasers as surface treatment protocols in the repair process and found out that Er,Cr:YSGG laser showed better repair bond strength values than Nd:YAG and CO_2 lasers without the formation of the smear layer [102].

When the efficacy of laser ablation is compared with other mechanical surface treatment protocols, Duran et al. proposed laser ablation as the surface treatment modality although superior repair bond strength values with sandblasting [108]. Murray et al. suggested laser treatment as an appropriate treatment option for enhanced repair bond strengths [109]; likewise, Rossato et al. found that laser and bur treatment had similar results when used in the repair process [113]. Oskoee et al. also found out that Er,Cr:YSGG laser treatment produced similar bond strength values with bur treatment in silorane-based resin composite repair approach [106]. Laser irradiation ablates the composite resin without smear layer production [107].

16.4.5 Chemical Bonding

While surface roughness enables micromechanical interlocking of the repair composite, intermediate materials, like adhesive resin, silane coupling agents, or flowable resin composite, are still necessary to promote surface wetting and subsequent formation of a durable bond between the aged and repair resin composite [13, 80, 93, 96]. In addition, a chemical bond may be achieved between resin and inorganic filler particles by application of special primers such as silane coupling agents [14]. According to Papacchini et al. use of a flowable hydrophobic resin composite as an intermediate material increased the repair bond strength of methacrylate-based composite resins [114].

Similarly, the adhesive systems enhance the bond between aged and the repair resin composite not only by infiltrating into the surface irregularities but also by their chemical affinity to the matrix and exposed filler particles [54, 55, 115]. Besides, every resin composite repair procedure involves enamel or dentin tissues; also, it is not clinically possible to avoid repair site from adhesive system contamination. The wettability of the treated aged resin composite by the adhesive resin is a fundamental prerequisite for the repair mechanism irrespective of the mechanism of adhesion (chemical, micromechanical interlocking, or a combination of both) since resin composites have high viscosity and low wetting potential complicating the repair mechanism [116]. Previous research confirmed the ability of the adhesive systems to promote optimized repair bond strengths [4, 68, 93, 96, 117]. However, the hydrophilicity of the intermediate material can compromise the longevity of the repair bond strength because hydrophilic adhesives tend to absorb more water over time and may undergo hydrolytic degradation [114, 118]. It has been confirmed that placing an extra layer of hydrophobic resin can improve the repair bond strength of methacrylate-based composite resins and decrease microleakage [119–121].

The three-step adhesive systems are considered as golden standard in adhesive technology when placing resin composite restorations [122, 123]. The superiority of these etch-and-rinse systems may be attributed to their less hydrophilic monomer constituents than the more acidic self-etching adhesives. Da Costa et al. reported early signs of degradation for hydrophilic self-etching adhesive repair bond compared with a hydrophobic three-step adhesive at 6 months [80]. Similarly, Eliasson et al. demonstrated a general reduction in mean tensile repair strength values after 12 months of storage in water in addition to thermocycling [117].

Nevertheless, it has been reported that self-etch adhesives may be an alternative treatment modality in the repair approach [124]. The acidic functional monomers provide a chemical bond between the inorganic constitutes of the aged and repair resin composite creating a continuous flow between the aged composite and the adhesive [125].

As stated previously, following mechanical surface treatment, chemical adhesion can be established using special primers or monomers that react with the surface of the material like the adhesive systems [126, 127]. The most common primer is a silane coupling agent that is also used in the fabrication of composites to bond the inorganic filler particles chemically to the resin matrix [67]. Silanes promote repair bond strength by enhancing surface energy that is a prerequisite for optimized wetting to obtain close contact between the resin composites [67]. The most commonly used silane in dental materials is a bifunctional molecule, 3-methacryloxypropyltri methoxysilane (MPS). MPS silanes consist of a methacrylate group that can react with the intermediate adhesive resin and composites, as well as a reactive silanol group that can form siloxane bonds with the alumina and/or silica present on the air-abraded or etched substrate surfaces [14].

Silane coupling agents are presently available as hydrolyzed or non-hydrolyzed. The hydrolyzed silanes are ready for use and should be applied as a separate step in the bonding procedure before the adhesive resin. The non-hydrolyzed silane has to be activated first with an acid, usually an acidic monomer (i.e., 10-methacryloxydecyldihydrogen phosphate (10-MDP)), which is present in the primer or adhesive resin [14].

Depending on the adhesive system, the silane coupling agent has to be mixed with the primer or adhesive resin. Many in vitro studies have shown significant positive effects on the use of silane coupling agents in composite repairs [51, 61, 62, 67, 93, 128]. However, Nassoohi et al. found that silane application resulted in the weakest bond strength [82]. Likewise, few researchers reported that the addition of silane to the bonding system might not significantly improve bond strength or even might reduce it [22, 34, 51, 61, 62].

The basic disadvantage of silanes is the hydrolytic instability which results in splitting the Si-O cation bridges over time. Therefore, the repair bond strength depends on weak Van der Waal forces rather than stronger covalent or ionic ones [67]. Besides, one-bottle hydrolyzed silane solutions have a relatively short shelf life and gradually become less reactive after opening of the bottle, preventing optimal adhesion [76]. Moreover, hydrolysis causes degradation of the bonding interface [76, 118, 129]. The 2-hydroxyethyl methacrylate (HEMA) content of the adhesive system in the interface is hydrophilic and attracts water leading to hydrolysis [76].

Barcellos et al. reported that surface roughening by mechanical treatment and subsequent silane application without further treatments resulted in reduced repair bond strength [60]. Imbery et al. suggested improved repair strength values when the aged resin composite surface was first silica coated and silanized and an adhesive system is applied [53]. However, Lima et al. suggested that similar repair bond strength values were obtained without the application of silanes [49].

The substantial interest in the polymerization process also led researchers to analyze the effect of light-curing units on the repair process.

Karaman and Gonulol concluded that currently available light-curing units (quartz-tungsten-halogen (QTH)), light-emitting diode (LED), and plasma arc curing (PAC)) performed similar repair bond strength values for methacrylate-based resin composites but suggested QTH or LED for polymerization of silorane-based resin composites [130]. However, as the clinician may not know the exact type of the aged resin composite, QTH or LED is recommended in any situation [130].

16.5 Effect of Existing Old Resin Composite

Although Specification No. 27 of American National Standards Institute/American Dental Association (ANSI/ADA) recommends the association of different resin composites, as long as they share a similar organic matrix, literature reports that the effectiveness of the repair procedures depend on the material to be repaired [57, 131], and it has been advised to repair resin composites with similar structured resin composites [132]. In fact, when performing a repair, the clinician is limited by the fact that the type and brand of the resin composite may not be known unless performed by the same clinician or not recorded. However, repair procedures between composites with different chemical composition, filler size, morphology, filler content, and distribution may yield variable results.

Studies have shown that it is generally advisable but not compulsory to combine identical composite resins for repair [58, 132–135].

As stated previously, the intimate adaptation between the old and the repair resin composite mostly depends on the surface roughness of the existing resin composite which can be influenced by different factors related to the nature of the material, such as the filler (type, shape, size, and distribution of the particles), the type of resin matrix, the degree of cure, and hardness [136–138].

Celik et al. in two consecutive studies, examined the quantitative microleakage and microtensile bond strength of resin composite restorations with different resin composite types (similar to the existing restoration or dissimilar one) and adhesive systems [89, 139]. The materials and methods section from the first study is summarized in Fig. 16.4. Mainly, occlusal cavities were prepared and restored with two different types of resin composite. After thermocycling, two parts of the restorations were drilled out to simulate repair. Different types of surface conditioning methods were employed, and the repaired restorations were re-thermocycled. The specimens were kept in basic fuchsin and sectioned mesiodistally to examine microleakage quantitatively (Fig. 16.5). The authors concluded that sandblasting produced the lowest microleakage values independent of the adhesive system and the preexisting resin composite [89].

The later research evaluated the microtensile bond strength of the previously tested setup, and the results were consistent with the previous research demonstrating that sandblasting produced the highest microtensile repair bond strength for dissimilar resin composite types independent of the adhesive system used [139].

16.5.1 Methacrylate-Based Resin Composite

Repair bond strength is affected by type, size, and amount of the filler of the existing resin composite [40, 44, 62]. As the filler parameter strongly determines the surface characteristics of a resin composite, this phenomenon acts as an issue in the repair process. In fact, identical filler amounts in existing and repair resin composite show better repair bond strength values than with different filler amounts. Larger filler particles in resin composite may provide more surface area for reaction with functional monomers in the adhesive systems [125].

Nanocomposites are claimed to have promising physico-mechanical properties with high proportion of filler particles. They are less susceptible to aging and more favorable to being repaired because they have a lower water sorption rate compared to other composites due to their high

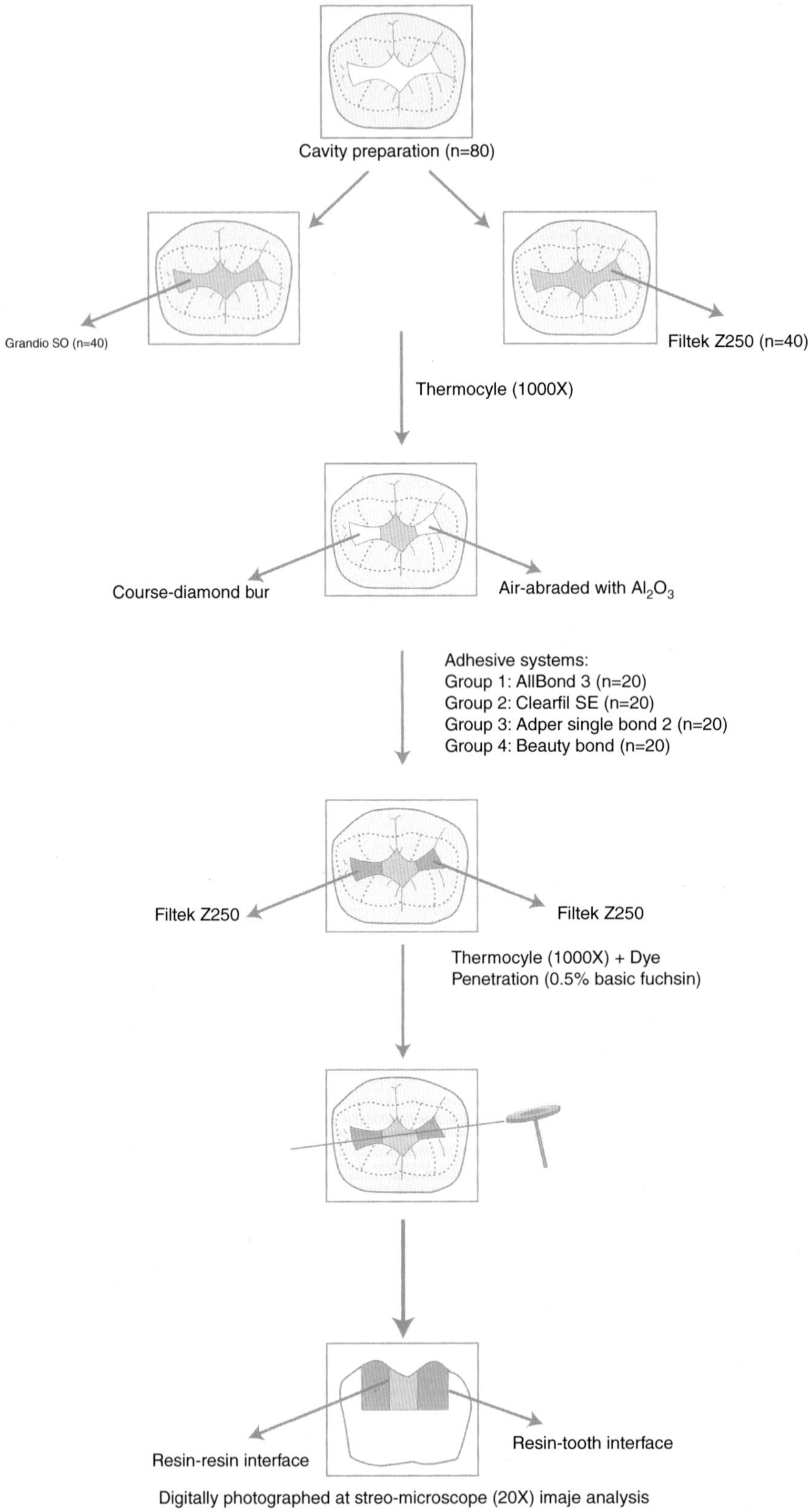

Fig. 16.4 Schematic representation of the research protocol

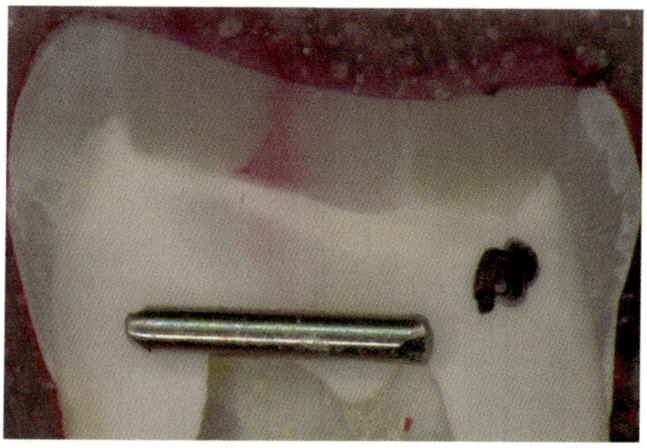

Fig. 16.5 A specimen exhibiting extensive microleakage at the repair interface

filler content [140, 141]. However, despite their broadening usage as esthetic materials, their repair bond strengths reported conflicting results [142]. Nassoohi et al. reported that microhybrid resin composite might have a better repair bond strength compared with nanocomposites, while nanofilled and nanohybrid types are less likely different from one another [82]. On the contrary, Özcan et al. found that nanofilled composites have better repair retention [142]. In fact, Rinastiti et al. emphasized the importance of the brand of the nanohybrid composites with one of the tested nanohybrid materials showed results similar to the microhybrid, while the other one showed slightly better results [143]. Loomans et al. [57] and Baena et al. [52] found that when repairing a nanohybrid composite, almost all repair procedures produced similar bond strength to the cohesive one. Moncada et al. reported that hybrid composites provide better repair strength than microfilled resins [133]. Rodrigues et al. did not observe differences between the repair bond strength of microhybrid and nanofilled resin composites (repaired with the same composite) after aluminum oxide air abrasion or other surface treatments [22].

Resins containing bisphenol glycidyl methacrylate (bis-GMA) have lower conversion rates compared with other matrices [144]. Therefore, bis-GMA-containing resins may have more unreacted carbon–carbon double bonds to chemically react with the repairing composite resulting in higher repair strengths than resins containing different matrices [124].

The importance of the age of the restoration on the repair bond strength of methacrylate-based composites was previously evaluated and found out that available vinyl groups for cross polymerization decrease affecting the clinical performance of repairs [145]. The age of an existing restoration mirrors the time that the restoration was exposed to water sorption, chemical degradation, and leaching of components. Besides the loss of unreacted double bonds, the potential for chemical bonding between the existing and repair composite layers decreases over time due to the diminished oxygen-inhibited layer and free radicals [146].

The effect of different surface treatment strategies was also evaluated on different types of resin composites. Kaneko et al. reported increased repair strength values after the air abrasion and adhesive application irrespective of the use of silane [34]. Thus, the knowledge of the material composition is crucial for the repair success since the microstructure influences the mechanical behavior of the repairs [22]. It should be emphasized that there is not an optimal surface treatment for all types of composites [57].

16.5.2 Silorane-Based Resin Composite

A silorane-based resin composite was the first non-methacrylate-based resin composite marketed for use in dentistry [147]. This epoxy-based resin contains an oxygen-containing ring molecule—oxiranes—and a siloxane molecule. It polymerizes with cationic ring-opening reaction rather than the linear chain reaction associated with conventional methacrylates [148]. The motivation of lying beneath the development of siloranes was to overcome the drawbacks of methacrylate-based resin composites like polymerization shrinkage and subsequent stress formation, water sorption, hydrolytic instability, and radical oxygen inhibition [149]. The polymerization of siloranes causes minimum reduction of the original distance between monomers with a volumetric shrinkage around 1%, which might generate less stress on the adhesive interface [148, 150, 151].

Silorane is considered a tetrafunctional molecule with greater molecular weight than other components used in most methacrylate-based materials. Although the degree of conversion of the material is smaller, components leach less than the methacrylate counterparts. However, epoxy groups polymerized by cationic mechanism may be less available for chemical reaction on the material surface than the polymeric products. When the silorane-based composites polymerize, an oxygen inhibition layer does not form as in methacrylate-based resin composites, because the cationic ring-opening process is not affected by the oxygen [152].

Silorane resin is highly hydrophobic because of the siloxane component. The adhesive system compatible with this hydrophobic system also contains hydrophobic dimethacrylate monomers (70–80 wt%) without hydrophilic HEMA monomer [153].

Thus, silorane-based restorations might be repaired with methacrylate-based composites if the dentist is not aware that the existing restoration is silorane-based. Therefore, it is of interest to evaluate the efficiency of other repair mechanisms involving methacrylate-based resin composites [154].

Most of the recent studies on repair of composites have included silorane-based restoratives [57, 145, 154–156]. Similar to methacrylate-based composites, it was concluded that there is no golden standard repair technique for silorane-based composites. However, Luhrs et al. demonstrated that the repair methods used for methacrylate-based composite resins could be also applied for silorane repair [81].

Laser treatment studies on the silorane-based resin composite surface pointed out that CO_2, Nd:YAG, and Er,Cr:YSGG lasers developed different ablation patterns which were accounted for different repair bond strengths. Oskoee et al. reported that these different patterns produced clinically acceptable bond strength values but Er,Cr:YSGG laser was found to be more efficient than the others [102]. Oskoee et al. also concluded that surface roughening either with Er,Cr:YSGG laser or diamond bur and subsequent application of the compatible adhesive system were adequate to obtain clinically acceptable repair bond strength values [106].

Bacchi et al. [131] and Kaneko et al. [34] reported that silorane-based composite had a lower repair bond strength than methacrylate-based ones. Besides, the repair bond strength was lower than the cohesive strength of the material [77, 152]. However, sandblasting and subsequent application of an adhesive system increased the repair bond strength of silorane-based resin composites [81, 131]. The lower repair potential of silorane resin can be explained by the lower reactivity of silorane groups after polymerization. However, repaired silorane-based resin composite produced similar repair bond strength values after 24 h and 2 years of storage [21].

Lima et al. confirmed that diamond bur and sandblasting with aluminum oxide can yield similar bond strength values of immediate bonding to silorane and an adhesive layer is crucial in the repair mechanism [49]. However, Hamano et al. did not demonstrate any additional value to repair bond strength of silorane by application of bonding agent [154].

Surprisingly, effective repair of methacrylate-based resin composite by silorane-based resin composite was suggested by many in vitro studies [4, 81, 145]. The vice versa was also suggested by Ivanovas et al. [145]. However, it was also showed that silorane-based resin composites yielded better results when used as a base material but was evidently a poor repair material [95, 132].

Previous studies reported that silane application was mandatory for the adhesion of methacrylate-based adhesives on silorane surfaces [4, 81, 143, 145, 157]; however, Wiegand et al. suggested that silane application is not necessary when silorane composite and its compatible silorane adhesive system were used in the repair mechanism [156].

Hamano et al. showed that silane did not contribute to an increase in the tensile strength of silorane-based composites repaired with methacrylate-based composites [154]. Since the silane agent did not adversely affect the bond strength of the silorane adhesive system, the routine application of silane for repair of composite restorations with unknown composite matrix could be recommended [156].

16.5.3 Fiber-Reinforced Resin Composite

Since there has been minimal achievement in improving the properties of the resin matrix for the last two decades, contemporary composite resin expertise has aimed to improve filler technology instead [158]. Composites reinforced with discontinuous fibers are known as short fiber-reinforced composites [159]. Fiber-reinforced resin composites have been shown to have adequate flexural properties and improved resistance to crack initiation and propagation [160–162]. Recently, a short fiber-reinforced resin composite was developed [163]. The composition of short-fiber-reinforced resin composite is different from that of conventional glass-filled resin composites [164]. The material has three basic components: (1) bis-GMA, TEGDMA, and PMMA forming a matrix called a semi-interpenetrating polymer network (semi-IPN); (2) the fillers that are composed of electrical (E) glass fibers, which improve the toughness of the resin matrix; and (3) inorganic particulate fillers. However, the material is indicated for use as a base material in high stress areas.

Although mechanical and structural characterization of these short-fiber-reinforced resin composites are well documented, dental literature is scarce about repair of short-fiber-reinforced resin composite materials [159]. Future research is essential for the validation of repair of short fiber-reinforced resin composites.

16.5.4 Dual-Cure Resin Composite

This type of resin composite materials was developed to overcome depth of cure problems [165] that can be faced with incremental technique [166]. Dual-cured resin composite buildup restorative materials utilize redox initiator systems and photoinitiators [167]. Polymerization begins with light activation on the surface of the material and continues by chemical activation in the deeper layers [168]. El-Deeb et al. suggested that this material can be repaired [169]. The repair strength of dual-cured core materials recovered 64–86% of their corresponding cohesive strength values, while the light-cured materials yielded a range between 76% and 81% of their corresponding cohesive strength values [47, 170, 171].

16.6 Clinical Success of Repaired Restorations

Although in vitro studies have generally revealed decreased repair bond strength, other studies have shown benefits of repairs on the longevity of the restoration [5]. This fact may indicate that there may not be a direct correlation to the clinical performance and longevity of the restoration [6, 23, 172, 173].

Many researchers proved that refurbishment and monitoring restoration defects increase the longevity of the defective restorations [13, 23, 172, 174]. On the other hand, in a systematic review, Cochrane Collaboration concluded that there is no scientific proof to state that repair of resin composites is advantageous [9]. As the literature contains no consensus by randomized clinical trials according to the Consolidated Standards of Reporting Trials (CONSORT), only available clinical trials enlighten the researchers' way to perform adequate and long-lasting repaired restorations [175].

Any clinical trial on the repair of resin composite should carefully report a repair action [14]. When the first repair is not considered a failure, longevity of restorations may increase significantly, and annual failure rate may even decrease to less than 1% [174, 176]. For example, Demarco et al. reported an annual failure rate of 1.9% of both replaced and repaired restorations; however, if the repaired restorations had not been considered failures, the annual failure rate would have dropped to 0.7% [176, 177]. Similarly, Opdam et al. demonstrated a similar reduction of annual failure rates from 1.83% to 0.72% with the same supposition [174].

Data available from recent in vivo studies confirm that resin composite repair can be a viable and long-term clinical procedure [13, 21, 80, 174, 176, 178].

Frencken et al. concluded that replaced and repaired restorations have the same or increased longevity [27]. Likewise, another randomized clinical trial on the performance of repaired composite restorations over a period of 10 years showed similar results to those that were replaced [178]. General dental practice-based prospective cohort studies have shown that repaired restorations have similar or increased longevity compared to replaced restorations [5, 172, 179, 180]. Some of these dental practice-based studies have found repairs to remain clinically acceptable up to 7-year observation periods [5, 16, 180].

Popoff et al. found that silorane-based resin composite provides clinically acceptable results when used as a repair material of methacrylate-based resin composite after 2 years of clinical service [181]. Although in vitro studies have shown lower values of polymerization shrinkage related to silorane-based composites, it is difficult to show the effects in clinical studies, where many different factors influence the final result [150, 151].

Fernandez et al. concluded that a simple procedure like repair doubles the longevity of a defective restoration [182]. The presence of secondary caries yielded better repair prognosis than restorations repaired because of fracture [174].

16.7 Clinical Recommendations and Conclusion

Decent diagnosis and treatment planning about a "defective" restoration are of fundamental importance in terms of restoration longevity. Although there are no sound data and guidelines derived from clinical trials in Cochrane Library, the repair of defected restorations is highly recommended by the scientific world if performed properly.

It is difficult to provide clear guidelines as every patient is unique and differences in diagnosing secondary caries, future caries risk, and oral hygiene habits may pose challenges to the clinician. The clinician should decide by taking into consideration individual circumstances with the patient's consent. Consequently, the repair concept should be included in dental education curricula; thus, prospective clinicians should diagnose defective restorations and decide on the treatment plan considering pros and cons of the "repair or replace" where appropriate.

Blum et al. proposed a clinical procedure for the repair of a direct resin composite restoration with one or more limited defects [7]. He advised preparation of the composite substrate or any exposed tooth tissue using an intraoral sandblaster or a fine-grit diamond bur, acid etching, application of silane primer and corresponding adhesive system, and subsequent application of resin composite.

Blunck documented working instructions of the International Academy of Adhesive Dentistry (IAAD) [183]. The IAAD recommends reducing the surface by diamond bur, air abrasion (50 μm aluminum oxide or 30 μm aluminum oxide coated with SiO_2) by protecting the adjacent teeth, acid etching the enamel parts of the cavity margins, applying a silane or a universal primer to the composite surface, and subsequent application of an adhesive system (preferably three-step adhesive system) before resin composite layering.

Loomans and Ozcan recommended roughening the existing resin composite surface with fine-grit diamond bur, etching the composite margins with 5–9.6% hydrofluoric acid or air abrasion, silane application, and subsequent adhesive system application before repair resin composite application [14].

References

1. Sunnegardh-Gronberg K, van Dijken JW, Funegard U, Lindberg A, Nilsson M. Selection of dental materials and longevity of replaced restorations in public dental health clinics in northern Sweden. J Dent. 2009;37(9):673–8. doi:10.1016/j.jdent.2009.04.010.
2. Statement on posterior resin-based composites. ADA Council on scientific affairs; ADA Council on dental benefit programs. J Am Dent Assoc. 1998;129(11):1627–8.

3. Burke FJ. Amalgam to tooth-coloured materials—implications for clinical practice and dental education: governmental restrictions and amalgam-usage survey results. J Dent. 2004;32(5):343–50. doi:10.1016/j.jdent.2004.02.003.
4. Maneenut C, Sakoolnamarka R, Tyas MJ. The repair potential of resin composite materials. Dent Mater. 2011;27(2):e20–7. doi:10.1016/j.dental.2010.09.006.
5. Gordan VV, Garvan CW, Blaser PK, Mondragon E, Mjor IA. A long-term evaluation of alternative treatments to replacement of resin-based composite restorations: results of a seven-year study. J Am Dent Assoc. 2009;140(12):1476–84.
6. Mjor IA, Gordan VV. Failure, repair, refurbishing and longevity of restorations. Oper Dent. 2002;27(5):528–34.
7. Blum IR, Lynch CD, Wilson NH. Factors influencing repair of dental restorations with resin composite. Clin Cosmet Investig Dent. 2014;6:81–7. doi:10.2147/CCIDE.S53461.
8. Lynch CD, Opdam NJ, Hickel R, Brunton PA, Gurgan S, Kakaboura A, et al. Guidance on posterior resin composites: academy of operative dentistry – European section. J Dent. 2014;42(4):377–83. doi:10.1016/j.jdent.2014.01.009.
9. Sharif MO, Catleugh M, Merry A, Tickle M, Dunne SM, Brunton P, et al. Replacement versus repair of defective restorations in adults: resin composite. Cochrane Database Syst Rev. 2014;2:CD005971. doi:10.1002/14651858.CD005971.pub3.
10. Tyas MJ, Anusavice KJ, Frencken JE, Mount GJ. Minimal intervention dentistry—a review. FDI Commission Project 1-97. Int Dent J. 2000;50(1):1–12.
11. Mjor IA, Shen C, Eliasson ST, Richter S. Placement and replacement of restorations in general dental practice in Iceland. Oper Dent. 2002;27(2):117–23.
12. Hickel R, Peschke A, Tyas M, Mjor I, Bayne S, Peters M, et al. FDI world dental federation—clinical criteria for the evaluation of direct and indirect restorations. Update and clinical examples. J Adhes Dent. 2010;12(4):259–72. doi:10.3290/j.jad.a19262.
13. Hickel R, Brushaver K, Ilie N. Repair of restorations—criteria for decision making and clinical recommendations. Dent Mater. 2013;29(1):28–50. doi:10.1016/j.dental.2012.07.006.
14. Loomans B, Ozcan M. Intraoral repair of direct and indirect restorations: procedures and guidelines. Oper Dent. 2016;41(S7):S68–78. doi:10.2341/15-269-LIT.
15. Staehle HJ, Wolff D, Frese C. More conservative dentistry: clinical long-term results of direct composite resin restorations. Quintessence Int. 2015;46(5):373–80. doi:10.3290/j.qi.a33718.
16. Blum IR, Jagger DC, Wilson NH. Defective dental restorations: to repair or not to repair? Part 1: direct composite restorations. Dent Update. 2011;38(2):78–80. 2-4
17. Hickel R, Roulet JF, Bayne S, Heintze SD, Mjor IA, Peters M, et al. Recommendations for conducting controlled clinical studies of dental restorative materials. Int Dent J. 2007;57(5):300–2.
18. Ismail AI, Pitts NB, Tellez M, Management S, Banerjee A, Authors of International Caries C, et al. The International Caries Classification and Management System (ICCMS) an example of a caries management pathway. BMC Oral Health. 2015;15(Suppl 1):S9. doi:10.1186/1472–6831-15-S1-S9.
19. Blum IR, Schriever A, Heidemann D, Mjor IA, Wilson NH. The repair of direct composite restorations: an international survey of the teaching of operative techniques and materials. Eur J Dent Educ. 2003;7(1):41–8.
20. Elderton RJ, Nuttall NM. Variation among dentists in planning treatment. Br Dent J. 1983;154(7):201–6.
21. Mobarak E, El-Deeb H. Two-year interfacial bond durability and nanoleakage of repaired silorane-based resin composite. Oper Dent. 2013;38(4):408–18. doi:10.2341/12-061-L.
22. Rodrigues SA Jr, Ferracane JL, Della BA. Influence of surface treatments on the bond strength of repaired resin composite restorative materials. Dent Mater. 2009;25(4):442–51. doi:10.1016/j.dental.2008.09.009.
23. Gordan VV, Shen C, Riley J 3rd, Mjor IA. Two-year clinical evaluation of repair versus replacement of composite restorations. J Esthet Restor Dent. 2006;18(3):144–153.; discussion 54. doi:10.1111/j.1708-8240.2006.00007.x.
24. Sharif MO, Catleugh M, Merry A, Tickle M, Dunne SM, Brunton P, et al. Replacement versus repair of defective restorations in adults: resin composite. Cochrane Database Syst Rev. 2010;2:CD005971. doi:10.1002/14651858.CD005971.pub2.
25. Sharif MO, Merry A, Catleugh M, Tickle M, Brunton P, Dunne SM, et al. Replacement versus repair of defective restorations in adults: amalgam. Cochrane Database Syst Rev. 2010;2:CD005970. doi:10.1002/14651858.CD005970.pub2.
26. Benn DK. Radiographic caries diagnosis and monitoring. Dentomaxillofac Radiol. 1994;23(2):69–72. doi:10.1259/dmfr.23.2.7835505.
27. Frencken JE, Peters MC, Manton DJ, Leal SC, Gordan VV, Eden E. Minimal intervention dentistry for managing dental caries - a review: report of a FDI task group. Int Dent J. 2012;62(5):223–43. doi:10.1111/idj.12007.
28. Turkun LS. The clinical performance of one- and two-step self-etching adhesive systems at one year. J Am Dent Assoc. 2005;136(5):656–64. quiz 83
29. Ermis RB, Temel UB, Cellik EU, Kam O. Clinical performance of a two-step self-etch adhesive with additional enamel etching in class III cavities. Oper Dent. 2010;35(2):147–55. doi:10.2341/09-089-C.
30. Fron H, Vergnes JN, Moussally C, Cazier S, Simon AL, Chieze JB, et al. Effectiveness of a new one-step self-etch adhesive in the restoration of non-carious cervical lesions: 2-year results

of a randomized controlled practice-based study. Dent Mater. 2011;27(3):304–12. doi:10.1016/j.dental.2010.11.006.
31. Perdigao J, Dutra-Correa M, Anauate-Netto C, Castilhos N, Carmo AR, Lewgoy HR, et al. Two-year clinical evaluation of self-etching adhesives in posterior restorations. J Adhes Dent. 2009;11(2):149–59.
32. Baracco B, Perdigao J, Cabrera E, Giraldez I, Ceballos L. Clinical evaluation of a low-shrinkage composite in posterior restorations: one-year results. Oper Dent. 2012;37(2):117–29. doi:10.2341/11-179-C.
33. Gordan VV, Riley JL 3rd, Geraldeli S, Rindal DB, Qvist V, Fellows JL, et al. Repair or replacement of defective restorations by dentists in the dental practice-based research network. J Am Dent Assoc. 2012;143(6):593–601.
34. Kaneko M, Caldas RA, Feitosa VP, Xediek Consani RL, Schneider LF, Bacchi A. Influence of surface treatments to repair recent fillings of silorane-and methacrylate-based composites. J Conserv Dent. 2015;18(3):242–6. doi:10.4103/0972-0707.157265.
35. Blum IR, Lynch CD, Schriever A, Heidemann D, Wilson NH. Repair versus replacement of defective composite restorations in dental schools in Germany. Eur J Prosthodont Restor Dent. 2011;19(2):56–61.
36. Blum IR, Lynch CD, Wilson NH. Teaching of the repair of defective composite restorations in Scandinavian dental schools. J Oral Rehabil. 2012;39(3):210–6. doi:10.1111/j.1365-2842.2011.02260.x.
37. Blum IR, Lynch CD, Wilson NH. Teaching of direct composite restoration repair in undergraduate dental schools in the United Kingdom and Ireland. Eur J Dent Educ. 2012;16(1):e53–8. doi:10.1111/j.1600-0579.2010.00674.x.
38. Schwendicke F, Frencken JE, Bjorndal L, Maltz M, Manton DJ, Ricketts D, et al. Managing carious lesions: consensus recommendations on carious tissue removal. Adv Dent Res. 2016;28(2):58–67. doi:10.1177/0022034516639271.
39. Vankerckhoven H, Lambrechts P, van Beylen M, Davidson CL, Vanherle G. Unreacted methacrylate groups on the surfaces of composite resins. J Dent Res. 1982;61(6):791–5.
40. Rinastiti M, Ozcan M, Siswomihardjo W, Busscher HJ. Immediate repair bond strengths of microhybrid, nanohybrid and nanofilled composites after different surface treatments. J Dent. 2010;38(1):29–38. doi:10.1016/j.jdent.2009.08.009.
41. Suzuki S, Ori T, Saimi Y. Effects of filler composition on flexibility of microfilled resin composite. J Biomed Mater Res B Appl Biomater. 2005;74(1):547–52. doi:10.1002/jbm.b.30235.
42. Ferracane JL. Hygroscopic and hydrolytic effects in dental polymer networks. Dent Mater. 2006;22(3):211–22. doi:10.1016/j.dental.2005.05.005.
43. Soderholm KJ, Zigan M, Ragan M, Fischlschweiger W, Bergman M. Hydrolytic degradation of dental composites. J Dent Res. 1984;63(10):1248–54.
44. Soderholm KJ, Roberts MJ. Variables influencing the repair strength of dental composites. Scand J Dent Res. 1991;99(2):173–80.
45. Lewis G, Johnson W, Martin W, Canerdy A, Claburn C, Collier M. Shear bond strength of immediately repaired light-cured composite resin restorations. Oper Dent. 1998;23(3):121–7.
46. Nakano Y, Yoshimura M, Koga T. Correlation between oral malodor and periodontal bacteria. Microbes Infect. 2002;4(6):679–83.
47. Fawzy AS, El-Askary FS, Amer MA. Effect of surface treatments on the tensile bond strength of repaired water-aged anterior restorative micro-fine hybrid resin composite. J Dent. 2008;36(12):969–76. doi:10.1016/j.jdent.2008.07.014.
48. Lucena-Martin C, Gonzalez-Lopez S. Navajas-Rodriguez de Mondelo JM. The effect of various surface treatments and bonding agents on the repaired strength of heat-treated composites. J Prosthet Dent. 2001;86(5):481–8.
49. Lima AF, Ferreira SF, Catelan A, Palialol AR, Goncalves LS, Aguiar FH, et al. The effect of surface treatment and bonding procedures on the bond strength of silorane composite repairs. Acta Odontol Scand. 2014;72(1):71–5. doi:10.3109/00016357.2013.804945.
50. Palasuk J, Platt JA, Cho SD, Levon JA, Brown DT, Hovijitra ST. Effect of surface treatments on microtensile bond strength of repaired aged silorane resin composite. Oper Dent. 2013;38(1):91–9. doi:10.2341/11-057-L.
51. Jafarzadeh Kashi TS, Erfan M, Rakhshan V, Aghabaigi N, Tabatabaei FS. An in vitro assessment of the effects of three surface treatments on repair bond strength of aged composites. Oper Dent. 2011;36(6):608–17. doi:10.2341/10-386-L.
52. Baena E, Vignolo V, Fuentes MV, Ceballos L. Influence of repair procedure on composite-to-composite microtensile bond strength. Am J Dent. 2015;28(5):255–60.
53. Imbery TA, Gray T, DeLatour F, Boxx C, Best AM, Moon PC. Evaluation of flexural, diametral tensile, and shear bond strength of composite repairs. Oper Dent. 2014;39(6):E250–60. doi:10.2341/13-299-L.
54. Kallio TT, Tezvergil-Mutluay A, Lassila LV, Vallittu PK. The effect of surface roughness on repair bond strength of light-curing composite resin to polymer composite substrate. Open Dent J. 2013;7:126–31. doi:10.2174/1874210601307010126.
55. Cavalcanti AN, De Lima AF, Peris AR, Mitsui FH, Marchi GM. Effect of surface treatments and bonding agents on the bond strength of repaired composites. J Esthet Restor Dent. 2007;19(2):90–98.; discussion 9. doi:10.1111/j.1708-8240.2007.00073.x.
56. Melo MA, Moyses MR, Santos SG, Alcantara CE, Ribeiro JC. Effects of different surface treatments and accelerated artificial aging on the bond strength of composite resin repairs. Braz Oral Res. 2011;25(6):485–91.

57. Loomans BA, Cardoso MV, Roeters FJ, Opdam NJ, De Munck J, Huysmans MC, et al. Is there one optimal repair technique for all composites? Dent Mater. 2011;27(7):701–9. doi:10.1016/j.dental.2011.03.013.
58. Ozcan M, Pekkan G. Effect of different adhesion strategies on bond strength of resin composite to composite-dentin complex. Oper Dent. 2013;38(1):63–72. doi:10.2341/11-482-L.
59. Gupta S, Parolia A, Jain A, Kundabala M, Mohan M, de Moraes Porto IC. A comparative effect of various surface chemical treatments on the resin composite-composite repair bond strength. J Indian Soc Pedod Prev Dent. 2015;33(3):245–9. doi:10.4103/0970-4388.160402.
60. Barcellos DCSV, Niu LN, Pashley DH, Franklin R, Tay FR, Cesar R, Pucci CR. Repair of composites: effect of laser and different surface treatments. Int J Adhesion & Adhesives. 2015;59:1–6.
61. Brosh T, Pilo R, Bichacho N, Blutstein R. Effect of combinations of surface treatments and bonding agents on the bond strength of repaired composites. J Prosthet Dent. 1997;77(2):122–6.
62. Furuse AY, da Cunha LF, Benetti AR, Mondelli J. Bond strength of resin-resin interfaces contaminated with saliva and submitted to different surface treatments. J Appl Oral Sci. 2007;15(6):501–5.
63. Bonstein T, Garlapo D, Donarummo J Jr, Bush PJ. Evaluation of varied repair protocols applied to aged composite resin. J Adhes Dent. 2005;7(1):41–9.
64. Chan KC, Boyer DB. Repair of conventional and microfilled composite resins. J Prosthet Dent. 1983;50(3):345–50.
65. Kupiec KA, Barkmeier WW. Laboratory evaluation of surface treatments for composite repair. Oper Dent. 1996;21(2):59–62.
66. Loomans BA, Cardoso MV, Opdam NJ, Roeters FJ, De Munck J, Huysmans MC, et al. Surface roughness of etched composite resin in light of composite repair. J Dent. 2011;39(7):499–505. doi:10.1016/j.jdent.2011.04.007.
67. Staxrud F, Dahl JE. Silanising agents promote resin-composite repair. Int Dent J. 2015;65(6):311–5. doi:10.1111/idj.12188.
68. Staxrud F, Dahl JE. Role of bonding agents in the repair of composite resin restorations. Eur J Oral Sci. 2011;119(4):316–22. doi:10.1111/j.1600-0722.2011.00833.x.
69. Van Meerbeek B, Yoshihara K, Yoshida Y, Mine A, De Munck J, Van Landuyt KL. State of the art of self-etch adhesives. Dent Mater. 2011;27(1):17–28. doi:10.1016/j.dental.2010.10.023.
70. Ozcan M. Evaluation of alternative intra-oral repair techniques for fractured ceramic-fused-to-metal restorations. J Oral Rehabil. 2003;30(2):194–203.
71. Loomans BA, Mine A, Roeters FJ, Opdam NJ, De Munck J, Huysmans MC, et al. Hydrofluoric acid on dentin should be avoided. Dent Mater. 2010;26(7):643–9. doi:10.1016/j.dental.2010.03.007.
72. Saracoglu A, Ozcan M, Kumbuloglu O, Turkun M. Adhesion of resin composite to hydrofluoric acid-exposed enamel and dentin in repair protocols. Oper Dent. 2011;36(5):545–53. doi:10.2341/10-312-L.
73. Asvesti C, Guadagni F, Anastasiadis G, Zakopoulou N, Danopoulou I, Zographakis L. Hydrofluoric acid burns. Cutis. 1997;59(6):306–8.
74. Ozcan M, Raadschelders J, Vallittu P, Lassilla L. Effect of particle deposition parameters on silica coating of zirconia using a chairside air-abrasion device. J Adhes Dent. 2013;15(3):211–4. doi:10.3290/j.jad.a29718.
75. Edelhoff D, Marx R, Spiekermann H, Yildirim M. Clinical use of an intraoral silicoating technique. J Esthet Restor Dent. 2001;13(6):350–6.
76. Lung CY, Matinlinna JP. Aspects of silane coupling agents and surface conditioning in dentistry: an overview. Dent Mater. 2012;28(5):467–77. doi:10.1016/j.dental.2012.02.009.
77. Da Silva S, Da Silva EM, Delphim MB, Poskus LT, Amaral CM. Influence of organic acids present in oral biofilm on the durability of the repair bond strength, sorption and solubility of resin composites. Am J Dent. 2015;28(6):367–72.
78. Hannig C, Laubach S, Hahn P, Attin T. Shear bond strength of repaired adhesive filling materials using different repair procedures. J Adhes Dent. 2006;8(1):35–40.
79. Cho SD, Rajitrangson P, Matis BA, Platt JA. Effect of Er,Cr:YSGG laser, air abrasion, and silane application on repaired shear bond strength of composites. Oper Dent. 2013;38(3):E1–9. doi:10.2341/11-054-L.
80. da Costa TR, Serrano AM, Atman AP, Loguercio AD, Reis A. Durability of composite repair using different surface treatments. J Dent. 2012;40(6):513–21. doi:10.1016/j.jdent.2012.03.001.
81. Luhrs AK, Gormann B, Jacker-Guhr S, Geurtsen W. Repairability of dental siloranes in vitro. Dent Mater. 2011;27(2):144–9. doi:10.1016/j.dental.2010.09.009.
82. Nassoohi N, Kazemi H, Sadaghiani M, Mansouri M, Rakhshan V. Effects of three surface conditioning techniques on repair bond strength of nanohybrid and nanofilled composites. Dent Res J (Isfahan). 2015;12(6):554–61.
83. Costa TR, Ferreira SQ, Klein-Junior CA, Loguercio AD, Reis A. Durability of surface treatments and intermediate agents used for repair of a polished composite. Oper Dent. 2010;35(2):231–7. doi:10.2341/09-216-L.
84. Yesilyurt C, Kusgoz A, Bayram M, Ulker M. Initial repair bond strength of a nano-filled hybrid resin: effect of surface treatments and bonding agents. J Esthet Restor Dent. 2009;21(4):251–60. doi:10.1111/j.1708-8240.2009.00271.x.
85. Mitsaki-Matsou H, Karanika-Kouma A, Papadoyiannis Y, Theodoridou-Pahine S. An in vitro study of the

tensile strength of composite resins repaired with the same or another composite resin. Quintessence Int. 1991;22(6):475–81.
86. Swift EJ Jr, LeValley BD, Boyer DB. Evaluation of new methods for composite repair. Dent Mater. 1992;8(6):362–5.
87. Roumanas ED. The frequency of replacement of dental restorations may vary based on a number of variables, including type of material, size of the restoration, and caries risk of the patient. J Evid Based Dent Pract. 2010;10(1):23–4. doi:10.1016/j.jebdp.2009.11.009.
88. Passos SP, Ozcan M, Vanderlei AD, Leite FP, Kimpara ET, Bottino MA. Bond strength durability of direct and indirect composite systems following surface conditioning for repair. J Adhes Dent. 2007;9(5):443–7.
89. Celik C, Cehreli SB, Arhun N. Resin composite repair: quantitative microleakage evaluation of resin-resin and resin-tooth interfaces with different surface treatments. Eur J Dent. 2015;9(1):92–9. doi:10.4103/1305-7456.149652.
90. Valente LL, Silva MF, Fonseca AS, Munchow EA, Isolan CP, Moraes RR. Effect of diamond bur grit size on composite repair. J Adhes Dent. 2015;17(3):257–63. doi:10.3290/j.jad.a34398.
91. Oliveira SS, Pugach MK, Hilton JF, Watanabe LG, Marshall SJ, Marshall GW Jr. The influence of the dentin smear layer on adhesion: a self-etching primer vs. a total-etch system. Dent Mater. 2003;19(8):758–67.
92. Tani C, Finger WJ. Effect of smear layer thickness on bond strength mediated by three all-in-one self-etching priming adhesives. J Adhes Dent. 2002;4(4):283–9.
93. Papacchini F, Dall'Oca S, Chieffi N, Goracci C, Sadek FT, Suh BI, et al. Composite-to-composite microtensile bond strength in the repair of a microfilled hybrid resin: effect of surface treatment and oxygen inhibition. J Adhes Dent. 2007;9(1): 25–31.
94. Joulaei M, Bahari M, Ahmadi A, Savadi OS. Effect of different surface treatments on repair micro-shear bond strength of silica- and zirconia-filled composite resins. J Dent Res Dent Clin Dent Prospects. 2012;6(4):131–7. doi:10.5681/joddd.2012.027.
95. Spyrou M, Koliniotou-Koumpia E, Kouros P, Koulaouzidou E, Dionysopoulos P. The reparability of contemporary composite resins. Eur J Dent. 2014;8(3):353–9. doi:10.4103/1305-7456.137647.
96. Rathke A, Tymina Y, Haller B. Effect of different surface treatments on the composite-composite repair bond strength. Clin Oral Investig. 2009;13(3):317–23. doi:10.1007/s00784-008-0228-2.
97. Burnett LH Jr, Shinkai RS, Eduardo CP. Tensile bond strength of a one-bottle adhesive system to indirect composites treated with Er:YAG laser, air abrasion, or fluoridric acid. Photomed Laser Surg. 2004;22(4):351–6. doi:10.1089/pho.2004.22.351.
98. Ozel Bektas O, Eren D, Herguner Siso S, Akin GE. Effect of thermocycling on the bond strength of composite resin to bur and laser treated composite resin. Lasers Med Sci. 2012;27(4):723–8. doi:10.1007/s10103-011-0958-2.
99. Kimyai S, Mohammadi N, Navimipour EJ, Rikhtegaran S. Comparison of the effect of three mechanical surface treatments on the repair bond strength of a laboratory composite. Photomed Laser Surg. 2010;28(Suppl 2):S25–30. doi:10.1089/pho.2009.2598.
100. Shahabi S, Chiniforush N, Juybanpoor N. Morphological changes of human dentin after erbium-doped yttrium aluminum garnet (Er:YAG) and carbon dioxide (CO2) laser irradiation and acid-etch technique: an scanning electron microscopic (SEM) evaluation. J Lasers Med Sci. 2013;4(1):48–52.
101. Chiniforush N, Nokhbatolfoghahaei H, Monzavi A, Pordel E, Ashnagar S. Surface treatment by different parameters of Erbium:Yttrium-Aluminum-Garnet (Er:YAG) laser: Scanning Electron Microscope (SEM) evaluation. J Lasers Med Sci. 2016;7(1):37–9. doi:10.15171/jlms.2016.08.
102. Alizadeh Oskoee P, Mohammadi N, Ebrahimi Chaharom ME, Kimyai S, Pournaghi Azar F, Rikhtegaran S, et al. Effect of surface treatment with Er;Cr:YSSG, Nd:YAG, and CO2 lasers on repair shear bond strength of a Silorane-based composite resin. J Dent Res Dent Clin Dent Prospects. 2013;7(2):61–6. doi:10.5681/joddd.2013.011.
103. Shiu P, De Souza-Zaroni WC, Eduardo Cde P, Youssef MN. Effect of feldspathic ceramic surface treatments on bond strength to resin cement. Photomed Laser Surg. 2007;25(4):291–6. doi:10.1089/pho.2007.2018.
104. van As G. Erbium lasers in dentistry. Dent Clin N Am. 2004;48(4):1017–1059., viii. doi:10.1016/j.cden.2004.06.001.
105. Iaria G. Clinical, morphological, and ultrastructural aspects with the use of Er:YAG and Er,Cr:YSGG lasers in restorative dentistry. Gen Dent. 2008;56(7):636–9.
106. Alizadeh Oskoee P, Kimyai S, Talatahari E, Rikhtegaran S, Pournaghi-Azar F, Sajadi OJ. Effect of mechanical surface treatment on the repair bond strength of the Silorane-based composite resin. J Dent Res Dent Clin Dent Prospects. 2014;8(2):61–6. doi:10.5681/joddd.2014.011.
107. Lizarelli Rde F, Moriyama LT, Bagnato VS. Ablation of composite resins using Er:YAG laser--comparison with enamel and dentin. Lasers Surg Med. 2003;33(2):132–9. doi:10.1002/lsm.10196.
108. Duran I, Ural C, Yilmaz B, Tatar N. Effects of Er:YAG laser pretreatment with different energy levels on bond strength of repairing composite materials. Photomed Laser Surg. 2015;33(6):320–5. doi:10.1089/pho.2014.3859.
109. Murray AK, Attrill DC, Dickinson MR. The effects of XeCl laser etching of Ni-Cr alloy on bond strengths

to composite resin: a comparison with sandblasting procedures. Dent Mater. 2005;21(6):538–44. doi:10.1016/j.dental.2004.07.021.

110. Etemadi A, Shahabi S, Chiniforush N, Pordel E, Azarbayejani Z, Heidari S. Scanning electron microscope (SEM) evaluation of composite surface irradiated by different powers of Er:YAG laser. J Lasers Med Sci. 2015;6(2):80–4.
111. Gokce B, Ozpinar B, Dundar M, Comlekoglu E, Sen BH, Gungor MA. Bond strengths of all-ceramics: acid vs laser etching. Oper Dent. 2007;32(2):173–8. doi:10.2341/06-52.
112. Tugut F, Akin H, Mutaf B, Akin GE, Ozdemir AK. Strength of the bond between a silicone lining material and denture resin after Er:YAG laser treatments with different pulse durations and levels of energy. Lasers Med Sci. 2012;27(2):281–5. doi:10.1007/s10103-010-0862-1.
113. Rossato DM, Bandeca MC, Saade EG, Lizarelli RFZ, Bagnato VS, Saad JRC. Influence of Er:YAG laser on surface treatment of aged composite resin to repair restoration. Laser Phys. 2009;19(11):2144–9. doi:10.1134/S1054660x09210105.
114. Papacchini F, Toledano M, Monticelli F, Osorio R, Radovic I, Polimeni A, et al. Hydrolytic stability of composite repair bond. Eur J Oral Sci. 2007;115(5): 417–24. doi:10.1111/j.1600-0722.2007.00475.x.
115. Hannig C, Hahn P, Thiele PP, Attin T. Influence of different repair procedures on bond strength of adhesive filling materials to etched enamel in vitro. Oper Dent. 2003;28(6):800–7.
116. Kim MJ, Kim YK, Kim KH, Kwon TY. Shear bond strengths of various luting cements to zirconia ceramic: surface chemical aspects. J Dent. 2011;39(11): 795–803. doi:10.1016/j.jdent.2011.08.012.
117. Eliasson ST, Tibballs J, Dahl JE. Effect of different surface treatments and adhesives on repair bond strength of resin composites after one and 12 months of storage using an improved microtensile test method. Oper Dent. 2014;39(5):E206–16. doi:10.2341/12-429-L.
118. Malacarne J, Carvalho RM, de Goes MF, Svizero N, Pashley DH, Tay FR, et al. Water sorption/solubility of dental adhesive resins. Dent Mater. 2006;22(10): 973–80. doi:10.1016/j.dental.2005.11.020.
119. Mousavinasab SM, Farhadi A, Shabanian M. Effect of storage time, thermocycling and resin coating on durability of dentin bonding systems. Dent Res J (Isfahan). 2009;6(1):29–37.
120. R P, Bs S, Arunagiri D, Manuja N. Influence of hydrophobic layer and delayed placement of composite on the marginal adaptation of two self-etch adhesives. J Conserv Dent. 2009;12(2):60–4. doi:10.4103/0972-0707.55619.
121. Pushpa R, Suresh BS. Marginal permeability of one step self-etch adhesives: effects of double application or the application of hydrophobic layer. J Conserv Dent. 2010;13(3):141–4. doi:10.4103/0972-0707.71646.
122. Manuja N, Nagpal R, Pandit IK. Dental adhesion: mechanism, techniques and durability. J Clin Pediatr Dent. 2012;36(3):223–34.
123. Van Meerbeek B, De Munck J, Yoshida Y, Inoue S, Vargas M, Vijay P, et al. Buonocore memorial lecture. Adhesion to enamel and dentin: current status and future challenges. Oper Dent. 2003;28(3): 215–35.
124. Teixeira EC, Bayne SC, Thompson JY, Ritter AV, Swift EJ. Shear bond strength of self-etching bonding systems in combination with various composites used for repairing aged composites. J Adhes Dent. 2005;7(2):159–64.
125. Yokokawa M, Rikuta A, Tsujimoto A, Tsuchiya K, Shibasaki S, Matsuyoshi S, et al. Influence of methyl mercaptan on the repair bond strength of composites fabricated using self-etch adhesives. Eur J Oral Sci. 2015;123(1):46–52. doi:10.1111/eos.12164.
126. Swift EJ Jr, Cloe BC, Boyer DB. Effect of a silane coupling agent on composite repair strengths. Am J Dent. 1994;7(4):200–2.
127. Brendeke J, Ozcan M. Effect of physicochemical aging conditions on the composite-composite repair bond strength. J Adhes Dent. 2007;9(4): 399–406.
128. Turner CW, Meiers JC. Repair of an aged, contaminated indirect composite resin with a direct, visible-light-cured composite resin. Oper Dent. 1993;18(5):187–94.
129. Lagouvardos PE, Pissis P, Kyritsis A, Daoukaki D. Water sorption and water-induced molecular mobility in dental composite resins. J Mater Sci Mater Med. 2003;14(9):753–9.
130. Karaman E, Gonulol N. Does the light source affect the repairability of composite resins? Braz Oral Res. 2014;28.
131. Bacchi A, Consani RL, Sinhoreti MA, Feitosa VP, Cavalcante LM, Pfeifer CS, et al. Repair bond strength in aged methacrylate- and silorane-based composites. J Adhes Dent. 2013;15(5):447–52. doi:10.3290/j.jad.a29590.
132. Baur V, Ilie N. Repair of dental resin-based composites. Clin Oral Investig. 2013;17(2):601–8. doi:10.1007/s00784-012-0722-4.
133. Moncada G, Angel P, Fernandez E, Alonso P, Martin J, Gordan VV. Bond strength evaluation of nanohybrid resin-based composite repair. Gen Dent. 2012;60(3):230–4.
134. Ozcan M, Barbosa SH, Melo RM, Galhano GA, Bottino MA. Effect of surface conditioning methods on the microtensile bond strength of resin composite to composite after aging conditions. Dent Mater. 2007;23(10):1276–82. doi:10.1016/j.dental.2006.11.007.
135. Sousa AB, Silami FD, da Garcia L, Naves LZ, de Pires-de-Souza F. Effect of various aging protocols and intermediate agents on the bond strength of repaired composites. J Adhes Dent. 2013;15(2):137–44. doi:10.3290/j.jad.a29513.

136. Jefferies SR. The art and science of abrasive finishing and polishing in restorative dentistry. Dent Clin N Am. 1998;42(4):613–27.
137. Marghalani HY. Effect of finishing/polishing systems on the surface roughness of novel posterior composites. J Esthet Restor Dent. 2010;22(2):127–38. doi:10.1111/j.1708-8240.2010.00324.x.
138. Park J, Chang J, Ferracane J, Lee IB. How should composite be layered to reduce shrinkage stress: incremental or bulk filling? Dent Mater. 2008;24(11):1501–5. doi:10.1016/j.dental.2008.03.013.
139. Celik C, Cehreli SB, Bagis B, Arhun N. Microtensile bond strength of composite-to-composite repair with different surface treatments and adhesive systems. J Adhes Sci Technol. 2015;28(13):1264–76.
140. Anfe TE, Agra CM, Vieira GF. Evaluation of sorption, solubility and staining of universal and silorane resin-based composites. Eur J Prosthodont Restor Dent. 2011;19(4):151–4.
141. Cavalcante LM, Schneider LF, Hammad M, Watts DC, Silikas N. Degradation resistance of ormocer- and dimethacrylate-based matrices with different filler contents. J Dent. 2012;40(1):86–90. doi:10.1016/j.jdent.2011.10.012.
142. Ozcan M, Corazza PH, Marocho SM, Barbosa SH, Bottino MA. Repair bond strength of microhybrid, nanohybrid and nanofilled resin composites: effect of substrate resin type, surface conditioning and ageing. Clin Oral Investig. 2013;17(7):1751–8. doi:10.1007/s00784-012-0863-5.
143. Rinastiti M, Ozcan M, Siswomihardjo W, Busscher HJ. Effects of surface conditioning on repair bond strengths of non-aged and aged microhybrid, nanohybrid, and nanofilled composite resins. Clin Oral Investig. 2011;15(5):625–33. doi:10.1007/s00784-010-0426-6.
144. Sideridou I, Tserki V, Papanastasiou G. Effect of chemical structure on degree of conversion in light-cured dimethacrylate-based dental resins. Biomaterials. 2002;23(8):1819–29.
145. Ivanovas S, Hickel R, Ilie N. How to repair fillings made by silorane-based composites. Clin Oral Investig. 2011;15(6):915–22. doi:10.1007/s00784-010-0473-z.
146. Ghivari S, Chandak M, Manvar N. Role of oxygen inhibited layer on shear bond strength of composites. J Conserv Dent. 2010;13(1):39–41. doi:10.4103/0972-0707.62635.
147. Burke FJ, Crisp RJ, James A, Mackenzie L, Pal A, Sands P, et al. Two year clinical evaluation of a low-shrink resin composite material in UK general dental practices. Dent Mater. 2011;27(7):622–30. doi:10.1016/j.dental.2011.02.012.
148. Eick JD, Kotha SP, Chappelow CC, Kilway KV, Giese GJ, Glaros AG, et al. Properties of silorane-based dental resins and composites containing a stress-reducing monomer. Dent Mater. 2007;23(8):1011–7. doi:10.1016/j.dental.2006.09.002.
149. Popoff DA, Santa Rosa TT, Ferreira RC, Magalhaes CS, Moreira AN, Mjor IA. Repair of dimethacrylate-based composite restorations by a silorane-based composite: a one-year randomized clinical trial. Oper Dent. 2012;37(5):E1–10. doi:10.2341/11-121-C.
150. Ilie N, Jelen E, Clementino-Luedemann T, Hickel R. Low-shrinkage composite for dental application. Dent Mater J. 2007;26(2):149–55.
151. Weinmann W, Thalacker C, Guggenberger R. Siloranes in dental composites. Dent Mater. 2005;21(1):68–74. doi:10.1016/j.dental.2004.10.007.
152. Tezvergil-Mutluay A, Lassila LV, Vallittu PK. Incremental layers bonding of silorane composite: the initial bonding properties. J Dent. 2008;36(7):560–3. doi:10.1016/j.jdent.2008.03.008.
153. Navarra CO, Cadenaro M, Armstrong SR, Jessop J, Antoniolli F, Sergo V, et al. Degree of conversion of Filtek Silorane adhesive system and Clearfil SE bond within the hybrid and adhesive layer: an in situ Raman analysis. Dent Mater. 2009;25(9):1178–85. doi:10.1016/j.dental.2009.05.009.
154. Hamano N, Ino S, Fukuyama T, Hickel R, Kunzelmann KH. Repair of silorane-based composites: microtensile bond strength of silorane-based composites repaired with methacrylate-based composites. Dent Mater J. 2013;32(5):695–701.
155. Giachetti L, Scaminaci Russo D, Baldini M, Goracci C, Ferrari M. Reparability of aged silorane with methacrylate-based resin composite: micro-shear bond strength and scanning electron microscopy evaluation. Oper Dent. 2012;37(1):28–36. doi:10.2341/10-397-L.
156. Wiegand A, Stawarczyk B, Buchalla W, Taubock TT, Ozcan M, Attin T. Repair of silorane composite—using the same substrate or a methacrylate-based composite? Dent Mater. 2012;28(3):e19–25. doi:10.1016/j.dental.2011.10.008.
157. Hamano N, Chiang YC, Nyamaa I, Yamaguchi H, Ino S, Hickel R, et al. Effect of different surface treatments on the repair strength of a nanofilled resin-based composite. Dent Mater J. 2011;30(4):537–45.
158. Ruddell DE, Maloney MM, Thompson JY. Effect of novel filler particles on the mechanical and wear properties of dental composites. Dent Mater. 2002;18(1):72–80.
159. Bijelic-Donova J, Garoushi S, Lassila LV, Keulemans F, Vallittu PK. Mechanical and structural characterization of discontinuous fiber-reinforced dental resin composite. J Dent. 2016;52:70–8. doi:10.1016/j.jdent.2016.07.009.
160. Xu HH, Schumacher GE, Eichmiller FC, Peterson RC, Antonucci JM, Mueller HJ. Continuous-fiber preform reinforcement of dental resin composite restorations. Dent Mater. 2003;19(6):523–30.
161. Drummond JL, Lin L, Al-Turki LA, Hurley RK. Fatigue behaviour of dental composite materials. J Dent. 2009;37(5):321–30. doi:10.1016/j.jdent.2008.12.008.

162. Omran TA, Garoushi S, Abdulmajeed AA, Lassila LV, Vallittu PK. Influence of increment thickness on dentin bond strength and light transmission of composite base materials. Clin Oral Investig. 2016. doi:10.1007/s00784-016-1953-6.
163. Garoushi S, Sailynoja E, Vallittu PK, Lassila L. Physical properties and depth of cure of a new short fiber reinforced composite. Dent Mater. 2013;29(8):835–41. doi:10.1016/j.dental.2013.04.016.
164. Tsujimoto A, Barkmeier WW, Takamizawa T, Watanabe H, Johnson WW, Latta MA, et al. Relationship between mechanical properties and bond durability of short fiber-reinforced resin composite with universal adhesive. Eur J Oral Sci. 2016;124(5):480–9. doi:10.1111/eos.12291.
165. Ariyoshi M, Nikaido T, Foxton RM, Tagami J. Influence of filling technique and curing mode on the bond strengths of composite cores to pulpal floor dentin. Dent Mater J. 2010;29(5):562–9.
166. Kournetas N, Tzoutzas I, Eliades G. Monomer conversion in dual-cured core buildup materials. Oper Dent. 2011;36(1):92–7. doi:10.2341/10-145-LR.
167. Taubock TT, Bortolotto T, Buchalla W, Attin T, Krejci I. Influence of light-curing protocols on polymerization shrinkage and shrinkage force of a dual-cured core build-up resin composite. Eur J Oral Sci. 2010;118(4):423–9. doi:10.1111/j.1600-0722.2010.00746.x.
168. Sunada N, Ishii R, Shiratsuchi K, Shimizu Y, Tsubota K, Kurokawa H, et al. Ultrasonic measurement of the effects of adhesive application and power density on the polymerization behavior of core build-up resins. Acta Odontol Scand. 2013;71(1):137–43. doi:10.3109/00016357.2011.654252.
169. El-Deeb HA, Ghalab RM, Elsayed Akah MM, Mobarak EH. Repair bond strength of dual-cured resin composite core buildup materials. J Adv Res. 2016;7(2):263–9. doi:10.1016/j.jare.2015.06.003.
170. El-Askary FS, El-Banna AH, van Noort R. Immediate vs delayed repair bond strength of a nanohybrid resin composite. J Adhes Dent. 2012;14(3):265–74. doi:10.3290/j.jad.a22716.
171. Frankenberger R, Kramer N, Sindel J. Repair strength of etched vs silica-coated metal-ceramic and all-ceramic restorations. Oper Dent. 2000;25(3):209–15.
172. Moncada G, Martin J, Fernandez E, Hempel MC, Mjor IA, Gordan VV. Sealing, refurbishment and repair of class I and class II defective restorations: a three-year clinical trial. J Am Dent Assoc. 2009;140(4):425–32.
173. Perriard J, Lorente MC, Scherrer S, Belser UC, Wiskott HW. The effect of water storage, elapsed time and contaminants on the bond strength and interfacial polymerization of a nanohybrid composite. J Adhes Dent. 2009;11(6):469–78. doi:10.3290/j.jad.a18141.
174. Opdam NJ, Bronkhorst EM, Loomans BA, Huysmans MC. Longevity of repaired restorations: a practice based study. J Dent. 2012;40(10):829–35. doi:10.1016/j.jdent.2012.06.007.
175. Sharif MO, Fedorowicz Z, Tickle M, Brunton PA. Repair or replacement of restorations: do we accept built in obsolescence or do we improve the evidence? Br Dent J. 2010;209(4):171–4. doi:10.1038/sj.bdj.2010.722.
176. Demarco FF, Correa MB, Cenci MS, Moraes RR, Opdam NJ. Longevity of posterior composite restorations: not only a matter of materials. Dent Mater. 2012;28(1):87–101. doi:10.1016/j.dental.2011.09.003.
177. Da Rosa Rodolpho PA, Donassollo TA, Cenci MS, Loguercio AD, Moraes RR, Bronkhorst EM, et al. 22-year clinical evaluation of the performance of two posterior composites with different filler characteristics. Dent Mater. 2011;27(10):955–63. doi:10.1016/j.dental.2011.06.001.
178. Fernandez EM, Martin JA, Angel PA, Mjor IA, Gordan VV, Moncada GA. Survival rate of sealed, refurbished and repaired defective restorations: 4-year follow-up. Braz Dent J. 2011;22(2):134–9.
179. Gordan VV, Riley JL 3rd, Blaser PK, Mondragon E, Garvan CW, Mjor IA. Alternative treatments to replacement of defective amalgam restorations: results of a seven-year clinical study. J Am Dent Assoc. 2011;142(7):842–9.
180. Gordan VV, Garvan CW, Richman JS, Fellows JL, Rindal DB, Qvist V, et al. How dentists diagnose and treat defective restorations: evidence from the dental practice-based research network. Oper Dent. 2009;34(6):664–73. doi:10.2341/08-131-C.
181. Popoff DA, de Magalhaes CS, de Freitas OW, Soares LA, de Almeida Santa Rosa TT, Ferreira RC, et al. Two-year clinical performance of dimethacrylate based composite restorations repaired with a silorane-based composite. J Adhes Dent. 2014;16(6):575–83. doi:10.3290/j.jad.a33196.
182. Fernandez E, Martin J, Vildosola P, Oliveira Junior OB, Gordan V, Mjor I, et al. Can repair increase the longevity of composite resins? Results of a 10-year clinical trial. J Dent. 2015;43(2):279–86. doi:10.1016/j.jdent.2014.05.015.
183. Blunck U. Pretreatment of composite resin surfaces for repair: why and how. J Adhes Dent. 2013;15(6):592. doi:10.3290/j.jad.a31110.

Clinical Longevity of Direct Resin Composite Restorations

17

Rafael R. Moraes, Maximiliano S. Cenci, and Luis Felipe J. Schneider

17.1 What Takes Place in the Mouth?

The tooth is finally restored and it looks good. Finishing and polishing procedures were accomplished. The patient leaves the office, and soon the restoration is subjected to all sorts of challenges, as illustrated in Fig. 17.1. What happens in the mouth over time? Over the first 24–48 h, the restorative complex (dental surface, bonded interface, bonding agent, and the resin composite itself) experiences a cascade of events. Hydration and hygroscopic effects due to the wet character of the environment take place. Thermal equilibrium is reached. Post-polymerization processes undergo within the polymer, also known as the "dark cure." The remaining unreacted monomers and other components start to leach out into the oral medium. Neutralization of acidic monomers, improved chemical interaction between the adhesive and dental tissues, and some degree of polymer relaxation occur. Color and translucency slightly change. Over a longer period of intraoral performance of composite restorations, the contact with tongue, food, and opposing dentition starts affecting surface roughness of the restoration.

Over the next few days, months, or years, biofilms of multiple composition and cariogenic abilities accumulate cyclically. Acids from bacteria chemically challenge the tooth, restorative, and bonded assembly. Interaction with proteins and countless enzymatic reactions take place. Tooth brushing, abrasion, and erosive challenges start to build up effects. Mechanical cyclic loading from chewing will dully impose stresses of different extents and magnitudes. In case of parafunctional activity, the magnitudes of occurring processes may be increased for a factor of two or three. Current resin-based materials do not offer smart features to respond to intraoral challenges on demand. Antimicrobial agents added to restoratives, for instance, still have to prove clinical efficiency. Load-oriented toughening mechanisms, such as in zirconia ceramics, are not present in conventional composites. The resin phase suffers from wear, while surface inorganic particles are worn off. The bonds between filler particles and polymer are hydrolytically challenged by water and strained by mechanical stresses. Restoration margins might show signs of breakdown; marginal staining likely occurs. The polymeric network becomes more brittle with micro-cracks growing within the structure. Fatigue is a matter of time as well as failures due to fracture or caries.

Is that scenario exaggerated? Do dental composites fail too often? Can we predict when failure

R.R. Moraes (✉) • M.S. Cenci
Graduate Program in Dentistry, School of Dentistry, Federal University of Pelotas, Pelotas, Brazil
e-mail: moraesrr@gmail.com

L.F.J. Schneider
Fluminense Federal University, Niterói, Brazil

Veiga de Almeida University, Rio de Janeiro, Brazil

V. Miletic (ed.), *Dental Composite Materials for Direct Restorations*,
http://doi.org/10.1007/978-3-319-60961-4_17

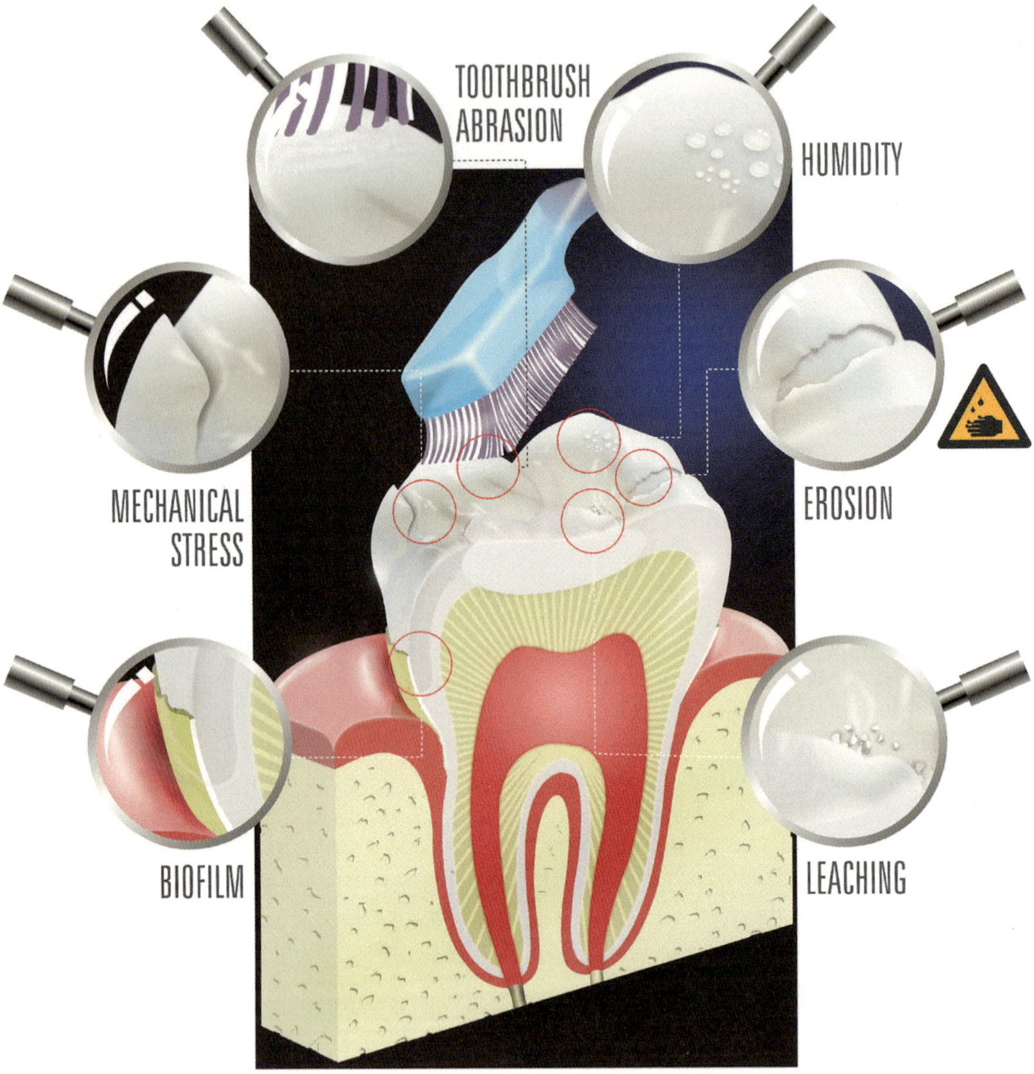

Fig. 17.1 Many intraoral aspects may affect the performance of resin composite restorations. Longevity depends on understanding how these aspects play together with clinical factors and pose risk to restoration failures

is going to happen or do something to postpone aging? This chapter is not intended to answer these questions specifically; the objectives are to discuss factors related to the clinical longevity of direct resin composite restorations and show that perhaps doing nothing in some cases when clinical signs of aging are present would be the best option. The chapter contains a review of recent data from clinical studies and discusses the meaning of clinical failures, the best restorative composite, the expected length of composite restorations, and answered/unanswered questions concerning the intraoral performance of restorations.

17.2 Factors Associated with Longevity

The literature was searched to gather updated information on the clinical longevity of resin composite restorations available in systematic reviews and meta-analyses. Data from 16 systematic reviews [1–16] including 221 studies, over 350,000 restorations placed in more than 14,000 patients were taken into account (Table 17.1). Many additional studies were reviewed in order to obtain a larger picture of factors affecting longevity. Specific parameters identified in those studies are addressed.

Table 17.1 Results from systematic reviews on the clinical performance of resin composite restorations

Author, year	Restoration type	Comparison	Estimates[a]			Follow-up, years	Main findings for composite restorations	Main reasons for failure	Factors associated with composite failure
			Studies	Patients	Restorations				
Afrashtehfar et al. (2016a) [1]	Posterior restorations in vital teeth	Remaining tooth structure	14	1903+	308,744	3–10	Failure rate was higher in teeth with less remaining structure; composites failed more than amalgam; direct restorations failed more than crowns	N.R.	Number of restored surfaces, restorative material, and technique
Afrashtehfar et al. (2016b) [2]	Posterior restorations in root-filled teeth	Remaining tooth structure, restorative material	5	955	1160	3–6	Teeth with more remaining tooth structure had better prognosis than teeth with less coronal structure	N.R.	Number of restored surfaces
Ahmed and Murbay (2016) [3]	Anterior restorations in worn teeth	N.R.	5	100	772	0.5–10	Survival rates were over 90% at 2.5 years and over 50% at 5 years; increasing overall vertical dimension resulted in posterior occlusion reestablishment in 91% of patients within 1.5 years	N.R.	N.R.
Alcaraz et al. (2014) [4]	Posterior restorations	Composite vs. amalgam	7	871	3010	5–7	Composites have higher risk of failure and secondary caries than amalgam	Caries, fracture, and restoration loss	Restorative material
Angeletaki et al. (2016) [5]	Inlays and onlays	Direct vs. indirect techniques	3	239	424	4.5–11	Both restorative techniques showed similar clinical performance	Caries and fracture (tooth or restoration)	None

(continued)

Table 17.1 (continued)

Author, year	Restoration type	Comparison	Estimates[a]			Follow-up, years	Main findings for composite restorations	Main reasons for failure	Factors associated with composite failure
			Studies	Patients	Restorations				
Astvaldsdottir et al. (2015) [6]	Class I and II	N.R.	8	420	910	4–12	Fractures and endodontic failures occurred mainly in the first 3 years of clinical service; failures due to caries predominated after 3 years	Caries, fracture, and restoration loss	N.R.
Chabouis et al. (2013) [7]	Inlays and onlays	Composite vs. ceramic	2	80	138	3–10	Ceramic inlays performed better than composite inlays in the short term	Fracture (tooth or restoration) and caries	Restorative material
Demarco et al. (2015) [8]	Class III and IV, veneers, reanatomization	Multiple factors	17	347+	1821	3–17	Annual failure rates varied from 0 to 4.1%, and survival rates varied from 53.4% to 100%; class III restorations generally had lower failures than the other types of restorations	Fracture (tooth or restoration), loss of restoration or anatomical form, esthetic reasons	Restoration type, patient retreatment risk
Heintze and Rousson (2012) [9]	Class I and II	Multiple factors	59	N.R.	8951	2–9	Performance of restorations was material dependent; more fractures and lower longevity in restorations applied without rubber dam; lower marginal discoloration when the enamel was phosphoric acid etched; no effect for enamel beveling	Bulk fractures and caries	Bonding strategy, restorative material, operative procedure

Heintze et al. (2015) [10]	Class III and IV, diastema closures	Multiple factors	21	N.R.	1722+	2–12	Performance of restorations was material dependent; polishing system did not affect clinical performance; class IV restorations showed more chippings and fractures; class III restorations placed without rubber dam had more adjacent caries; hybrids performed better than microfills; no effect for enamel beveling	Bulk fractures and caries	Cavity type, restorative material, bonding strategy
Magno et al. (2016) [11]	Class I and II	Silorane vs. methacrylate-based composites	11	423	920	0–5	Silorane and methacrylate-based composites showed similar clinical behavior	Fracture (tooth or restoration)	None
Moraschini et al. (2015) [12]	Class I and II	Composite vs. amalgam	8	1453+	3486	1–10	Average annual failure rate was 3.2%; amalgam restorations performed better than composite restorations	Fracture (tooth or restoration) and caries	N.R.
Nguyen et al. (2015) [13]	Class I and II	Laminate (sandwich) vs. nonlaminate techniques	13	492+	1097	Up to 7	Laminate and nonlaminate restorations performed similarly, irrespective of the base material (glass-ionomer cement or flowable resin composite)	N.R.	N.R.

(continued)

Table 17.1 (continued)

Author, year	Restoration type	Comparison	Estimates[a]			Follow-up, years	Main findings for composite restorations	Main reasons for failure	Factors associated with composite failure
			Studies	Patients	Restorations				
Opdam et al. (2014) [14]	Class I and II	N.R.	12	N.R.	2816	6–22	Endodontic failures were predominant in the first year of clinical service; annual failure rates varied from 1.2% (5 years) to 4.6% (10 years)	Caries and fracture (tooth or restoration)	Patient caries risk, presence of lining cement, number of restored surfaces, composite filler loading
Van de Sande et al. (2016) [15]	Posterior restorations	Patient-related factors	27	8523+	25,859	3–21	Younger patients influenced negatively restorations survival; more failures in men; more failures in high-caries-risk patients; annual failure rates between 0.3% and 6.3% (5 years)	N.R.	Patient age, gender, caries risk, and parafunctional habits
Veiga et al. (2016) [16]	Class I and II with or without cusp involvement	Direct vs. indirect techniques	9	207+	483+	2–11	Both restorative techniques showed similar clinical performance	Fracture (tooth or restoration)	None

N.R. not reported
[a]Many studies were not able to report precisely the number of patients, restorations, and dropouts

17.2.1 Cavity Size, Tooth Position, and Presence of Endodontic Treatment

For a long time, the cavity size has been indicated as one of the major factors influencing longevity. This means that Class II restorations fail more often than Class I, as Class IV fail more often than Class III restorations. In general terms, the less restorative material placed to replace tooth tissues, the lower the effects of intraoral aging. Likewise, the shorter the length of the bonded interface, the lower the bonding degradation, marginal staining, or gap formation. Even if the overall effect of the cavity size is a summation of all those events, or not related to any, the fact is that lower surface and cavity volume occupied by the composite are associated with better dissipation of the mechanical stresses to the dental structure. A more sound dental structure means higher resistance to deformation and crack propagation. The composite shows less signs of intraoral degradation, and the treatment lasts longer. Particularly important for longevity is the maintenance of surrounding enamel margins, low ratio of isthmus to intercuspal width, and preservation of marginal ridges [9, 17–19]. It has been shown that appropriate shape (contour) at proximal restoration surfaces in cervico-occlusal direction may result in stronger, better supported marginal ridges compared to straight surfaces [20]. The tooth position in the mouth or tooth type also affect restoration longevity, with restorations in premolars usually showing better performance than those in molars [21–23] due to the increased loads molar teeth have to withstand.

The presence of endodontic treatment is another factor that the literature indicates to affect the longevity of resin composite restorations. The annual failure rates for non-vital restored teeth are up to three times higher the failure rates for vital teeth [18, 24, 25]. One study showed that less than 20% restorations in endodontically treated teeth had survived after 10 years of clinical service [24]. There is evidence that even resin composite veneers have a lower risk of failure in vital teeth than in non-vital teeth [26]. The presence of endodontic treatment means increased removal of dental tissues, affecting the overall strength of the restored structure. Therefore, being as far as possible from the pulp is relevant, which means being conservative in caries excavation, mitigating pulpal injury, and maintaining more coronal dentin. A recent study in children showed that complete caries removal leads to more pulp exposure than selective partial caries removal [27]. A clinical trial with a 3-year follow-up showed that partial caries removal reduces the risk of endodontic complications [28]. Systematic reviews indicate that restorations in either vital or root-filled teeth with more coronal dentin have better clinical prognosis [1, 2]. Dentin, having up to six times the enamel toughness [29], resists crack propagation better than enamel. The dentin-enamel junction is another important structure that should be maintained since cracks navigating through the dental structure usually stop when they reach that junction [29]. All these aspects explain why unrestored teeth fractures are not as common as fractures in restored teeth and why restorations in endodontically treated teeth fail more often. To date, it is still correct to state that no restorative material is able to replace enamel and dentin; thus, their maximal preservation is of utmost importance [30]. This is in line with the principles of minimally invasive dentistry.

17.2.2 Restorative Technique

The effect of variables related to the restorative technique has been addressed in clinical studies, including the use of direct versus indirect composites, beveling or not the enamel margins, the type of polishing system employed, and the use of rubber dam for tooth isolation. These four variables, in most studies, were shown not to affect significantly the clinical outcomes of resin composite restorations [5, 9, 10, 13, 16]. However, further evaluation is needed for each of these variables. The comparison of direct and indirect techniques, for instance, needs to take into account less removal of tooth structure in direct restorations and the better anatomical shaping (occlusal and proximal) and improved polymer curing in indirect procedures. Considering the current evidence on the similar clinical performance of either technique, direct restorations seem preferable due to the increased time consumed and costs associated with indirect techniques. Final decisions should be based on operator and patient preferences. Chair time for patients, for instance, could be longer for placing four direct restorations in a single session than using two sessions for placing the same four indirect restorations prepared using a stone cast mold or CAD-CAM procedures. Additionally, the literature discloses that indirect restorations are better indicated for large rehabilitations in which the dentition has to be restored extensively, in cases where optimal form and esthetics are required and in cases in which a direct restoration is too difficult for the operator to make [31].

Enamel beveling, a procedure often associated with esthetical prerequisites, was shown not to influence longevity of restorations in either anterior or posterior teeth [9, 10]. Beveling could be linked with increased longevity, for instance, if able to reduce the marginal discoloration of restorations usually (and incorrectly) associated with recurrent caries (refer to Sect. 17.3 for in-depth discussion). In anterior teeth, beveling could improve longevity by masking the cavity finish line and enhancing esthetics. But the literature evidence does not seem to corroborate those assumptions. One study showed that beveling was associated with reduced deterioration of the anatomical form in the anterior teeth, but it had no effect on the frequency of marginal discoloration or longevity [10]. The effects of using good bonding materials and techniques seem to be more pronounced. The bevel size used in the studies might have influenced the outcomes [10], but the current literature cannot confirm that effect yet. Regarding the polishing system, a systematic review of clinical studies [10] showed that it did not affect color match or surface texture of restorations. A recent systematic review of in vitro studies [32] showed that the combination polishing system-resin composite might influence the outcomes of surface roughness and gloss for a given resin composite, but this effect is not evident in clinical studies, perhaps due to surface abrasive and erosive challenges in the mouth. None of the systematic review articles addressed here indicates esthetics as a main reason for failure of restorations, probably because the vast majority of data derive from studies including mainly posterior restorations.

Regarding restoration technique, the variable that might raise more controversy is the use of rubber dam for tooth isolation. It is true that one of the systematic reviews showed more fractures and reduced longevity in restorations applied without rubber dam [9]. The authors conclude their study indicating that if the clinical situation allows it, the isolation with rubber dam is preferable. However, the efficiency of the "relative isolation" method used in each included study cannot be evaluated for comparison. If good isolation from moisture and contaminants using cotton rolls and appropriate suction is achieved, perhaps the use of a rubber dam sheet itself is of minor significance. Although few clinical studies address this topic as their main research question, the annual failure rates of resin composite restorations in studies placing resin composites with or without using rubber dam isolation are similar. For instance, in a study reporting up to 22 years survival of posterior resin composites, all restorations were placed under rubber dam isolation [21]. Whereas in a study reporting a 27-year follow-up of posterior composites, restorations were placed using cotton rolls and suction device [33]. The results of these two studies and the systematic reviews addressed here indicate that resin composite restorations can be successfully placed using different methods to isolate the operative field provided that humidity and contamination are under control. Using appropriate suction device and working with the aid of a dental nurse are even more important for achieving good isolation from humidity in case rubber dam is not used.

17.2.3 Cavity Lining and Bonding Strategy

One systematic review [13] compared resin composite restorations with and without lining using flowable resin composite or glass-ionomer cement. The authors did not find any effect of lining but stated that long-term evidence was insufficient. Another systematic review, which included clinical studies with follow-ups of at least 6 years, in contrast indicated that the presence of a glass-ionomer cement liner or base had a negative influence on survival of posterior resin composite restorations [14]. The authors further explained that the effect disappeared when two large practice-based studies were excluded from the analysis, indicating that operator variables were likely present. A study by the same group [22] had already indicated that the so-called sandwich restorations have a failure risk about four times higher than total-etch composite restorations, with fracture as the main reason for failure. Available scientific data suggest that thin glass-ionomer lining does not affect adversely clinical longevity of composite restorations. Conversely, thicker glass-ionomer base, such as in sandwich restorations, increases the risk for negative effects due to lower strength and higher sensitivity to fatigue of glass ionomers than resin composites. A recent study on clinical longevity showed similar performance up to 18 years for restorations placed with and without glass-ionomer cement lining [34]. This reinforces the assumption that operator variables might be more significant for the performance of restorations than the presence of a glass-ionomer layer itself.

The effect of bonding strategy on the clinical longevity of Class V restorations has been the focus of much research [35]. Based on these studies, the current gold standard dental adhesive technique is the use of a mild two-step, self-etch adhesive system with selective phosphoric acid enamel etching should the cavity present enamel margins. There is no reason to think the gold standard technique for bonding other restoration classes differs from the recommended strategy for Class V restorations. A recent network meta-analysis showed that the effect of the bonding agent in posterior restorations is less pronounced as compared with cervical restorations [36]. In contrast, two systematic reviews [9, 10] reported that the bonding strategy was associated with anterior and posterior resin composite restoration failures. In both studies, the absence of enamel acid etching was associated with increased failure rates. Explanation relies mainly on the accelerated marginal staining when the enamel was not acid etched. Although it is known that marginal staining does not mean marginal caries, the presence of stained margins is likely to induce some practitioners to replace restorations even when no other signs of secondary caries are present. This topic is further addressed in Sect. 17.3. Postoperative sensitivity, often related to the performance of resin composite restorations, is not a frequent cause for restoration replacement. The occurrence of postoperative sensitivity in recent clinical literature is low and more often associated with the adhesive bonding strategy or restorative approach itself [37, 38], although a recent systematic review indicated that the adhesive strategy does not influence the risk and intensity of postoperative sensitivity in posterior teeth [39]. Strategies to stabilize the dental adhesive interface (e.g., inhibition of dentin matrix metalloproteinases, collagen crosslinking, alternative bonding techniques), which show fairly good results in vitro, still lack evidence of clinical applicability and relevance.

17.2.4 Patient's Risks

Few studies address patients' risks as variables and their influence on the clinical performance of composite restorations. One systematic review [15] covered this specific aspect and observed mainly that patient age, gender, caries risk, and parafunctional habits may affect the longevity of resin composite restorations. In that study, restorations in younger patients and men showed more failures. These findings could be related to increased risk for caries in younger patients and occlusal stress in men. The results of two retrospective studies with large sample sizes [24, 40], in contrast, indicated higher failure rates in elder patients. Explanation for that finding might be multifactorial, including the influence of repeated restorative interventions in elder patients, in addition to dietary and salivary flow differences. One thing that should not be underestimated is that resin composite restorations placed in patients with high risk for occlusal stress are likely to fracture eventually due to the harsh mechanical conditions they have to withstand daily. No dental restorative material is fatigue-proof. This discussion will not cover the tricky clinical treatment or attenuation of occlusal stress issues, but patients and professionals should be aware of the increased risk for failures.

A retrospective clinical study evaluated the performance of direct resin composite restorations in patients with severe tooth wear requiring an increase of the occlusal vertical dimension and observed that restoration failures occurred mainly due to fractures [41]. Resin composites have the advantage of being more prone to repairs than any other restorative material, either direct or indirect. In addition, in patients with higher risk for occlusal stress, the viscoelasticity of resin composites is advantageous over more stiff and brittle restoratives (e.g., ceramics), which will be more prone to catastrophic, unrepairable failures.

The literature clearly shows that restorations fail more often in high caries-risk than low caries-risk individuals [15, 25, 42, 43]. In fact, patients with high caries risk will more often develop new caries lesions (including caries lesions adjacent to restorations) as compared with low-risk patients. Sometimes secondary caries may be accounted for restoration failure, whereas the professional and patient failed to address patient's high caries risk. Current evidence acknowledges that sugar-related feeding habits are the main cause of higher incidence of caries in general population [44]. The presence of marginal gaps is arguably a significant factor in the development of caries adjacent to restorations [45, 46]. Nonetheless, there is clinical evidence that resin composite restorations showed an increased risk for secondary caries compared to amalgam restorations [47]. The presence of a glass-ionomer lining is believed to reduce the risk for secondary caries due to fluoride release, but one clinical study indicated that the occurrence of secondary caries depended on the caries-risk level of the patient and not on the presence of lining [22]. In Sect. 17.3, we discuss that the misdiagnosis of secondary caries due to the presence of marginal staining (or "microleakage") might lead to increased failure rates supposedly due to secondary caries.

17.2.5 Operator

It would be naive to believe that the professional who is in charge of the diagnosis, treatment indication, cavity preparation, and application of materials and techniques is not a significant factor in restoration longevity. The operator experience and post-graduation training have been associated, for instance, with the choice of restorative materials and techniques applied clinically [48, 49].

A recent study addressed the clinical performance of resin composite restorations placed in 24 practices by 67 operators working solo, in small groups (2 or 3 professionals) or larger practices [24]. The annual failure rates for restorations with follow-ups of at least 12 years varied between 2.6% and 7.9%, which means a two to three times greater difference between operators in the long term. The failure rates of restorations placed solo or in small group practices were lower in comparison with larger practices in the same study. There is also evidence that the type of practice may influence caries treatment thresholds among clinicians [50]. Higher failure rates for restorations placed by less experienced dentists (years since graduation) also were reported [24, 43]. Another study showed shorter intervals from placement of restorations to re-intervention for older dentists, whereas dentist's gender had no relationship with time from restoration to re-intervention [51]. Interestingly, the same study showed that the older the patient, the older the dentist is likely to be.

The operator is so important that changing dentists has been associated with increased risk of restoration re-interventions [40, 51, 52]. This could be a result of a large variability in diagnosis and decision-making among clinicians. In addition, this result is likely an indication that the new dentist more strictly judges the previous work of an unknown colleague than the same dentist might judge their own previous work [53]. In that scenario, less re-intervention occurs, and restorations may last longer if checkup appointments are conducted by the same professional. There is a widespread trend for clinical ability to place good-looking restorations, hands-on courses, and lectures on how to place undetectable restorations. However, there is no clinical evidence whether or not restoration morphology, anatomy, and shade matching affect longevity. The way the restorations look is of course important, especially in anterior teeth, but it is just unlikely that beautiful restorations last longer than restorations that do not look as perfect. It seems nowadays that the way restorations look are sometimes more important to the dentist than to patients. This is particularly relevant considering the number of professionals who share their "work of excellence" online as a marketing strategy for attracting patients to their practice or dentists to their "how-to-do" courses. Data from one clinical study [54] indicated that anterior restorations are more prone to failure due to esthetic problems than posterior restorations; however, the failure rates were low in both regions.

17.2.6 Other Factors

The failure rates of state-of-the-art restorative techniques and materials are low compared to the frequent failures reported in the past, e.g., due to wear, a problem that is not considered to be clinically significant anymore. In a scenario of relatively good long-term clinical performance, other factors influencing restoration longevity may become more prevalent, including patient demographic, socioeconomic, and behavioral variables. Dental caries being associated with social determinants [55], for instance, suggests that restoration longevity should also be associated to the same factors. Two papers have reported an increased risk of restoration failure with increasing number of restored teeth per patient [56, 57]. Children with gingivitis were shown to have almost three times higher risk of restoration failure [27]. The periodontal pocket depth was found to be a significant factor in the survival of restored endodontically treated teeth [58]. These findings suggest oral hygiene conditions playing a role in restoration longevity. Another study in a birth cohort showed the presence of posterior restorations and higher number of restored surfaces associated with higher prevalence of gingival bleeding and dental calculus around teeth [59].

Restorations placed in dental practices located in areas with low socioeconomic status showed higher failure rates than practices located in richer areas [24]. Secondary caries was not reported as a main reason for failure in studies with patients from private clinics with higher economic status [21, 54]. Evidence from population-based studies [60, 61] indicates that the type of payment of dental services is associated with dentists' choice of restorative materials and that patient's socioeconomic characteristics affected restoration failures more than clinical variables. Other findings available in the literature show that people in the poorest population strata had more restoration failures [61], that restorations last longer in charge-payer patients compared with nonpayers [40], and that there is a relationship between restoration survival and practice attendance frequency [51]. In the latter study [51], it is interesting to notice that restorations in less frequent attenders performed better than those in more frequent attenders, which suggests that visiting the dentist too often might pose an increased risk for overtreatment. This could also be related to the fact that re-intervention in a restoration might be considered something usual for patients, since no large procedures are required and treatments are usually not that expensive. By comparison, the same patient would likely complain or require more information about a re-intervention involving an implant, which required a surgical and more expensive procedure, than a simple composite restoration.

17.3 The Meaning of Clinical Failures

One thing usually not addressed in studies on the longevity of dental restorations is the meaning of clinical failures. For instance, do failures due to fracture indicate that the restorative materials are not yet strong or tough enough? Are the failure rates due to secondary caries overestimated due to caries misdiagnosis? Do the "dentist's eye" and decision-making process interfere with the overall failure rates? Most clinical studies report that fractures and caries are the main reasons for failure of resin composite restorations, but usually no or insufficient details are given regarding the criteria and methods used in caries diagnostics or regarding the extension and origin of fractures. In addition, clinical studies usually do not differentiate failures according to, e.g., (1) the cause of initial restoration placement (caries, fracture, replacement), (2) the number of previous restorative procedures on the same tooth, (3) specific patient risks, or (4) additional details regarding clinical aspects taken into account in failure diagnoses.

A recent study showed an interesting result comparing clinical studies on the performance of resin composite restorations published between 1995–2005 and 2006–2016 [62]. The authors observed that while the incidence of secondary caries was similar between the two periods, fractures involving the tooth structure increased almost seven times in the latter decade, in addition to a decrease in postoperative sensitivity, unsatisfactory marginal adaptation, and wear. These findings could be interpreted in two ways: (1) improvements in restorative materials and techniques (including adhesives and photoactivation procedures) had a positive impact on the longevity, and (2) the positive clinical results of resin composites likely led to an increase in their use in many clinical cases, including large posterior restorations, increasing the rates of restored tooth fractures. The main reasons for failure of resin composite restorations are analyzed in the next section.

17.3.1 Fractures

Fractures of tooth, restoration, or both are reported in almost 100% of studies as a reason for failure of resin composite restorations. Fractures are a result of the cyclic mechanical loading that the restorative complex is subjected to constantly in the mouth. Not only resin composite restorations fail due to fracture but also amalgam fillings, onlays, crowns, fixed partial dentures, implant-supported dentures, and so on. Fatigue is the main reason for long-term failures, with all aspects presented in Fig. 17.1 contributing to intraoral deterioration of the restorative complex. Constant mechanical stimulation of varied intensity and duration leads to crack growth within the restored structure, which does not have the same toughening mechanisms of sound teeth. This results in a gradual deterioration in strength over time, meaning that the load a restoration can withstand after years of clinical service is much lower than in the first few days after placement. This explains why patients usually report that restorations failed when they were eating bread, for instance, aside from other reasons. Early failures, in contrast, are not explained by fatigue. Studies show that fractures might happen when the patient bites very hard small objects [63], but this is not the case for every clinical fracture. Short-term fractures may also occur due to technical errors during clinical procedure, such as mistakes in cavity preparation and leaving voids within the composite or in the final anatomical form of the restoration. Minor fractures and chippings with good repair prognosis often are observed in the short term.

In some situations, usually in the long-term and in larger restorations, the fracture will not only break the restoration but also involve a portion of the surrounding tooth structure. This is why cavity preparations should be made as conservative as possible to preserve sound tooth structure and reduce the risk of generating fractures with poorer repair prognosis. With all that in mind, would stronger resin composites have longer clinical durability? Probably not, since fatigue will still be in place. In addition, no restorative material is able to reproduce the way enamel and dentin interact with each other and the natural toughening mechanisms that oppose crack growth. Tooth morphology and the hierarchical structure of dental hard tissues generate a microstructural mechanism of damage resistance [64] that is the main reason for uncommon catastrophic fractures in young and sound teeth. In case stronger restorative resin composites are used, fractures would still be observed (take the example of zirconia-based ceramics) and perhaps involving more often and more severely the remaining tooth structure. This would likely lead to worse prognoses in re-restoring fractured teeth. A good example is amalgam, which is so strong that sometimes an amalgam restoration remains intact, while the surrounding tooth structure fractures. Long-term amalgam fractures often involve an entire tooth free surface or a cusp, sometimes even with crack lines extending to the root portion.

17.3.2 Secondary Caries

Untreated caries is the most prevalent human disease [65], and studies indicate that patients with high caries risk may have two to three times higher risk of restoration failure due to secondary caries than low-risk patients [14, 15]. However, the results of two meta-analyses indicated that the frequency of caries adjacent to restorations is low in most studies, with a median prevalence around 2.5% after 10 years [9, 10].

The presence of marginal gaps was traditionally associated with the development of caries lesions adjacent to resin composite restorations. Gaps and other marginal irregularities could indeed facilitate biofilm accumulation and lead to marginal staining. In most cases, however, the presence of stained margins does not lead to marginal caries, especially in occlusal areas. It has been shown that caries is about eight times more frequent at the gingival margin than at the occlusal margin of resin composite restorations [9, 66]. However, studies usually do not indicate a clear difference between existing caries and marginal restoration defects associated with active cavity-wall caries lesion. In addition, variability in caries diagnoses has been raised as a potential bias in clinical studies [14]. This makes even harder to detect whether misdiagnosis of secondary caries is leading to increased failure rates. Clinical evidence indicates that the presence of marginal staining increases with the clinical service time of restorations [9, 10, 67]. In fact, the prevalence of marginal staining is up to seven times higher than that of caries adjacent to restorations [9, 10], and it is almost impossible to make dental restorations margins free of staining in the long term. This finding raises a question about the existence of marginal gaps and other irregularities, particularly when they lead to marginal staining, being incorrectly associated with secondary caries. With all that in mind, it can be assumed that the overall prevalence of secondary caries in the literature is grossly overestimated.

Take the example of restorations shown in Fig. 17.2. Many dentists would be inclined to intervene in those situations when, in reality, there is nothing else than marginal staining. These restorations were placed up to 10 years before the pictures were taken. Had the dentists who saw those patients along the years been less conservative, the longevity of those restorative treatments would have been decreased. It is common to hear from clinicians that a “restoration was replaced because it was suffering from marginal leakage,” despite the evidence from caries research indicating that marginal gaps and marginal staining are not interrelated in the development of secondary caries [68, 69]. In that scenario, it is likely that many restorations are daily judged clinically as “failing due to caries” when, in reality, they only had pigmented margins, with no clinical significance except for esthetic concerns in anterior teeth. This means that the diagnosis and clinical assessment of secondary caries are, in fact, a risk factor for increased failure rates. If the clinicians judge marginal staining as a sign of marginal caries without taking into account other clinical variables (sensitivity to stimuli, clinical and radiographic signs of a progressing caries lesion), the failure rates would be higher. This should be considered with much attention by clinicians and educators.

17.3.3 Esthetics

Patient complaints about restoration esthetics are definitely a reason for intervention. However, intervening in situations when the patient does not complain but it is the dentist who feels the

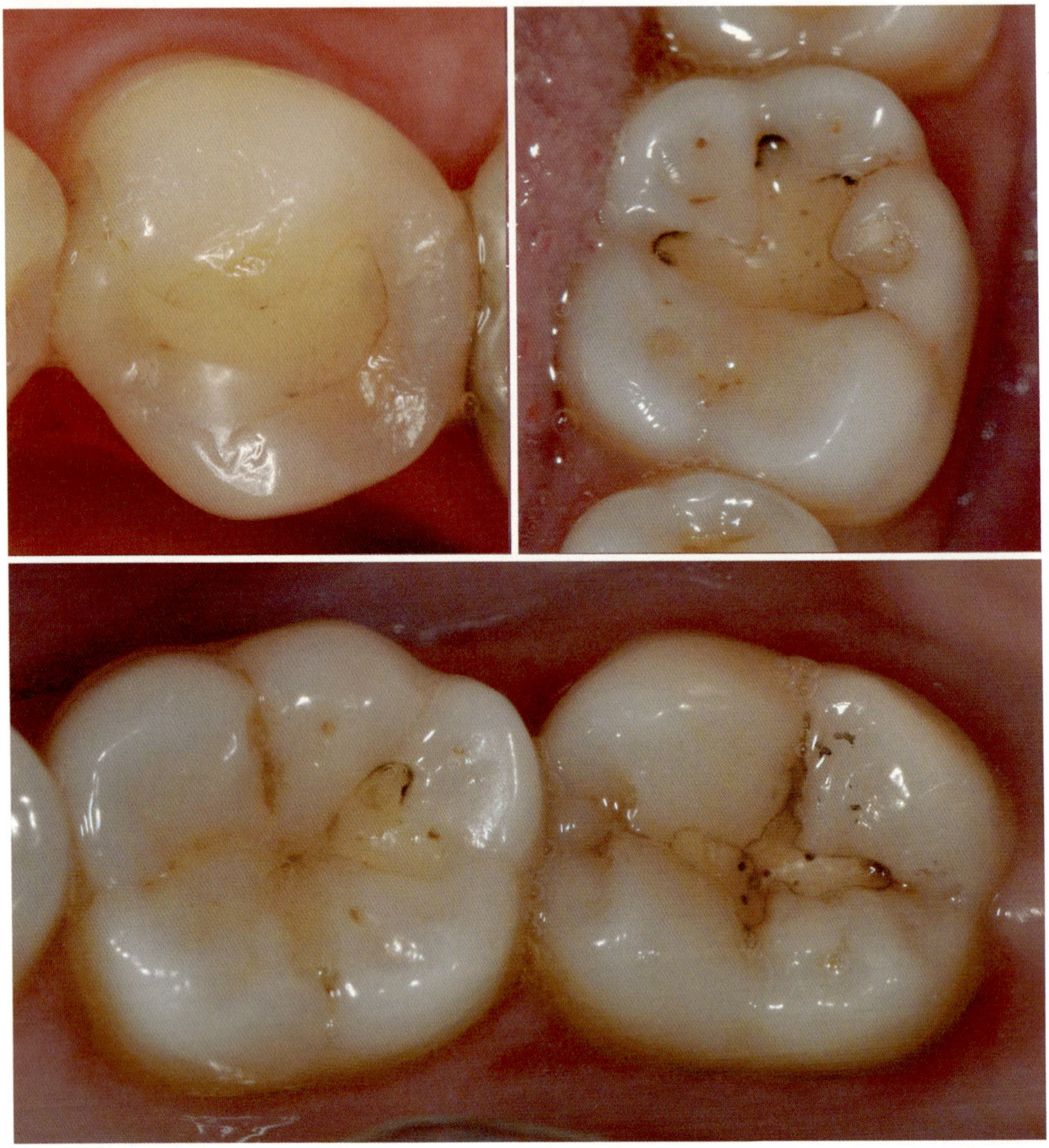

Fig. 17.2 Clinical photographs showing restorations that are clinically acceptable but with signs of marginal degradation or staining, which per se should not be the reason for intervention

restoration could look prettier should be considered overtreatment. Resin composite restorations in anterior teeth, as expected, present more failures due to esthetic problems than posterior teeth [54]. Esthetic failures in resin composite restorations might be related to several factors: marginal staining (here a good example when marginal staining is clinically significant), changes in resin composite color or translucency over time (likely an effect of pigment absorption and intrinsic discoloration), or loss of anatomical form. Although it is known that resin composites do not have the same color stability as ceramics, for instance, failures of resin composite restorations due to esthetics are not reported very often in the literature. One systematic review showed that failures due to unacceptable esthetics are more common in situations when esthetics was the primary reason for placing the original restoration [8]. Current restorative resin composites show improved color stability as compared with older materials, particularly due to improvements in curing efficiency and stability of photoinitiators. Therefore, despite the challenge in achieving excellent results in terms of shade and shape matching with adjacent teeth in anterior restorations, failures due to esthetics alone are not much prevalent in clinical studies. Cultural differences between continents and countries regarding patients' esthetic issues should be considered, and failure rates in anterior restorations could vary largely depending on that aspect.

17.3.4 Differences in Early and Long-Term Failures

As stated before, there are differences between short- and long-term restoration failures. Early failures, for instance, are usually related to chippings and other minor fractures, most likely resulting from the technical procedures of placing the resin composite restorations, an experience that have been entitled "stressful" [70]. Larger fractures are more frequent in the long term, in this case associated with fatigue of the restorative complex and more often involving the surrounding dental structure. Long-term fractures are usually more severe than early fractures, particularly in endodontically treated teeth. Endodontic complications, in contrast, are more prevalent in the first years of clinical service [6, 14], likely owing to incorrect diagnosis of pulpal viability or associated with injuries to the dentin-pulp complex during cavity preparation. Studies also have linked partial caries removal during caries excavation with lower prevalence of endodontic complications [27, 28]. With regard to secondary caries, most clinical studies show that it is a prevalent reason for failure in resin composite restorations only after 2 or 3 years of clinical service [6, 9], although failures could happen earlier in high caries-risk patients. Overall, provided that care is taken in the diagnosis and operative procedures, large failures in resin composite restorations are unlikely to happen in the short term. In the long term, generally failures are more likely to take place, although many current clinical studies indicate that under excellent clinical conditions resin composite restorations could last for decades [21, 33]. The selection of the restorative materials also has implications in restoration failures, as discussed in Sect. 17.4.

17.4 How Long Should We Expect Dental Restorations to Last?

This is a popular question among clinicians and patients. Patients want treatments that last forever; professionals know there is no such thing. Clinical failures are tricky to anticipate, though. One of the aims of this chapter is to leave the message that perhaps the question should be, "Within these clinical conditions, what are the factors playing a major role in restoration longevity?" In that scenario, expectations on the longevity of resin composite restorations would be more realistic. To be fair, perhaps, we could be demanding a little too much from a restorative procedure that is carried out in loco, in a timely fashion, under suboptimal placement conditions as compared with other restorative health treatments. If one looks at Table 17.2, the survival, success, and failure rates of crowns, fixed partial dentures, endodontic treatments, implants, or even hip and ankle replacements are somewhat similar to dental resin composite restorations. By the way, patients who underwent restorative therapies in the hips, knees, or ankles are told to bear in mind that these structures should not be overloaded and that longevity depends on it. Moreover, even with extreme care, the longevity of these treatments is not guaranteed, and re-intervention is often needed. Since dentists do not make the same sort of recommendation to patients with restored teeth, it is expected from patients to understand even without saying that the harsh conditions imposed by the oral environment are likely to trigger failures. Good communication between the professional and patient is always important.

Another good question is whether the annual failure rates for resin composite restorations

Table 17.2 Clinical longevity of selected restorative health treatments

Treatment	Clinical longevity	References
Resin composite restorations	Survival rates between 85% and 95% after 5 years	Demarco et al. (2012) [18]
Dental crowns	Survival rates between 90.7% and 96.6% after 5 years	Sailer et al. (2015) [71]
Dental implants	Survival rates between 77% and 97.4% after 10 years	Hultin et al. (2007) [72]
Fixed partial dentures	Survival rates between 81% and 93.8% after 10 years	Tan et al. (2004) [73]
Endodontic treatments	Success rates between 81% and 87% after 6+ years	Torabinejad et al. (2007) [74]
Total hip replacement	Success rates between 80% and 95% after 10 years	Corbett et al. (2010) [75]
Total ankle arthroplasty	Survival rate between 69.0% and 87.6% after 5 years	Haddad et al. (2007) [76]

reported in clinical studies are realistic, usually between 1% and 4% [8, 18]. Most studies are carried out under optimal clinical conditions (e.g., university settings), with restorations placed solo or by a few experienced operators, usually in low-risk patients. The restorative environment in the everyday practice is far less controlled; higher failure rates for resin composite restorations can be expected particularly when patients with all sorts of risks are treated and restorations of assorted complexity placed. By comparison, the same could happen with the longevity of crowns, implants, or knee replacements. If one looks at failure rates reported for restorations placed by multiple inexperienced operators in high caries-risk patients, for instance, survival rates as low as 58% after 3 years can be found [27]. In endodontically treated teeth, restorations might fail two or three times more frequently than restorations in vital teeth [18]. There are several other aspects that could influence longevity, as discussed previously. Therefore, given a precise or average number of years a resin composite restoration might last is not just tricky but misleading. One should not aim to predict how many years the restoration would be in place without the need of re-intervention but rather understand the circumstances involved in the durability of restorative treatments.

17.4.1 What Is the Best Restorative Resin Composite?

In the complex scenario described here for predicting the longevity of restorative treatments, choosing the "best" restorative material is a challenging task. In theoretical terms, the restorative resin composite should be selected based on the results reported in clinical studies. However, a service period of at least 3 or 5 years would be needed to draw initial conclusions on clinical performance, but the resin composite material might not be available on the market anymore after these years. Therefore, one could believe that the selection should be based on its mechanical strength, abrasion and wear resistance, handling conditions, versatility, optical properties, and so on. Although this is correct, some clinical studies failed in observing significant differences between composites that theoretically differ significantly in mechanical properties, for instance [77–79]. One study observed differences in the clinical performance within two composites after 22 years of clinical service, whereas these differences were absent in the first 17 years [21]. For sure, 17 or 22 years are really long-lasting restorative treatments, and not all restorations are expected to last that long. However, the data from this study and others highlight that, under good clinical conditions and taking into account the factors associated with longevity, resin composite restorations might have low failure rates. This does not mean that care selecting a resin composite should be neglected; rather, it highlights that the clinical behavior of direct restorations is reliable provided that many factors are taken into account.

As far as the resin composite material is concerned, hybrids and microhybrids (often called nanohybrids) are the gold standard materials considering restoration longevity [9, 10, 14, 18]. This is corroborated by the results of clinical studies showing that even resin composites available on the market one or two decades ago had a quality standard sufficient to fulfill most clinical requirements [9, 10, 21, 33, 54]. Although some studies reported differences in clinical performance of distinct resin composites [14, 21, 54], these differences are usually minor if hybrid resin composites were used. One study showed recently that hybrid composites could be indeed considered universal restoratives since good clinical performance was observed for anterior and posterior restorations in the long term [54]. With that in mind, it can be stated that most gold standard resin composites available on the market are of sufficient quality to generate treatments with similar clinical longevity. Therefore, selection of material could be based on specific handling characteristics, consistencies, optical qualities, and other clinical features related to the use of materials according to preferences of the professional. It should be kept in mind that efforts in diagnosis, planning, treatment indication, observation of occlusal aspects, biofilm control, and follow-ups are essential in order to obtain durable restorations. The effect of operator skills and experience and the use of gold standard adjunctive materials (e.g., bonding agents), techniques, and equipment are also relevant, as discussed in this chapter.

17.4.2 Answered and Unanswered Questions on Longevity

Table 17.3 lists aspects that are known, based on current clinical literature, to affect or not the longevity of resin composite restorations. At the same time that new evidence has emerged in the literature in recent years, there are still questions not clearly answered that warrant further investigation.

Table 17.3 Answered and unanswered questions concerning the clinical performance of composite restorations

What is known	What still warrants investigation
• Resin composite is the material of choice for restoring posterior teeth • Hybrids and microhybrids (or nanohybrids) are the gold standard resin composites regarding longevity of restorations • The composite type or brand has a minor effect on longevity provided that up-to-date materials are used • The number of restored surfaces is one of the most important parameters affecting the performance of restorations • Patient risks play a major role on longevity, even more important than materials and techniques • Direct and indirect composite restorations have similar performance and longevity but may differ in clinical applicability • Acid etching the enamel with phosphoric acid is still the gold standard in the bonding technique • Enamel beveling does not affect the clinical performance • The use of rubber dam seems not decisive provided that good isolation with cotton and suction may be achieved • Restorations in endodontically treated teeth fail more often than restorations in vital teeth • Repair is a viable alternative over replacing restorations with minor failures • Marginal staining is not marginal caries and "marginal leakage" does not lead to secondary caries	• How frequent are clinical failures due to "secondary caries" associated with misdiagnosis of caries? • What is the role of mechanical loading on the formation of caries adjacent to restorations? • What is the effect of suboptimal photoactivation procedures on clinical failures? • What is the effect of failed bonded interfaces on restoration longevity? • Is there still room for improving restorative composites based on the methacrylate technology? • Are expensive resin composites cost-effective? • Why do clinical studies usually discard patients "from the real word," with all sorts of risks? • In case of large coronal tooth destruction, are indirect restorations more cost-effective than direct composite restorations?

17.5 Concluding Remarks

This chapter addressed the factors that might affect the clinical longevity of resin composite restorations. State-of-the-art techniques and materials for placing resin composite restorations, in both anterior and posterior teeth, show acceptable survival rates in clinical studies. In that scenario, other factors affecting the longevity of resin composite restorations arise, including patient risks and demographic, socioeconomic, and behavioral variables. Clinical studies still report that fractures and secondary caries are the main reasons for restoration failure.

Strategies that could be taken into account to increase the clinical longevity and predictability (or reduce the disappointment with failures) of resin composite restorative treatments are listed below:

- Understand the aging process of teeth and restorations. Keep in mind that placing a restoration is not a cure. If the patient presents high caries risk, for instance, behavioral, dietary, and other aspects should be addressed.
- Take into account all patient's risks (caries, occlusal stress) when discussing the treatment with the patient. These patients should have more frequent monitoring of existing restorations.
- Work in an operative field isolated from humidity and other contaminants.
- Be conservative in removing carious dentin, and do not enlarge the cavity unnecessarily; pay particular attention not to lead to pulp injury and not involve additional walls and marginal ridges in the preparation. Marginal enamel and the dentin-enamel junction should be preserved as much as possible.
- If lining a restoration with glass-ionomer cement or flowable resin composite, the lining thickness should not exceed 1 mm.
- If the cavity has enamel margins, etch the enamel with phosphoric acid. In dentin, mild two-step self-etch adhesives are preferable. There is no reason to bevel the enamel for improved restoration longevity.
- Be sure to have an appropriate proximal contour of the restoration and contact with adjacent teeth.
- In case of minor restoration failures, be skeptical in indicating complete restoration replacement, and take into consideration the possibility of repairing or refurbishing the restoration.
- Also in case of minor restoration failures such as marginal degradation, loss of color match, or marginal staining, if there is no complaint from the patient, consider doing nothing except monitoring the restoration.
- Keep a detailed and accurate record of the reasons for restoration placement, changes over time, and reasons for new interventions.
- Be less enthusiastic in digging and filling when assessing restorations clinically. Training in caries diagnosis, particularly secondary caries, might be essential in that aspect. Professionals that are stricter in intervening in existing restorations may have longer-lasting treatment results.

References

1. Afrashtehfar KI, et al. Failure of single-unit restorations on root filled posterior teeth: a systematic review. Int Endod J. 2016.
2. Afrashtehfar KI, et al. Failure rate of single-unit restorations on posterior vital teeth: a systematic review. J Prosthet Dent. 2016.
3. Ahmed KE, Murbay S. Survival rates of anterior composites in managing tooth wear: systematic review. J Oral Rehabil. 2016;43(2):145–53.
4. Alcaraz MG, et al. Direct composite resin fillings versus amalgam fillings for permanent or adult posterior teeth. Cochrane Database Syst Rev. 2014;3:CD005620.
5. Angeletaki F, et al. Direct versus indirect inlay/onlay composite restorations in posterior teeth. A systematic review and meta-analysis. J Dent. 2016;53:12–21.
6. Astvaldsdottir A, et al. Longevity of posterior resin composite restorations in adults – a systematic review. J Dent. 2015;43(8):934–54.
7. Chabouis HF, Smail Faugeron V, Attal JP. Clinical efficacy of composite versus ceramic inlays and onlays: a systematic review. Dent Mater. 2013;29(12):1209–18.
8. Demarco FF, et al. Anterior composite restorations: a systematic review on long-term survival and reasons for failure. Dent Mater. 2015;31(10):1214–24.
9. Heintze SD, Rousson V. Clinical effectiveness of direct class II restorations - a meta-analysis. J Adhes Dent. 2012;14(5):407–31.

10. Heintze SD, Rousson V, Hickel R. Clinical effectiveness of direct anterior restorations--a meta-analysis. Dent Mater. 2015;31(5):481–95.
11. Magno MB, et al. Silorane-based composite resin restorations are not better than conventional composites - a meta-analysis of clinical studies. J Adhes Dent. 2016;18(5):375–86.
12. Moraschini V, et al. Amalgam and resin composite longevity of posterior restorations: a systematic review and meta-analysis. J Dent. 2015;43(9):1043–50.
13. Nguyen KV, et al. Clinical performance of laminate and non-laminate resin composite restorations: a systematic review. Aust Dent J. 2015;60(4):520–7.
14. Opdam NJ, et al. Longevity of posterior composite restorations: a systematic review and meta-analysis. J Dent Res. 2014;93(10):943–9.
15. van de Sande FH, et al. Restoration survival: revisiting Patients' risk factors through a systematic literature review. Oper Dent. 2016;41(S7):S7–S26.
16. Veiga AM, et al. Longevity of direct and indirect resin composite restorations in permanent posterior teeth: a systematic review and meta-analysis. J Dent. 2016;54:1–12.
17. Burke FJ. Tooth fracture in vivo and in vitro. J Dent. 1992;20(3):131–9.
18. Demarco FF, et al. Longevity of posterior composite restorations: not only a matter of materials. Dent Mater. 2012;28(1):87–101.
19. Shahrbaf S, et al. The effect of marginal ridge thickness on the fracture resistance of endodontically-treated, composite restored maxillary premolars. Oper Dent. 2007;32(3):285–90.
20. Loomans BA, et al. The effect of proximal contour on marginal ridge fracture of class II composite resin restorations. J Dent. 2008;36(10):828–32.
21. Da Rosa Rodolpho PA, et al. 22-year clinical evaluation of the performance of two posterior composites with different filler characteristics. Dent Mater. 2011;27(10):955–63.
22. Opdam NJ, et al. Longevity and reasons for failure of sandwich and total-etch posterior composite resin restorations. J Adhes Dent. 2007;9(5):469–75.
23. Van Nieuwenhuysen JP, et al. Long-term evaluation of extensive restorations in permanent teeth. J Dent. 2003;31(6):395–405.
24. Laske M, et al. Longevity of direct restorations in Dutch dental practices. Descriptive study out of a practice based research network. J Dent. 2016;46:12–7.
25. van de Sande FH, et al. Patient risk factors' influence on survival of posterior composites. J Dent Res. 2013;92(7 Suppl):78S–83S.
26. Coelho-de-Souza FH, et al. Direct anterior composite veneers in vital and non-vital teeth: a retrospective clinical evaluation. J Dent. 2015;43(11):1330–6.
27. Casagrande L, et al. Longevity and associated risk factors in adhesive restorations of young permanent teeth after complete and selective caries removal: a retrospective study. Clin Oral Investig. 2016;21(3):847–55.
28. Maltz M, et al. Randomized trial of partial vs. stepwise caries removal: 3-year follow-up. J Dent Res. 2012;91(11):1026–31.
29. Söderholm KJ. *Fracture of dental materials*. In: Belov A, editor. *Applied fracture mechanics*: InTech; 2012. p. 109–42.
30. Tyas MJ, et al. Minimal intervention dentistry—a review. FDI Commission project 1-97. Int Dent J. 2000;50(1):1–12.
31. Opdam N, Frankenberger R, Magne P. From 'Direct versus Indirect' toward an integrated restorative concept in the posterior dentition. Oper Dent. 2016;41(S7):S27–34.
32. Kaizer MR, et al. Do nanofill or submicron composites show improved smoothness and gloss? A systematic review of in vitro studies. Dent Mater. 2014;30(4):e41–78.
33. Pallesen U, van Dijken JW. A randomized controlled 27 years follow up of three resin composites in class II restorations. J Dent. 2015;43(12):1547–58.
34. van de Sande FH, et al. 18-year survival of posterior composite resin restorations with and without glass ionomer cement as base. Dent Mater. 2015;31(6):669–75.
35. Van Meerbeek B, et al. Relationship between bond-strength tests and clinical outcomes. Dent Mater. 2010;26(2):e100–21.
36. Schwendicke F, et al. Directly placed restorative materials: review and network meta-analysis. J Dent Res. 2016;95(6):613–22.
37. Perdigao J, et al. One-year clinical performance of self-etch adhesives in posterior restorations. Am J Dent. 2007;20(2):125–33.
38. Perdigao J, Geraldeli S, Hodges JS. Total-etch versus self-etch adhesive: effect on postoperative sensitivity. J Am Dent Assoc. 2003;134(12):1621–9.
39. Reis A, et al. Does the adhesive strategy influence the post-operative sensitivity in adult patients with posterior resin composite restorations? A systematic review and meta-analysis. Dent Mater. 2015;31(9):1052–67.
40. Burke FJ, Lucarotti PS, Holder RL. Outcome of direct restorations placed within the general dental services in England and Wales (part 2): variation by patients' characteristics. J Dent. 2005;33(10):817–26.
41. Hamburger JT, et al. Clinical performance of direct composite restorations for treatment of severe tooth wear. J Adhes Dent. 2011;13(6):585–93.
42. Opdam NJ, et al. 12-year survival of composite vs. amalgam restorations. J Dent Res. 2010;89(10):1063–7.
43. Sunnegardh-Gronberg K, et al. Selection of dental materials and longevity of replaced restorations in public dental health clinics in northern Sweden. J Dent. 2009;37(9):673–8.
44. Peres MA, et al. Sugar consumption and changes in dental caries from childhood to adolescence. J Dent Res. 2016;95(4):388–94.
45. Cenci MS, et al. Relationship between gap size and dentine secondary caries formation assessed

in a microcosm biofilm model. Caries Res. 2009;43(2):97–102.
46. Kuper NK, et al. Gap size and wall lesion development next to composite. J Dent Res. 2014;93(7 Suppl):108S–13S.
47. Kuper NK, et al. The influence of approximal restoration extension on the development of secondary caries. J Dent. 2012;40(3):241–7.
48. Demarco FF, et al. Anterior composite restorations in clinical practice: findings from a survey with general dental practitioners. J Appl Oral Sci. 2013;21(6):497–504.
49. Nascimento GG, et al. Do clinical experience time and postgraduate training influence the choice of materials for posterior restorations? Results of a survey with Brazilian general dentists. Braz Dent J. 2013;24(6):642–6.
50. Kakudate N, et al. Restorative treatment thresholds for proximal caries in dental PBRN. J Dent Res. 2012;91(12):1202–8.
51. Lucarotti PS, Holder RL, Burke FJ. Outcome of direct restorations placed within the general dental services in England and Wales (part 3): variation by dentist factors. J Dent. 2005;33(10):827–35.
52. Bogacki RE, et al. Survival analysis of posterior restorations using an insurance claims database. Oper Dent. 2002;27(5):488–92.
53. Gordan VV, et al. The decision to repair or replace a defective restoration is affected by who placed the original restoration: findings from the National Dental PBRN. J Dent. 2014;42(12):1528–34.
54. Baldissera RA, et al. Are there universal restorative composites for anterior and posterior teeth? J Dent. 2013;41(11):1027–35.
55. Thomson WM. Dental caries experience in older people over time: what can the large cohort studies tell us? Br Dent J. 2004;196(2):89–92. discussion 87
56. Opdam NJ, et al. A retrospective clinical study on longevity of posterior composite and amalgam restorations. Dent Mater. 2007;23(1):2–8.
57. Soncini JA, et al. The longevity of amalgam versus compomer/composite restorations in posterior primary and permanent teeth: findings from the New England Children's amalgam trial. J Am Dent Assoc. 2007;138(6):763–72.
58. Skupien JA, et al. Survival of restored Endodontically treated teeth in relation to periodontal status. Braz Dent J. 2016;27(1):37–40.
59. Demarco FF, et al. Multilevel analysis of the association between posterior restorations and gingival health in young adults: a population-based birth cohort0. J Clin Periodontol. 2013;40(12):1126–31.
60. Correa MB, et al. Amalgam or composite resin? Factors influencing the choice of restorative material. J Dent. 2012;40(9):703–10.
61. Correa MB, et al. Do socioeconomic determinants affect the quality of posterior dental restorations? A multilevel approach. J Dent. 2013;41(11):960–7.
62. Alvanforoush N, et al. A comparison between published clinical success of direct resin composite restorations in vital posterior teeth in 1995–2005 and 2006–2016 periods. Aust Dent J. 2016;62(2):132–45.
63. Popowics TE, Rensberger JM, Herring SW. The fracture behaviour of human and pig molar cusps. Arch Oral Biol. 2001;46(1):1–12.
64. Chai H, et al. Remarkable resilience of teeth. Proc Natl Acad Sci U S A. 2009;106(18):7289–93.
65. Marcenes W, et al. Global burden of oral conditions in 1990–2010: a systematic analysis. J Dent Res. 2013;92(7):592–7.
66. Mjor IA. The location of clinically diagnosed secondary caries. Quintessence Int. 1998;29(5):313–7.
67. Gaengler P, Hoyer I, Montag R. Clinical evaluation of posterior composite restorations: the 10-year report. J Adhes Dent. 2001;3(2):185–94.
68. Cenci MS, et al. Effect of microleakage and fluoride on enamel-dentine demineralization around restorations. Caries Res. 2008;42(5):369–79.
69. Mjor IA. Clinical diagnosis of recurrent caries. J Am Dent Assoc. 2005;136(10):1426–33.
70. Ferracane JL. Buonocore lecture. Placing dental composites—a stressful experience. Oper Dent. 2008;33(3):247–57.
71. Sailer I, et al. All-ceramic or metal-ceramic tooth-supported fixed dental prostheses (FDPs)? A systematic review of the survival and complication rates. Part I: single crowns (SCs). Dent Mater. 2015;31(6):603–23.
72. Hultin M, Komiyama A, Klinge B. Supportive therapy and the longevity of dental implants: a systematic review of the literature. Clin Oral Implants Res. 2007;18(Suppl 3):50–62.
73. Tan K, et al. A systematic review of the survival and complication rates of fixed partial dentures (FPDs) after an observation period of at least 5 years. Clin Oral Implants Res. 2004;15(6):654–66.
74. Torabinejad M, et al. Outcomes of root canal treatment and restoration, implant-supported single crowns, fixed partial dentures, and extraction without replacement: a systematic review. J Prosthet Dent. 2007;98(4):285–311.
75. Corbett KL, et al. Population-based rates of revision of primary total hip arthroplasty: a systematic review. PLoS One. 2010;5(10):e13520.
76. Haddad SL, et al. Intermediate and long-term outcomes of total ankle arthroplasty and ankle arthrodesis. A systematic review of the literature. J Bone Joint Surg Am. 2007;89(9):1899–905.
77. Kramer N, Garcia-Godoy F, Frankenberger R. Evaluation of resin composite materials. Part II: in vivo investigations. Am J Dent. 2005;18(2):75–81.
78. Pallesen U, Qvist V. Composite resin fillings and inlays. An 11-year evaluation. Clin Oral Investig. 2003;7(2):71–9.
79. Turkun LS, Aktener BO, Ates M. Clinical evaluation of different posterior resin composite materials: a 7-year report. Quintessence Int. 2003;34(6):418–26.

Part VII

Future Perspectives

Future Perspectives for Dental Composites

18

Marcela Carrilho and Paulo H.P. D'Alpino

18.1 Introduction

It has been suggested that soon there will be a day when dental restoratives would be no longer inert materials that merely fill the space left by cavity preparation, but instead, once placed in intimate contact, should stimulate dental tissues regeneration and/or be themselves self-mending. Although this day has not come yet, in an overview of this book chapter, one can grasp that such expectation may not be so far from fulfillment. The literature is plentiful of reports recounting new approaches to the manufacturing of biocompatible and structurally sufficient materials that can be applied to replace or repair dental, oral, and craniofacial tissues, focusing on clinical efficiency and usefulness (for deeper overview, readers are advised to consult the special issue of *Journal Dental Research* entirely dedicated to this subject – *Special Issue on Novel Materials* [1]). The intention of the present chapter is not to exhaust the subject but rather provide some brushstrokes about the state of the art and future perspectives of bioactive restorative materials.

M. Carrilho • P.H.P. D'Alpino (✉)
Biomaterials in Dentistry/Biotechnology and Innovation in Health Programs, Universidade Anhanguera de São Paulo (UNIAN-SP), São Paulo, SP, Brazil
e-mail: paulodalpino@yahoo.com

The term *bioactive restoratives* could be simply characterized by what its etymology enunciates, that is, these are materials that while restoring the damaged structures should exert a biological effect on their tissues and surroundings with which they are in contact. Perhaps in its least literal definition, restorative bioactivity includes many of the different therapies that biologically intend to stimulate dentin-pulp complex regeneration and/or healing. The dentin-pulp complex regeneration encompasses a cascade of cellular events in a variety of stages that are directly related with these tissues, which include synthesizing process, homeostasis, and function. Accordingly, these metabolic cascades are triggered, sustained, and strongly controlled by different signaling molecules secreted from the cells or sequestered in the extracellular matrix of dentin-pulp complex (Fig. 18.1).

It is consensually accepted that within the dentin-pulp complex, the burden of dental turnover and remodeling would rely entirely on the cellular and molecular contribution of the pulp. Differently, dentin has been regarded as a relatively static mineralized connective tissue that exhibits minor physiological remodeling activity after having reached its maturation. In fact, the assumed stillness of dentin reflects a clinical perception/conduct that has been limiting the therapies of dentin regeneration to procedures that simply replace the lost structure with synthetic materials, without exploring the actual bioactive potential of this tissue.

V. Miletic (ed.), *Dental Composite Materials for Direct Restorations*,
http://doi.org/10.1007/978-3-319-60961-4_18

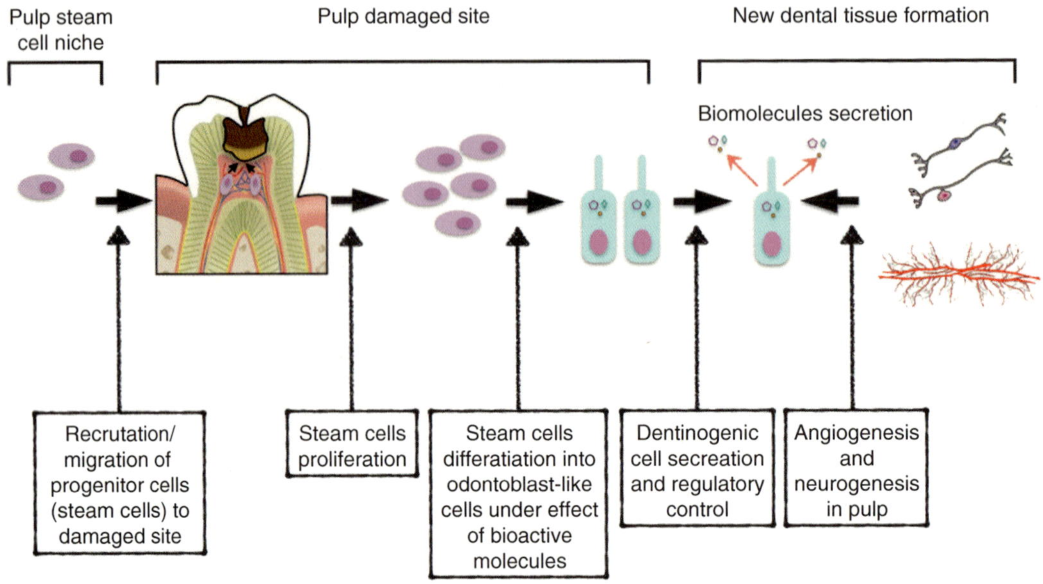

Fig. 18.1 Schematic illustrating a potential cascade of biological steps associated with healing events during dentin-pulp regeneration [Adapted from Smith et al. Exploiting the Bioactive Properties of the Dentin-Pulp Complex in Regenerative Endodontics. J Endod 2016;42:47–56]

For about four decades, scientists have been focusing their attention toward profiling the molecular identity of dentin [2]. Despite numerous restrictions imposed by the analytical methods when characterizing molecules in mineralized connective tissues, significant advances in terms of identification and partially understanding of dentin molecular frame were recently attained. Non-collagenous structural proteins, peptides, several enzymes, growth factors, chemokines, cytokines, and other extracellular matrix molecules were already found present in mature sound dentin [3–10]. Regardless of the fact that these molecules have accessed dentin by means of the dentinal fluid and/or have remained immobilized in the dentin after its matrix mineralization, the presence of these molecules in mature dentin suggests that they would have a biological function, which could be, for instance, involved in the signaling cascade of events that promotes tissue regeneration.

Many of the bioactive molecules present in dentin-pulp complex seem to have the potential to influence stem cell niches, even though our current perception of these interactions is still unclear. It was shown that the growth of pulp cells on a layer of isolated pulp extracellular matrix decreased their proliferation rate, while the expression of a stem cell-like phenotype was noticeably favored [11]. Moreover, when these cells were grown in mineralizing-inducing conditions, the pulp matrix allowed improved mineralization [12]. It was demonstrated, in fact, that the undifferentiated state of mesenchymal stem cells could be prolonged in culture when these cells were harvested on an extracellular matrix that mimicked their native niche [13]. Together, these studies suggest that the niche with its rich array of attachment and bioactive molecules has the ability to maintain stem cells at their maximum differentiation potential and this could be definitive to promote tissue regeneration in a temporal mode [2].

A consistent number of studies have investigated the biological function of isolated molecules in dentin-pulp regeneration [14], but in realistic terms, the tissue damage microenvironment will indeed display a multitude of local dissolved bioactive molecules; this implicates that the outline and actual interplay of these molecules may differ significantly from those conditions wherein their functions were separately analyzed [15]. Furthermore, despite the broad range of bioactive molecules found within the pulp tissue, their long-standing bioavailability may be restricted by a faster turnover rate of the pulpal extracellular matrix and the fact that this font may be severely jeopardized in cases of pulpal necrosis. Accordingly, dentin emerges as a reservoir of growth factors and other bioactive molecules with decisive roles in healing and repairing.

It would be interesting (or perhaps mandatory), therefore, for bioactive agents/materials to mirror themselves on and take advantage of bioactive molecules intrinsically constituting the dentin organic matrix and temporarily inactivated due to, for example, their interaction with other extracellular matrix components, sheltered in this mineralized structure. Theoretically, as occurring in caries and erosion processes, the demineralization of dentin matrix could facilitate the release and somehow activate dentin bioactive molecules [2], hence allowing them to participate of innate regenerative events. Taking this into account, one should consider that a fundamental prerequirement for an exogenous bioactive molecule or biomaterial would be that of being dotted with the ability to release and/or activate the tissue constitutive bioactive molecules.

Dental biomimetic regenerative approaches/materials are surely more promising and thrilling than simply getting accommodated with classical, well-established techniques for dentin-pulp protection/sealing and other restorative procedures. However, several are the drawbacks actually affronted by bioactive molecules/biomaterials currently assigned as therapeutic promoters for the regeneration of damaged dentin-pulp complex [2, 16, 17]. For instance, a number of delivery and technical critical aspects must be carefully considered when synthesizing and characterizing these materials. In order to exert a biological reparative function, bioactive molecules would need to be present and/or released in optimal and sustained concentrations and, at the same time, should overcome physical obstacles that would impede or restrain their interaction with labile endogenous molecules (i.e., from the tissue) that cue or contribute for the tissue regenerative cascade [14]. In addition, agents/biomaterials designed to bioengineer lost tissue should have a biocompatible matrix (little or no degradable) in order to offer structure for a new tissue to grow within, following a well-established spatial morphology. These agents include exogenous bioactive molecules/ions that encompass themselves a function or are able to chemoattract endogenous bioactive molecules via cellular recruitment from the site that, in turn, could in materialistic terms promote regeneration to engender a new living tissue [2, 17, 18] (Fig. 18.2).

Several studies have now brought to light the impending capability of various agents and bio-

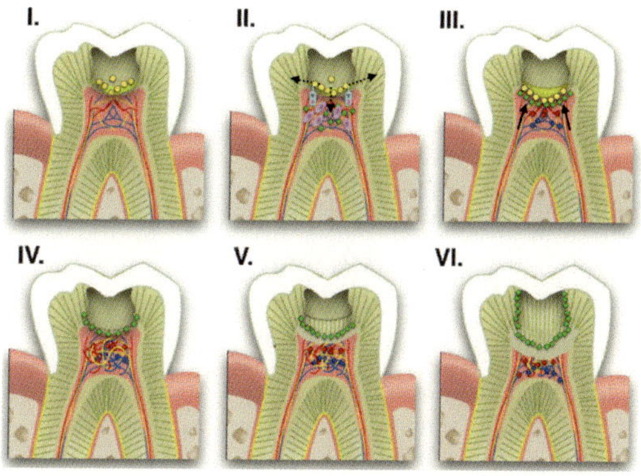

Fig. 18.2 Schematic illustrating the ideal activity that restorative biomaterials should exert on dentin-pulp complex, stimulating the release of endogenous bioactive ions and molecules to promote full tissue regeneration. **I.** Placement of the restorative biomaterial that can serve as scaffold with antimicrobial, chemoattracting, and tissue growth-stimulating properties (represented as *yellow spheres* within the restorative biomaterial). **II.** Tissue disinfection, stem cell proliferation, differentiation into odontoblasts under action of endogenous bioactive molecules (represented as *green diamonds*). **III.** Chemoattraction of endogenous (from pulp and dentin – *green diamonds*) bioactive molecules toward the site of the injured tissue **IV.** Pulp angiogenesis, pulp neurogenesis, and dentinogenesis under activated endogenous bioactive molecules (*diamonds red* and *blue*). **V.** Maintenance of the biological cascade to complete dentin-pulp regeneration. **VI.** Full dentin-pulp complex regeneration. [In other not to overcharge the schemes, from stage III to IV cells were not represented, but they will be indeed acting in the whole process of tissue regeneration. Represented structures are out of scale]

materials to release and expose bioactive molecules from dentin to stimulate stem cell behavior [19–26]. In fact, this is actually a quite triumph since it represents the first step in the complex and long sequence of other events to support a tissue regenerative excursion. There is still certainly much to be learned about both the cell-matrix interactions controlling the pulp stem cell behavior and all derived consequences from this, so that the recreation of dentin-pulp tissue could be completed on a macroscale terms. The good news is, from an evolutionary perspective, the understanding of multi-varied mechanisms underpinning the dentin-pulp complex self-regeneration properties has been greatly benefited thanks to the ongoing transdisciplinary revolution experienced in science and the technological advances of analytical resources achieved over the past decade. Thus, we speculate that the future of bioactive bioengineering restorative materials to support dentin-pulp regeneration will be nothing short of extraordinary.

18.2 General Application of Marketed Bioactive Materials in Dentistry

In a recent review, Sonarkar & Rucheet, in 2015, aimed to establish differences between the terms that have been used to define materials and their properties [27]. Thus, these authors defined bioactive as being a material that may have an "effect on or eliciting a response from living tissue, organisms or cell such as inducing the formation of hydroxyapatite" [27]. The term bioinductive was described as "the property of a material to induce a response in a biological system." Biomaterial was then defined as "any substance, surface, or construct that interacts with biological systems," and, finally, biomimetics was described as being an interdisciplinary field in which principles from different scientific areas are applied for "synthesizing similar products by artificial mechanisms that mimic normal structures" [27]. Based on this description and conducting a brief and pragmatic consultancy to the literature, one may find miscellaneous clinical conditions wherein dental materials, which are branded and commercialized as bioactive, have been indicated; such as:

- Pulp capping material: besides the well-known calcium hydroxide, varied cements present bioactive action and include mineral trioxide aggregate (MTA) [28], calcium-enriched mixture (CEM), Biodentine, inert material (isobutyl cyanoacrylate and tricalcium phosphate ceramic) [29], and also the resin cement MTYA1-Ca filler [30].
- To treat dental hypersensitivity by leaching ions that occlude dentinal tubules and favor remineralization of hard tooth tissues: sol-gel-derived bioactive glass (BAG) ceramic containing silver ions (Ag-BG) [31].
- As luting cements: the water-based calcium aluminate cement (marked Ceramir C&B luting cement) comprises the properties of both calcium aluminate and glass-ionomer cements [32, 33], is presented in a power-liquid, triturated capsule delivery system [34], and is claimed to present favorable mechanical and rheological properties, as well as biocompatibility.
- As scaffold that helps in regeneration of bone tissue cement: sol-gel-derived bioactive glass (BAG), releasing both calcium and phosphorus ions leading to hydroxyapatite production [35].
- For endodontic root repair: calcium phosphate, a novel endodontic cement (NEC), releases both calcium and phosphorus ions leading to hydroxyapatite production [36].
- As restorative material: liners and restorative materials that are manufactured to release bioactive ions and stimulate pulp regeneration and dentin mineralization [37, 38].

18.3 Past, Present, and Future Bioactive Restoratives

Possibly, the first sign in dentistry that a restorative could be "active" rather than simply and inert/biocompatible material is exemplified by the use of calcium hydroxides for temporary restorations and/or expectant treatments. For many years, calcium hydroxides have been used in close contact with exposed and/or injured pulp tissue. It functions on a very local and minute scale, enhancing the replacement of only small portions of the hard tissue lost to disease [18]. The use of calcium hydroxides as definite restorative is, moreover, rigorously restricted by many of their inherent characteristics: high solubility, low resistance to chemical degradation, low cohesive strength, lack of aesthetic properties [39, 40] and potential caustic degradation effects on exposed collagen, denaturing them [41] as well as increasing their water absorption and swelling [42, 43], altogether contributing to reduced tooth mechanical properties [44].

Another class of non-inert, biocompatible materials with a bioengineering potential has appeared with the development of conventional glass-ionomer cements (GICs). This class of material is defined as acid-base cements because they are by-products' reaction of weak polymeric acids with powdered glasses of basic character [45]. Although the appellation "glass-ionomer" has accompanied these materials' identification since the earliest reports, it is not technically appropriate. The proper term to identify these materials, according to the International Organization for Standardization (ISO), is "glass polyalkenoate cement" [46], but the term "glass-ionomer" was widely accepted as a clinical nickname [47]; GICs are considered to have an innate bioactivity because they have shown to develop an interfacial ion-exchange layer with tooth structures [48–50] eliciting a specific biological response. Accordingly, GICs release ions (fluoride, sodium, phosphate, and silicate) into surrounding aqueous media at levels at which they are biologically beneficial, enhancing, for instance, tissue remineralization [51]. Under acidic conditions, GICs may reduce the pH of the surrounding storage medium [51]. In parallel, GICs are also capable of taking up oral fluid ions, such as calcium and phosphate, and in consequence become harder [52]. GICs remain as the only material with true capacity to establish chemical adherence to dental tissues. For all these properties, we can easily conclude that these materials reflect and actually have permitted a shift in terms of dental material philosophy.

GICs are versatile materials with a variety of clinical uses in contemporary dentistry, including restoration of deciduous teeth [53, 54], anterior class III and V restorations [55, 56], cementation of crowns and orthodontic appliances [57, 58], restorations of non-carious teeth with minimal preparation [59], temporary cementation of crowns and other indirect restorations [60], restoration of teeth via the sandwich technique [61, 62], and for atraumatic restorative therapy [63–65]. Better performance of GICs as direct restoratives are reported when using their high-viscosity and non-excessively low-cost versions. However, two of the critical issues most commonly associated with such relatively aesthetic material are their apparent inability to provide a therapeutic remineralization of caries-affected dentin [66], poor wear strength, and inadequate surface properties [67, 68] and high potential to absorb moisture [69]. Thus, despite being less soluble, more biocompatible, and more cohesively and chemically resistant than calcium hydroxide cements, the GICs have shown to promote the dental tissues regeneration in scales that are also locally restricted to tissue injury [48–50].

Improvements in the formulation of conventional GICs have led to the development of hybrid materials that contain varied amounts of resin monomers. Thus, if the material sets predominantly via an acid-base reaction without depending on photoactivation, it is then regarded as a resin-modified glass-ionomer cement (RMGIC). Differently, that is, if the setting reaction is mainly based on the photoactivation of resin monomers, the material is more likely a polyacid-modified resin composite (compomer) and does not fit into the class of glass-ionomer cements [70]. The advantages of RMGICs over conventional GICs include a dual-curing mode (light activated and self-curing), higher flexural strength, and better handling properties, apart the fact that they are capable of bonding to composite materials [70–72].

Bioactive glasses and ceramics have been combined to GICs and RMGICs to challenge these materials' ability to function as matrices for the slow release of active species [73]. Likewise, chlorhexidine is another additive used to explore the potentiality of GICs and RMGICs as biological scaffolds [74]. The rationale behind the addition of bioactive glasses/ceramics or chlorhexidine to restorative glass-ionomers is clearly an attempt to interfere with the process of dentin mineralization and to control responses of the dentin organic matrix [70].

The addition of several other agents in dental glass-ionomers is in fact an up-to-date subject driving the scientists' attention [75–78]. Such interest in evaluating the benefits of the incorporation of active substances in the basic formula of glass-ionomer cements strongly suggests that the bioengineering capacity of this class of materials has not been totally exhausted and should not be definitely discarded.

Apart from glass-ionomers, there are currently on the market several cavity liners and restorative materials that claim to be able to help rebuilding and remineralizing affected tooth structure, preventing the teeth from acid attack. These materials could be reunited into the macro group of composites, which exhibit any capacity to release bioactive agents. As most of pathologies affecting the dental organ leads to a variable extension, the tooth demineralization, and because fluoride products have been systematically used for over 60 years to control or combat such tissue demineralization, manufactures of self-claimed bioactive composites have been practically betting most of their tokens to produce fluoride-releasing materials.

Resin composites may contain fluoride in a range of modes, such as inorganic salts, leachable glasses, or organic fluoride [79]. As a consequence, the amount and the velocity of fluorides release can be directly influenced by the type, size, and degree of silanization of the fluoridated filler, as well as by the type of resin matrix and the material porosity [80–84]. Moreover, the leaching rate of fluorides from resin composites was enhanced by the hydrophilicity and acidic nature of the polymer matrix wherein they are found incorporated [85]. The levels of fluoride release from resin composites are mostly much lower compared to those leached out from conventional or resin modified glass-ionomers [85–91]. Critical reviews that evaluated the effectiveness of these fluoride-releasing restorative composites have not shown consistent and conclusive outcomes [79], and higher fluoride release from filling materials seemed to result only in superficially increased remineralization of underlying demineralized dentin [92].

It is believed that remineralization may be truly promoted by a slow release of calcium and phosphate ions concentration from materials onto the fluid that baths dental hard tissues, followed by the precipitation of new calcium-phosphate mineral on these tissues surface [93, 94]. Calcium phosphates (CaP) are of significant interest to the biomedical and dental fields as they participate in both normal and pathological process of mineralization and demineralization of biological fluids and tissues' organic matrices [95–97]. Among different forms of calcium phosphates, amorphous calcium phosphate (ACP) is a unique noncrystalline compound that, due to its thermodynamic instability in aqueous environments, spontaneously transforms into crystalline orthophosphates, mainly hydroxyapatites (OH-Ap) [98]. The conversion of ACP into OH-Ap depends directly on the microenvironment chemistry it is found; thereby the presence of inorganic ions or organic molecules that can adsorb on the ACP surface will affect both the crystallinity and the Ca/PO_4 ratio of formed OH-Ap [99, 100]. Actually, OH-Ap is a thermodynamically stable form of CaP in neutral and basic environments and, as we know, the major mineral component constituting dental hard tissues. Thus, it might be hypothesized that once exposed to oral fluids, ACP-filled composites will release Ca and PO_4 ions (natural building blocks of tooth minerals) and with this create supersaturation conditions for the regeneration of injured tooth structures.

Concerned about these issues, novel resin composites for tooth direct restoration started being manufactured and doped with calcium phosphate particles. Studies evaluating these new formulations have been so far mostly concentrated on detecting whether the incorporation of calcium-phosphate particles could interfere with basic properties of nonfunctionalized resin composites

[101–105]. It is known that the osteoconductivity and biocompatibility of calcium phosphate-based biomaterials designed for dental and/or orthopedic bone tissue regeneration vary as a function of the type of calcium phosphate [101]. In general, when using ACP or DPCD (dicalcium phosphate dihydrate) particles, the outcomes revealed that resin matrix degree of conversion was not affected [102, 103], while mechanical properties tend not to be affected [105] or, even, be fairly enhanced [102, 103]. On the other hand, when calcium phosphate-containing composites were challenged in water-supersaturated environments, they exhibited a higher rate of water sorption [104, 106], which naturally reflects on these materials' integrity and on their mechanical strength [104, 106]. If the calcium phosphate included in the composite is in the ACP form, the excess of water uptake will further alter the kinetics of OH-Ap conversion, ultimately affecting the remineralizing capacity of the material [104].

Light-cure methyl methacrylate-based copolymers and their calcium phosphate-containing composites were shown to achieve high degree of vinyl conversion when diluting hydrophilic comonomers, such as HEMA (≥28 mass %) and TEGDMA (between 14 and 22 mass %), which are included in the resin at relatively high content [102, 104]. This is a positive aspect considering that it indicates a reduction in the amount of available unreacted (and toxic) monomers that these composites may potentially leach out. Conversely, as a consequence of a higher degree of vinyl conversion, experimental resin composites doped with ACP particles were shown to undergo high shrinkage upon polymerization [103, 104], which might definitely affect the performance of restorations built up with these materials.

Although still scant, in vitro protocols have been verifying the remineralizing potentiality of calcium phosphate-containing composites over demineralized human enamel specimens that underwent pH cycling regimens [101, 107]. Using a quantitative microradiography technique, these studies concluded that the experimental calcium phosphate-based composites efficiently established mineral ionic transfer throughout the body of the in vitro caries lesions, hence restoring on enamel surface the previously lost mineral content. An important detail is that such rematerializing effect was, as expected, solely localized and did not differ significantly from that of exerted by a fluoride control rematerializing solution [101].

The chemical structure/property relationships of monomers, compositional differences among polymers and photo-initiation molecules, as well as the achievable degree of monomer conversion, are fundamental factors that determine the potential toxicity of the polymeric composites and, obviously, of the composites containing bioactive agents. In vitro cytotoxicity tests comparing experimental composites functionalized with bioactive particles and the representative commercial controls urge as they are good predictors of the new material's suitability for the intended applications and should be one of the main parameters when considering their recommendation for clinical trials.

The concept of a "smart" material capable of reacting with the dental tissues to promote their regeneration is very tempting and should be massively encouraged [106]. Considering the biomaterials classification purposed by *Sonarkar and Rucheet* [27], it can be concluded that some of current direct restorative materials have shown their involvement in biomimetic processes in vitro and then could be categorized between those with bioactive and bioinductive properties, but have not yet proven to be able to regenerate and recreate dental injured tissues in a macroscale or to provide significant predictability when tested in animal models or in humans.

18.4 Concluding Remarks

The future for regenerative dentistry offers not only consistent challenges but also exciting promises. Successful bioactive restorative materials will need likely to contain nano-sized additives that deliver the essential components or additional molecules and ions, combining all desirable properties, that is, to be antimicrobial, to stimulate tissue growth and tissue remineralization. Thus, it is expected that the nanotechnology approach to manufacture ion-releasing particles, tubes, and fibers for delivering appropriate growth or antimicrobial agents will keep serving biomaterials scientists and industry in the development of efficient bioactive materials. A goal to be definitely achieved with bioactive regenerative materials is to recreate the entire tooth structures in a realistic scale, that is, in human subjects; however, essential short-term goals along that clinical and scientific course should be primarily resolved. The authors consider that future research should concentrate on the disinfection of damaged dentin-pulp tissue through an accurate and controlled delivery of antibiotic drugs, followed by programmed release of other molecules, which may activate and release the endogenous bioactive molecules (i.e., peptides, several enzymes, growth factors, chemokines, cytokines) to truly support a successful and functional regeneration of the dentin-pulp complex. For this reason, better understanding of the molecules involved and the cellular behavior necessary for dentin-pulp complex repair should keep guiding new therapeutic avenues for exploitation. More than ever, advances in biomaterials' development and added value will be increasingly and unavoidably dependent on the transdisciplinary activity between biological (at molecular and cellular levels) and physical (biophysics and bioengineering) sciences, and technology branches.

References

1. Ferracane JL, Giannobile WV. Special issue on novel materials. J Dent Res. 2014;93:1185–336.
2. Smith AJ, Duncan HF, Diogenes A, Simon S, Cooper PR. Exploiting the bioactive properties of the dentin-pulp complex in regenerative endodontics. J Endod. 2016;42:47–56.
3. Tersariol IL, Geraldeli S, Minciotti CL, Nascimento FD, Paakkonen V, Martins MT, et al. Cysteine cathepsins in human dentin-pulp complex. J Endod. 2010;36:475–81.
4. Boukpessi T, Menashi S, Camoin L, Tencate JM, Goldberg M, Chaussain-Miller C. The effect of stromelysin-1 (MMP-3) on non-collagenous extracellular matrix proteins of demineralized dentin and the adhesive properties of restorative resins. Biomaterials. 2008;29:4367–73.
5. Sulkala M, Tervahartiala T, Sorsa T, Larmas M, Salo T, Tjaderhane L. Matrix metalloproteinase-8 (MMP-8) is the major collagenase in human dentin. Arch Oral Biol. 2007;52:121–7.
6. Smith AJ, Lesot H. Induction and regulation of crown dentinogenesis: embryonic events as a template for dental tissue repair? Crit Rev Oral Biol Med. 2001;12:425–37.
7. Thomadakis G, Ramoshebi LN, Crooks J, Rueger DC, Ripamonti U. Immunolocalization of bone morphogenetic protein-2 and -3 and osteogenic protein-1 during murine tooth root morphogenesis and in other craniofacial structures. Eur J Oral Sci. 1999;107:368–77.
8. Helder MN, Karg H, Bervoets TJ, Vukicevic S, Burger EH, D'Souza RN, et al. Bone morphogenetic protein-7 (osteogenic protein-1, OP-1) and tooth development. J Dent Res. 1998;77:545–54.
9. Tjaderhane L, Larjava H, Sorsa T, Uitto VJ, Larmas M, Salo T. The activation and function of host matrix metalloproteinases in dentin matrix breakdown in caries lesions. J Dent Res. 1998;77:1622–9.
10. Finkelman RD, Mohan S, Jennings JC, Taylor AK, Jepsen S, Baylink DJ. Quantitation of growth factors IGF-I, SGF/IGF-II, and TGF-beta in human dentin. J Bone Miner Res. 1990;5:717–23.
11. Smith JG, Smith AJ, Shelton RM, Cooper PR. Dental pulp cell behavior in biomimetic environments. J Dent Res. 2015;94:1552–9.
12. Booth C, Potten CS. Gut instincts: thoughts on intestinal epithelial stem cells. J Clin Invest. 2000;105:1493–9.
13. Chen XD. Extracellular matrix provides an optimal niche for the maintenance and propagation of mesenchymal stem cells. Birth Defects Res C Embryo Today. 2010;90:45–54.
14. Murray PE, Garcia-Godoy F, Hargreaves KM. Regenerative endodontics: a review of current status and a call for action. J Endod. 2007;33:377–90.
15. Simon S, Smith AJ, Berdal A, Lumley PJ, Cooper PR. The MAP kinase pathway is involved in odontoblast stimulation via p38 phosphorylation. J Endod. 2010;36:256–9.
16. Tziafas D, Smith AJ, Lesot H. Designing new treatment strategies in vital pulp therapy. J Dent. 2000;28:77–92.
17. Albuquerque MT, Valera MC, Nakashima M, Nor JE, Bottino MC. Tissue-engineering-based strategies for regenerative endodontics. J Dent Res. 2014;93:1222–31.
18. Ferracane JL, Giannobile WV. Novel biomaterials and technologies for the dental, oral, and craniofacial structures. J Dent Res. 2014;93:1185–6.
19. Galler KM, Buchalla W, Hiller KA, Federlin M, Eidt A, Schiefersteiner M, et al. Influence of root canal disinfectants on growth factor release from dentin. J Endod. 2015;41:363–8.
20. Tomson PL, Grover LM, Lumley PJ, Sloan AJ, Smith AJ, Cooper PR. Dissolution of bio-active dentine matrix components by mineral trioxide aggregate. J Dent. 2007;35:636–42.

21. Galler KM, D'Souza RN, Federlin M, Cavender AC, Hartgerink JD, Hecker S, et al. Dentin conditioning codetermines cell fate in regenerative endodontics. J Endod. 2011;37:1536–41.
22. Martin DE, De Almeida JF, Henry MA, Khaing ZZ, Schmidt CE, Teixeira FB, et al. Concentration-dependent effect of sodium hypochlorite on stem cells of apical papilla survival and differentiation. J Endod. 2014;40:51–5.
23. Trevino EG, Patwardhan AN, Henry MA, Perry G, Dybdal-Hargreaves N, Hargreaves KM, et al. Effect of irrigants on the survival of human stem cells of the apical papilla in a platelet-rich plasma scaffold in human root tips. J Endod. 2011;37:1109–15.
24. Duncan HF, Smith AJ, Fleming GJ, Cooper PR. Histone deacetylase inhibitors epigenetically promote reparative events in primary dental pulp cells. Exp Cell Res. 2013;319:1534–43.
25. Graham L, Cooper PR, Cassidy N, Nor JE, Sloan AJ, Smith AJ. The effect of calcium hydroxide on solubilisation of bio-active dentine matrix components. Biomaterials. 2006;27:2865–73.
26. Murray PE, Smith AJ, Garcia-Godoy F, Lumley PJ. Comparison of operative procedure variables on pulpal viability in an ex vivo model. Int Endod J. 2008;41:389–400.
27. Sonarkar S, Purba R. Bioactive materials in conservative dentistry. Int J Contemp Dent Med Rev. 2015;2015:1–4.
28. Chen L, Shen H, Suh BI. Bioactive dental restorative materials: a review. Am J Dent. 2013;26:219–27.
29. Mehta AB, Kumari V, Jose R, Izadikhah V. Remineralization potential of bioactive glass and casein phosphopeptide-amorphous calcium phosphate on initial carious lesion: an in-vitro pH-cycling study. J Conserv Dent. 2014;17:3–7.
30. Sabbagh J, Ryelandt L, Bacherius L, Biebuyck JJ, Vreven J, Lambrechts P, et al. Characterization of the inorganic fraction of resin composites. J Oral Rehabil. 2004;31:1090–101.
31. Rath SN, Brandl A, Hiller D, Hoppe A, Gbureck U, Horch RE, et al. Bioactive copper-doped glass scaffolds can stimulate endothelial cells in co-culture in combination with mesenchymal stem cells. PLoS One. 2014;9:e113319.
32. Parirokh M, Torabinejad M. Mineral trioxide aggregate: a comprehensive literature review – Part III: clinical applications, drawbacks, and mechanism of action. J Endod. 2010;36:400–13.
33. Asgary S, Eghbal MJ, Parirokh M, Torabzadeh H. Sealing ability of three commercial mineral trioxide aggregates and an experimental root-end filling material. Iran Endod J. 2006;1:101–5.
34. Asgary S, Eghbal MJ, Parirokh M, Ghoddusi J, Kheirieh S, Brink F. Comparison of mineral trioxide aggregate's composition with Portland cements and a new endodontic cement. J Endod. 2009;35:243–50.
35. Asgary S, Eghbal MJ, Parirokh M, Ghoddusi J. Effect of two storage solutions on surface topography of two root-end fillings. Aust Endod J. 2009;35:147–52.
36. Amini Ghazvini S, Abdo Tabrizi M, Kobarfard F, Akbarzadeh Baghban A, Asgary S. Ion release and pH of a new endodontic cement, MTA and Portland cement. Iran Endod J. 2009;4:74–8.
37. Qureshi A, E S, Nandakumar, Pratapkumar, Sambashivarao. Recent advances in pulp capping materials: an overview. J Clin Diagn Res. 2014;8:316–21.
38. Chatzistavrou X, Fenno JC, Faulk D, Badylak S, Kasuga T, Boccaccini AR, et al. Fabrication and characterization of bioactive and antibacterial composites for dental applications. Acta Biomater. 2014;10:3723–32.
39. Powers JM, Wataha JC. Cements. Dental materials properties and manipulation. 10th ed. St. Louis, Missouri: Elsevier; 2014. p. 248.
40. Sakagushi RL, Powers JM. Craig's restorative dental materials. 13th ed. St. Louis, Missouri: Elsevier; 2012.
41. Sun Y, Chen WL, Lin SJ, Jee SH, Chen YF, Lin LC, et al. Investigating mechanisms of collagen thermal denaturation by high resolution second-harmonic generation imaging. Biophys J. 2006;91:2620–5.
42. Bowes JH. The swelling of collagen in alkaline solutions; swelling in solutions of bivalent bases. Biochem J. 1950;46:530–2.
43. Kemp GD, Tristram GR. The preparation of an alkali-soluble collagen from demineralized bone. Biochem J. 1971;124:915–9.
44. Andreasen JO, Farik B, Munksgaard EC. Long-term calcium hydroxide as a root canal dressing may increase risk of root fracture. Dental Traumatol. 2002;18:134–7.
45. Mount GJ. Color atlas of glass Ionomer cement. 2nd ed. Martin Dunitz: London, UK; 2002.
46. ISO. Dentistry - water-based cements Part 1 Powder/liquid acid-base cements. In: IOf S, editor. ISO 9917–1: Dental water based cements. Switzerland: International Organization for Standardization; 2007.
47. McLean JW, Nicholson JW, Wilson AD. Proposed nomenclature for glass-ionomer dental cements and related materials. Quintessence Int. 1994;25:587–9.
48. Sennou HE, Lebugle AA, Gregoire GL. X-ray photoelectron spectroscopy study of the dentin-glass ionomer cement interface. Dent Mater. 1999;15:229–37.
49. Watson TF, Atmeh AR, Sajini S, Cook RJ, Festy F. Present and future of glass-ionomers and calcium-silicate cements as bioactive materials in dentistry: biophotonics-based interfacial analyses in health and disease. Dent Mater. 2014;30:50–61.
50. Yiu CK, Tay FR, King NM, Pashley DH, Sidhu SK, Neo JC, et al. Interaction of glass-ionomer cements with moist dentin. J Dent Res. 2004;83:283–9.
51. Nicholson JW, Czarnecka B, Limanowska-Shaw H. The long-term interaction of dental cements with lactic acid solutions. J Mater Sci Mater Med. 1999;10:449–52.
52. Okada K, Tosaki S, Hirota K, Hume WR. Surface hardness change of restorative filling materials stored in saliva. Dent Mater. 2001;17:34–9.

53. de Amorim RG, Leal SC, Frencken JE. Survival of atraumatic restorative treatment (ART) sealants and restorations: a meta-analysis. Clin Oral Investig. 2012;16:429–41.
54. Mijan MC, de Amorim RG, Mulder J, Frencken JE, Leal SC. Exfoliation rates of primary molars submitted to three treatment protocols after 3.5 years. Community Dent Oral Epidemiol. 2015;43:232–9.
55. Abdalla AI, Alhadainy HA, Garcia-Godoy F. Clinical evaluation of glass ionomers and compomers in Class V carious lesions. Am J Dent. 1997;10:18–20.
56. van Dijken JW. 3-year clinical evaluation of a compomer, a resin-modified glass ionomer and a resin composite in Class III restorations. Am J Dent. 1996;9:195–8.
57. Leevailoj C, Platt JA, Cochran MA, Moore BK. In vitro study of fracture incidence and compressive fracture load of all-ceramic crowns cemented with resin-modified glass ionomer and other luting agents. J Prosthet Dent. 1998;80:699–707.
58. Pascotto RC, Navarro MF, Capelozza Filho L, Cury JA. In vivo effect of a resin-modified glass ionomer cement on enamel demineralization around orthodontic brackets. Am J Orthod Dentofacial Orthop. 2004;125:36–41.
59. Peumans M, De Munck J, Mine A, Van Meerbeek B. Clinical effectiveness of contemporary adhesives for the restoration of non-carious cervical lesions. A systematic review. Dent Mater. 2014;30:1089–103.
60. Terata R, Nakashima K, Kubota M. Effect of temporary materials on bond strength of resin-modified glass-ionomer luting cements to teeth. Am J Dent. 2000;13:209–11.
61. McLean JW, Powis DR, Prosser HJ, Wilson AD. The use of glass-ionomer cements in bonding composite resins to dentine. Br Dent J. 1985;158:410–4.
62. Andersson-Wenckert IE, van Dijken JW, Kieri C. Durability of extensive Class II open-sandwich restorations with a resin-modified glass ionomer cement after 6 years. Am J Dent. 2004;17:43–50.
63. Frencken JE, Makoni F, Sithole WD. ART restorations and glass ionomer sealants in Zimbabwe: survival after 3 years. Community Dent Oral Epidemiol. 1998;26:372–81.
64. Zanata RL, Fagundes TC, Freitas MC, Lauris JR, Navarro MF. Ten-year survival of ART restorations in permanent posterior teeth. Clin Oral Investig. 2011;15:265–71.
65. da Mata C, Allen PF, McKenna G, Cronin M, O'Mahony D, Woods N. Two-year survival of ART restorations placed in elderly patients: a randomised controlled clinical trial. J Dent. 2015;43:405–11.
66. De Munck J, Van Landuyt K, Peumans M, Poitevin A, Lambrechts P, Braem M, et al. A critical review of the durability of adhesion to tooth tissue: methods and results. J Dent Res. 2005;84:118–32.
67. Peutzfeldt A, Garcia-Godoy F, Asmussen E. Surface hardness and wear of glass ionomers and compomers. Am J Dent. 1997;10:15–7.
68. Zafar MS, Ahmed N. Effects of wear on hardness and stiffness of restorative dental materials. Life Sci J. 2014;11:11–8.
69. Um CM, Oilo G. The effect of early water contact on glass-ionomer cements. Quintessence Int. 1992;23:209–14.
70. Pegoraro TA, da Silva NR, Carvalho RM. Cements for use in esthetic dentistry. Dent Clin N Am. 2007;51:453–71.
71. Xie D, Brantley WA, Culbertson BM, Wang G. Mechanical properties and microstructures of glass-ionomer cements. Dent Mater. 2000;16:129–38.
72. Moshaverinia A, Roohpour N, Chee WWL, Schricker SR. A review of powder modifications in conventional glass-ionomer dental cements. J Mater Chem. 2011;21:1319–28.
73. Yli-Urpo H, Vallittu PK, Narhi TO, Forsback AP, Vakiparta M. Release of silica, calcium, phosphorus, and fluoride from glass ionomer cement containing bioactive glass. J Biomater Appl. 2004;19:5–20.
74. Palmer G, Jones FH, Billington RW, Pearson GJ. Chlorhexidine release from an experimental glass ionomer cement. Biomaterials. 2004;25:5423–31.
75. Chen S, Gururaj S, Xia W, Engqvist H. Synthesis of Ag doped calcium phosphate particles and their antibacterial effect as additives in dental glass ionomer cements. J Mater Sci Mater Med. 2016;27:172.
76. Felemban NH, Ebrahim MI. Effects of adding silica particles on certain properties of resin-modified glass-ionomer cement. Eur J Dent. 2016;10:225–9.
77. Pinheiro SL, Azenha GR, Milito FDE, Democh YM. Antimicrobial capacity of casein phosphopeptide/amorphous calcium phosphate and enzymes in glass ionomer cement in dentin carious lesions. Acta Stomatol Croat. 2015;49:104–11.
78. Zainuddin N, Karpukhina N, Law RV, Hill RG. Characterisation of a remineralising Glass Carbomer(R) ionomer cement by MAS-NMR spectroscopy. Dent Mater. 2012;28:1051–8.
79. Wiegand A, Buchalla W, Attin T. Review on fluoride-releasing restorative materials – fluoride release and uptake characteristics, antibacterial activity and influence on caries formation. Dent Mater. 2007;23:343–62.
80. Xu X, Burgess JO. Compressive strength, fluoride release and recharge of fluoride-releasing materials. Biomaterials. 2003;24:2451–61.
81. Dijkman GE, de Vries J, Lodding A, Arends J. Long-term fluoride release of visible light-activated composites in vitro: a correlation with in situ demineralisation data. Caries Res. 1993;27:117–23.
82. Xu HH, Eichmiller FC, Antonucci JM, Flaim GM. Single-crystalline ceramic whisker-reinforced carboxylic acid-resin composites with fluoride release. Oper Dent. 2000;25:90–7.
83. Xu HH, Eichmiller FC, Antonucci JM, Schumacher GE, Ives LK. Dental resin composites containing ceramic whiskers and precured glass ionomer particles. Dent Mater. 2000;16:356–63.

84. Arends J, Dijkman GE, Dijkman AG. Review of fluoride release and secondary caries reduction by fluoridating composites. Adv Dent Res. 1995;9:367–76.
85. Asmussen E, Peutzfeldt A. Long-term fluoride release from a glass ionomer cement, a compomer, and from experimental resin composites. Acta Odontol Scand. 2002;60:93–7.
86. Karantakis P, Helvatjoglou-Antoniades M, Theodoridou-Pahini S, Papadogiannis Y. Fluoride release from three glass ionomers, a compomer, and a composite resin in water, artificial saliva, and lactic acid. Oper Dent. 2000;25:20–5.
87. Attar N, Onen A. Fluoride release and uptake characteristics of aesthetic restorative materials. J Oral Rehabil. 2002;29:791–8.
88. Vermeersch G, Leloup G, Vreven J. Fluoride release from glass-ionomer cements, compomers and resin composites. J Oral Rehabil. 2001;28:26–32.
89. Preston AJ, Mair LH, Agalamanyi EA, Higham SM. Fluoride release from aesthetic dental materials. J Oral Rehabil. 1999;26:123–9.
90. Carvalho AS, Cury JA. Fluoride release from some dental materials in different solutions. Oper Dent. 1999;24:14–9.
91. Preston AJ, Agalamanyi EA, Higham SM, Mair LH. The recharge of esthetic dental restorative materials with fluoride in vitro-two years' results. Dent Mater. 2003;19:32–7.
92. Exterkate RA, Damen JJ, ten Cate JM. Effect of fluoride-releasing filling materials on underlying dentinal lesions in vitro. Caries Res. 2005;39:509–13.
93. Xu HH, Weir MD, Sun L, Moreau JL, Takagi S, Chow LC, et al. Strong nanocomposites with Ca, PO(4), and F release for caries inhibition. J Dent Res. 2010;89:19–28.
94. Xu HH, Moreau JL, Sun L, Chow LC. Novel CaF(2) nanocomposite with high strength and fluoride ion release. J Dent Res. 2010;89:739–45.
95. Wang L, Nancollas GH. Pathways to biomineralization and biodemineralization of calcium phosphates: the thermodynamic and kinetic controls. Dalton Trans. 2009:21:2665–72.
96. Dorozhkin S. Calcium orthophosphates in nature, biology and medicine. Materials. 2009;2:399–498.
97. Dorozhkin SV. Calcium orthophosphate-based biocomposites and hybrid biomaterials. J Mater Sci. 2009;44:2343–87.
98. Hench LL. Bioceramics and the origin of life. J Biomed Mater Res. 1989;23:685–703.
99. Dorozhkin SV. Amorphous calcium (ortho)phosphates. Acta Biomater. 2010;6:4457–75.
100. Eanes ED. Amorphous calcium phosphate. Monogr Oral Sci. 2001;18:130–47.
101. Bienek DR, Tutak W, Skrtic D. Bioactive polymeric materials for tissue repair. J Funct Biomater. 2017;8:4.
102. Alania Y, Chiari MD, Rodrigues MC, Arana-Chavez VE, Bressiani AH, Vichi FM, et al. Bioactive composites containing TEGDMA-functionalized calcium phosphate particles: degree of conversion, fracture strength and ion release evaluation. Dent Mater. 2016;32:e374–e81.
103. Marovic D, Sariri K, Demoli N, Ristic M, Hiller KA, Skrtic D, et al. Remineralizing amorphous calcium phosphate based composite resins: the influence of inert fillers on monomer conversion, polymerization shrinkage, and microhardness. Croat Med J. 2016;57:465–73.
104. Skrtič D, Antonucci JM. Bioactive polymeric composites for tooth mineral regeneration: physicochemical and cellular aspects. J Funct Biomater. 2011;2:271–307.
105. Xie X, Wang L, Xing D, Arola DD, Weir MD, Bai Y, et al. Protein-repellent and antibacterial functions of a calcium phosphate rechargeable nanocomposite. J Dent. 2016;52:15–22.
106. Ferracane JL. Resin composite-state of the art. Dent Mater. 2011;27:29–38.
107. Langhorst SE, O'Donnell JN, Skrtic D. In vitro remineralization of enamel by polymeric amorphous calcium phosphate composite: quantitative microradiographic study. Dent Mater. 2009;25:884–91.

Part VIII

Appendix

19 Clinical Application of Dental Composites for Direct Restorations

Eduardo Souza Jr.

19.1 Case 1: Teeth Remodeling Using Direct Resin Composite

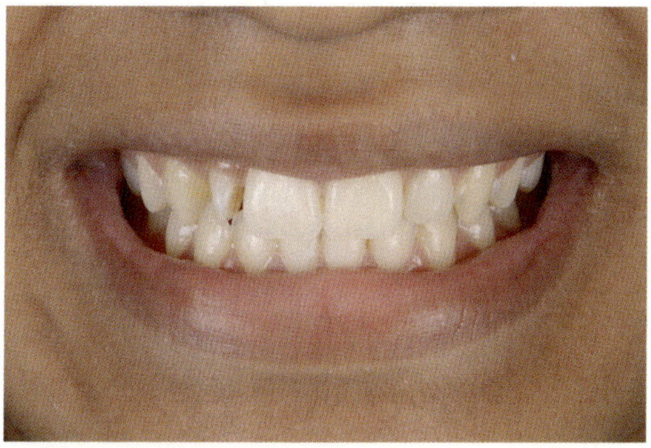

Fig. 19.1 Preoperative smile of the patient showing a conoid lateral incisor. In these cases, the professional needs to close diastemas and remodel the buccal surface

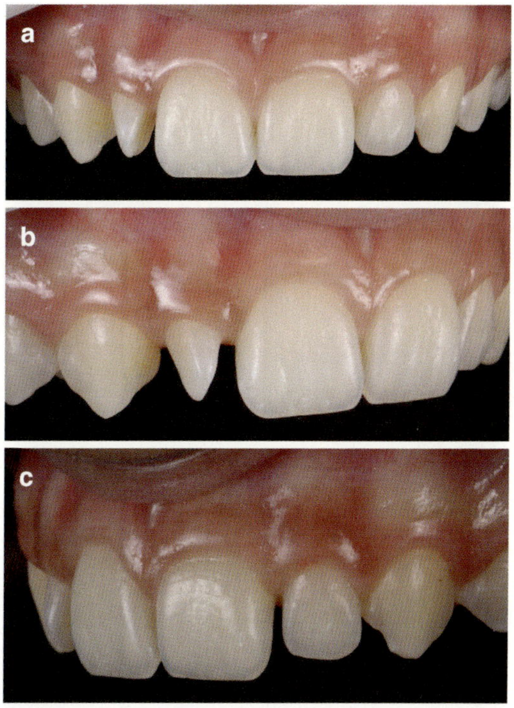

Fig. 19.2 (a–c) Preliminary intraoral view of maxillary anterior teeth. The patient presented lateral conoid and diastema

E. Souza Jr.
FAIPE University—FAIPE, Cuiabá, Mato Grosso, Brazil
e-mail: edujcsj@gmail.com

V. Miletic (ed.), *Dental Composite Materials for Direct Restorations*, http://doi.org/10.1007/978-3-319-60961-4_19

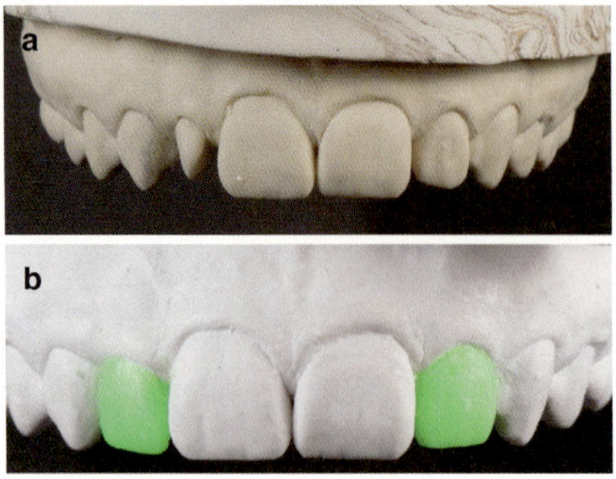

Fig. 19.3 (**a**, **b**) Initial stone cast and wax-up

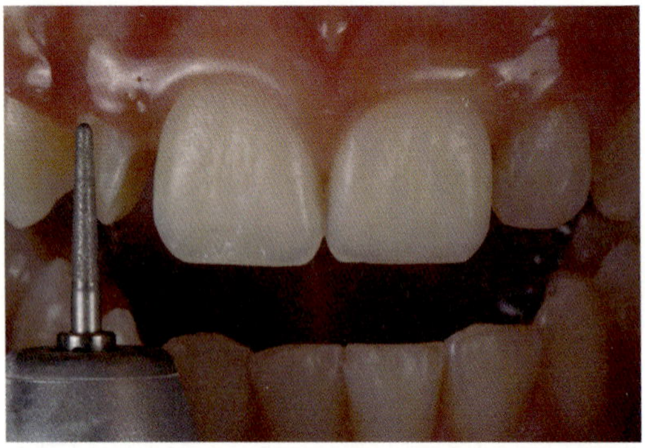

Fig. 19.4 Tooth preparation of the buccal surface of the lateral incisor

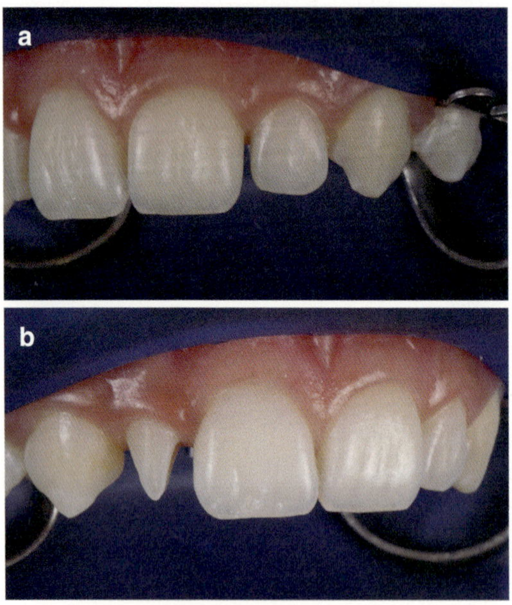

Fig. 19.5 (**a**, **b**) Rubber dam modified isolation for the restoration procedure of the lateral incisors

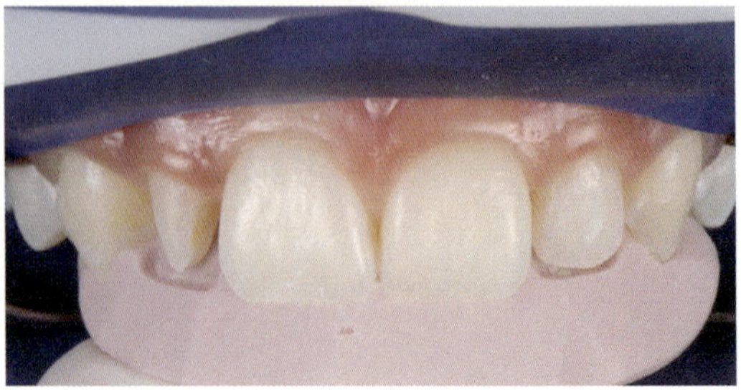

Fig. 19.6 A silicone index was made to guide the palatal and incisal layering

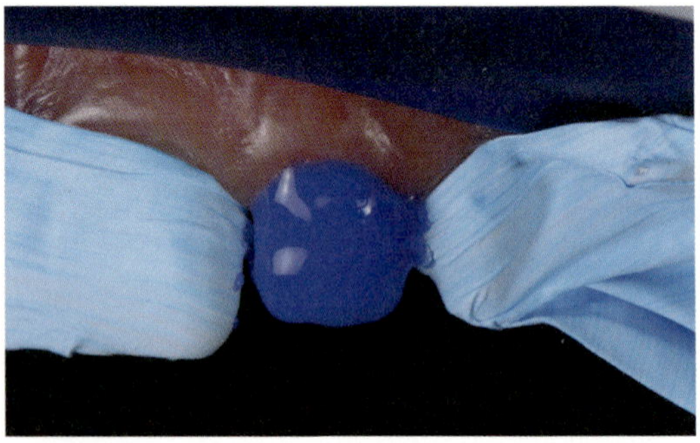

Fig. 19.7 The tooth 22 was acid etched with 37% phosphoric acid for 15 s, thoroughly rinsed with water for 15 s, and air-dried

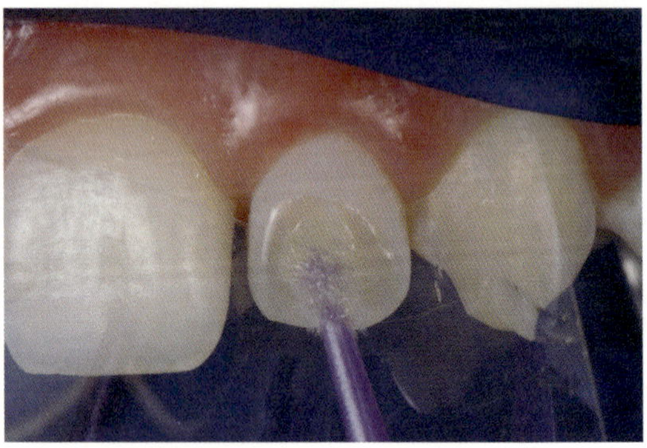

Fig. 19.8 The adhesive system was applied and gently air-dried

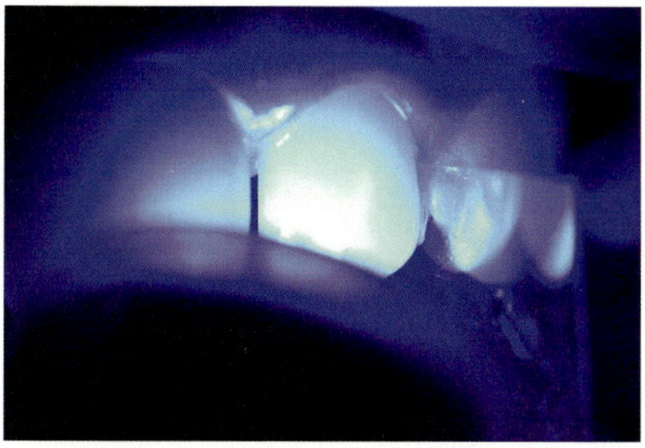

Fig. 19.9 Photoactivation of the adhesive system for 20 s, using a third-generation LED (Bluephase N, Ivoclar Vivadent, Schaan, Liechtenstein)

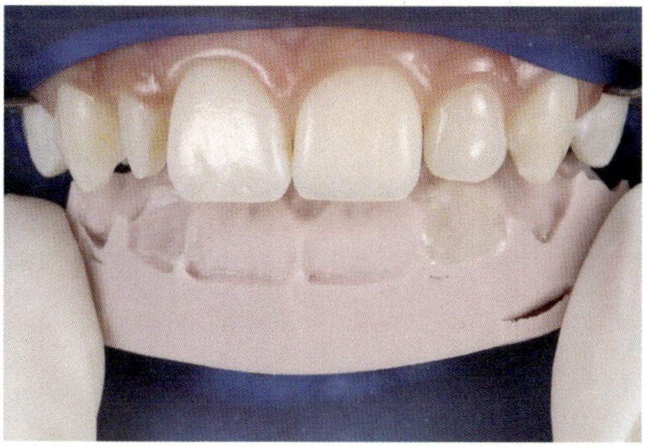

Fig. 19.10 Composite placed on the silicone index to reconstruct the palatal wall of the lateral incisor

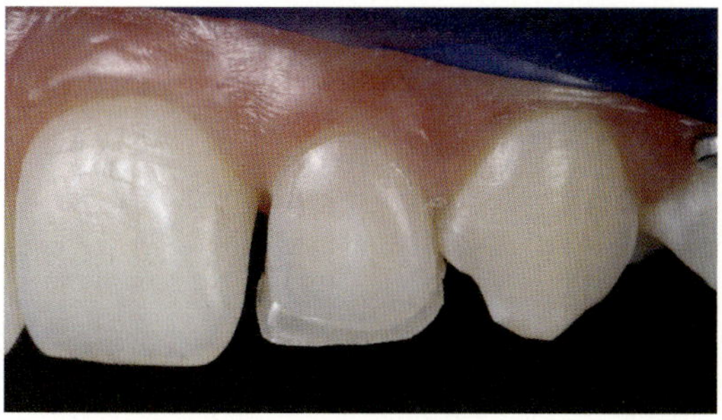

Fig. 19.11 Palatal wall using the resin composite shade A2E (Opallis, FGM, Joaçaba, Brazil)

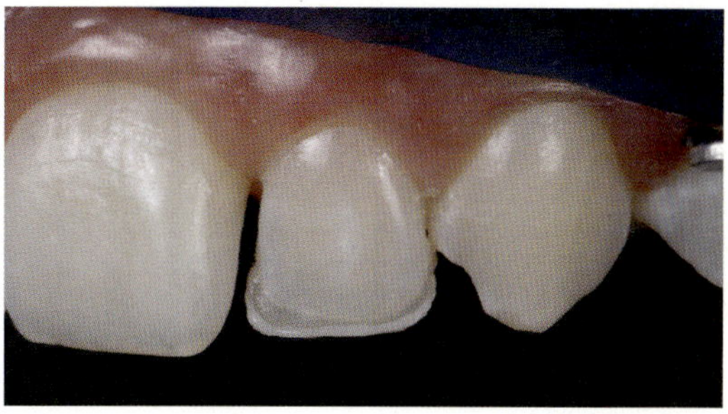

Fig. 19.12 Incisal edge (opaque halo) made from an opaque resin composite, shade OP (Opallis, FGM)

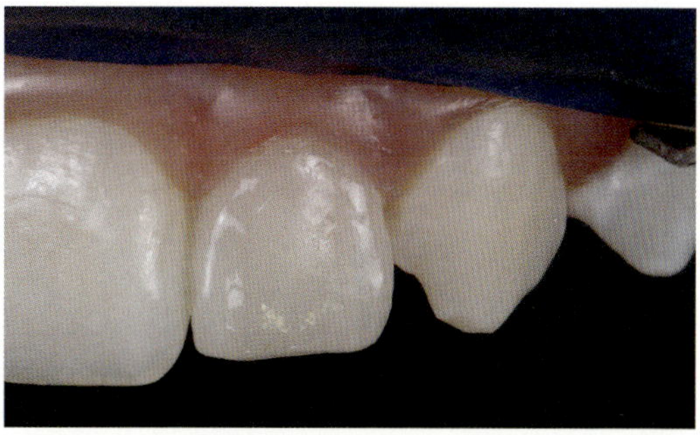

Fig. 19.13 Buccal wall made using the resin shade EA1 (Opallis, FGM)

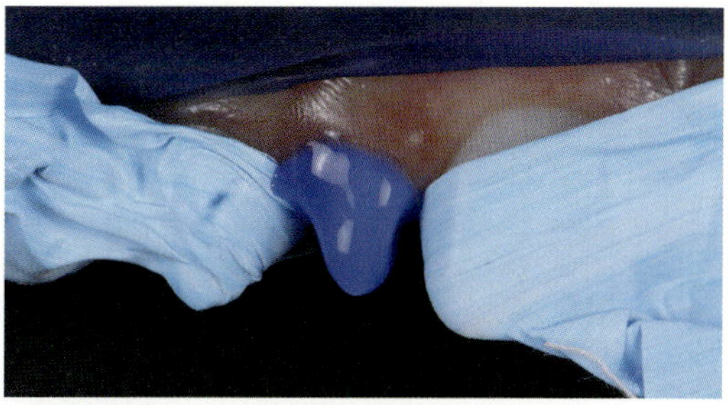

Fig. 19.14 The tooth 12 was acid etched with 37% phosphoric acid for 15 s thoroughly rinsed with water for 15 s and air-dried

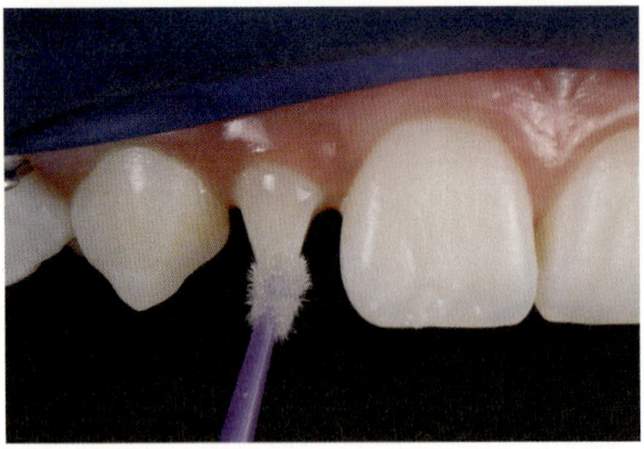

Fig. 19.15 The adhesive system was applied and gently air-dried

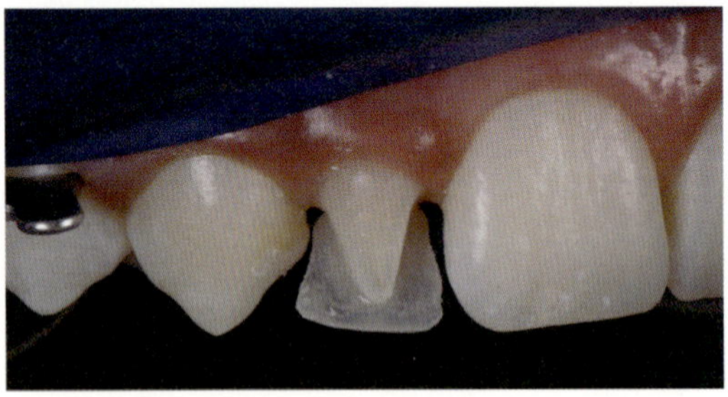

Fig. 19.16 Palatal wall of tooth 12 was made using the resin composite shade A2E (Opallis, FGM, Joaçaba, Brazil)

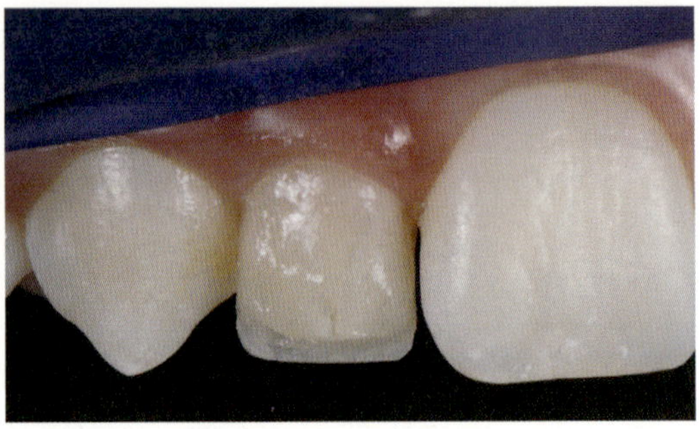

Fig. 19.17 Placement of the dentin composite shade DA2 (Opallis, FGM)

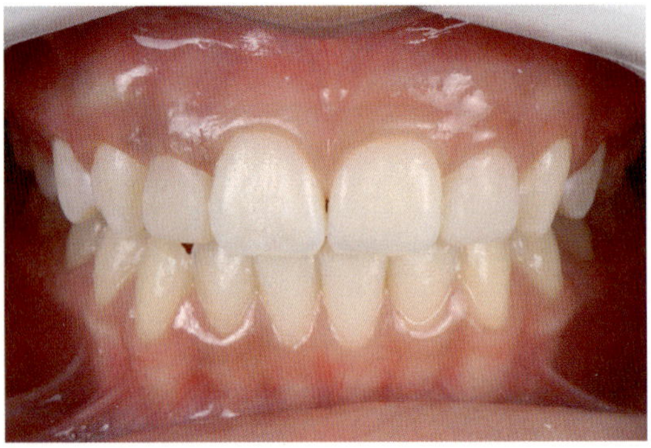

Fig. 19.18 Composites layering complete, without finishing and polishing procedures

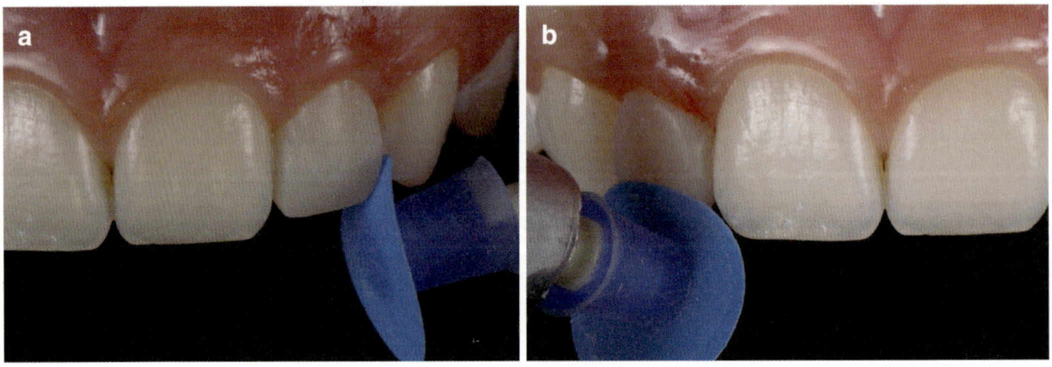

Fig. 19.19 (**a**, **b**) Finishing procedure using abrasive disks. It is important in order to determine the area of light reflection and the proximal rounded areas

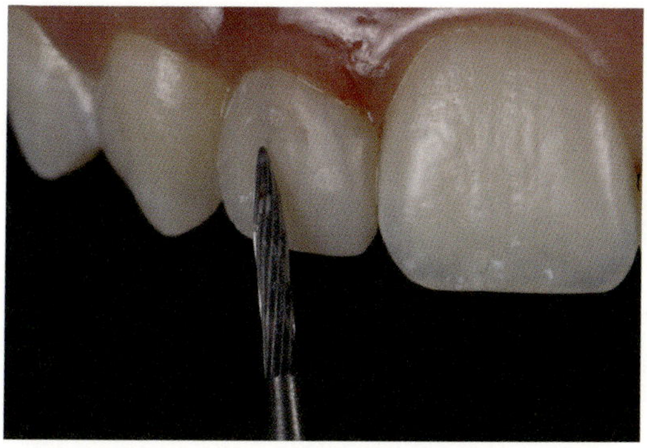

Fig. 19.20 Defining the developmental groove and secondary anatomy using a multiblade bur (H48L—Komet)

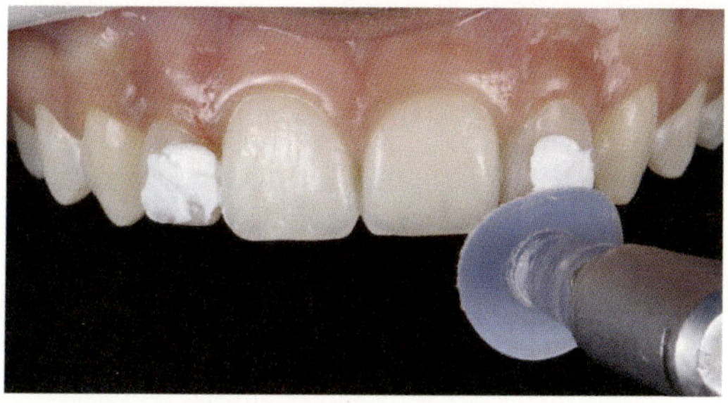

Fig. 19.21 Initial polishing using a felt disk in association with aluminum oxide polishing paste (Enamelize, Cosmedent, USA)

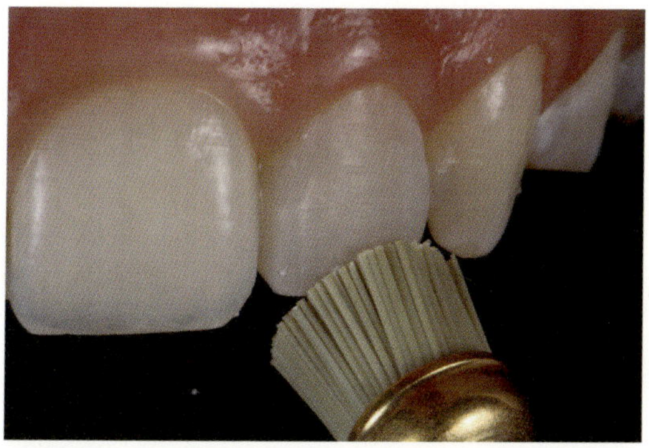

Fig. 19.22 Final polishing using a silicon carbide brush (Astrobrush, Ivoclar Vivadent). This brush is used dry and promotes a final luster, similar to tooth enamel

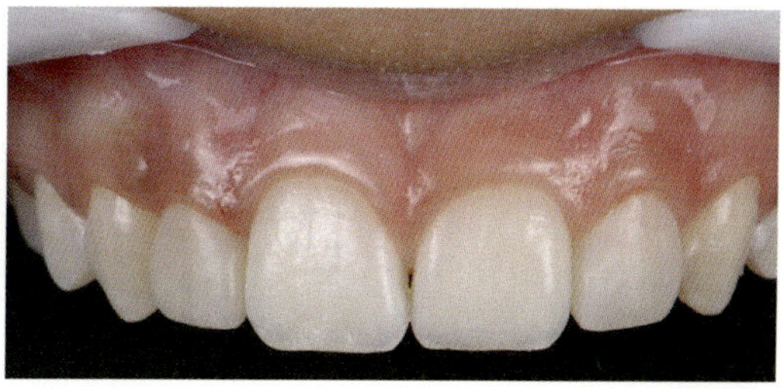

Fig. 19.23 Final aspect of the restored teeth. Note the natural shape and color of the direct resin composite restorations

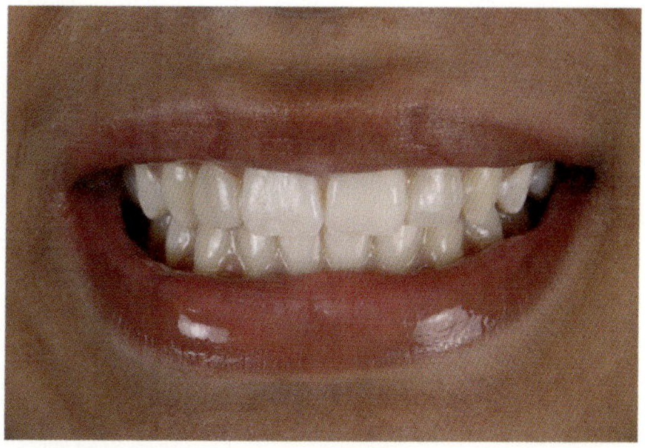

Fig. 19.24 Final smile of the patient, showing natural appearance of the lateral incisors

19.2 Case 2: Diastema Closure in the Anterior Region

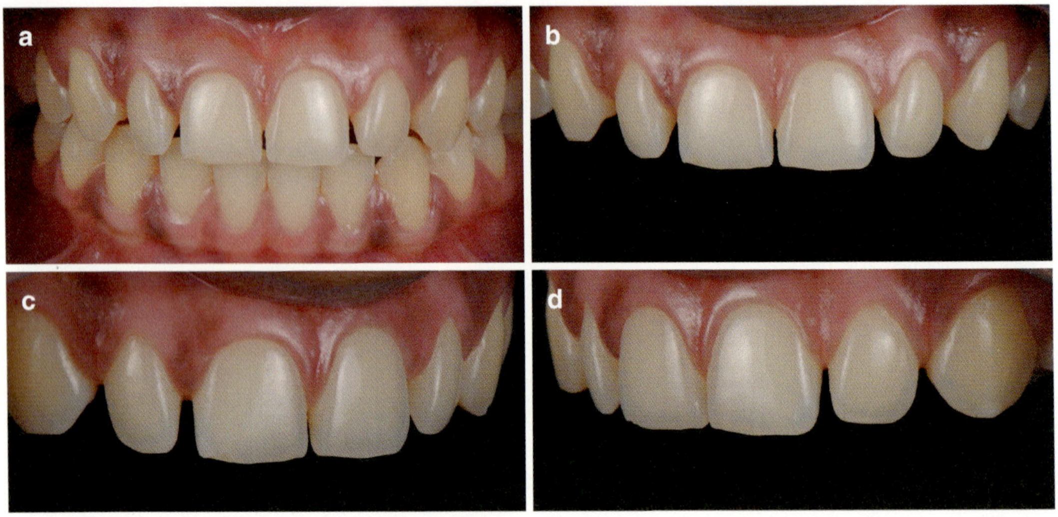

Fig. 19.25 (**a–d**) Preoperative situation. Note the presence of diastemas from canine to canine

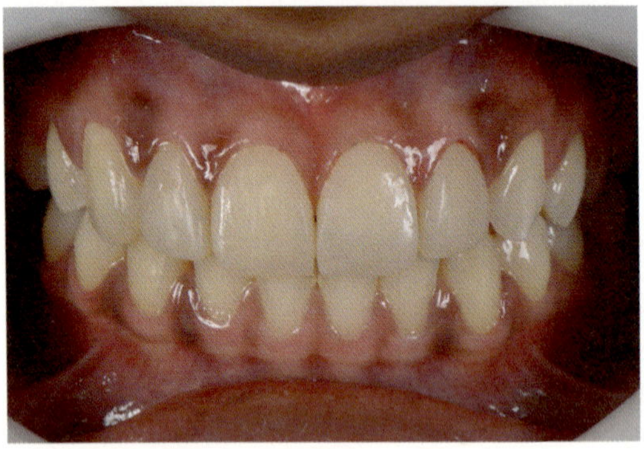

Fig. 19.26 Final aspect after the resin composite restoration, without finishing and polishing

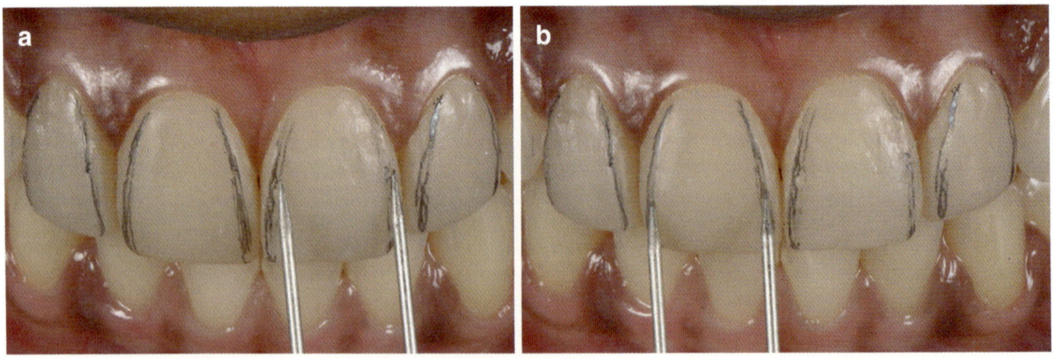

Fig. 19.27 (**a**, **b**) Determination of the transition angles (mesial and distal), using a metal compass, which will establish the reflection area and curved areas of the buccal surface

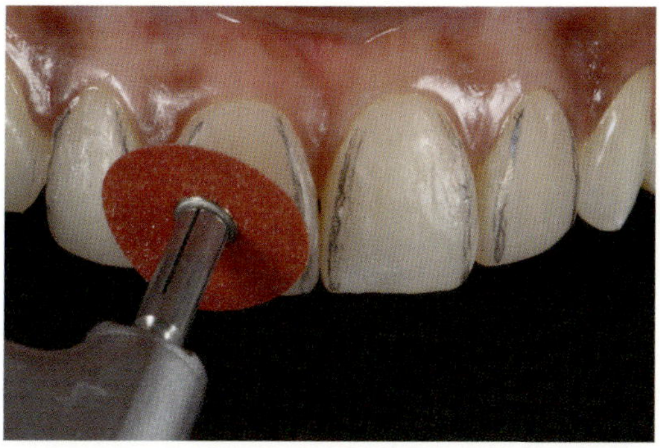

Fig. 19.28 Use of abrasive disks (Sof-Lex Pop On, 3M ESPE), in order to smooth the buccal surface and determine the transition angles

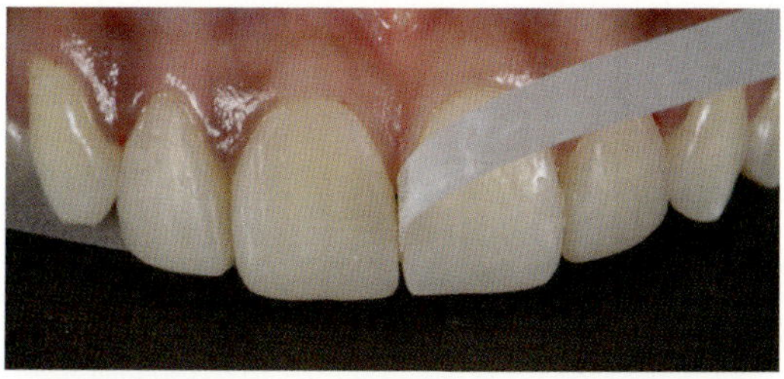

Fig. 19.29 Interproximal sandpaper strips to guarantee the mesial and distal contours and contact point

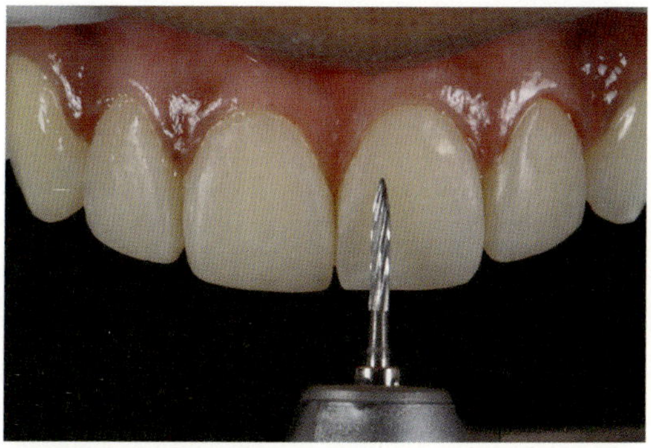

Fig. 19.30 Initial shape finishing, using a multiblade carbide bur to define the developmental grooves and secondary anatomy using a multiblade bur (H48L—Komet)

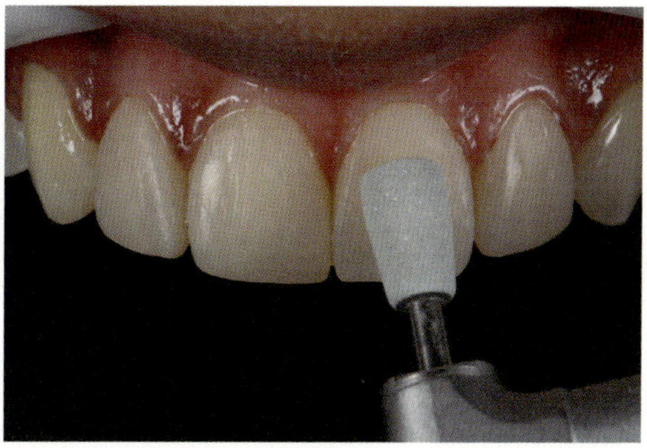

Fig. 19.31 Use of a rubber cup (Astropol, Ivoclar Vivadent) to smooth the secondary anatomy made with the multiblade carbide bur

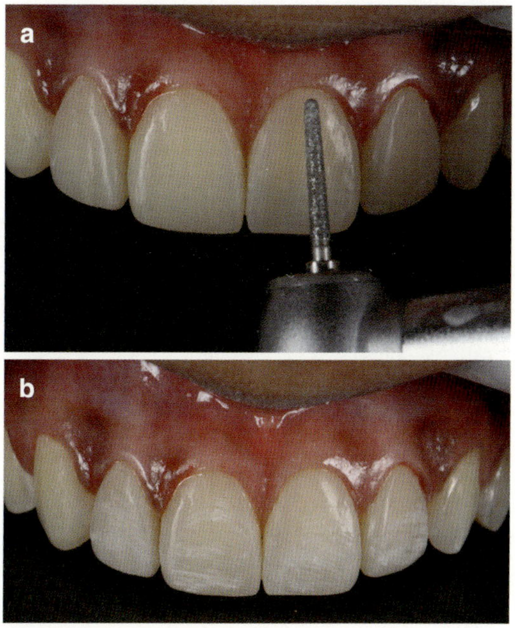

Fig. 19.32 (**a**, **b**) Horizontal textures made using a conventional diamond bur, in horizontal movements

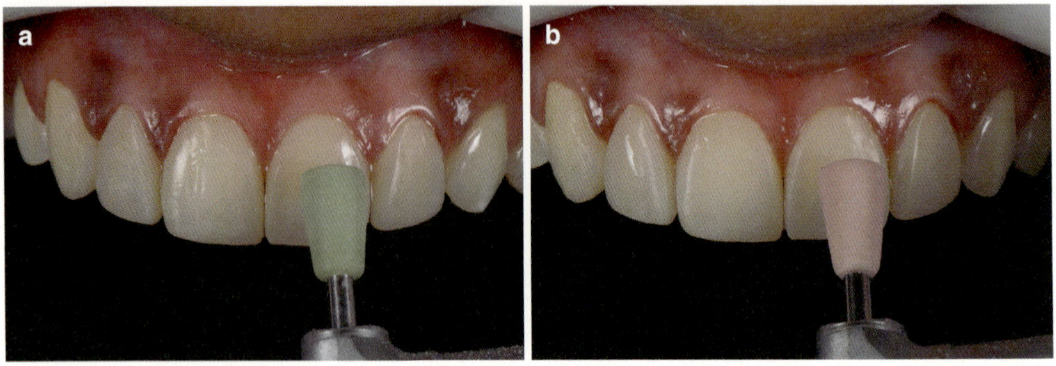

Fig. 19.33 (**a**, **b**) Use of rubber cups (medium and fine, Astropol, Ivoclar Vivadent) to polish the restoration

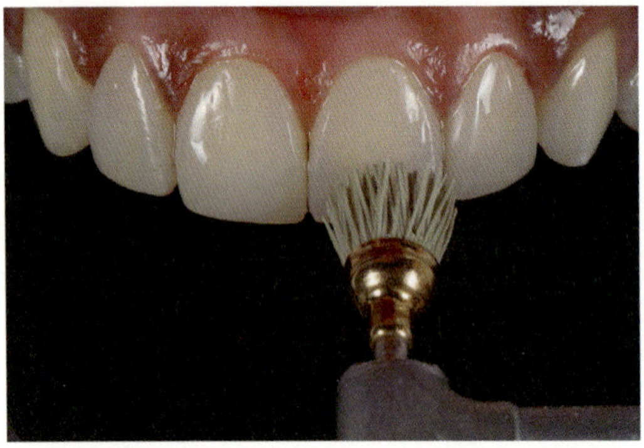

Fig. 19.34 Polishing procedure using the silicon carbide brush (Astrobrush, Ivoclar Vivadent)

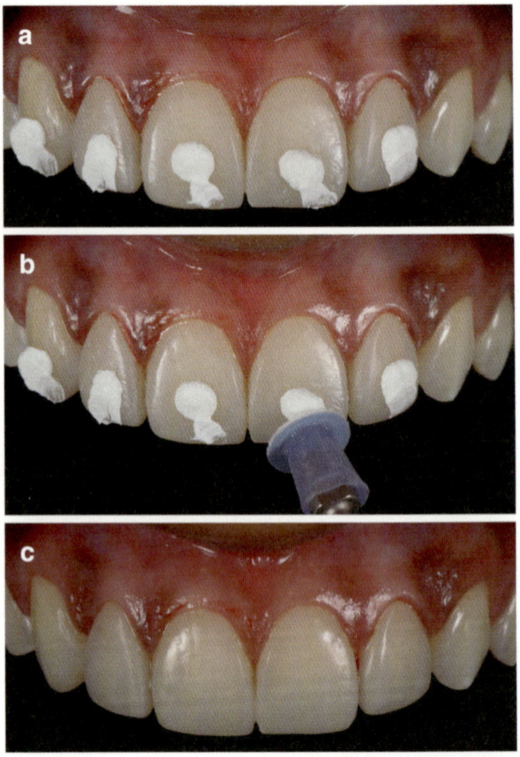

Fig. 19.35 (**a–c**) The final polishing step is aluminum oxide paste associated to felt disks. This last step of polishing promotes a shiny and smooth composite surface

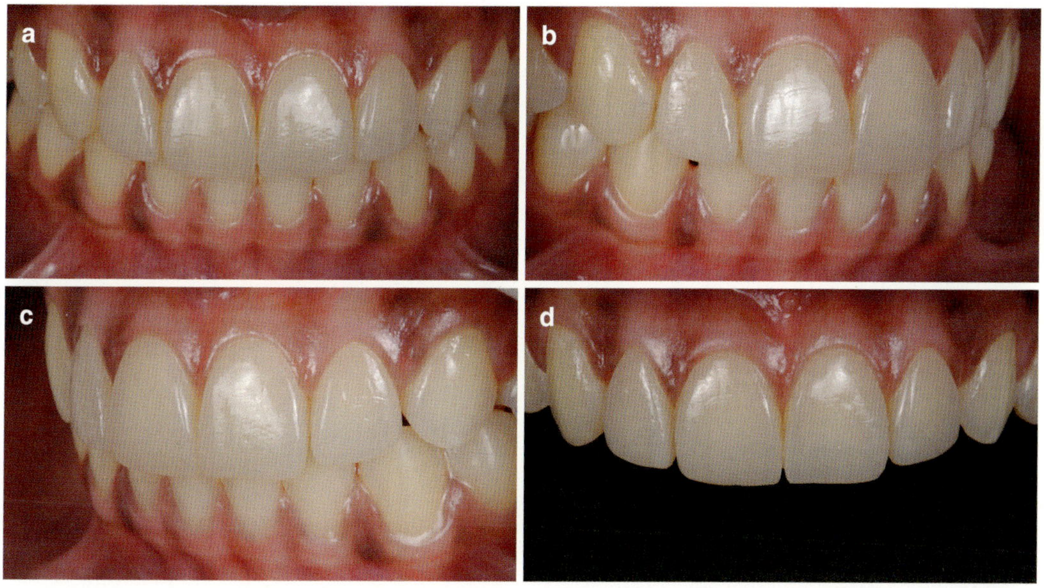

Fig. 19.36 (**a–d**) Note the esthetic and natural aspect of the teeth, showing perfect integration between soft and hard tissues, leading to a successful treatment

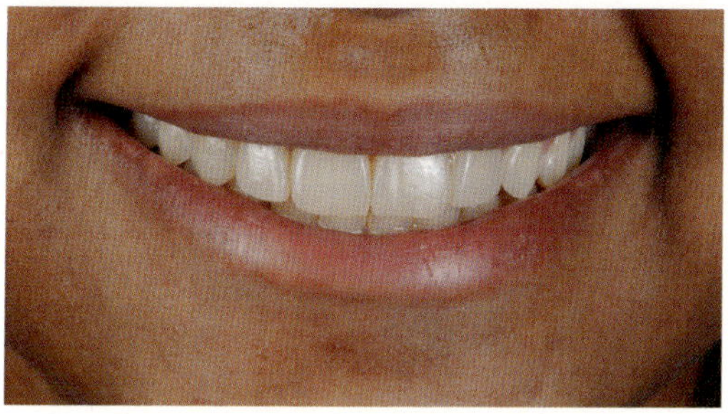

Fig. 19.37 Final smile of the patient showing natural appearance and esthetics

19.3 Case 3: Class I Restoration of a Lower Molar Using a Two-Shade Technique

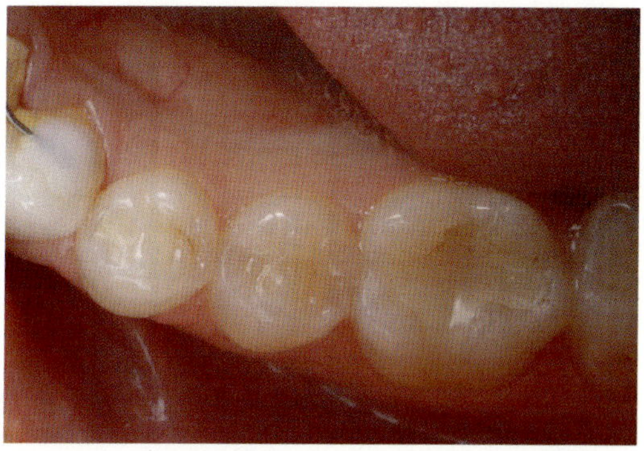

Fig. 19.38 Initial aspect of an old resin composite restoration

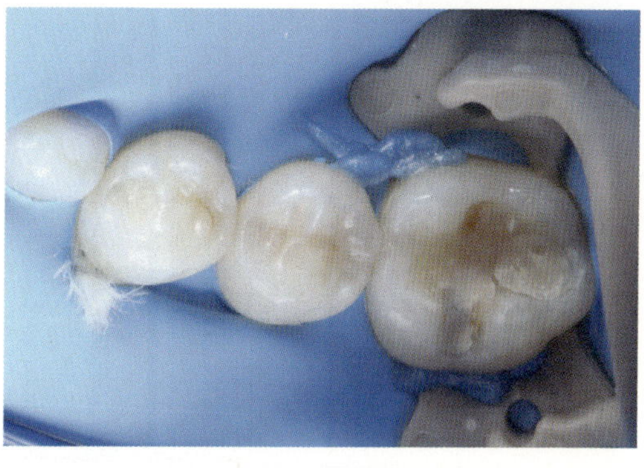

Fig. 19.39 Class I cavity preparation

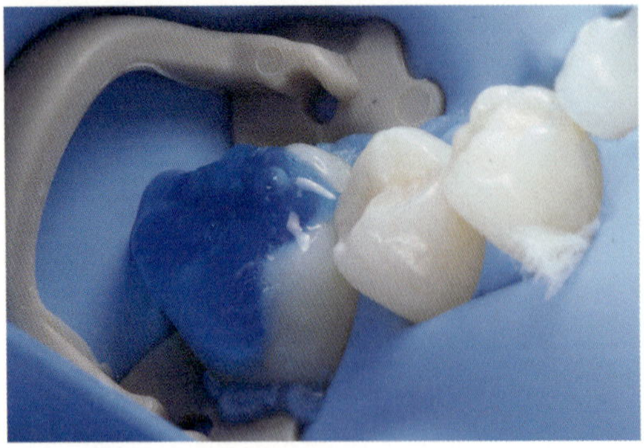

Fig. 19.40 Acid etching using 37% phosphoric acid (power etching, BM4, Brazil)

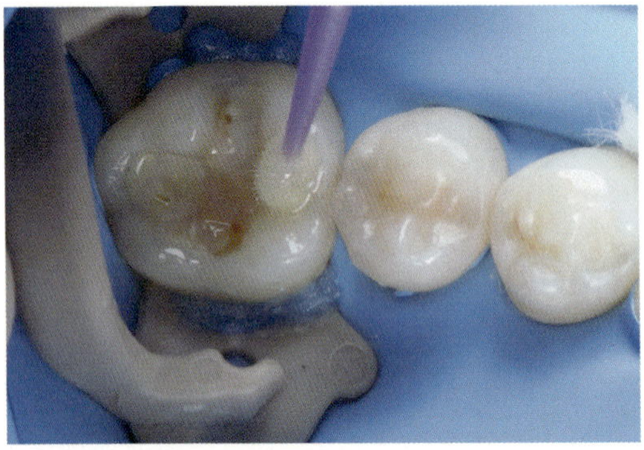

Fig. 19.41 Application of a three-step total etch adhesive system—primer application (OptiBond FL Primer, Kerr, CA, USA)

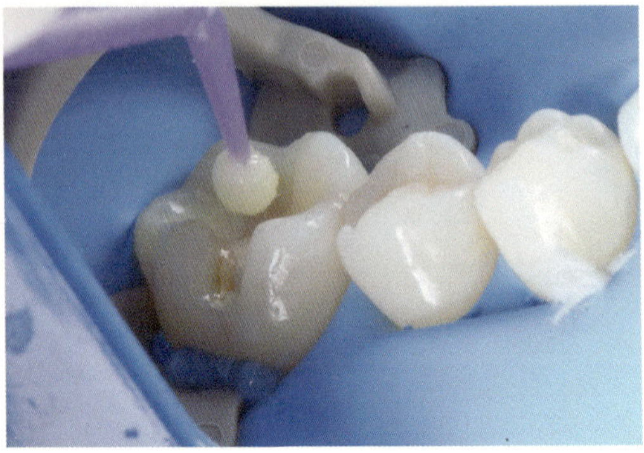

Fig. 19.42 Application of a three-step total etch adhesive system—bond application (OptiBond FL Primer, Kerr, CA, USA)

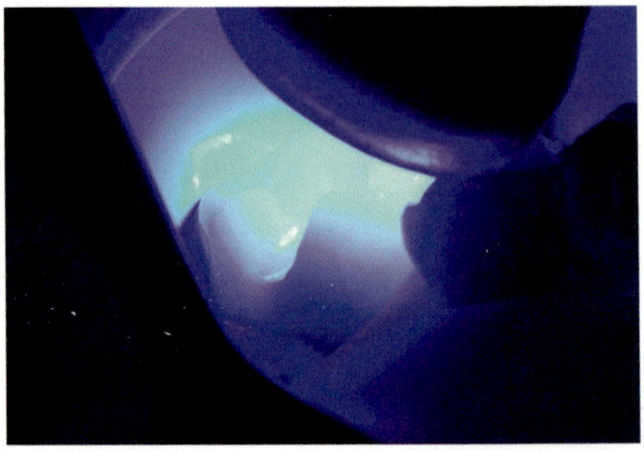

Fig. 19.43 Photoactivation of the bonding agent using a third-generation LED unit (Bluephase Style, Ivoclar Vivadent)

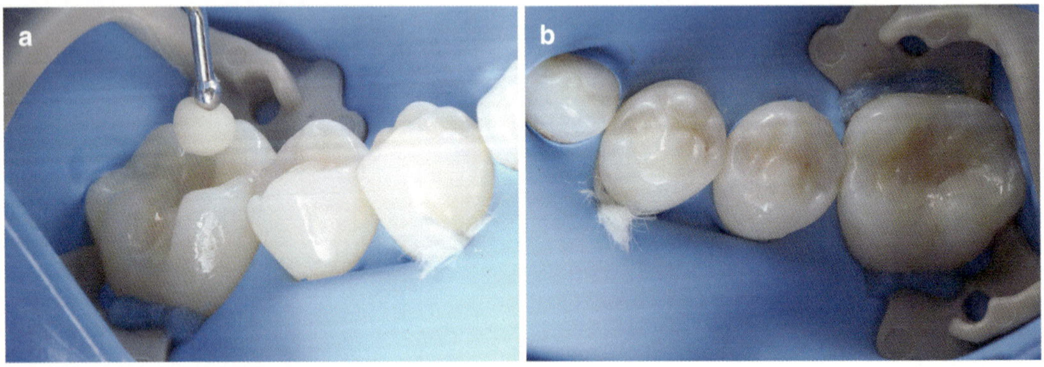

Fig. 19.44 (**a**, **b**) Placement of a body shade composite resin (Filtek Z350 XT A3B, 3M ESPE, St Paul, MN, USA). This layer will rule as a translucent dentin, before the insertion of the enamel layer

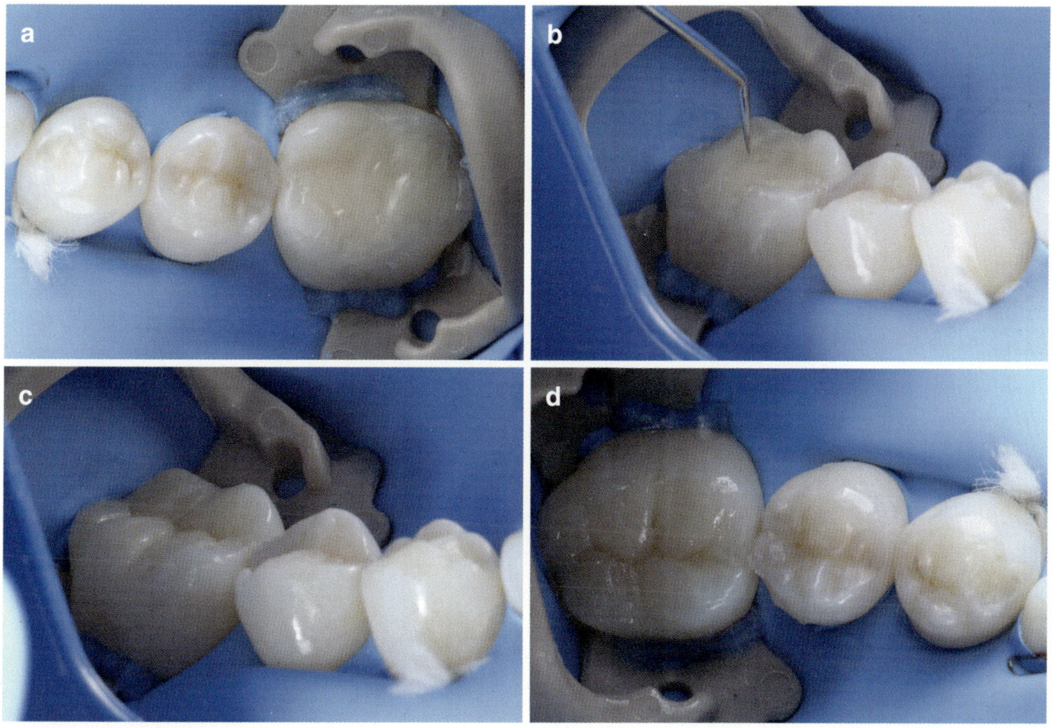

Fig. 19.45 (**a–d**) Placement, adaptation, and sculpting of the enamel shade composite resin (Filtek Z350XT A2E, 3M ESPE, USA)

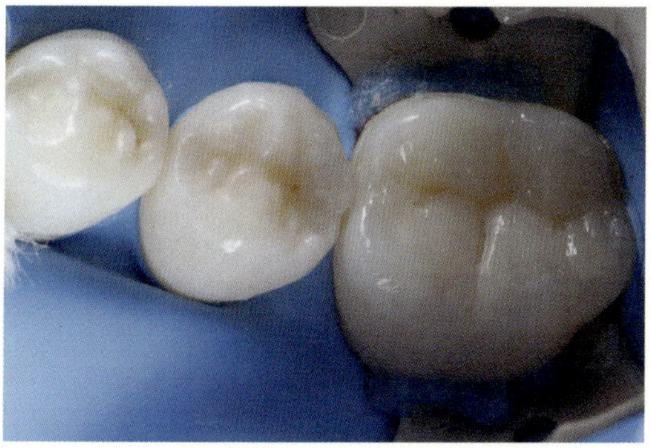

Fig. 19.46 Restoration after the photopolymerization procedure

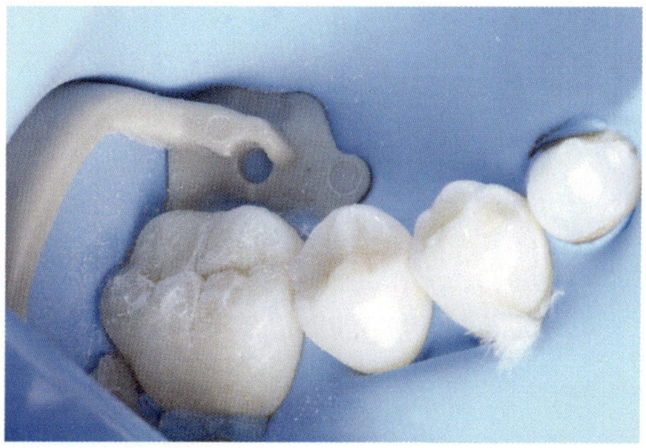

Fig. 19.47 Finishing procedure using a multiblade carbide bur

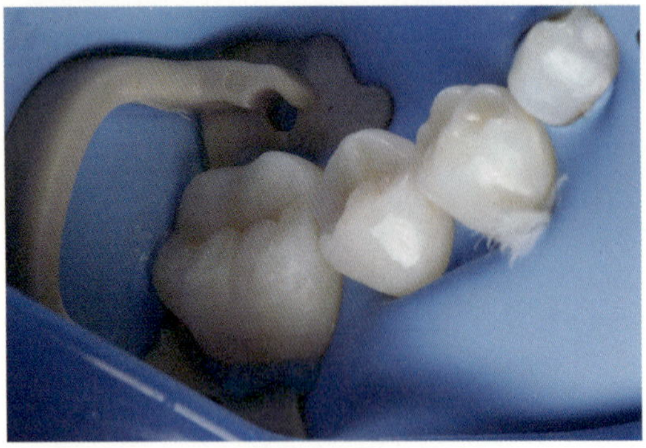

Fig. 19.48 Final aspect of the restoration, after polishing with a silicon carbide brush (Astrobrush, Ivoclar Vivadent)

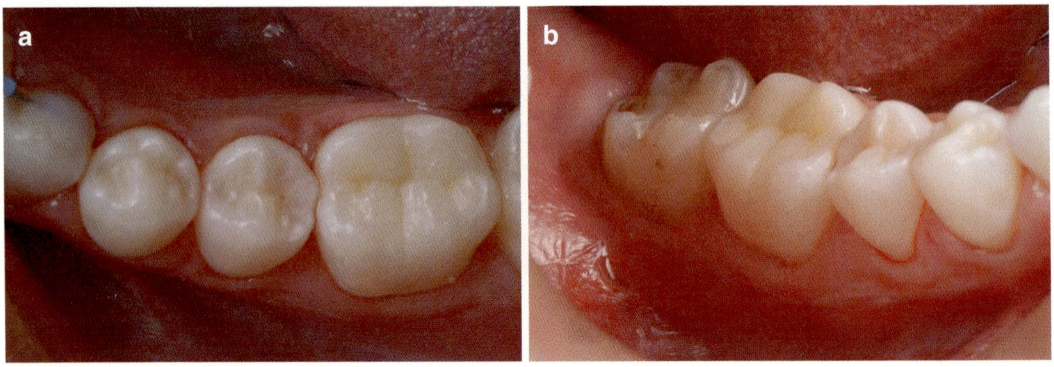

Fig. 19.49 (**a**, **b**) One-week follow-up of the class I composite restoration. Note the natural aspect of shape and color of the restoration

19.4 Case 4: Class I Restoration of an Upper Molar Using a Three-Shade Technique with Characterization Tints

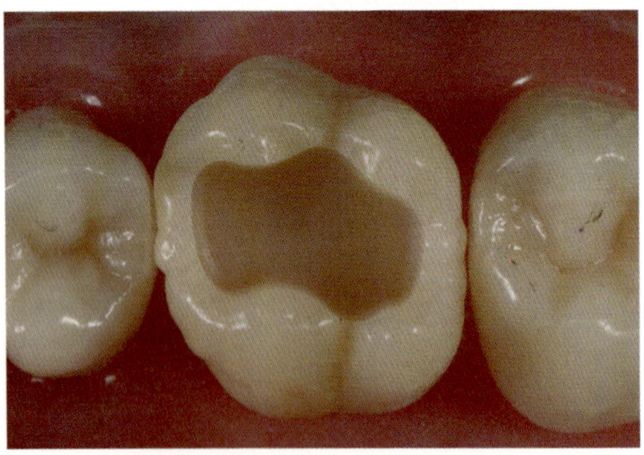

Fig. 19.50 Class I cavity of a first upper molar

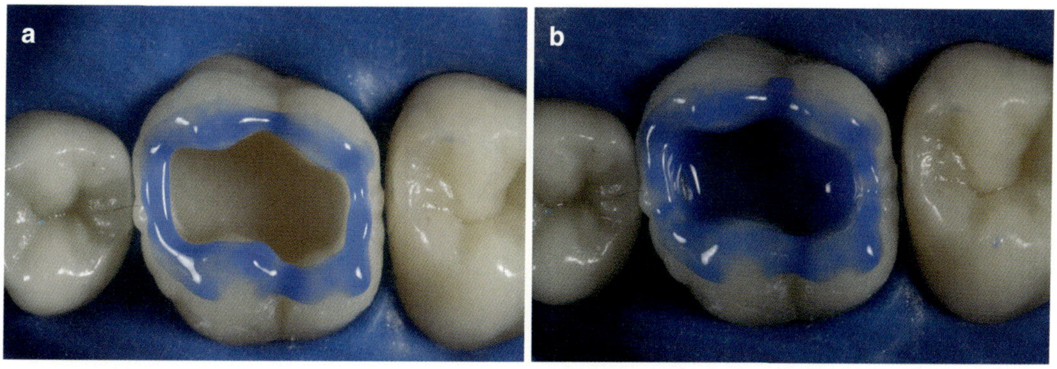

Fig. 19.51 (**a**, **b**) Acid etching using 37% phosphoric acid (power etching, BM4, Brazil). Enamel can be etched for 30 s and dentin for 15 s

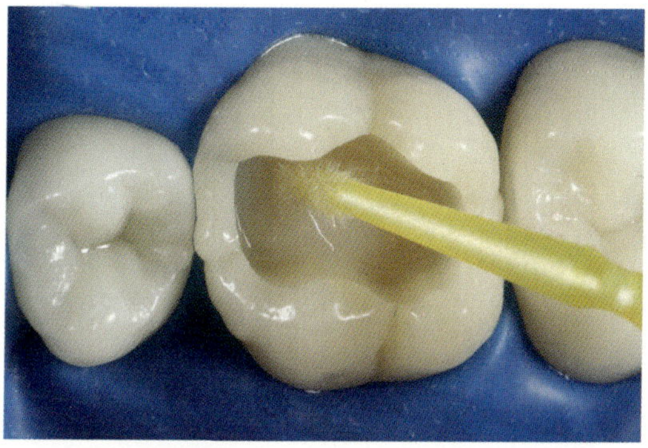

Fig. 19.52 Application of a conventional two-step adhesive system (Ybond Mono, Yller Biomateriais, Brazil). The adhesive is light-cured

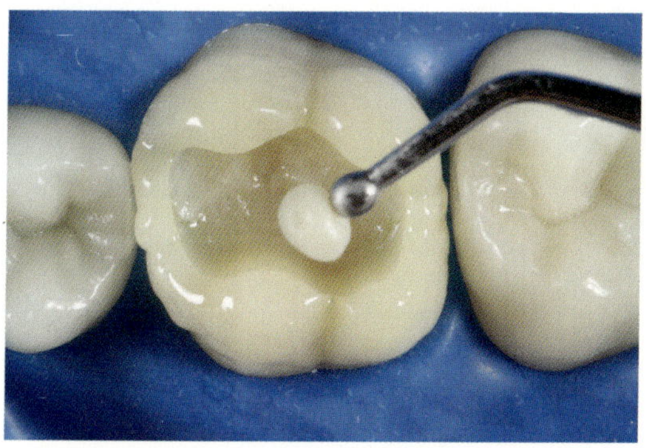

Fig. 19.53 Layering using the three-layer technique. The first layer is a resin composite dentin shade (A3.5 D, Tetric N-Ceram, Ivoclar Vivadent)

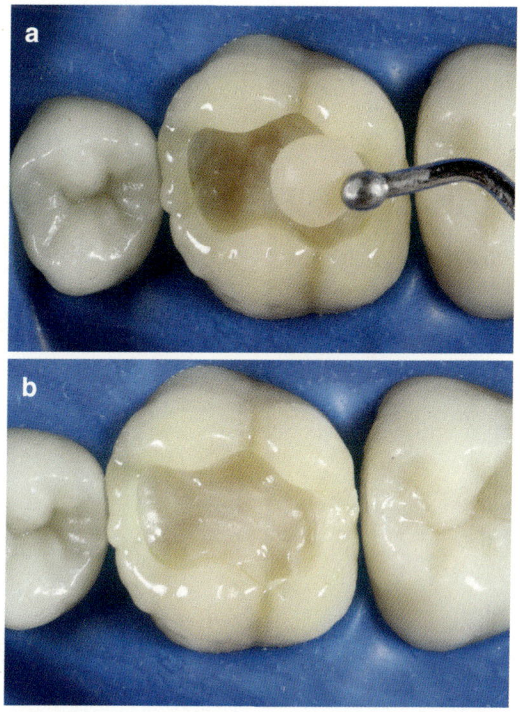

Fig. 19.54 (**a**–**d**) Insertion of an increment of chromatic enamel (A3E, Tetric N-Ceram, Ivoclar Vivadent). After the adaptation of this increment, using a thin edge instrument, like SD2 (Golgran Millennium, Brazil), the cusps will be divided, guiding the future occlusal anatomy

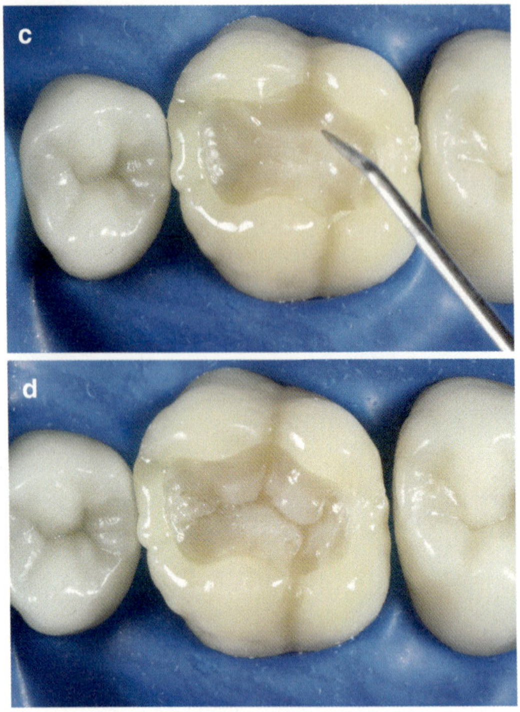

Fig. 19.54 (continued)

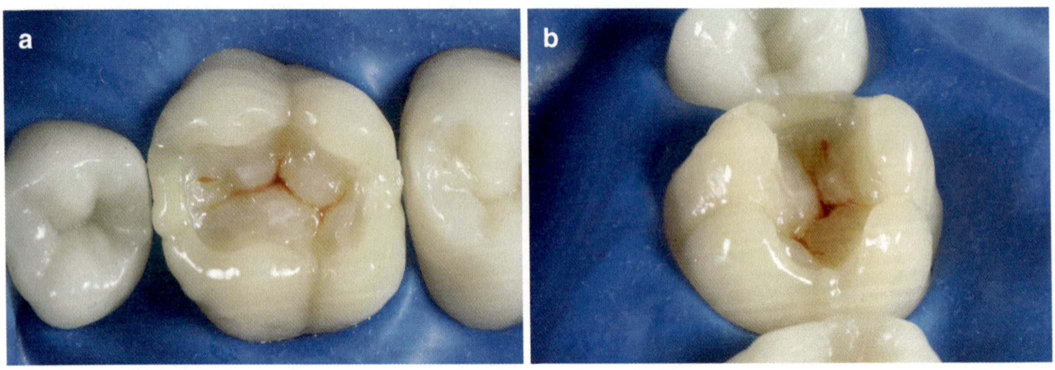

Fig. 19.55 (**a**, **b**) Application of intrinsic tints (white, ocher, and brown) to simulate the naturally stained sulcus condition

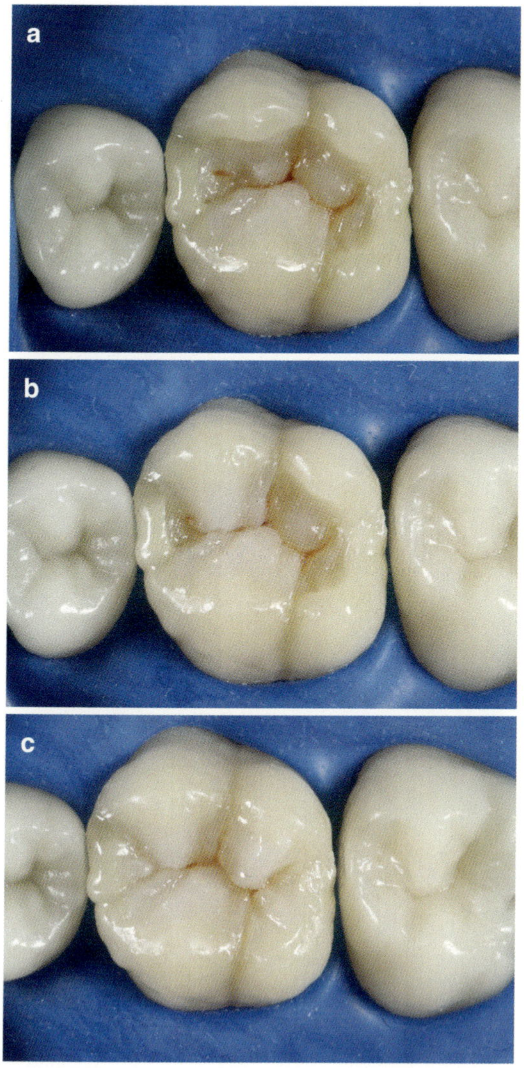

Fig. 19.56 (**a–c**) Placement of the last composite layer, using achromatic enamel shade composite (Bleach L, Tetric N-Ceram, Ivoclar Vivadent). In this step, using the achromatic resin composite, the cusps will be built-up in sequence, until the occlusal anatomy is completed

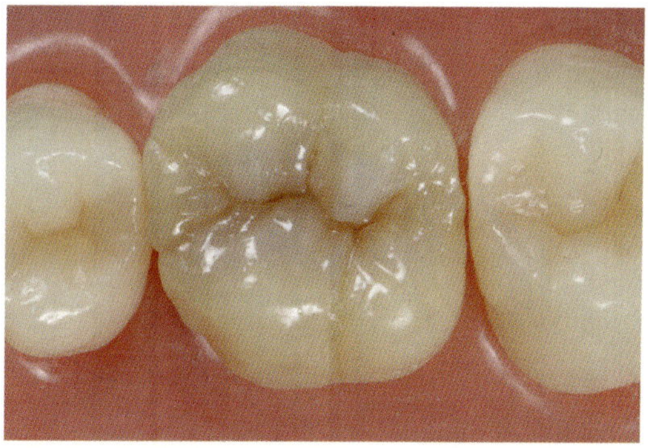

Fig. 19.57 Final restoration, showing a natural aspect of the first upper molar

Printed by Printforce, the Netherlands